Straight A's
in
Pathophysiology

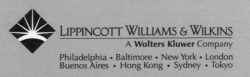

LIPPINCOTT WILLIAMS & WILKINS
A **Wolters Kluwer** Company

Philadelphia • Baltimore • New York • London
Buenos Aires • Hong Kong • Sydney • Tokyo

STAFF

Publisher
Judith A. Schilling McCann, RN, MSN

Senior Acquisitions Editor
Elizabeth Nieginski

Editorial Director
David Moreau

Clinical Director
Joan M. Robinson, RN, MSN

Senior Art Director
Arlene Putterman

Editorial Project Manager
Jaime Stockslager Buss

Clinical Project Manager
Carol A. Saunderson, RN, BA, BS

Editors
Rita Breedlove, Laura Bruck,
Karen Comerford, Jo Donofrio,
Diane Labus, Brenna H. Mayer,
Liz Schaeffer, Libby Tucker

Clinical Editors
Tamara M. Kear, RN, MSN CNN;
Pamela Kovach, RN, BSN

Copy Editors
Kimberly Bilotta (supervisor),
Scotti Cohn, Tom DeZego, Amy Furman,
Shana Harrington, Kelly Pavlovsky,
Dorothy P. Terry, Pamela Wingrod

Designer
Matie Anne Patterson (project manager)

Digital Composition Services
Diane Paluba (manager),
Joyce Rossi Biletz, Donna S. Morris

Manufacturing
Patricia K. Dorshaw (director),
Beth J. Welsh

Editorial Assistants
Megan L. Aldinger, Karen J. Kirk,
Linda K. Ruhf

Indexer
Barbara Hodgson

The clinical treatments described and recommended in this publication are based on research and consultation with nursing, medical, and legal authorities. To the best of our knowledge, these procedures reflect currently accepted practice. Nevertheless, they can't be considered absolute and universal recommendations. For individual applications, all recommendations must be considered in light of the patient's clinical condition and, before administration of new or infrequently used drugs, in light of the latest package-insert information. The authors and publisher disclaim any responsibility for any adverse effects resulting from the suggested procedures, from any undetected errors, or from the reader's misunderstanding of the text.

STRPATHO011105–020708

**Library of Congress
Cataloging-in-Publication Data**

Straight A's in pathophysiology.
     p. ; cm.
   Includes bibliographical references and index.
   1. Physiology, Pathological 2. Nursing—Study and teaching.
   I. Lippincott Williams & Wilkins.
   [DNLM: 1. Pathology—Examination Questions.
QZ 18.2 S896 2006]
  RB113.S85 2006
  616.07'076—dc22
ISBN13: 978-1-58255-449-5
ISBN10: 1-58255-449-8 (alk. paper)   2005022096

Contents

Advisory board

Contributors and consultants

Katrina D. Allen, RN, MSN, CCRN
Nursing Instructor, Faulkner State Community College, Bay Minette, Ala.

Kim Cooper, RN, MS
Nursing Department Program Chair, Ivy Tech State College, Terre Haute, Ind.

Lillian Craig, RN, MSN, FNP, CS
FNP Internal Medicine, Instructor of Nursing, Oklahoma Panhandle State University, Goodwell

Ken W. Edmisson, RNC, ND, EdD, FNP
Associate Professor, Middle Tennessee State University, Murfreesboro

Charla K. Hollin, RN, BSN
Nursing Program Director, Rich Mountain Community College, Mena, Ark.

Bernadette Madara, APRN, BC, EdD
Associate Professor-Nursing, Southern Connecticut State University, New Haven

Dana Reeves, MSN, RN
Assistant Professor, University of Arkansas College of Health Sciences, Fort Smith

Doris J. Rosenow, CCRN, PhD, CNS-M-S
Associate Professor, Texas A&M International University, Laredo

How to use this book

Straight A's is a multivolume study guide series developed especially for nursing students. Each volume provides essential course material in a unique two-column design. The easy-to-read interior outline format offers a succinct review of key facts as presented in leading textbooks on the subject. The bulleted exterior columns provide only the most crucial information, allowing for quick, efficient review right before an important quiz or test.

Special features appear in every chapter to make information accessible and easy to remember. **Learning objectives** encourage the student to evaluate knowledge before and after study. **Chapter overview** highlights the chapter's major concepts. Within the outlined text, color is used to highlight critical information and key points. Key points may include cardinal signs and symptoms, current theories, important steps in a nursing procedure, critical assessment findings, crucial nursing interventions, or successful therapies and treatments. The NCLEX®-style questions found in **NCLEX checks** at the end of each chapter offer additional opportunities to review material and assess knowledge gained before moving on to new information.

Other features appear throughout the book to facilitate learning. **Time-out for teaching** highlights key areas to address when teaching patients. **Go with the flow** charts promote critical thinking. Lastly, a brand-new Windows-based software program (see CD-ROM on inside back cover) poses more than 250 multiple-choice and alternate-format NCLEX-style questions in random order to assess your knowledge.

The *Straight A's* volumes are designed as learning tools, not as primary information sources. When read conscientiously as a supplement to class attendance and textbook reading, *Straight A's* can enhance understanding and help improve test scores and final grades.

Foreword

Pathophysiology is a challenging course of study for many nursing students; however, knowledge of the critical concepts inherent in this subject is essential to provide competent care to patients in all health care settings. The study of pathophysiology forms a framework for professional nursing practice and is the bedrock of our practice. Choosing a review book that provides the student with clear explanations of the essential concepts and a user-friendly organizational approach can be challenging for educators. Moreover, educators should provide a review book that motivates students to learn and analyze concepts without causing cognitive overload from extraneous information.

Straight A's in Pathophysiology is a great addition to the *Straight A's* series because it presents pathophysiology in a straightforward format that is user friendly and is written in a manner that's simple to understand. Its no-nonsense approach to learning this often-dreaded subject matter is refreshing and original. The outline format streamlines learning by providing important information without complicated explanations. Furthermore, for students who are short on time or are just interested in a quick review of the material, this extraordinary review book presents a more succinct synopsis of pathophysiology essentials in the outer columns. This distinctive format is like having two books in one.

Systematically presented, each chapter in *Straight A's in Pathophysiology* provides the student with well-written learning outcomes, a concise chapter overview, definitions of commonly seen clinical concepts, and descriptions of physiological disorders. Familiar disorders are further broken down into clear and important parts: definition, underlying pathophysiology, causes, physiological changes displayed by the patient, complications associated with the specific disorder, findings from diagnostic analyses, treatment modalities, and essential nursing interventions. Clear and uncomplicated images enhance the students' learning of specific concepts described in the text. Each chapter ends with a list of key learning points.

Students who are eager to begin their preparation for the NCLEX will be pleased to find *NCLEX checks* test questions at the end of each chapter. These tests allow the learner to assess retention of material learned from the chapter by providing NCLEX-style questions, including alternate-format questions, correct answers, and rationales for correct and incorrect answer options. In addition to the more than 125 questions in the book, readers will find more than 250 NCLEX-style questions on the CD in the back of the book, further enhancing their NCLEX review.

Students aren't the only ones who will benefit from this unique review book. Nurse-educators can formulate case studies from the concepts presented in the textbook and then use the *NCLEX checks* in the classroom or online learning environment.

In summary, *Straight A's in Pathophysiology* is a well-written textbook that students will use as a learning guide and reference throughout their student tenures and nursing careers and that educators will reach for to support learning strategies used in the classroom setting. This one-of-a-kind review book not only streamlines the presentation of pathophysiologic concepts but also promotes self-regulated learning and critical thinking. And, without a doubt, once students have used *Straight A's in Pathophysiology,* they will ask for other *Straight A's* textbooks to complement their studies.

Margaret M. Maag, RN, MSN, EdD
Assistant Professor
University of San Francisco, School of Nursing

1

Cardiovascular system

LEARNING OBJECTIVES

After studying this chapter, you should be able to:

● Describe the relationship between presenting signs and symptoms and the pathophysiologic changes of various cardiovascular disorders.

● Identify conditions that impede cardiac output.

● List probable causes of various cardiovascular disorders.

● Identify nursing interventions for various cardiovascular disorders.

● Write teaching goals for a patient with a cardiovascular disorder.

● Identify medications that can improve or control cardiac dysfunction.

CHAPTER OVERVIEW

The cardiovascular system includes the heart and blood vessels. It delivers oxygenated blood and other essential products, such as hormones, enzymes, and electrolytes, to tissues. This system also removes carbon dioxide from the lungs and transports metabolic waste products to other organs for excretion.

Caring for a patient with a cardiovascular disorder requires an understanding of the pathophysiologic changes that occur and the signs and symptoms such changes produce. This chapter reviews key pathophysiologic concepts related to the cardiovascular system, and then outlines the underlying pathophysiology, causes, pathophysiologic changes, complications, diagnostic test findings, treatment approaches, and nursing considerations associated with common cardiovascular disorders.

PATHOPHYSIOLOGIC CONCEPTS

Key facts about aneurysm

- Outpouching or dilation of a blood vessel or heart wall
- Can occur in the abdominal aorta, thoracic aorta, cerebral artery, and femoral and popliteal arteries

● **Aneurysm**
  - Abnormal outpouching or dilation of a blood vessel or wall of the heart
  - Can result from various conditions
    - Atherosclerotic plaque formation
    - Loss of elastin and collagen in vessel wall
    - Congenital abnormalities in media of arterial wall
    - Trauma
    - Infections
    - Syphilis
  - Can occur in various locations
    - Abdominal aorta, between renal arteries and iliac branches
    - Thoracic aorta (ascending, transverse, or descending)
    - Cerebral artery, at arterial junction in circle of Willis
    - Femoral and popliteal arteries
  - False aneurysm
    - Hematoma from trauma to a vessel or cardiac wall
    - Unlike aneurysm, no continuous blood flow through affected area

Key facts about shunts

- Are congenital

Left-to-right
- Deliver oxygenated blood back to right side of heart or to lungs
- Increase pulmonary blood flow

Right-to-left
- Add deoxygenated blood to systemic circulation
- Lead to hypoxia and cyanosis

● **Cardiac shunt**
  - Creates an inappropriate link between pulmonary and systemic circulations
  - Causes blood to flow from area of high pressure to area of low pressure, or from area of high resistance to area of low resistance
  - Left-to-right shunt
    - Is congenital (called an *acyanotic* defect)
    - Occurs with an atrial or a ventricular defect, which allows blood to partially bypass valves, thus mixing oxygenated and deoxygenated blood together
    - Occurs with a patent ductus arteriosus, which causes blood to flow from the aorta to the pulmonary circulation
    - Delivers oxygenated blood back to right side of heart or to lungs
    - Increases pulmonary blood flow because blood is continually recirculated to lungs
    - Leads to increased pressure and volume within the pulmonary vessels
    - Can cause hypertrophy and failure because pressure and volume back up into right ventricle
  - Right-to-left shunt
    - Is congenital (called a *cyanotic* defect)
    - Involves blood flowing from right side of heart to left (such as in tetralogy of Fallot) or from the pulmonary artery directly into the systemic circulation through a patent ductus arteriosus
    - Adds deoxygenated blood to systemic circulation
    - Leads to hypoxia and cyanosis
    - Commonly manifests as fatigue, increased respiratory rate, clubbing of fingers and toes (hypertrophic osteoarthropathy), and polycythemia

Key facts about thrombus

- Blood clot
- Forms anywhere within vascular system
- May cause blood vessel occlusion or embolus

● **Thrombus**
  - Blood clot that consists of platelets, fibrin, red blood cells (RBCs), and white blood cells (WBCs)

- Forms anywhere within vascular system
- Conditions that promote thrombus formation (Virchow's triad)
  - Endothelial injury—attracts platelets and other inflammatory mediators, which may stimulate clot formation
  - Sluggish blood flow—allows platelets and clotting factors to accumulate and adhere to blood vessel walls
  - Increased coagulability—promotes clot formation
- May cause blood vessel occlusion or embolus

● Embolus

- Substance that circulates through the bloodstream from one location in body to another
- Most are blood clots from a thrombus
- May contain other substances
  - Pieces of tissue
  - Air or nitrogen bubble
  - Amniotic fluid
  - Fat
  - Bacteria
  - Tumor cells
    Atherosclerotic debris
  - Bits of bone marrow
  - Foreign substance
- Venous embolus
  - Originates in venous circulation
  - Travels to right side of heart and pulmonary circulation
  - Eventually lodges in capillary
- Arterial embolus
  - Originates in left side of heart from arrhythmias, valvular heart disease, myocardial infarction (MI), heart failure, or endocarditis
  - May lodge in organs (such as brain, kidneys) or extremities

● Release of cardiac enzymes and proteins

- Triggered by damaged heart muscle and impaired integrity of cell membrane
- Involves the cardiac enzymes creatine kinase (CK), lactate dehydrogenase (LD), and aspartate aminotransferase (AST)
- Involves the proteins troponin T, troponin I, and myoglobin
- Leads to characteristic rising and falling of cardiac values

● Stenosis

- Narrowing of a blood vessel or heart valve
- Stenosis of a blood vessel
  - Involves decreased blood flow to tissues and organs due to narrowed blood vessels
  - Causes tissues and organs to become ischemic and function abnormally
  - May cause necrosis and death of involved tissues
- Stenosis of the heart valve
  - Occurs when blood accumulates in the chamber behind the stenosed valve
  - Results in increased chamber pressure due to resistance of the stenosed valve
  - May result in hypertrophy of the cardiac wall

Key facts about embolus

- Circulates through the bloodstream
- Typically is a blood clot
- May contain other substances, such as tissue, fat, and tumor cells

Key facts about cardiac enzyme and protein release

- Triggered by damaged heart muscle and impaired integrity of cell membrane
- Causes cardiac values to rise and fall in characteristic patterns

Key facts about stenosis

- Narrowing of a blood vessel or heart valve
- In blood vessel, leads to ischemia of distal tissues and organs
- In heart, leads to heart failure

– If on the left side of heart, increases pulmonary venous pressure and pulmonary congestion, leading to right-sided heart failure
– If on the right side of heart, leads to systemic venous congestion

● **Valve insufficiency**
  • Occurs when valve leaflets don't completely close
  • May affect vein or heart valves
  • Venous valve insufficiency
    – Leaflets close improperly
    – Blood flows backward and pools above, causing valve to weaken and become incompetent
    – Veins eventually become distended, resulting in varicose veins, chronic venous insufficiency, and venous stasis ulcers
    – Blood clots may form as blood flow becomes sluggish
  • Cardiac valve insufficiency
    – Incompetent heart valves allow blood to flow in both directions through valve
    – Volume of pumped blood increases
    – Involved heart chambers dilate to accommodate increased volume

AORTIC INSUFFICIENCY

● **Definition**
  • Incomplete closure of aortic valve
  • Usually results from postinflammatory scarring or retraction of valve leaflets

● **Underlying pathophysiology**
  • Blood flows back into the left ventricle during diastole, causing increased left ventricular diastolic pressure
  • Volume overload, dilatation and, eventually, hypertrophy of the left ventricle result
  • Excess fluid volume leads to increased left atrial and pulmonary vascular pressure

● **Causes**
  • Ankylosing spondylitis
  • Atherosclerosis
  • Chest trauma
  • Connective tissue disorder (as in Marfan's syndrome)
  • Endocarditis
  • Hypertension
  • Prosthetic valve malfunction
  • Rheumatic fever
  • Syphilis
  • Ventricular septal defect

● **Pathophysiologic changes**
  • Exertional dyspnea, orthopnea, and paroxysmal nocturnal dyspnea due to increased pulmonary venous pressure and cardiac dysfunction
  • Fatigue, exercise intolerance, pulmonary congestion, left-sided heart failure, pulsating nail beds (Quincke's sign), and an S_3 heart sound resulting from left ventricular dysfunction

---

Key facts about valve insufficiency

- Occurs when valve leaflets don't completely close
- May affect veins or heart valves
- Damages involved veins or cardiac chambers

Key facts about aortic insufficiency

- Incomplete closure of aortic valve
- Causes blood to flow back into left ventricle during diastole
- Leads to left ventricular hypertrophy and increased left atrial and pulmonary vascular pressures

Key pathophysiologic changes in aortic insufficiency

- Exertional and nocturnal dyspnea and orthopnea
- Angina
- Murmur

- Angina resulting from inadequate coronary perfusion
- Palpitations due to a hyperdynamic and tachycardic left ventricle
- Widened pulse pressure resulting from low diastolic pressure
- Diastolic blowing murmur heard at the left sternal border caused by regurgitant blood flow

- **Complications**
  - Left-sided heart failure
  - Pulmonary edema
  - Myocardial ischemia

- **Diagnostic test findings**
  - Cardiac catheterization detects a reduction in arterial diastolic pressure, aortic insufficiency, other valvular abnormalities, and increased left ventricular end-diastolic pressure
  - Chest X-rays reveal left ventricular enlargement and pulmonary venous congestion
  - Echocardiography reveals left ventricular enlargement, dilation of the aortic annulus and left atrium, thickening of the aortic valve, and alterations in mitral valve movement (indirect indication of aortic valve disease)
  - Electrocardiography (ECG) shows sinus tachycardia, left axis deviation, left ventricular hypertrophy, and left atrial hypertrophy (in severe disease)

- **Treatment**
  - Oxygen to increase oxygenation in acute episodes
  - Dobutamine (Dobutrex) to reduce afterload in acute episodes
  - Vasodilators to reduce systolic load and regurgitant volume
  - Digoxin (Lanoxin, Digitek), low-sodium diet, and a diuretic to treat left-sided heart failure
  - Nitroglycerin (NitroQuick, Nitrostat) to relieve angina
  - Valve replacement with prosthetic valve to remove diseased aortic valve
  - Prophylactic antibiotics before and after surgery or dental care to prevent endocarditis

- **Nursing considerations**
  - Watch closely for signs of heart failure or pulmonary edema
  - Watch for adverse effects of drug therapy
  - Teach the patient about diet restrictions, medications, and the importance of consistent follow-up care
  - After surgery
    - Watch for hypotension, arrhythmias, and thrombus formation
    - Monitor vital signs, arterial blood gas (ABG) values, intake, output, daily weight, blood chemistries, chest X-rays, and pulmonary artery catheter readings

AORTIC STENOSIS

- **Definition**
  - Narrowing of aortic valve
  - Classified as acquired or rheumatic
  - Characterized by angina pectoris, dyspnea, palpitations, and syncope

Key diagnostic test results for aortic insufficiency
- Echocardiogram: Thickening of aortic valve
- Cardiac catheterization: Increased left-ventricular end-diastolic pressure

Key treatments for aortic insufficiency
- Vasodilators
- Digoxin
- Diuretics and low-sodium diet
- Valve replacement (if severe)

Key nursing considerations for aortic insufficiency
- Watch closely for signs and symptoms of heart failure or pulmonary edema.
- Monitor blood pressure, pulse, and weight regularly.
- Postoperatively, watch for hypotension, arrhythmias, and thrombus formation.

Key facts about aortic stenosis
- Narrowing of aortic valve
- May be acquired or rheumatic
- Impedes blood flow
- Can result in left-sided heart failure

Common causes of aortic stenosis

- Congenital aortic bicuspid valve
- Idiopathic fibrosis and calcification
- Rheumatic fever

Key pathophysiologic changes in aortic stenosis

- Systolic murmur
- Exertional dyspnea
- Angina

Key diagnostic test results for aortic stenosis

- Cardiac catheterization: Increased left-ventricular end-diastolic pressure
- Chest X-ray: Dilated aorta

Key treatments for aortic stenosis

- Periodic echocardiography
- Cardiac glycosides
- Low-sodium diet
- Diuretics
- Prophylactic antibiotics before and after surgery or dental care

● **Underlying pathophysiology**
- Aortic valve stenosis impedes forward blood flow
- The left ventricle requires greater pressure to open the narrowed aortic valve
- The added workload increases myocardial oxygen demands
- Diminished cardiac output reduces coronary artery blood flow, leading to ischemia of the left ventricle
- Left ventricular hypertrophy and failure result

● **Causes**
- Atherosclerosis
- Congenital aortic bicuspid valve
- Idiopathic fibrosis and calcification
- Rheumatic fever

● **Pathophysiologic changes**
- Exertional dyspnea due to abnormal diastolic function
- Angina resulting from increased oxygen needs of the hypertrophic myocardium and diminished oxygen delivery secondary to coronary vessel compression
- Syncope due to systemic vasodilation or arrhythmias
- Pulmonary congestion resulting from left-sided heart failure
- Harsh, rasping, crescendo-decrescendo systolic murmur resulting from forced blood flow across stenotic valve

● **Complications**
- Cardiac arrhythmias, especially atrial fibrillation
- Infective endocarditis
- Left-sided heart failure
- Left ventricular hypertrophy
- Right-sided heart failure
- Sudden death

● **Diagnostic test findings**
- Cardiac catheterization reveals a pressure gradient across the valve (indicating obstruction) and increased left ventricular end-diastolic pressures
- Chest X-rays show dilation of the aorta, valvular calcification, left ventricular enlargement, and pulmonary vein congestion
- Echocardiography shows a thickened aortic valve and left ventricular wall, possibly coexistent with mitral valve stenosis
- ECG shows left ventricular hypertrophy

● **Treatment**
- Periodic noninvasive evaluation, such as echocardiography, to monitor severity of valve narrowing
- Cardiac glycosides, such as digoxin, to control atrial fibrillation and to prevent or treat heart failure
- Low-sodium diet and diuretics to treat left-sided heart failure
- Prophylactic antibiotics before and after surgery or dental care to prevent endocarditis
- Percutaneous balloon aortic valvuloplasty to reduce the degree of stenosis
- Aortic valve replacement to replace the diseased valve

TIME-OUT FOR TEACHING

Topics for cardiac patients

Be sure to include these points in your teaching plan for patients with cardiovascular disorders:

- explanation of disease process and goals of treatment
- explanation of medication regimen, including instructions for over-the-counter and herbal preparations; dose, frequency, and time of administration; drug effects; and possible adverse reactions
- need to balance rest with activities
- need to ensure good sleep hygiene to prevent fatigue and strain on cardiac reserve (maintaining a regular bedtime, avoiding stimulants or alcohol before bed, avoiding reading or watching television in bed)
- proper use and maintenance of oxygen therapy equipment, as needed
- need for a low-fat, low-cholesterol diet (with sodium and fluid restrictions, if required) to promote cardiac health and prevent complications
- importance of cardiac rehabilitation or recommended exercise program to enhance aerobic capacity
- need to weigh himself daily first thing in the morning to monitor risk of fluid retention and heart failure and to call the physician if he experiences a 3 lb (1.4 kg) or more gain in 24 hours
- importance of complying with follow-up laboratory testing and physician visits.

TOP 4

Patient teaching topics for cardiac patients

1. Disease process and goals of treatment
2. Medication regimen
3. Diet restrictions
4. Importance of balancing rest with activities

Nursing considerations
- Watch closely for signs of heart failure or pulmonary edema
- Watch for adverse effects of drug therapy
- Teach the patient about diet restrictions, medications, and the importance of consistent follow-up care (see *Topics for cardiac patients*)
- After surgery
  - Watch for hypotension, arrhythmias, and thrombus formation
  - Monitor vital signs, ABG values, intake, output, daily weight, blood chemistries, chest X-rays, and pulmonary artery catheter readings

Key nursing considerations for aortic stenosis

- Watch for signs and symptoms of heart failure or pulmonary edema.
- Instruct patient about diet and medication therapies.
- Postoperatively, watch for hypotension, arrhythmias, and thrombus formation.

BUERGER'S DISEASE

Definition
- Inflammatory, nonlipid occlusive condition that impairs circulation to the legs, feet and, occasionally, hands
- Sometimes called *thromboangiitis obliterans*
- Rare; incidence highest in young and middle-aged men

Underlying pathophysiology
- Polymorphonuclear leukocytes infiltrate the walls of small and medium-sized arteries and veins
- Thrombus develops in the vascular lumen, eventually occluding and obliterating portions of the small vessels, resulting in decreased blood flow to the feet and legs
- Diminished blood flow may produce ulceration and, eventually, gangrene

Key facts about Buerger's disease

- Inflammatory, nonlipid occlusive condition
- Impairs circulation to legs, feet and, occasionally, hands
- Linked to smoking

Key pathophysiologic changes in Buerger's disease

- Intermittent claudication of in-step
- Impaired peripheral pulses

Key diagnostic test results for Buerger's disease

- Doppler ultrasonography: Diminished peripheral vessel circulation
- Arteriography: Lesions in arteries (rules out atherosclerosis)

Key treatments for Buerger's disease

- Exercise program
- Analgesics
- Lumbar sympathectomy (if severe)

● **Causes**
- Unknown
- Linked to smoking (suggesting a hypersensitivity reaction to nicotine)

● **Pathophysiologic changes**
- Intermittent claudication of the instep (due to decreased blood flow) that's aggravated by exercise and relieved by rest
- Impaired peripheral pulses from vasoconstriction and impaired blood flow
- Initially: coldness, cyanosis, and numbness in feet during exposure to low temperatures
- Later: redness, heat, and tingling due to vascular wall hyperactivity

● **Complications**
- Diminished pulses in distal extremities
- Sensitivity to cold in the extremities
- Possible muscle atrophy
- Pain in the digits
- Ulceration and gangrene (fingertip ulcerations if the hands are affected)

● **Diagnostic findings**
- Doppler ultrasonography reveals diminished circulation in the peripheral vessels
- Arteriography locates lesions in arteries and rules out atherosclerosis
- Plethysmography detects decreased circulation in the peripheral vessels
- Venography locates occlusions in veins and rules out thrombophlebitis, varicose veins

● **Treatment**
- Exercise programs that use gravity to fill and drain the blood vessels to promote adequate circulation
- Antibiotics for secondary infection
- Analgesics to control pain
- In severe disease, a lumbar sympathectomy to increase blood supply to the skin
- Amputation for nonhealing ulcers, intractable pain, or gangrene

● **Nursing considerations**
- Encourage the patient to stop smoking permanently to enhance the effectiveness of treatment; if necessary, refer him to a self-help group to stop smoking
- Caution the patient to avoid precipitating factors, such as emotional stress, exposure to extreme temperatures, and trauma
- Teach proper foot care
  - Stress the importance of wearing well-fitting shoes and cotton or wool socks
  - Show the patient how to inspect his feet daily for cuts, abrasions, and signs of skin breakdown, such as redness and soreness
  - Remind the patient to seek medical attention immediately after trauma
- Enforce bed rest for the patient with ulcers and gangrene
  - Provide a padded footboard or bed cradle to prevent pressure from bed linens
  - Protect the feet with soft padding

- Assess rehabilitative needs if the patient has undergone amputation
  - Address concerns regarding changes in body image
  - Refer the patient to physical therapists, occupational therapists, and social service agencies, as needed
- Provide emotional support; if necessary, refer the patient for psychological counseling to help him cope with restrictions imposed by this chronic disease
- Teach the patient about effects, proper usage, and adverse effects of prescribed medications

CARDIAC ARRHYTHMIAS

● **Definition**
  - Instances of abnormal electrical conduction or automaticity that change the heart's rate and rhythm
  - Vary in severity from asymptomatic and not medically treated to catastrophic
  - Generally classified according to origin (ventricular or supraventricular) (see *Types of cardiac arrhythmias,* pages 10 to 15)

● **Underlying pathophysiology**
  - Altered automaticity resulting from partial depolarization may increase the intrinsic rate of the sinoatrial node or latent pacemakers, or may induce ectopic pacemakers to reach threshold and depolarize
  - Formation of abnormal circuits within the conduction fibers leads to back-channel reentry of escape beats, or abnormal electrical conduction

● **Causes**
  - Acid-base imbalances
  - Cellular hypoxia
  - Congenital defects
  - Connective tissue disorders
  - Degeneration of the conductive tissue
  - Drug toxicity
  - Electrolyte imbalances
  - Emotional stress
  - Hypertrophy of the heart muscle
  - Myocardial ischemia or infarction
  - Organic heart disease

● **Pathophysiologic changes**
  - Angina resulting from inadequate coronary artery circulation
  - Dyspnea from inadequate cardiac contractility, which can lead to heart failure
  - Dizziness, weakness, and syncope resulting from impaired cerebral oxygenation due to poor cardiac force and volume
  - Reduced urine output resulting from decreased renal perfusion due to reduced cardiac output

● **Complications**
  - Heart failure
  - MI
  - Sudden cardiac death
  - Thromboembolism

(Text continues on page 16.)

Key nursing considerations for Buerger's disease
- Caution patient to avoid precipitating factors (stress, smoking, extreme temperatures, trauma).
- Teach proper foot care.

Key facts about cardiac arrhythmias
- Instances of abnormal electrical conduction or automaticity
- Alter heart rate and rhythm
- Classified by origin: ventricular or supraventricular

Key pathophysiologic changes in cardiac arrhythmias
- Angina
- Dyspnea
- Dizziness
- Reduced urine output

Types of cardiac arrrhythmias

This chart reviews common cardiac arrhythmias and outlines their features, causes, and treatments. Use a normal electrocardiogram strip, if available, to compare normal cardiac rhythm configurations with the rhythm strips below. Characteristics of normal sinus rhythm include:
- ventricular and atrial rates of 60 to 100 beats/minute
- regular and uniform QRS complexes and P waves
- PR interval of 0.12 to 0.20 second
- QRS duration less than 0.12 second
- identical atrial and ventricular rates, with constant PR intervals.

ARRHYTHMIA	FEATURES

Sinus tachycardia

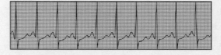

- Atrial and ventricular rhythms regular
- Rate > 100 beats/minute; rarely, > 160 beats/minute
- Normal P wave preceding each QRS complex

Sinus bradycardia

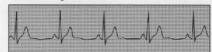

- Atrial and ventricular rhythms regular
- Rate < 60 beats/minute
- Normal P waves preceding each QRS complex

Paroxysmal supraventricular tachycardia

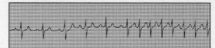

- Atrial and ventricular rhythms regular
- Heart rate > 160 beats/minute; rarely exceeds 250 beats/minute
- P waves regular but aberrant; difficult to differentiate from preceding T wave
- P wave preceding each QRS complex
- Sudden onset and termination of arrhythmia

Atrial flutter

- Atrial rhythm regular; rate 250 to 400 beats/minute
- Ventricular rate variable, depending on degree of AV block (usually 60 to 100 beats/minute)
- No P waves, atrial activity appears as fibrillatory waves (F waves); sawtooth configuration common in lead II
- QRS complexes uniform in shape, but usually irregular in rate

CAUSES	TREATMENT
• Normal physiologic response to fever, exercise, anxiety, pain, dehydration; may also accompany shock, left ventricular failure, cardiac tamponade, hyperthyroidism, anemia, hypovolemia, pulmonary embolism, and anterior wall myocardial infarction (MI) • May also occur with atropine, epinephrine, isoproterenol, quinidine, caffeine, alcohol, cocaine, amphetamine, and nicotine use	• Correction of underlying cause • Beta-adrenergic blocker or calcium channel blocker
• Normal, in well-conditioned heart, as in an athlete • Increased intracranial pressure; increased vagal tone due to straining during defecation, vomiting, intubation, or mechanical ventilation; sick sinus syndrome; hypothyroidism; and inferior wall MI • May also occur with anticholinesterase, beta-adrenergic blocker, digoxin, and morphine use	• Correction of underlying cause • For low cardiac output, dizziness, weakness, altered level of consciousness, or low blood pressure; advanced cardiac life support (ACLS) protocol for administration of atropine • Temporary or permanent pacemaker • Dopamine or epinephrine infusion
• Intrinsic abnormality of atrioventricular (AV) conduction system • Physical or psychological stress, hypoxia, hypokalemia, cardiomyopathy, congenital heart disease, MI, valvular disease, Wolff-Parkinson-White syndrome, cor pulmonale, hyperthyroidism, and systemic hypertension • Digoxin toxicity; use of caffeine, marijuana, or central nervous system stimulants	• If patient is unstable, immediate cardioversion • If patient is stable, vagal stimulation, Valsalva's maneuver, and carotid sinus massage. • If cardiac function is preserved, treatment priority: calcium channel blocker, beta-adrenergic blocker, digoxin, and cardioversion; then consider procainamide, amiodarone, or sotolol if each preceding treatment is ineffective in rhythm conversion. • If the ejection fraction is less than 40% or if the patient is in heart failure, treatment order: digoxin, amiodarone, then diltiazem.
• Heart failure, tricuspid or mitral valve disease, pulmonary embolism, cor pulmonale, inferior wall MI, and pericarditis • Digoxin toxicity	• If patient is unstable with a ventricular rate > 150 beats/minute, immediate cardioversion • If patient is stable, follow ACLS protocol for cardioversion and drug therapy, which may include calcium channel blockers, beta-adrenergic blockers, or antiarrhythmics • Anticoagulation therapy may also be necessary • Radiofrequency ablation to control rhythm

(continued)

Types of cardiac arrrhythmias *(continued)*

ARRHYTHMIA	FEATURES
Atrial fibrillation 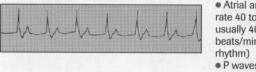	• Atrial rhythm grossly irregular; rate > 400 beats/minute • Ventricular rhythm grossly irregular • QRS complexes of uniform configuration and duration • PR interval indiscernible • No P waves, atrial activity appears as erratic, irregular, baseline fibrillatory waves (F waves)
Junctional rhythm 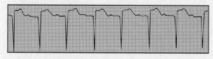	• Atrial and ventricular rhythms regular; atrial rate 40 to 60 beats/minute; ventricular rate usually 40 to 60 beats/minute (60 to 100 beats/minute is accelerated junctional rhythm) • P waves preceding, hidden within (absent), or after QRS complex; usually inverted if visible • PR interval (when present) < 0.12 second • QRS complex configuration and duration normal, except in aberrant conduction
First-degree AV block 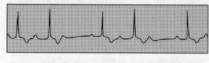	• Atrial and ventricular rhythms regular • PR interval > 0.20 second • P wave precedes QRS complex • QRS complex normal
Second-degree AV block Mobitz I (Wenckebach) 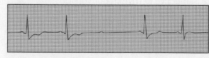	• Atrial rhythm regular • Ventricular rhythm irregular • Atrial rate exceeds ventricular rate • PR interval progressively, but only slightly, longer with each cycle until QRS complex disappears (dropped beat); PR interval shorter after dropped beat
Second-degree AV block Mobitz II 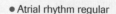	• Atrial rhythm regular • Ventricular rhythm regular or irregular, with varying degree of block • P-P interval constant • QRS complexes periodically absent
Third-degree AV block (complete heart block)	• Atrial rhythm regular • Ventricular rhythm regular and rate slower than atrial rate • No relation between P waves and QRS complexes • No constant PR interval • QRS duration normal (junctional pacemaker) or wide and bizarre (ventricular pacemaker)

CAUSES	TREATMENT
• Heart failure, chronic obstructive pulmonary disease, thyrotoxicosis, constrictive pericarditis, ischemic heart disease, sepsis, pulmonary embolus, rheumatic heart disease, hypertension, mitral stenosis, atrial irritation, or complication of coronary bypass or valve replacement surgery • Nifedipine and digoxin use	• If patient is unstable with a ventricular rate > 150 beats/minute, immediate cardioversion • If patient is stable, follow ACLS protocol and drug therapy, which may include calcium channel blockers, beta-adrenergic blockers, or antiarrhythmics • Anticoagulation therapy may also be necessary • In some patients with refractory atrial fibrillation uncontrolled by drugs, radiofrequency catheter ablation
• Inferior wall MI or ischemia, hypoxia, vagal stimulation, and sick sinus syndrome • Acute rheumatic fever • Valve surgery • Digoxin toxicity	• Correction of underlying cause • Atropine for symptomatic slow rate • Pacemaker insertion if patient doesn't respond to drugs • Discontinuation of digoxin if appropriate
• May be seen in healthy persons • Inferior wall MI or ischemia, hypothyroidism, hypokalemia, and hyperkalemia • Digoxin toxicity; use of quinidine, procainamide, beta-adrenergic blockers, calcium channel blockers, or amiodarone	• Correction of underlying cause • Possibly atropine if severe symptomatic bradycardia develops • Cautious use of digoxin, calcium channel blockers, and beta-adrenergic blockers
• Inferior wall MI, cardiac surgery, acute rheumatic fever, and vagal stimulation • Digoxin toxicity; use of propranolol, quinidine, or procainamide	• Treatment of underlying cause • Atropine or temporary pacemaker for symptomatic bradycardia • Discontinuation of digoxin if appropriate
• Severe coronary artery disease, anterior wall MI, and acute myocarditis • Digoxin toxicity	• Temporary or permanent pacemaker • Atropine, dopamine, or epinephrine for symptomatic bradycardia • Discontinuation of digoxin if appropriate
• Inferior or anterior wall MI, congenital abnormality, rheumatic fever, hypoxia, postoperative complication of mitral valve replacement, postprocedure complication of radiofrequency ablation in or near AV nodal tissue, Lev's disease (fibrosis and calcification that spreads from cardiac structures to the conductive tissue), and Lenègre's disease (conductive tissue fibrosis) • Digoxin toxicity	• Atropine, dopamine, or epinephrine for symptomatic bradycardia • Temporary or permanent pacemaker

(continued)

Types of cardiac arrrhythmias *(continued)*

ARRHYTHMIA	FEATURES
Premature ventricular contraction (PVC) 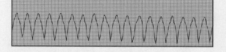	• Atrial rhythm regular • Ventricular rhythm irregular • QRS complex premature, usually followed by a complete compensatory pause • QRS complex wide and distorted, usually > 0.14 second • Premature QRS complexes occurring alone, in pairs, or in threes, alternating with normal beats; focus from one or more sites • Ominous when clustered, multifocal, with R wave on T pattern
Ventricular tachycardia 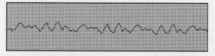	• Ventricular rate 100 to 220 beats/minute, rhythm usually regular • QRS complexes wide, bizarre, and independent of P waves • P waves not discernible • May start and stop suddenly
Ventricular fibrillation 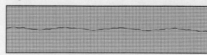	• Ventricular rhythm and rate chaotic and rapid • QRS complexes wide and irregular; no visible P waves
Asystole	• No atrial or ventricular rate or rhythm • No discernible P waves, QRS complexes, or T waves

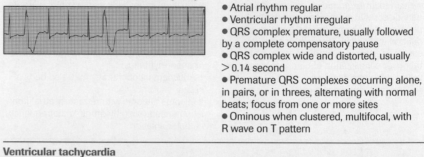

CAUSES	TREATMENT
• Heart failure; old or acute MI, ischemia, or contusion; myocardial irritation by ventricular catheter or a pacemaker; hypercapnia; hypokalemia; hypocalcemia; and hypomagnesemia • Drug toxicity (digoxin, aminophylline, tricyclic antidepressants, beta-adrenergic blockers, isoproterenol, or dopamine) • Caffeine, tobacco, or alcohol use • Psychological stress, anxiety, pain, or exercise	• If warranted, procainamide, amiodarone, or lidocaine I.V. • Treatment of underlying cause • Discontinuation of drug causing toxicity • Potassium chloride I.V. if PVC induced by hypokalemia • Magnesium sulfate I.V. if PVC induced by hypomagnesemia
• Myocardial ischemia, MI, or aneurysm; coronary artery disease; rheumatic heart disease; mitral valve prolapse; heart failure; cardiomyopathy; ventricular catheters; hypokalemia; hypercalcemia; hypomagnesemia; and pulmonary embolism • Digoxin, procainamide, epinephrine, or quinidine toxicity • Anxiety	• With pulse: If hemodynamically stable with monomorphic QRS complexes administration of procainamide, sotalol, amiodarone, or lidocaine (follow ACLS protocol); if drugs are ineffective, cardioversion • If polymorphic QRS complexes and normal QT interval, administer beta-adrenergic blockers, lidocaine, amiodarone, procainamide, or sotalol (follow ACLS protocol); if drug is unsuccessful, cardioversion • If polymorphic QRS and QT interval is prolonged, magnesium I.V., then overdrive pacing if rhythm persists; may also administer isoproterenol, phenytoin, or lidocaine • If pulseless, initiate cardiopulmonary resuscitation (CPR); follow ACLS protocol for defibrillation, endotracheal (ET) intubation, and administration of epinephrine or vasopressin, followed by amiodarone or lidocaine and, if ineffective, magnesium sulfate or procainamide • Implanted cardioverter defibrillator if recurrent ventricular tachycardia
• Myocardial ischemia, MI, untreated ventricular tachycardia, R-on-T phenomenon, hypokalemia, hyperkalemia, hypercalcemia, hypoxemia, alkalosis, electric shock, and hypothermia • Digoxin, epinephrine, or quinidine toxicity	• CPR; follow ACLS protocol for defibrillation, ET intubation, and administration of epinephrine or vasopressin, amiodarone, or lidocaine and, if ineffective, magnesium sulfate or procainamide • Implanted cardioverter defibrillator if risk for recurrent ventricular fibrillation
• Myocardial ischemia, MI, aortic valve disease, heart failure, hypoxia, hypokalemia, severe acidosis, electric shock, ventricular arrhythmia, AV block, pulmonary embolism, heart rupture, cardiac tamponade, hyperkalemia, and electromechanical dissociation • Cocaine overdose	• Continue CPR, follow ACLS protocol for ET intubation, transcutaneous pacing, and administration of epinephrine and atropine.

Key diagnostic test results for cardiac arrhythmias

- ECG: Arrhythmia
- Electrophysiologic testing: Mechanism of the arrhythmia (can also be used for treatment)

Key nursing considerations for cardiac arrhythmias

- Assess an unmonitored patient for rhythm disturbances and assess for possible causes and effects.
- When life-threatening arrhythmias develop, rapidly assess level of consciousness, respirations, and pulse rate.
- Initiate CPR if indicated.

Key facts about cardiac tamponade

- Rapid increase in intrapericardial pressure
- Caused by fluid accumulation in pericardial sac
- Obstructs blood flow into ventricles
- Decreases cardiac output

● **Diagnostic test findings**
- ECG identifies arrhythmias, ischemia, and infarction that may result in arrhythmias
- Laboratory testing identifies electrolyte abnormalities, acid-base abnormalities, or drug toxicities that may cause arrhythmias
- Holter monitoring, event monitoring, and loop recording can detect arrhythmias and the effectiveness of drug therapy during a patient's daily activities
- Exercise testing may detect exercise-induced arrhythmias
- Electrophysiologic testing identifies the mechanism of an arrhythmia and the location of accessory pathways and assesses the effectiveness of antiarrhythmic drugs, radiofrequency ablation, and implanted cardioverter-defibrillators

● **Treatment**
- Varies according to the type of arrhythmia (see *Types of cardiac arrhythmias*, pages 10 to 15)

● **Nursing considerations**
- Assess an unmonitored patient for rhythm disturbances
- Document arrhythmias in a monitored patient, and assess for possible causes and effects
- When life-threatening arrhythmias develop, rapidly assess level of consciousness, respirations, and pulse rate
- Initiate cardiopulmonary resuscitation (CPR) if indicated

CARDIAC TAMPONADE

● **Definition**
- Rapid increase in intrapericardial pressure caused by fluid accumulation in the pericardial sac
- Impaired diastolic filling of the heart

● **Underlying pathophysiology**
- Progressive accumulation of fluid in the pericardial sac causes compression of the heart chambers
- Compression of the heart chambers obstructs blood flow into the ventricles and reduces the amount of blood pumped out with each contraction
- With each contraction more fluid accumulates, decreasing cardiac output

● **Causes**
- Acute MI
- Chronic renal failure in which dialysis is required
- Connective tissue disorders (such as rheumatoid arthritis, Marfan's syndrome, systemic lupus erythematosus, rheumatic fever, vasculitis, and scleroderma)
- Adverse drug reaction to procainamide (Pronestyl), hydralazine (Apresoline), minoxidil (Loniten), isoniazid (Nydrazid), penicillin (Wycillin, Pen Vee K), methysergide maleate (Sansert), or daunorubicin (Cerubidine)
- Effusion, possibly from cancer, bacterial infections, tuberculosis (TB) and, rarely, acute rheumatic fever
- Hemorrhage from nontraumatic causes (such as anticoagulant therapy in patients with pericarditis or rupture of the heart or great vessels)

- Hemorrhage from trauma (such as gunshot or stab wounds to the chest or perforation by the catheter during cardiac or central venous catheterization or after cardiac surgery)
- Idiopathic causes (Dressler's syndrome)
- Viral or postirradiation pericarditis

Pathophysiologic changes

- Elevated central venous pressure (CVP) due to increased jugular venous pressure
- Muffled heart sounds caused by fluid in the pericardial sac, which is unable to distend
- Diaphoresis and cool, clammy skin caused by decreased venous return and cardiac output
- Weak, rapid pulse in response to decreased cardiac output
- Cough, dyspnea, orthopnea, and tachycardia resulting from lung compression caused by an expanding pericardial sac and the inability to move blood from the pulmonary vasculature into the compromised left ventricle

Complications

- Cardiogenic shock
- Death

Diagnostic test findings

- Chest X-rays show a slightly widened mediastinum and possible cardiomegaly; the cardiac silhouette may be goblet-shaped
- ECG shows various changes
  - A low-amplitude QRS complex and electrical alternans are present
  - An alternating beat-to-beat change occurs in the amplitude of the P wave, QRS complex, and T wave
  - Generalized ST-segment elevation is noted in all leads
  - Changes produced by acute pericarditis may appear
- Pulmonary artery catheterization reveals increased right atrial pressure, right ventricular diastolic pressure, and CVP
- Echocardiography reveals pericardial effusion with signs of right ventricular and atrial compression

Treatment

- Supplemental oxygen to improve oxygenation
- Continuous ECG and hemodynamic monitoring in an intensive care unit to detect complications and monitor effects of therapy
- Pericardiocentesis (needle aspiration of the pericardial cavity)
  - Reduces fluid in the pericardial sac
  - Improves systemic arterial pressure and cardiac output
  - May include leaving a catheter in the pericardial space and attaching it to a drainage container to allow for continuous fluid drainage
- Pericardial window (surgical creation of an opening) to remove accumulated fluid from the pericardial sac
- Pericardiectomy (resection of a portion or all of the pericardium) to allow full connection with the pleura if repeated pericardiocentesis fails to prevent recurrence
- Trial volume loading with crystalloids, such as I.V. normal saline solution, to maintain systolic blood pressure

---

Key pathophysiologic changes in cardiac tamponade

- Elevated CVP
- Muffled heart sounds
- Diaphoresis and cool, clammy skin
- Cough, dyspnea, and tachycardia

Key diagnostic test results for cardiac tamponade

- Echocardiography: Pericardial effusion
- Pulmonary artery catheterization: Increased central venous, right atrial, and right ventricular diastolic pressures

Key treatments for cardiac tamponade

- Continuous ECG and hemodynamic monitoring
- Pericardiocentesis
- Pericardial window
- Pericardiectomy
- Inotropic drugs

- Inotropic drugs, such as isoproterenol (Isuprel) or dopamine (Intropin), to improve myocardial contractility until fluid in the pericardial sac can be removed
- Possible blood transfusion or a thoracotomy to drain reaccumulating fluid or to repair bleeding sites (in traumatic injury)
- Administration of protamine sulfate (a heparin antagonist) to stop bleeding in heparin-induced tamponade
- Administration of vitamin K to stop bleeding in warfarin-induced tamponade

● **Nursing considerations**
- If the patient needs pericardiocentesis, monitor vital signs, hemodynamics, and ECG
- Watch for a decrease in CVP and a concomitant increase in blood pressure, which indicate cardiac compression
- Watch for complications, such as ventricular fibrillation, vasovagal response, or coronary artery or cardiac chamber puncture
- Give prescribed medications

CARDIOGENIC SHOCK

● **Definition**
- Diminished cardiac output that severely impairs tissue perfusion
- Sometimes called pump failure

● **Underlying pathophysiology**
- Left ventricular dysfunction initiates a series of compensatory mechanisms that attempt to increase cardiac output
- As cardiac output decreases, aortic and carotid baroreceptors activate sympathetic nervous system responses
- Sympathetic system responses increase heart rate, left ventricular filling pressure, and peripheral resistance to flow to enhance venous return to the heart
- Actions initially stabilize but gradually cause deterioration as oxygen demands increase on already compromised coronary arteries and cardiac muscle
- These events consist of a cycle of low cardiac output, sympathetic compensation, myocardial ischemia, and even lower cardiac output (see *Cardiogenic shock*)

● **Causes**
- Acute mitral or aortic insufficiency
- End-stage cardiomyopathy
- Cardiac tamponade
- MI
- Myocardial ischemia
- Myocarditis
- Papillary muscle dysfunction
- Ventricular aneurysm
- Ventricular arrhythmias
- Ventricular septal defect

● **Pathophysiologic changes**
- Tachycardia and bounding pulse due to sympathetic stimulation
- Restlessness, irritability, and tachypnea resulting from cerebral hypoxia
- Cool, pale skin resulting from vasoconstriction

Key nursing considerations for cardiac tamponade
- Closely monitor blood pressure, CVP, and heart sounds.
- Monitor for ventricular fibrillation, vasovagal response, or cardiac puncture.

Key facts about cardiogenic shock
- Refers to markedly decreased cardiac output
- Severely impairs tissue perfusion
- Involves a cycle of low cardiac output, sympathetic compensation, myocardial ischemia, and even lower cardiac output

Key pathophysiologic changes in cardiogenic shock
- Tachycardia
- Restlessness
- Cool, pale skin
- Hypotension
- Reduced urine output

GO WITH THE FLOW

Cardiogenic shock

This flowchart shows what happens during cardiogenic shock.

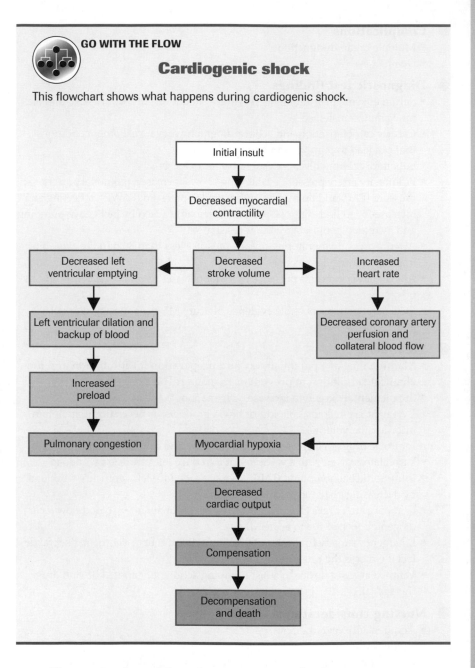

- Hypotension due to failure of compensatory mechanisms
- Narrowed pulse pressure resulting from reduced stroke volume
- Weak, rapid, thready pulse due to decreased cardiac output
- Reduced urine output resulting from poor renal perfusion
- Cyanosis due to hypoxia
- Unconsciousness and absent reflexes due to reduced cerebral perfusion, acid-base imbalance, or electrolyte abnormalities
- Slow, shallow, or Cheyne-Stokes respirations resulting from weakening of patient; respiratory center depression

Key diagnostic test results for cardiogenic shock

- Serum enzyme measurements: Elevated CK, LD, AST, and alanine aminotransferase levels
- Laboratory testing: Elevated troponin levels
- ABG analysis: Metabolic and respiratory acidosis and hypoxia
- ECG: Evidence of acute MI, ischemia, or ventricular aneurysm

Key treatments for cardiogenic shock

- Mechanical ventilation
- Supplemental oxygen
- Inotropic drugs
- Vasodilators given with a vasopressor
- IABP

Key nursing considerations for cardiogenic shock

- Closely monitor vital signs and hemodynamic parameters.
- Check for a patent airway and adequate circulation.
- Initiate emergency response team and begin CPR, if necessary.
- Monitor for cardiac arrhythmias.

● **Complications**
- Multiple organ dysfunction
- Death

● **Diagnostic test findings**
- Serum enzyme measurements reveal elevated levels of CK, LD, AST, and alanine aminotransferase
- Cardiac catheterization and echocardiography may reveal other conditions that can lead to pump dysfunction and failure
- Laboratory testing reveals elevated troponin levels
- Pulmonary artery pressure monitoring shows increased pulmonary artery pressure (PAP) and pulmonary artery wedge pressure (PAWP), reflecting an increase in left end-diastolic pressure (preload) caused by ineffective pumping and increased peripheral vascular resistance
- Arterial pressure monitoring reveals pressure less than 80 mm Hg caused by impaired ventricular ejection
- ABG analysis indicates presence of metabolic and respiratory acidosis and hypoxia
- ECG demonstrates possible evidence of acute MI, ischemia, or ventricular aneurysm

● **Treatment**
- Maintenance of a patent airway and preparation for intubation and mechanical ventilation to prevent or manage respiratory distress
- Supplemental oxygen to increase oxygenation
- I.V. fluids, crystalloids, colloids, or blood products, as necessary, to maintain intravascular volume
- Inotropic drugs to increase heart contractility and cardiac output
- Vasodilators given with a vasopressor to reduce left ventricle's workload
- Intra-aortic balloon pump (IABP) therapy to reduce left ventricle's workload by decreasing systemic vascular resistance
- Coronary artery revascularization to restore coronary artery blood flow if cardiogenic shock is due to acute MI
- Emergency surgery to repair papillary muscle rupture or ventricular septal defect if either is the cause of cardiogenic shock
- Ventricular assist device to assist pumping action of heart if IABP and drug therapy fail

● **Nursing considerations**
- Administer oxygen therapy
- Follow IABP protocols and policies
- Assess continuous hemodynamic parameters with pulmonary artery catheter monitoring
- Monitor the patient for cardiac arrhythmias
- Plan nursing care to allow frequent rest periods for the patient
- Provide as much privacy as possible
- Allow the patient's family to visit and comfort him as much as possible
- Check for a patent airway and adequate circulation
- Perform CPR if blood pressure and heart rate are absent

CARDIOMYOPATHY

● **Definition**
- Disease of the heart muscle fibers
- Occurs in three main forms: dilated, hypertrophic obstructive, and restrictive

● **Underlying pathophysiology**
- Dilated cardiomyopathy
  - Extensively damaged myocardial muscle fibers reduce contractility of the left ventricle
  - As systolic function declines, cardiac output falls
  - The sympathetic nervous system is stimulated to increase heart rate and contractility
  - When compensatory mechanisms can no longer maintain cardiac output, the heart begins to fail
- Hypertrophic obstructive cardiomyopathy
  - The hypertrophied ventricle becomes stiff, noncompliant, and unable to relax during ventricular filling
  - Ventricular filling time is further reduced as a result of tachycardia
  - Reduced ventricular filling leads to low cardiac output
- Restrictive cardiomyopathy
  - Left ventricular hypertrophy and endocardial fibrosis and thickening stiffen the ventricle, thus reducing its ability to relax and fill during diastole
  - Failure of the myocardium to contract completely during systole causes decreased cardiac output

● **Causes**
- Dilated cardiomyopathy
  - Viral or bacterial infections
  - Hypertension
  - Peripartum syndrome related to toxemia
  - Ischemic heart disease
  - Valvular disease
  - Drug hypersensitivity
  - Chemotherapy
  - Cardiotoxic effects of drugs or alcohol
- Hypertrophic obstructive cardiomyopathy
  - Autosomal-dominant trait
  - Hypertension
- Restrictive cardiomyopathy
  - Idiopathic
  - Associated with other diseases, heart transplant, mediastinal radiation, or carcinoid heart disease

● **Pathophysiologic changes**
- Shortness of breath, orthopnea, dyspnea on exertion, paroxysmal nocturnal dyspnea, fatigue, and dry cough at night related to left-sided heart failure
- Peripheral edema, hepatomegaly, jugular vein distention, and weight gain resulting from right-sided heart failure
- Peripheral cyanosis and tachycardia resulting from low cardiac output
- Irregular pulse due to atrial fibrillation

Key facts about cardiomyopathy

- Dilated: Damaged myocardial muscle fibers reduce contractility of the left ventricle
- Hypertrophic obstructive: Ventricle becomes stiff and noncompliant, reducing ventricular filling time
- Restrictive: Left ventricular hypertrophy and endocardial fibrosis and thickening stiffen the ventricle, reducing fill during diastole

Common causes of cardiomyopathy

- Uncontrolled hypertension
- Viral or bacterial infections
- Cardiotoxic effects of chemotherapy or other drugs
- Severe valvular disease

Key pathophysiologic changes in cardiomyopathy

- Dyspnea
- Peripheral edema
- Fatigue
- Tachycardia
- Dry cough at night

- Angina due to inability of intramural coronary arteries to supply enough blood to meet increased oxygen demands of hypertrophied heart
- Systolic ejection murmur along left sternal border and at apex resulting from mitral insufficiency
- Fatigue, dyspnea, orthopnea, chest pain, edema, liver engorgement, peripheral cyanosis, pallor, and S_3 or S_4 gallop rhythms caused by heart failure
- Systolic murmurs resulting from mitral and tricuspid insufficiency

Complications

- Dilated cardiomyopathy
  - Intractable heart failure
  - Arrhythmias
  - Emboli
- Hypertrophic obstructive cardiomyopathy
  - Dyspnea
  - Fatigue
  - Signs of heart failure
  - Sudden cardiac death
- Restrictive cardiomyopathy
  - Heart failure
  - Arrhythmia
  - Systemic or pulmonary embolization
  - Sudden death

Diagnostic test findings

- Echocardiography confirms dilated cardiomyopathy
- Chest X-ray may reveal associated cardiomegaly
- Cardiac catheterization and biopsy can be definitive in cases of hypertrophic cardiomyopathy
- Radionuclide studies may reveal left ventricular dilation and reduced ejection fraction

Treatment

- Dilated cardiomyopathy
  - Angiotensin-converting enzyme (ACE) inhibitors to promote vasodilation and reduce afterload
  - Diuretics to reduce fluid retention
  - Digoxin (Digitek, Lanoxin) to improve myocardial contractility in patients who don't respond to diuretics
  - Hydralazine and isosorbide dinitrate (Isordil) to promote vasodilation
  - Beta-adrenergic blockers (atenolol [Tenormin], metoprolol [Toprol XL], nadolol [Corgard], propranolol [Inderal]) to treat New York Heart Association (NYHA) class II or III heart failure
  - Antiarrhythmics or an implantable cardioverter-defibrillator (ICD) to control arrhythmias
  - Pacemaker insertion to correct arrhythmias
  - Biventricular pacemaker for cardiac resynchronization therapy if patient has certain criteria
    - Presence of symptoms despite optimal drug therapy
    - QRS duration of 0.13 second or more
    - Ejection fraction of 35% or less
    - NYHA class III or IV heart failure

Common complications of cardiomyopathy

- Intractable heart failure
- Arrhythmias
- Sudden cardiac death

Key diagnostic test results for cardiomyopathy

- Echocardiography: Dilated cardiomyopathy
- Cardiac catheterization and biopsy: Hypertrophic cardiomyopathy

Key treatments for cardiomyopathy

Dilated
- ACE inhibitors
- Diuretics
- Digoxin
- Antiarrhythmics or an ICD
- Beta-adrenergic blockers

Hypertrophic obstructive
- Beta-adrenergic blockers
- Antiarrhythmics
- Anticoagulants
- Cardioversion

Restrictive
- Deferoxamine
- Digoxin
- Diuretics
- Low-sodium diet
- Oral vasodilators

- Revascularization (such as coronary artery bypass graft [CABG] surgery) to manage dilated cardiomyopathy caused by ischemia
- Valvular repair or replacement to manage dilated cardiomyopathy from valve dysfunction
- Heart transplantation for patients who don't respond to medical therapy
- Lifestyle modifications (smoking cessation; low-fat, low-sodium diet; physical activity; abstinence from alcohol) to reduce symptoms and improve quality of life
- Hypertrophic obstructive cardiomyopathy
  - Beta-adrenergic blockers to relax obstructing muscle, thereby slowing heart rate, reducing myocardial oxygen demands, increasing ventricular filling, and increasing cardiac output
  - Antiarrhythmic drugs, such as amiodarone (Cordarone), to reduce arrhythmias
  - Cardioversion to treat atrial fibrillation
  - Anticoagulants, such as warfarin (Coumadin), to reduce the risk of systemic embolism with atrial fibrillation
  - Verapamil (Calan) or diltiazem (Cardizem) to reduce septal stiffness and diastolic pressures
  - ICD to treat ventricular arrhythmias
  - Ventricular myotomy or myectomy (resection of hypertrophied septum) to ease outflow tract obstruction and relieve symptoms
- Restrictive cardiomyopathy
  - Deferoxamine (Desferal) to bind iron due to hemochromatosis
  - Digoxin, diuretics, and restricted sodium diet to ease symptoms of heart failure
  - Oral vasodilators, such as isosorbide dinitrate and hydralazine, to decrease afterload and facilitate ventricular ejection

● **Nursing considerations**
- Alternate periods of rest with required activities of daily living
- Provide active or passive range-of-motion (ROM) exercises
- Administer oxygen because oxygen consumption increases
- Check serum potassium levels for hypokalemia, especially if therapy includes cardiac glycosides
- Teach the patient about his medications and potential adverse reactions

CORONARY ARTERY DISEASE

● **Definition**
- Narrowing of coronary arteries due to atherosclerosis
- Results in heart disease
- Primary effect: loss of oxygen and nutrients to myocardial tissue because of diminished coronary blood flow
- Also known as CAD

● **Underlying pathophysiology**
- Increased blood levels of low-density lipoprotein (LDL) irritate or damage the inner layer of coronary vessels
- LDL enters the vessel after damaging the protective barrier, accumulates, and forms a fatty streak

---

Key nursing considerations for cardiomyopathy

- Help patient balance rest and activity.
- Administer oxygen therapy as required.
- Regularly check laboratory values, especially potassium.

Key facts about CAD

- Narrowing of coronary arteries due to atherosclerosis
- Develops when increased blood levels of LDL damage coronary vessels and form fatty streaks
- Progresses when smooth muscle cells engulf fatty streaks, produce fibrous tissue, and stimulate calcium deposition, creating a CAD lesion
- Results in heart disease

- Smooth muscle cells move to the inner layer to engulf the fatty substance, produce fibrous tissue, and stimulate calcium deposition
- This cycle continues, resulting in transformation of the fatty streak into fibrous plaques, and eventually a coronary artery disease (CAD) lesion evolves
- Oxygen deprivation forces the myocardium to shift from aerobic to anaerobic metabolism, leading to accumulation of lactic acid and reduction of cellular pH
- A combination of hypoxia, reduced energy availability, and acidosis rapidly impairs left ventricular function
- Strength of contractions in the affected myocardial region is reduced because the fibers shorten inadequately, resulting in less force and velocity
- Wall motion is abnormal in the ischemic area, resulting in less blood being ejected from the heart with each contraction

Causes
- Atherosclerosis
- Congenital defects
- Coronary artery spasm
- Dissecting aneurysm
- Infectious vasculitis
- Syphilis

Pathophysiologic changes
- Substernal or precordial chest pain resulting from myocardial ischemia (may radiate to left arm, neck, jaw, or shoulder blade)
- Shortness of breath from decreased oxygenation due to ischemia
- Diaphoresis and pallor caused by the sympathetic nervous system's response to ischemia

Complications
- Arrhythmias
- Ischemic cardiomyopathy
- MI

Diagnostic test findings
- ECG during angina may show ischemic changes
- Exercise stress testing has two purposes
  - It reveals ST-segment changes during exercise or pharmacologic stress, indicating ischemia
  - It determines a safe level of exercise for patients who are instructed to increase activity
- Coronary angiography reveals the location and degree of coronary artery stenosis or obstruction, collateral circulation, and the condition of the artery beyond the narrowing
- Intravascular ultrasound may be used to determine the extent of coronary and lumenal narrowing and further define the location and characteristics of the patient's coronary anatomy
- Myocardial perfusion imaging with thallium-201 may be performed during treadmill exercise to detect ischemic areas of the myocardium
  - Ischemic areas appear as "cold spots," which normalize during rest, indicating viable tissue
- Stress echocardiography may show abnormal wall motion in ischemic areas

• Pharmacologic myocardial perfusion imaging in arteries with stenosis shows a decrease in blood flow proportional to the percentage of occlusion

● **Treatment**
  • Nitrates to reduce myocardial oxygen consumption
  • Beta-adrenergic blockers to reduce the heart's workload and oxygen demands by reducing heart rate and peripheral resistance to blood flow
  • Calcium channel blockers to prevent coronary artery spasm
  • Antiplatelet drugs to minimize platelet aggregation and the risk of coronary occlusion
  • Antilipemic drugs to reduce serum cholesterol or triglyceride levels
  • Antihypertensive drugs to control hypertension
  • CABG surgery to restore blood flow by bypassing an occluded artery using another vessel
  • Minimally invasive surgery, using fiber-optic cameras inserted through small cuts in the chest, to correct blockages in one or two accessible arteries
  • Angioplasty to relieve occlusion in patients without calcification and partial occlusion
  • Laser angioplasty to correct occlusion by vaporizing fatty deposits
  • Rotational atherectomy (removal of arterial plaque with a rotating shaver or high-speed "burr" device)
  • Stent placement to maintain patency in a reopened artery
  • Drug-eluting stent placement (currently being used in clinical trials)
    – Keeps the reopened artery open
    – Minimizes the risk of restenosis in the stent
  • Lifestyle modifications (smoking cessation, regular exercise, stress management, maintaining an ideal body weight, following a low-fat, low-sodium diet) to reduce further progression of the CAD

● **Nursing considerations**
  • Provide appropriate care during anginal episodes
    – Monitor blood pressure and heart rate
    – Obtain an ECG during anginal episodes and before administering nitroglycerin or other nitrates
    – Record duration of pain, amount of medication required to relieve the pain, and accompanying symptoms
  • **Keep nitroglycerin available for immediate use**
  • **Instruct the patient to call immediately whenever he feels chest, arm, or neck pain**
  • Before cardiac catheterization, explain the procedure to the patient
  • Provide appropriate care after catheterization
    – **Monitor the catheter site for bleeding**
    – **Check for distal pulses**
    – Make sure the patient drinks plenty of fluids to counter the diuretic effect of the dye
    – Assess potassium levels
  • If the patient is scheduled for surgery, explain the procedure to the patient and his family
  • After surgery, monitor blood pressure, intake and output, breath sounds, chest tube drainage, and ECG, watching for signs of ischemia and arrhythmias

Key treatments for CAD
● Nitrates
● Beta-adrenergic blockers
● Calcium channel blockers
● Antiplatelet drugs
● Antilipemic drugs
● Lifestyle modifications

Key nursing considerations for CAD
● Intervene as needed with nitroglycerin or morphine during acute episodes.
● Instruct patient to call immediately whenever he feels chest, arm, or neck pain.
● Inform patient about cardiac procedures ordered.
● After cardiac catheterization, monitor site for bleeding and check distal pulses.

Key facts about endocarditis

- Infection of endocardium, heart valves, or cardiac prosthesis
- Develops when fibrin and platelets on valve tissue engulf circulating bacteria or fungi, creating vegetation that covers valve surfaces and spreads to chordae tendineae and endothelium

Predisposing factors for endocarditis

- I.V. drug abuse
- Presence of prosthetic heart valve
- Mitral valve prolapse

Key pathophysiologic changes in endocarditis

- Fever
- Cough
- Pleuritic pain
- Heart murmur
- Neurologic defects

- Before discharge, stress the need to follow the prescribed drug regimen, exercise program, and diet

ENDOCARDITIS

● Definition
- Infection of the endocardium, heart valves, or cardiac prosthesis

● Underlying pathophysiology
- Fibrin and platelets cluster on valve tissue, engulfing bacteria or fungi that catch on to valves as they circulate in the bloodstream
- The collection of microorganisms, fibrin, and platelets forms vegetation that can cover the valve surfaces and spread to the chordae tendineae, the endothelial lining of the heart chambers, or the endothelium of the great vessels leading to and from the heart
- Deformities and destruction of valvular tissue occur and may extend to the chordae tendineae, causing them to rupture, and leading to valvular insufficiency
- Pieces of the vegetative growth may break off and form emboli that travel to the spleen, kidneys, central nervous system (CNS), or lungs

● Causes
- Results from bacterial or fungal invasion
- Most common predisposing conditions
  - I.V. drug abuse
  - Presence of a prosthetic heart valve
  - Mitral valve prolapse (especially in males with a systolic murmur)
  - Rheumatic heart disease
- Other predisposing conditions
  - Coarctation of the aorta
  - Tetralogy of Fallot
  - Subaortic and valvular aortic stenosis
  - Ventricular septal defects
  - Pulmonary stenosis
  - Connective tissue disorders, such as Marfan's syndrome or systemic lupus erythematosus
  - Degenerative heart disease, especially calcific aortic stenosis
  - Syphilitic aortic valve (rarely)

● Pathophysiologic changes
- Fever and chills due to bacterial infection
- Heart murmur due to turbulent blood flow
- Hematuria, pyuria, flank pain, and decreased urine output resulting from renal infarction
- Cough, pleuritic pain, pleural friction rub, dyspnea, and rales resulting from pulmonary infarction
- Pain in the left upper quadrant radiating to the left shoulder, and abdominal rigidity resulting from splenic infarction
- Hemiparesis, aphasia, or other neurologic deficits due to cerebral infarction from emboli

Complications
- Acute renal failure
- Aortic root abscesses
- Arthritis
- Brain abscess
- Cardiac arrhythmia
- Cerebral emboli
- Glomerulonephritis
- Heart failure
- Meningitis
- Myocardial abscess
- New cardiac murmur
- Pericarditis
- Septic pulmonary infarct
- Death

Diagnostic test findings
- Three or more blood cultures in a 24- to 48-hour period (each from a separate venipuncture) can identify the causative organism in up to 90% of patients
- WBC count and differential are normal or elevated
- Complete blood count (CBC) and anemia panel show normocytic, normochromic anemia in subacute infective endocarditis
- Erythrocyte sedimentation rate (ESR) and serum creatinine levels are elevated
- Serum rheumatoid factor is positive in about one-half of all patients with endocarditis after the disease is present for 6 weeks
- Urinalysis shows proteinuria and microscopic hematuria
- Echocardiography may identify valvular damage in up to 80% of patients with valve disease
- ECG may show atrial fibrillation and other arrhythmias that accompany valvular disease

Treatment
- Antimicrobial therapy (combination of penicillin and an aminoglycoside, usually gentamicin [Garamycin, Jenamicin]) for 4 to 6 weeks
- Supportive treatment (bed rest, aspirin for fever and aches, sufficient fluid intake)
- Corrective surgery
  - For patients with severe valvular damage, especially aortic or mitral insufficiency, if refractory heart failure develops
  - For replacement of an infected prosthetic valve

Nursing considerations
- Administer antibiotics on time to maintain consistent blood levels
- Observe for signs of infiltration or inflammation at the venipuncture site
  - These signs (redness, swelling, heat) are possible complications of long-term I.V. drug administration
  - To reduce the risk of complications, rotate venous access sites
- Watch for signs of embolization (hematuria, pleuritic chest pain, left upper quadrant pain, or paresis), a common occurrence during the first 3 months of treatment

Key diagnostic test results for endocarditis
- Blood cultures: Causative organism
- Echocardiography: Valvular damage

Key treatments for endocarditis
- Antimicrobial therapy
- Supportive treatment

Key nursing considerations for endocarditis
- Administer antibiotics on time to maintain consistent blood levels.
- Monitor for embolic effects.
- Observe for signs of heart failure.

- Monitor the patient's renal status (blood urea nitrogen [BUN] levels, creatinine clearance, and urine output) for signs of renal emboli or evidence of drug toxicity
- Observe for signs of heart failure, such as dyspnea, tachypnea, tachycardia, crackles, jugular vein distention, edema, and weight gain
- Teach the patient and his family about the disease and the need for prolonged treatment
- Make sure the patient who's susceptible to endocarditis understands the need for prophylactic antibiotics before, during, and after dental work, childbirth, and urologic, GI, or gynecologic procedures
- Teach the patient to recognize signs and symptoms of endocarditis that should be reported to the physician immediately

HEART FAILURE

Definition
- Syndrome that occurs when the heart can't pump enough blood to meet the body's metabolic needs
- Results in intravascular and interstitial volume overload and poor tissue perfusion
- May be classified according to side of heart affected (left- or right-side heart failure) (see *What happens in heart failure*)

Underlying pathophysiology
- Left-sided heart failure
  - Pumping ability of the left ventricle fails
  - Cardiac output falls
  - Blood backs up into the left atrium and lungs, causing pulmonary congestion
- Right-sided heart failure
  - Right ventricular contractility is ineffective
  - Blood backs up into the right atrium and the peripheral circulation
  - Peripheral edema develops and the kidneys and other organs become engorged

Causes
- Anemia
- Arrhythmias
- Atherosclerosis with MI
- Constrictive pericarditis
- Emotional stress
- Hypertension
- Increased salt or water intake
- Infections
- Mitral or aortic insufficiency
- Mitral stenosis secondary to rheumatic heart disease, constrictive pericarditis, or atrial fibrillation
- Myocarditis
- Pregnancy
- Pulmonary embolism

Key facts about heart failure
- Heart can't pump enough blood to meet the body's metabolic needs

Left-sided heart failure
- Occurs when pumping ability of left ventricle fails
- Results in pulmonary congestion because blood backs up into left atrium and lungs

Right-sided heart failure
- Develops because right ventricular contractility is ineffective
- Causes blood to back up into right atrium and peripheral circulation

Common causes of heart failure
- Atherosclerosis with MI
- Increased salt or water intake
- Mitral stenosis secondary to rheumatic heart disease, constrictive pericarditis, or atrial fibrillation

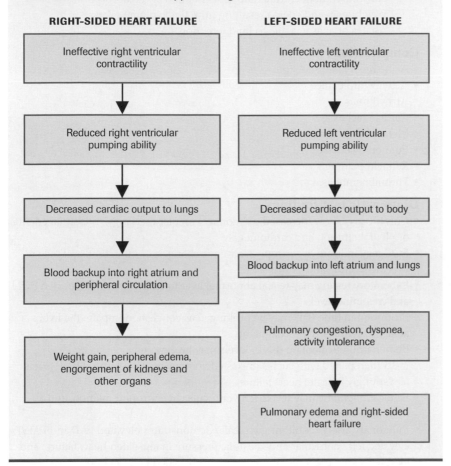

GO WITH THE FLOW

What happens in heart failure

This flowchart shows what happens in right-sided and left-sided heart failure.

RIGHT-SIDED HEART FAILURE

Ineffective right ventricular contractility

↓

Reduced right ventricular pumping ability

↓

Decreased cardiac output to lungs

↓

Blood backup into right atrium and peripheral circulation

↓

Weight gain, peripheral edema, engorgement of kidneys and other organs

LEFT-SIDED HEART FAILURE

Ineffective left ventricular contractility

↓

Reduced left ventricular pumping ability

↓

Decreased cardiac output to body

↓

Blood backup into left atrium and lungs

↓

Pulmonary congestion, dyspnea, activity intolerance

↓

Pulmonary edema and right-sided heart failure

- Thyrotoxicosis
- Ventricular and atrial septal defects

Pathophysiologic changes

- Left-sided heart failure
  - Dyspnea, orthopnea, paroxysmal nocturnal dyspnea, nonproductive cough, and crackles due to pulmonary congestion
  - Fatigue resulting from reduced oxygenation
  - Inability to increase cardiac output in response to physical activity
  - Tachycardia due to sympathetic stimulation
  - Cool, pale skin related to peripheral vasoconstriction
  - S_3 due to rapid ventricular filling
  - S_4 resulting from atrial contraction against the noncompliant ventricle
- Right-sided heart failure

Key pathophysiologic changes in heart failure

Left-sided heart failure
- Dyspnea
- Crackles
- S_3 and S_4

Right-sided heart failure
- Elevated jugular vein distention
- Weight gain
- Edema

– Elevated jugular vein distention, positive hepatojugular reflux, and hepatomegaly from venous congestion
– Right upper quadrant pain resulting from liver engorgement
– Anorexia, fullness, and nausea due to congestion of the liver and intestines
– Nocturia from nocturnal fluid redistribution and reabsorption
– Weight gain and edema resulting from fluid volume excess
– Ascites or anasarca due to fluid retention

● **Complications**
  • Acute renal failure
  • Activity intolerance
  • Arrhythmias
  • Cardiac cachexia
  • Metabolic impairment
  • Pulmonary edema
  • Renal impairment
  • Thromboembolism

● **Diagnostic test findings**
  • Chest X-rays show increased pulmonary vascular markings, interstitial edema, or pleural effusion and cardiomegaly
  • ECG may indicate hypertrophy, ischemic changes, or infarction, and may reveal tachycardia and extrasystoles
  • Laboratory testing may reveal abnormal liver function tests and elevated BUN and creatinine levels
  • Prothrombin time (PT) may be prolonged as congestion impairs the liver's ability to synthesize procoagulants
  • Brain natriuretic peptide (BNP) levels may be elevated
    – When paired with such signs as edematous ankles, elevated BNP levels strongly indicate heart failure
  • Echocardiography may reveal left ventricular hypertrophy, dilation, and abnormal contractility
  • Pulmonary artery monitoring typically demonstrates elevated PAP and PAWP, elevated left ventricular end-diastolic pressure in left-sided heart failure, and elevated right atrial pressure or CVP in right-sided heart failure
  • Radionuclide ventriculography may reveal an ejection fraction less than 40%; in diastolic dysfunction, the ejection fraction may be normal

● **Treatment**
  • ACE inhibitors to reduce angiotensin II production, thus reducing preload and afterload
  • Cardiac glycoside (digoxin) to increase myocardial contractility, improve cardiac output, reduce ventricular volume, and decrease ventricular stretch
  • Diuretics to reduce fluid volume overload and venous return
  • Beta-adrenergic blockers to prevent remodeling in the patient with NYHA class II or III heart failure caused by left ventricular systolic dysfunction (see *Classifying heart failure*)
  • Inotropic therapy with dobutamine (Dobutrex) or milrinone (Primacor) for acute treatment of exacerbated heart failure

---

Key diagnostic test results for heart failure

● Chest X-rays: Increased pulmonary vascular markings, interstitial edema, or pleural effusion and cardiomegaly
● Echocardiography: Cardiac enlargement and abnormal contractility
● Pulmonary artery monitoring: Elevated PAP and PAWP, elevated left ventricular end-diastolic pressure in left-sided heart failure, elevated right atrial pressure or CVP in right-sided heart failure

Key treatments for heart failure

● ACE inhibitors
● Cardiac glycosides
● Diuretics
● Beta-adrenergic blockers
● Lifestyle modifications
● Nitrates

Classifying heart failure

The New York Heart Association classification is a universal gauge of heart failure severity based on physical limitations.

CLASS I: MINIMAL
- No limitations
- Ordinary physical activity doesn't cause undue fatigue, dyspnea, palpitations, or angina

CLASS III: MODERATE
- Markedly limited physical activity
- Comfortable at rest
- Less than ordinary activity produces symptoms

CLASS II: MILD
- Slightly limited physical activity
- Comfortable at rest
- Ordinary physical activity results in fatigue, palpitations, dyspnea, or angina

CLASS IV: SEVERE
- Unable to perform physical activity without discomfort
- Angina or symptoms of cardiac inefficiency may develop at rest

---

- Nesiritide (Natrecor), a human B-type natriuretic peptide, to augment diuresis and decrease afterload for acute management of exacerbated heart failure
- Diuretics, nitrates, morphine (MSIR, Avinza, Roxanol), and oxygen to treat pulmonary edema
- Lifestyle modifications (weight loss, limited sodium and alcohol intake, reduced fat intake, smoking cessation, stress reduction, participation in an exercise program) to reduce symptoms of heart failure
- CABG surgery or angioplasty for heart failure due to CAD
- Heart transplantation for the patient who experiences limitations or repeated hospitalizations after receiving aggressive medical treatment

● **Nursing considerations**
- Place the patient in Fowler's position and give supplemental oxygen to optimize gas exchange
- Monitor daily weight to detect peripheral edema and other signs and symptoms of fluid overload
- Frequently monitor BUN, creatinine, and serum potassium, sodium, chloride, and magnesium levels
- Provide continuous cardiac monitoring during acute and advanced stages
- Assist the patient with ROM exercises
- Apply antiembolism stockings and check regularly for calf pain and tenderness
- Advise the patient to avoid foods high in sodium
- Encourage the patient to participate in an outpatient cardiac rehabilitation program
- Explain that the potassium lost through diuretic therapy may need to be replaced by taking a prescribed potassium supplement and eating high-potassium foods
- Teach medication dosage, administration, potential adverse effects, and monitoring needs

Key nursing considerations for heart failure

- Monitor weight daily.
- Monitor electrolyte levels.
- Inform patient about therapeutic and adverse effects of prescribed medications.
- Teach patient signs and symptoms of heart failure.

Key facts about hypertension

- Refers to systolic blood pressure higher than 139 mm Hg and diastolic blood pressure higher than 89 mm Hg
- May be essential (primary) or secondary
- Is explained by several theories

Modifiable risk factors for hypertension

- Diabetes mellitus
- Excessive alcohol consumption
- High intake of sodium and saturated fat
- Obesity
- Sedentary lifestyle
- Stress
- Tobacco use

Key pathophysiologic changes in hypertension

- Dizziness
- Fatigue
- Edema
- Vision changes

- Teach the patient signs and symptoms to report
  - Irregular pulse (less than 60 beats/min)
  - Dizziness, blurred vision
  - Shortness of breath, persistent dry cough, palpitations, increased fatigue, paroxysmal nocturnal dyspnea
  - Swollen ankles, decreased urine output, rapid weight gain (3 to 5 lb [1.5 to 2.5 kg] in 1 week)

HYPERTENSION

Definition
- Intermittent or sustained elevation of blood pressure
  - Systolic blood pressure higher than 139 mm Hg
  - Diastolic blood pressure higher than 89 mm Hg
- Occurs as two major types
  - Essential (primary)
  - Secondary
- Can be labeled malignant—a severe, fulminant form of hypertension common to both types

Underlying pathophysiology
- Several theories explain how hypertension develops
  - Changes in the arteriolar bed cause increased peripheral vascular resistance
  - Abnormally increased tone in the sympathetic nervous system that originates in the vasomotor system centers causes increased peripheral vascular resistance
  - Renal or hormonal dysfunction results in increased blood volume
  - An increase in arteriolar thickening caused by genetic factors leads to increased peripheral vascular resistance
  - Abnormal renin release causes the formation of angiotensin II, which constricts the arteriole and increases blood volume

Causes
- Exact cause unknown; several risk factors identified
- Modifiable risk factors
  - Diabetes mellitus
  - Excessive alcohol consumption
  - High intake of sodium and saturated fat
  - Obesity
  - Sedentary lifestyle
  - Stress
  - Tobacco use
- Nonmodifiable risk factors
  - Advancing age
  - Family history
  - Race (most common in blacks)

Pathophysiologic changes
- Elevated blood pressure due to vasoconstriction
- Bruits resulting from stenosis or aneurysm

- Dizziness, confusion, and fatigue from decreased tissue perfusion due to vasoconstriction of blood vessels
- Blurry vision resulting from retinal damage
- Nocturia due to increased blood flow to kidneys and increased glomerular filtration
- Edema resulting from increased capillary pressure

Complications
- Hypertensive crisis, peripheral arterial disease, dissecting aortic aneurysm, CAD, angina, MI, heart failure, arrhythmias, and sudden death
- Renal failure
- Transient ischemic attacks, stroke, retinopathy, and hypertensive encephalopathy

Diagnostic test findings
- Urinalysis suggests various conditions
  - Presence of protein, casts, RBCs, or WBCs suggests renal disease
  - Presence of catecholamines is associated with pheochromocytoma
  - Presence of glucose suggests diabetes
- Laboratory testing reveals elevated BUN and serum creatinine levels, suggestive of renal disease; or hypokalemia, indicating adrenal dysfunction (primary hyperaldosteronism)
- CBC may reveal other causes of hypertension, such as polycythemia or anemia
- Excretory urography shows renal atrophy, indicating chronic renal disease
  - One kidney smaller than the other suggests unilateral renal disease
- ECG detects left ventricular hypertrophy or ischemia
- Chest X-rays may show cardiomegaly
- Echocardiography may reveal left ventricular hypertrophy

Treatment
- Lifestyle modifications (weight reduction, moderation of alcohol intake, regular physical exercise, diet low in saturated fat and sodium, smoking cessation)
- Correction of the underlying cause and control of hypertensive effects (secondary hypertension)
- Adequate calcium, magnesium, and potassium intake
- Drug therapy, including diuretics, beta-adrenergic blockers, calcium channel blockers, ACE inhibitors, alpha-adrenergic blockers, and aldosterone antagonists

Nursing considerations
- Encourage the patient to establish a daily routine for taking his medications
- Instruct the patient to report adverse drug effects
- Advise the patient to avoid high-sodium antacids and over-the-counter cold and sinus medications, which contain harmful vasoconstrictors
- Help the obese patient develop a weight-loss nutrition plan
  - Explain the need to avoid high-sodium foods and table salt
- Help the patient examine and modify his lifestyle
- When routine blood pressure screening reveals elevated pressure, make sure the cuff size is appropriate for the patient's upper arm circumference
  - Take pressure readings in both arms while the patient is lying, sitting, and standing

Key diagnostic test results for hypertension
- ECG: Left ventricular enlargement or ischemia
- Chest X-ray: Cardiac enlargement
- Laboratory testing: Elevated renal blood levels (renal origin) or decreased potassium level (adrenal origin)

Key treatments for hypertension
- Lifestyle modifications
- Correction of underlying cause
- Diuretics and other medications

Key nursing considerations for hypertension
- Instruct patient about diet and medication restrictions.
- Instruct patient about techniques for maintaining optimal weight.
- Ensure accurate blood pressure measurement at home and in medical facilities.

HYPOVOLEMIC SHOCK

● **Definition**
- Circulatory dysfunction and inadequate tissue perfusion caused by reduced intravascular blood volume
- Prognosis depends on early recognition and prompt treatment

● **Underlying pathophysiology**
- Fluid is lost from the intravascular space
- Venous return to the heart is reduced
- Ventricular filling is decreased, which leads to a drop in stroke volume
- Cardiac output falls, causing reduced perfusion to tissues and organs
- Tissue anoxia prompts a shift in cellular metabolism from aerobic to anaerobic pathways; this produces an accumulation of lactic acid, resulting in metabolic acidosis

● **Causes**
- Blood loss, hemothorax
- Burns
- Fluid shifts as with ascites
- GI fluid loss
- Peritonitis
- Renal loss (diabetic ketoacidosis, diabetes insipidus, adrenal insufficiency)

● **Pathophysiologic changes**
- Tachycardia related to sympathetic stimulation
- Restlessness, irritability, and tachypnea resulting from cerebral hypoxia
- Reduced urine output and cool, pale, clammy skin due to reduced fluid volume or vasoconstriction
- Hypotension resulting from failure of compensatory mechanisms
- Narrowed pulse pressure and weak, rapid, thready pulse due to reduced stroke volume and decreased cardiac output
- Shallow respirations due to overall weakening
- Reduced urine output due to poor renal perfusion
- Cyanosis resulting from hypoxia
- Metabolic acidosis due to tissue anoxia

● **Complications**
- Acute respiratory distress syndrome
- Acute tubular necrosis and renal failure
- Disseminated intravascular coagulation (DIC)
- Multiple organ dysfunction

● **Diagnostic test findings**
- Laboratory testing reveals decreased hematocrit, hemoglobin level, RBCs, and platelets, and elevated serum potassium, sodium, LD, creatinine, and BUN
- Urine specific gravity and urine osmolality are increased
- ABG analysis shows decreased pH and partial pressure of arterial oxygen (Pao_2), and increased partial pressure of arterial carbon dioxide ($Paco_2$)
- Aspiration of gastric contents through a nasogastric tube may reveal internal bleeding
- Occult blood tests are positive

Key facts about hypovolemic shock
- Refers to circulatory dysfunction and inadequate tissue perfusion
- Caused by reduced intravascular blood volume
- If profuse, can quickly lead to tissue anoxia

Key pathophysiologic changes in hypovolemic shock
- Tachycardia
- Restlessness
- Hypotension
- Reduced urine output

Key diagnostic test results for hypovolemic shock
- ABG analysis: Decreased pH and Pao_2; increased $Paco_2$
- CBC: Decreased hemoglobin level, hematocrit, and RBC and platelet counts
- Invasive hemodynamic monitoring: Reduced pressures

- Coagulation studies show coagulopathy from DIC
- Gastroscopy and X-rays help identify internal bleeding sites
- Invasive hemodynamic monitoring shows reduced CVP, right atrial pressure, PAP, PAWP, and cardiac output

Treatment
- Maintenance of patent airway and preparation for intubation and mechanical ventilation to prevent or manage respiratory distress
- Supplemental oxygen to increase oxygenation
- Pneumatic antishock garment to control internal and external hemorrhage by direct pressure
- Fluids, such as normal saline or lactated Ringer's solution, to restore filling pressures
- Packed RBCs to restore blood loss and improve blood's oxygen-carrying capacity (hemorrhagic shock)

Nursing considerations
- Check for a patent airway and adequate circulation
- Perform CPR if blood pressure and heart rate are absent
- Obtain blood type and crossmatch, as ordered
- Give prescribed I.V. solutions or blood products
- Insert an indwelling urinary catheter
- Give prescribed oxygen to reduce cardiac workload and increase gas exchange
- Monitor vital signs and peripheral pulses, cardiac rhythm, coagulation studies, CBC, electrolyte measurements, ABG levels, intake and output, and hemodynamics
- Teach the patient about prescribed medications and their possible adverse effects

MITRAL INSUFFICIENCY

Definition
- Inadequate closing of the mitral valve
- Backflow of blood from the left ventricle to the right atrium during systole (insufficiency)

Underlying pathophysiology
- Blood from the left ventricle flows back into the left atrium during systole, causing the atrium to enlarge to accommodate the backflow
- Left ventricle dilates to accommodate the increased volume of blood from the atrium and to compensate for diminishing cardiac output
- Ventricular hypertrophy and increased end-diastolic pressure result in increased PAP, eventually leading to left- and right-sided heart failure

Causes
- Hypertrophic obstructive cardiomyopathy
- Mitral valve prolapse
- MI
- Rheumatic heart disease
- Ruptured chordae tendineae
- Transposition of great arteries

Key treatments for hypovolemic shock
- Maintenance of patent airway
- Supplemental oxygen
- Fluid replacement
- Blood replacement

Key nursing considerations for hypovolemic shock
- Check airway and circulation and initiate CPR if necessary.
- Transfuse blood products and fluids as indicated.
- Monitor vital signs, hemodynamic parameters, ABG levels, and laboratory test results.
- Maintain an intake and output record.

Key facts about mitral insufficiency
- Inadequate closing of mitral valve
- Causes blood from left ventricle to flow back into left atrium during systole
- Increases volume of blood in atrium, which leads to dilation of left ventricle
- Can lead to heart failure

Key pathophysiologic changes in mitral insufficiency

- Dyspnea
- Peripheral edema
- Angina
- Holosystolic murmur

Key diagnostic test results for mitral insufficiency

- Echocardiography: Abnormal valve leaflet motion, left atrial enlargement
- Cardiac catheterization: Increased left ventricular end-diastolic volume and pressure, increased atrial pressure and PAWP, decreased cardiac output

Key treatments for mitral insufficiency

- Digoxin
- Diuretics and low-sodium diet
- ACE inhibitors
- Anticoagulants
- Prophylactic antibiotics

Key nursing considerations for mitral insufficiency

- Monitor vital signs, pulse oximetry, cardiac rhythm, pulmonary artery catheter readings, and intake and output.
- Teach patient about dietary restrictions and prescribed medications.

● **Pathophysiologic changes**
- Orthopnea, dyspnea, fatigue, peripheral edema, jugular vein distention, tachycardia, pulmonary congestion, and pulmonary edema due to left ventricular dysfunction
- Angina resulting from inadequate coronary artery circulation
- Holosystolic murmur at the apex due to regurgitant blood flow

● **Complications**
- Arrhythmias
- Endocarditis
- Heart failure
- Pulmonary edema
- Thromboembolism

● **Diagnostic test findings**
- Cardiac catheterization reveals mitral insufficiency with increased left ventricular end-diastolic volume and pressure, increased atrial pressure and PAWP, and decreased cardiac output
- Chest X-rays show left atrial and ventricular enlargement and pulmonary venous congestion
- Echocardiography shows abnormal valve leaflet motion and left atrial enlargement
- ECG may show left atrial and ventricular hypertrophy, sinus tachycardia, and atrial fibrillation

● **Treatment**
- Digoxin, low-sodium diet, diuretics, vasodilators and, especially important, ACE inhibitors to treat left-sided heart failure
- Oxygen (in acute situations) to increase oxygenation
- Anticoagulants to prevent thrombus formation around diseased or replaced valves
- Prophylactic antibiotics before and after surgery or dental care to prevent endocarditis
- Nitroglycerin to relieve angina
- Annuloplasty or valvuloplasty to reconstruct or repair a damaged valve
- Prosthetic valve replacement when repair isn't possible

● **Nursing considerations**
- Give prescribed oxygen
- Watch for signs of heart failure or pulmonary edema
- Monitor vital signs, pulse oximetry, cardiac rhythm, pulmonary artery catheter readings, and intake and output
- Monitor for adverse effects of drug therapy
- Teach the patient about dietary restrictions and prescribed medications

MITRAL STENOSIS

● **Definition**
- Narrowing of the mitral valve orifice

● **Underlying pathophysiology**
- Valve leaflets become diffusely thickened by fibrosis and calcifications

- Mitral commissures and the chordae tendineae fuse and shorten, the valvular cusps become rigid, and the valve's apex becomes narrowed
- Blood flow is obstructed from the left atrium to the left ventricle, resulting in incomplete emptying
- Left atrial volume and pressure increase, and the atrial chamber dilates
- Increased resistance to blood flow causes pulmonary hypertension, right ventricular hypertrophy and, eventually, right-sided heart failure and reduced cardiac output

Causes
- Atrial myxoma
- Congenital anomalies
- Endocarditis
- Rheumatic fever

Pathophysiologic changes
- Dyspnea on exertion, paroxysmal nocturnal dyspnea, orthopnea, weakness, fatigue, and palpitations due to cardiac dysfunction
- Peripheral edema, jugular vein distention, hepatomegaly, tachycardia, crackles, and pulmonary edema resulting from heart failure
- Opening snap and diastolic murmur due to turbulent blood flow over the stenotic valve

Complications
- Cardiac arrhythmias, especially atrial fibrillation
- Thromboembolism

Diagnostic test findings
- Cardiac catheterization reveals several abnormalities
  - A diastolic pressure gradient is across the valve
  - Left atrial pressure and PAWP are elevated (greater than 15 mm Hg) with severe pulmonary hypertension
  - Pressure on the right side of the heart is elevated (with decreased cardiac output)
  - Contraction of the left ventricle is abnormal
- Chest X-rays show left atrial and ventricular enlargement, enlarged pulmonary arteries, and mitral valve calcification
- Echocardiography shows thickened mitral valve leaflets and left atrial enlargement
- ECG detects left atrial hypertrophy, atrial fibrillation, right ventricular hypertrophy, and right axis deviation

Treatment
- Digoxin, low-sodium diet, diuretics, vasodilators and, especially, ACE inhibitors to treat left-sided heart failure
- Oxygen (in acute situations) to increase oxygenation
- Anticoagulants to prevent thrombus formation around diseased or replaced valves
- Prophylactic antibiotics before and after surgery or dental care to prevent endocarditis
- Nitrates to relieve angina
- Beta-adrenergic blockers or digoxin to slow ventricular rate in atrial fibrillation or atrial flutter

Key facts about mitral stenosis
- Results from valve leaflets thickened by fibrosis and calcification
- Causes shortened and fused mitral commissures and chordae tendinae, rigid valvular cusps, and narrowed valve apex
- Obstructs blood flow from left atrium to left ventricle

Key pathophysiologic changes in mitral stenosis
- Dyspnea on exertion
- Orthopnea
- Fatigue
- Peripheral edema
- Pulmonary edema
- Opening snap and diastolic murmur

Key diagnostic test results for mitral stenosis
- Echocardiography: Thickened mitral valve leaflets, left atrial enlargement
- Cardiac catheterization: Abnormal pressure gradient across valve and abnormal contractility of left venticle

Key treatments for mitral stenosis
- ACE inhibitors, cardiac glycosides, and diuretics
- Prophylactic antibiotics
- Anticoagulants
- Valve repair or replacement (if severe)

Key nursing considerations for mitral stenosis

- Check for hypersensitivity reaction to antibiotics.
- Teach patient signs and symptoms to report to physician.
- Instruct patient about use of prophylactic antibiotics.
- Inform patient about therapeutic and adverse effects of prescribed medications.

Key facts about MI

- Reduced blood flow through one or more occluded coronary arteries, causing myocardial ischemia and necrosis
- Can cause irreversible myocardial cell damage and muscle necrosis if ischemia lasts longer than 45 minutes

Key pathophysiologic changes in MI

- Persistent, crushing substernal chest pain that may radiate
- Shortness of breath
- Perspiration
- Anxiety
- Nausea and vomiting

- Cardioversion to convert atrial fibrillation to sinus rhythm
- Balloon valvuloplasty to enlarge the orifice of the stenotic mitral valve
- Prosthetic valve replacement when repair isn't possible

Nursing considerations

- Check for hypersensitivity reaction to antibiotics
- Stress the importance of bed rest
- Place the patient in an upright position to relieve dyspnea, if needed
- Provide a low-sodium diet
- Monitor vital signs and hemodynamics, and intake and output
- Monitor the patient for signs and symptoms of thromboembolism, adverse drug reactions, and cardiac arrhythmias
- Teach the patient about dietary restrictions
- Teach the patient about his prescribed medications and their potential adverse effects
- Make sure the patient understands the need for prophylactic antibiotics before, during, and after dental work, childbirth, and urologic, GI, or gynecologic procedures
- Teach the patient signs and symptoms to report to the physician
  - Irregular pulse (more than 100 beats/minute), skipped beats, or palpitations
  - Chest discomfort or pain, even if it's relieved by resting
  - Sudden shortness of breath (at rest or with exertion), increased fatigue, or paroxysmal nocturnal dyspnea
  - Swollen ankles, decreased urine output, rapid weight gain (3 to 5 lb [1.5 to 2.5 kg] in 1 week)

MYOCARDIAL INFARCTION

Definition

- Reduced blood flow through one or more coronary arteries, causing myocardial ischemia and necrosis
- Infarction site depends on the vessels involved

Underlying pathophysiology

- One or more coronary arteries becomes occluded
- If coronary occlusion causes ischemia lasting longer than 45 minutes, irreversible myocardial cell damage and muscle necrosis occur.
- Every MI has a central area of hypoxic injury
  - Transmural infarction involves the full thickness of the cardiac wall
  - Subendocardial infarction involves the inner half of the myocardium
- Injured tissue is potentially viable and may be salvaged if circulation is restored, or it may progress to necrosis

Causes

- Atherosclerosis
- Coronary artery stenosis or spasm
- Platelet aggregation
- Thrombosis

Pathophysiologic changes

- Persistent, crushing substernal chest pain

Pinpointing myocardial infarction

Depending on their locations, ischemia and infarction cause changes in specific electrocardiogram leads.

TYPES OF MYOCARDIAL INFARCTION	LEADS
Inferior	II, III, aV_F
Anterior	V_3, V_4
Septal	V_1, V_2
Lateral	I, aV_L V_5, V_6
Anterolateral	I, aV_L, V_3 to V_6
Posterior	V_1 or V_2
Right ventricular	V_{1R} to V_{4R}

- Caused by coronary artery occlusion
- May radiate to the left arm, jaw, neck, or shoulder blades
- Cool extremities, shortness of breath, hypotension, and fatigue due to impaired myocardial function
- Perspiration, anxiety, hypertension, and feeling of impending doom resulting from pain or sympathetic stimulation
- Nausea and vomiting due to pain or vagal stimulation

Complications
- Arrhythmias
- Cardiogenic shock
- Extensions of the original infarction
- Heart failure causing pulmonary edema
- Mural thrombi causing cerebral or pulmonary emboli
- Myocardial rupture
- Pericarditis
- Rupture of the atrial or ventricular septum, ventricular wall, or valves
- Ventricular aneurysms
- Death

Diagnostic test findings
- Serial 12-lead ECG reveals characteristic changes
  - Serial ST-segment depression is apparent in non–Q-wave MI
  - ST-segment is elevated in Q-wave MI
- ECG can also identify the location of MI, arrhythmias, hypertrophy, and pericarditis (see *Pinpointing myocardial infarction*)
- Serial cardiac enzymes and proteins (specifically creatine kinase MB [CK-MB], the proteins troponin T and I, and myoglobin) may show a characteristic rise and fall (see *Release of cardiac enzymes and proteins,* page 40)
- Laboratory testing reveals elevated WBC count, C-reactive protein level, and ESR due to inflammation

Common complications of MI
- Arrhythmias
- Cardiogenic shock
- Heart failure

Key diagnostic test results for MI
- Serial 12-lead ECG: ST-segment depression in non–Q-wave MI, ST-segment elevation in Q-wave MI
- Serial cardiac enzymes and proteins: Rising and falling of CK-MB, troponins T and I, and myoglobin levels

Cardiac enzymes and proteins

- Myoglobin – quickest; least specific
- CK-MB – also used to assess success of reperfusion therapy
- Troponins I and T – most specific
- LD_1-LD_2 – slowest

Release of cardiac enzymes and proteins

Because they're released by damaged tissue, serum proteins and isoenzymes (catalytic proteins that vary in concentration in specific organs) can help identify the compromised organ and assess the extent of damage. After acute myocardial infarction, cardiac enzymes and proteins rise and fall in a characteristic pattern, as shown here.

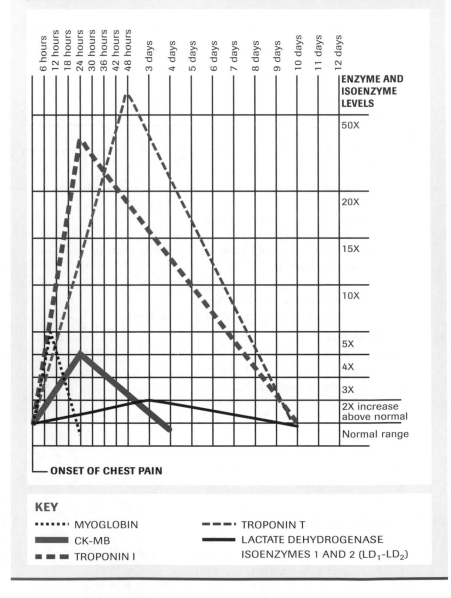

KEY
········· MYOGLOBIN
▬▬▬ CK-MB
■ ■ ■ TROPONIN I
‑ ‑ ‑ TROPONIN T
▬▬▬ LACTATE DEHYDROGENASE ISOENZYMES 1 AND 2 (LD_1-LD_2)

- Echocardiography shows ventricular wall motion abnormalities and may detect septal or papillary muscle rupture
- Nuclear imaging using sestamibi, thallium-201, and technetium 99m can be used to identify areas of infarction and viable muscle cells
- Cardiac catheterization may be used

– It can identify the involved coronary artery
– It can provide information on ventricular function and pressure and volumes within the heart

Treatment

- Thrombolytic therapy (unless contraindicated) within 3 hours of onset of symptoms to restore vessel patency and minimize necrosis
- Percutaneous transluminal coronary angioplasty (PTCA) to open blocked or narrowed arteries
- Oxygen administration to increase oxygenation of blood
- Sublingual nitroglycerin to relieve intermittent chest pain
    – Contraindicated if systolic blood pressure is less than 90 mm Hg or heart rate is less than 50 or greater than 100 beats/minute
- Morphine to relieve pain
- Aspirin to inhibit platelet aggregation
- I.V. heparin (heparin sodium injection) for patients who have received tissue plasminogen activator to promote patency in affected coronary artery
- Lidocaine (Xylocaine), transcutaneous pacing patches or transvenous pacemaker, defibrillation, or epinephrine to combat arrhythmias
- I.V. nitroglycerin for 24 to 48 hours to reduce afterload and preload and prevent chest pain in patients without hypotension, bradycardia, or excessive tachycardia
- Glycoprotein IIb/IIIa inhibitors to reduce platelet aggregation
    – Used in patients with continued unstable angina or acute chest pain
    – Used after invasive cardiac procedures

Nursing considerations

- Assess and record the severity and duration of pain, and administer analgesics
- Avoid I.M. injections
    – Absorption from the muscle is unpredictable
    – Bleeding is likely if the patient is receiving fibrinolytic therapy
- Check the patient's blood pressure after giving nitroglycerin, especially after the first dose
- Frequently monitor ECG to detect rate changes or arrhythmias
    – Place rhythm strips in the patient's chart periodically for evaluation
- **During episodes of chest pain, obtain 12-lead ECG, blood pressure, and pulmonary artery catheter measurements and monitor them for changes**
- Watch for signs and symptoms of fluid retention, such as crackles, cough, tachypnea, and edema
- Auscultate for adventitious breath sounds, S_3 or S_4 gallops, and new-onset heart murmurs
- Provide a stool softener to prevent straining during defecation, which causes vagal stimulation and may slow the heart rate
- Assist the patient with ROM exercises
- If the patient is completely immobilized by a severe MI, reposition him every 2 hours
- Measure for and apply antiembolism stockings to help prevent venostasis and thrombophlebitis
- Provide emotional support to the patient, and help reduce stress and anxiety
- Teach the patient about drug therapy and other treatment measures to promote compliance

Key treatments for MI

- Thrombolytic therapy
- PTCA
- Oxygen administration
- Nitroglycerin
- Morphine

Key nursing considerations for mitral stenosis

- Assess pain, vital signs, and ECG findings.
- During episodes of chest pain, obtain 12-lead ECG, blood pressure, and pulmonary artery catheter measurements and monitor them for changes.
- Inform patient about benefits of cardiac rehabilitation.
- Teach patient postinfarction precautions regarding chest pain, diet, activity, and medications.

– Thoroughly explain drug dosages
– Warn about adverse drug effects
– Advise the patient to watch for and report signs of toxicity
- Review dietary restrictions with the patient (low-sodium or low-fat and low-cholesterol diets)
- Counsel the patient about resuming sexual activity progressively
- Advise the patient to report typical and atypical chest pain
    – Postinfarction syndrome may develop
    – Associated chest pain must be differentiated from recurrent MI, pulmonary infarct, or heart failure
- Stress the need to stop smoking, if applicable
- Encourage the patient to participate in a cardiac rehabilitation program

MYOCARDITIS

● **Definition**
- Focal or diffuse inflammation of the cardiac muscle (myocardium)
- May be acute or chronic
- Usually involves spontaneous recovery without residual defects

● **Underlying pathophysiology**
- An infectious organism triggers an autoimmune, cellular, and humoral reaction
- Inflammation may lead to hypertrophy, fibrosis, and inflammatory changes of the myocardium and conduction system
- Heart muscle weakens and contractility is reduced

● **Causes**
- Bacterial infections, such as diphtheria, TB, typhoid fever, tetanus, and staphylococcal, pneumococcal, and gonococcal infections
- Fungal infections
- Helminthic infections such as trichinosis
- Hypersensitive immune reactions, including acute rheumatic fever and postcardiotomy syndrome
- Parasitic infections
- Radiation therapy
- Toxins, such as lead, chemicals, and cocaine
- Chronic alcoholism
- Viral illnesses, such as coxsackievirus A and B and, possibly, poliomyelitis, influenza, Epstein-Barr virus, human immunodeficiency virus, cytomegalovirus, measles, mumps, rubeola, rubella, and adenoviruses and echoviruses

● **Pathophysiologic changes**
- Fatigue, dyspnea, palpitations, and fever caused by systemic infection
- Tachycardia due to a compensatory sympathetic response
- S_3 and S_4 gallops as a result of heart failure
- Pericardial friction rub due to pericarditis

● **Complications**
- Arrhythmias and sudden death

Key facts about myocarditis
- Focal or diffuse inflammation of cardiac muscle
- Develops when an infectious organism triggers an autoimmune, cellular, and humoral reaction

Key pathophysiologic changes in myocarditis
- Fatigue
- Dyspnea
- Tachycardia
- Palpitations

- Chronic valvulitis (when it results from rheumatic fever)
- Dilated cardiomyopathy
- Heart failure
- Pericarditis
- Recurrence of myocarditis
- Ruptured myocardial aneurysm
- Thromboembolism

Diagnostic test findings
- Laboratory testing detects elevated levels of CK, CK-MB, troponin I, troponin T, AST, and LD
- Antibody titers may be elevated; for example, antistreptolysin-O titer is elevated in rheumatic fever
- ECG shows diffuse ST-segment and T-wave abnormalities, conduction defects, supraventricular arrhythmias, and ventricular extrasystoles
- Chest X-rays show an enlarged heart and pulmonary vascular congestion
- Echocardiography may demonstrate some degree of left ventricular dysfunction
- Radionuclide scanning identifies inflammatory and necrotic changes characteristic of myocarditis
- Laboratory cultures of stool, throat specimens, and other body fluids may identify bacterial or viral causes of infection
- Endomyocardial biopsy may confirm the diagnosis, but a negative biopsy doesn't exclude it

Treatment
- Antibiotics to treat bacterial infections
- Antipyretics to reduce fever and decrease stress on the heart
- Bed rest to reduce oxygen demands and the heart's workload
- Restricted activity to minimize myocardial oxygen consumption
- Supplemental oxygen therapy, sodium restriction, and diuretics to decrease fluid retention
- ACE inhibitors and digoxin to increase myocardial contractility in patients with heart failure
- Antiarrhythmic drugs, such as quinidine (Quinidex Extentabs) or procainamide, to treat arrhythmias
- Anticoagulant drug therapy to prevent thromboembolism
- Corticosteroids and immunosuppressants to combat life-threatening complications such as intractable heart failure (controversial)
- Cardiac assist devices or transplantation as a last resort in severe cases that resist treatment

Nursing considerations
- Assess the patient's cardiovascular status frequently, watching for signs of heart failure
- Observe for signs of digoxin toxicity
  - Certain factors, such as electrolyte imbalance or hypoxia, may potentiate toxicity
- Stress the importance of bed rest
- During recovery, recommend that the patient resume normal activities slowly

Key diagnostic test results for myocarditis
- Laboratory testing: Elevated CK, CK-MB, troponins I and T, AST, and LD levels
- Antibody titers: Possibly elevated
- ECG: Diffuse ST-segment and T-wave abnormalities, conduction defects, supraventricular arrhythmias

Key treatments for myocarditis
- Antibiotics and antipyretics
- Bed rest
- Oxygen therapy
- Anticoagulants
- ACE inhibitors and digoxin (for patients with heart failure)

Key nursing considerations for myocarditis
- Assess patient's cardiovascular status frequently, watching for signs of heart failure.
- Instruct patient to gradually resume activities.

Key facts about pericarditis

- Inflammation of pericardium
- Characterized by dense, fibrous pericardial thickening
- Chemical mediators released, resulting in extracellular edema

Key pathophysiologic changes in pericarditis

- Pericardial friction rub
- Sharp, sudden pain, usually starting over the sternum and radiating to the neck, shoulders, back, and arm
- Mild fever
- Muffled and distant heart sounds

Key diagnostic test results for pericarditis

- ECG: Diffuse ST-segment elevation, diminished QRS segments when pericardial effusion exists, arrhythmias
- Echocardiography: An echo-free space between ventricular wall and pericardium; reduced pumping action of heart

PERICARDITIS

- **Definition**
  - Inflammation of the pericardium
  - Can be fibrous or effusive, with purulent, serous, or hemorrhagic exudate
  - Characterized by dense, fibrous pericardial thickening

- **Underlying pathophysiology**
  - Pericardial tissue is damaged by bacteria or another substance that releases chemical mediators of inflammation into surrounding tissue
  - Friction occurs as the inflamed layers rub against each other
  - Chemical mediators dilate blood vessels and increase vessel permeability
  - Vessel walls leak fluids and proteins, causing extracellular edema

- **Causes**
  - Bacterial, fungal, or viral infection
  - Cardiac trauma
  - Drugs, such as hydralazine or procainamide
  - High-dose radiation
  - Hypersensitivity or autoimmune disease
  - Idiopathic factors
  - Neoplasm
  - TB
  - Uremia

- **Pathophysiologic changes**
  - Pericardial friction rub and sharp, typically sudden, pain (usually starting over the sternum and radiating to the neck, shoulders, back, and arm) related to roughened, inflamed, irritated pericardial membranes
  - Shallow, rapid respirations due to pleuritic pain
  - Mild fever resulting from inflammation
  - Dyspnea, orthopnea, tachycardia, and other signs of heart failure due to pericardial effusion
  - Muffled and distant heart sounds from fluid buildup
  - Fluid retention, ascites, hepatomegaly, jugular vein distention, and other signs of chronic right-sided heart failure from increased systemic venous pressure
  - May be benign and self-limiting if idiopathic

- **Complications**
  - Pericardial effusion
  - Cardiac tamponade

- **Diagnostic test findings**
  - ECG shows various conditions
    - A diffuse ST-segment elevation reflects the inflammatory process
    - QRS segments may be diminished when pericardial effusion exists
    - Arrhythmias, such as atrial fibrillation and sinus arrhythmias, may occur
  - Laboratory testing detects various abnormalities
    - ESR is elevated as a result of the inflammatory process
    - WBC count may be normal or elevated, especially in infectious pericarditis
    - BUN may detect uremia as a cause
    - Blood cultures identify an infectious cause

- Antistreptolysin-O titers are positive if pericarditis is due to rheumatic fever
- Purified protein derivative skin test is positive if pericarditis is due to TB
- Echocardiography may show an echo-free space between the ventricular wall and the pericardium, and reduced pumping action of the heart
- Chest X-rays may vary
  - They may appear normal with acute pericarditis
  - The cardiac silhouette may be enlarged and bottle-shaped because of fluid accumulation if pleural effusion is present

Treatment
- Bed rest as long as fever and pain persist to reduce metabolic needs
- Treatment of the underlying cause, if it can be identified
- Nonsteroidal anti-inflammatory drugs (NSAIDs), such as aspirin and indomethacin (Indocin), to relieve pain and reduce inflammation
- Corticosteroids
  - Used if NSAIDs are ineffective and no infection exists
  - Must be administered cautiously because episodes may recur when therapy is discontinued
- Antibacterial, antifungal, or antiviral therapy if an infectious cause is suspected
- Pericardiocentesis to remove excess fluid from the pericardial space
- For recurrent pericarditis, partial pericardectomy to create a window that allows fluid to drain into the pleural space
- For constrictive pericarditis, total pericardectomy to permit adequate filling and contraction of the heart

Nursing considerations
- Assess pain in relation to respiration and body position to distinguish pericardial pain from myocardial ischemic pain
- Place the patient in an upright position to relieve dyspnea and chest pain
- Administer analgesics and oxygen as needed
- Inform the patient with acute pericarditis that his condition is temporary and treatable
- Monitor the patient for signs of cardiac compression, cardiac tamponade, and pericardial effusion
  - Decreased blood pressure
  - Increased CVP
  - Pulsus paradoxus
- Explain tests and treatments to the patient

RAYNAUD'S DISEASE

Definition
- Disorder of the small blood vessels that feed the skin
- Precipitated by exposure to cold or stress
- Occurs bilaterally
- Usually affects the hands or, less commonly, the feet

Underlying pathophysiology
- Vascular wall hyperactivity occurs due to cold
- Vasomotor tone is increased due to sympathetic stimulation

Key treatments for pericarditis
- Bed rest
- Antibacterial, antifungal, or antiviral therapy (if an infectious cause is suspected)
- NSAIDs and corticosteroids
- Surgery (if severe)

Key nursing considerations for pericarditis
- Monitor pain, dyspnea, and vital signs.
- Monitor for decreased blood pressure, increased CVP, and pulsus paradoxus.
- Administer analgesics and oxygen as needed.

Key facts about Raynaud's disease
- Disorder of the small blood vessels that feed the skin
- Results in vascular wall hyperactivity and increased vasomotor tone
- Characterized by bilateral involvement of hands and, occasionally, feet

- An antigen-antibody immune response occurs (most probable theory)

● Causes
- Primary disease
  - Unknown
  - Risk factor: family history
- Secondary disease
  - Arterio-occlusive disease
  - Collagen vascular disease
  - Exposure to heavy metals
  - Myxedema
  - Previous damage from cold exposure
  - Pulmonary hypertension
  - Serum sickness
  - Smoking
  - Some antimigraine and beta-adrenergic blocker drugs
  - Thoracic outlet syndrome
  - Trauma
  - Risk factor: family history

● Pathophysiologic changes
- Bilateral, white skin in the fingers after exposure to cold or stress as vasoconstriction or vasospasm reduces blood flow
- Possible blue skin in the fingers because of increased oxygen loss back to the veins due to sluggish blood flow
- Cold and numbness or tingling, possibly occurring during the vasoconstrictive phase because of ischemia
- Red skin, possibly with throbbing, aching pain, swelling, or tingling during the hyperemic phase as the extremities are warmed and blood flow returns
- Possible trophic changes as a result of ischemia in longstanding disease
  - Sclerodactyly (tight skin over osteoporitic phalanges with atrophied subcutaneous tissue)
  - Ulcerations
  - Chronic paronychia (chronic bacterial or fungal infection of the nail base)

● Complications
- Amputation
- Cutaneous gangrene
- Ischemia

● Diagnostic test findings
- Antinuclear antibody (ANA) titer is used to identify autoimmune disease as an underlying cause of Raynaud's disease
  - Further tests must be performed if the ANA titer is positive
- Arteriography rules out arterial occlusive disease
- Doppler ultrasonography may show reduced blood flow if symptoms result from arterial occlusive disease

● Treatment
- Avoidance of triggers, such as cold, and mechanical or chemical injury
- Smoking cessation and avoidance of decongestants and caffeine to reduce vasoconstriction
- Maintaining warm body temperature to reduce vasoconstriction

- Calcium channel blockers, such as nifedipine (Procardia), diltiazem, and nicardipine (Cardene), to produce vasodilation and prevent vasospasm
- Adrenergic blockers, such as phenoxybenzamine (Dibenzyline) or reserpine (Serpasil), which may improve blood flow to fingers and toes
- Biofeedback and relaxation exercises to reduce stress and improve circulation
- Sympathectomy to prevent ischemic ulcers by promoting vasodilation (necessary in less than 25% of patients)
- Amputation, if ischemia causes ulceration and gangrene

● Nursing considerations

- Caution the patient against exposure to the cold
- Tell the patient to wear mittens or gloves in cold weather, when handling cold items, or when defrosting the freezer
- Advise the patient to avoid stressful situations and to stop smoking
- Instruct the patient to inspect skin frequently and to seek immediate care for signs of skin breakdown or infection
- Teach the patient about prescribed medications, their proper use, and their adverse effects
- Provide psychological support to allay the patient's fear of amputation and disfigurement

RHEUMATIC FEVER AND RHEUMATIC HEART DISEASE

● Definition

- Acute rheumatic fever
  - Systemic inflammatory disease of childhood
  - Develops after infection of the upper respiratory tract with group-A streptococcus (GAS)
  - Mainly involves the heart, joints, CNS, skin, and subcutaneous tissues
- Rheumatic heart disease
  - Cardiac and valvular manifestations of rheumatic fever
  - Includes pancarditis (myocarditis, pericarditis, and endocarditis) during the early acute phase and chronic valve disease in the later phase

● Underlying pathophysiology

- Infection leads to a hypersensitivity reaction in which antibodies produced to combat streptococci affect many connective tissues of the body
- Antigens of GAS bind to receptors in the heart, muscle, brain, and synovial joints, causing an autoimmune response
- Antibodies may attack healthy body cells by mistake because the bacterial antigens are similar to the body's own cells

● Causes

- GAS pharyngitis

● Pathophysiologic changes

- Rheumatic fever
  - Polyarthritis or migratory joint pain caused by inflammation
  - Subcutaneous nodules
    - Firm, movable, and nontender
    - About 3 mm to 2 cm in diameter

– Erythema marginatum skin rash
- Found on trunk and upper part of extremities
- Ring-shaped or snakelike appearance
- Usually near tendons or bony prominences of joints
- May last a few days to several weeks
– Carditis with dyspnea and chest pain
– Sydenham's chorea (rapid jerky movements)
- May develop up to 6 months after the original streptococcal infection
- Changes associated with mild chorea
  - Hyperirritability
  - Deterioration in handwriting
  - Inability to concentrate
- Changes associated with severe chorea
  - Purposeless, nonrepetitive, involuntary muscle spasms
  - Poor muscle coordination
  - Muscle weakness
– Temperature of at least 100.4° F (38° C) due to infection and inflammation
• Rheumatic heart disease
– If pericarditis exists, pericardial friction rub caused by inflamed pericardial membranes rubbing against one another
– Chest pain, typically pleuritic, due to inflammation and irritation of the pericardial membranes
– Dyspnea, tachypnea, nonproductive cough, bibasilar crackles, and edema due to heart failure in severe rheumatic carditis

● Complications
• Destruction of the mitral and aortic valves
• Pancarditis (pericarditis, myocarditis, and endocarditis)
• Heart failure

● Diagnostic test findings
• Jones criteria are used to standardize diagnosis (see *Jones criteria for diagnosing rheumatic fever*)
• Laboratory testing detects an elevated WBC count and elevated ESR during the acute phase
• Hemoglobin level and hematocrit may show slight anemia due to suppressed erythropoiesis during inflammation
• C-reactive protein may be positive, especially during the acute phase
• Cardiac enzyme levels may be increased in severe carditis
• Antistreptolysin-O titer may be elevated in 95% of patients within 2 months of onset.
• Throat cultures may continue to show the presence of GAS; however, the streptococci usually occur in small numbers
• Chest X-rays may show normal heart size or cardiomegaly, pericardial effusion, or heart failure
• Echocardiography provides various findings
– It can detect valvular damage and pericardial effusion
– It can measure chamber size
– It can provide information on ventricular function
• Cardiac catheterization provides information on valvular damage and left ventricular function

---

Key pathophysiologic changes in rheumatic heart disease

• Pleuritic chest pain
• Dyspnea or tachypnea
• Cough

Key diagnostic test results for rheumatic fever and rheumatic heart disease

• Laboratory testing: Elevated WBC count; elevated ESR during acute phase
• Throat culture: Presence of GAS
• Echocardiography: Valve damage, pericardial effusion, efficiency of left ventricle

Jones criteria for diagnosing rheumatic fever

The Jones criteria are used to standardize the diagnosis of rheumatic fever. Diagnosis requires that the patient have either two major criteria, or one major criterion and two minor criteria, plus evidence of a previous group A-hemolytic streptococcal infection.

MAJOR CRITERIA
- Carditis
- Migratory polyarthritis
- Sydenham's chorea
- Subcutaneous nodules
- Erythema marginatum

MINOR CRITERIA
- Fever
- Arthralgia
- Elevated acute phase reactants
- Prolonged PR interval

● Treatment
- Prompt treatment of GAS pharyngitis with antibiotics
- Salicylates to relieve fever and pain and minimize joint swelling
- Corticosteroids for carditis or if salicylates fail to relieve pain and inflammation
- Strict bed rest for about 5 weeks for patients with active carditis
- Bed rest, sodium restriction, ACE inhibitors, digoxin, and diuretics to treat heart failure
- Corrective surgery, such as commissurotomy (separation of adhered valves or surrounding tissues), valvuloplasty, or valve replacement for severe mitral or aortic valvular dysfunction that causes persistent heart failure
- Secondary prevention of rheumatic fever
  - Monthly I.M. injections of penicillin G benzathine or daily doses of oral penicillin V (Bicillin L-A) or sulfadiazine (Veetids) beginning after the acute phase subsides
  - Treatment for at least 5 years or until age 21, whichever is longer
- Prophylactic antibiotics for dental work and other invasive or surgical procedures to prevent endocarditis

● Nursing considerations
- Teach the patient about the disease and the need for prolonged antibiotic therapy to promote compliance with the prescribed therapy
- Check for antibiotic allergies, especially to penicillins and cephalosporins, before administering drugs from these classes
- Instruct the patient and his family to report early signs of heart failure, such as dyspnea and a hacking, nonproductive cough
- Stress the need for bed rest during the acute phase and suggest appropriate, physically undemanding diversions
- If the patient is a child, address parental concerns
  - Help parents overcome feelings of guilt they may have about their child's illness
  - If the child has severe carditis, help the parents prepare for permanent changes in the child's lifestyle
  - Instruct the parents to watch for and immediately report signs of recurrent streptococcal infection (sore throat, fever, flulike complaints)
- Promote good dental hygiene to prevent infection

Key treatments for rheumatic fever
- Antibiotics
- Anti-inflammatory agents

Key treatment for secondary prevention of rheumatic heart disease
- Monthly I.M. injections of penicillin G benzathine or daily doses of oral penicillin V or sulfadiazine beginning after the acute phase subsides

Key nursing considerations for rheumatic fever and rheumatic heart disease
- Teach patient about the disease process and treatment.
- Instruct patient about signs and symptoms of heart failure and recurrent streptococcal infection.
- Check carefully for antibiotic allergies before drug administration.

SEPTIC SHOCK

Key facts about septic shock

- Has two phases: hyperdynamic (warm) and hypodynamic (cold)
- Develops when chemical mediators respond to an invading organism
- Leads to low systemic vascular resistance and increased cardiac output (which eventually decreases)
- Progresses to functional hypovolemia and increased capillary permeability
- Results in mutisystem dysfunction syndrome and death

Key pathophysiologic changes in septic shock

- Chills
- Fever
- Tachycardia
- Tachypnea
- Decreased urine output
- Restlessness
- LOC deterioration

Common complications of septic shock

- Renal failure
- Heart failure
- DIC
- Death

● **Definition**
- Inadequate tissue perfusion, metabolic changes, and circulatory collapse in response to infection
- Developed by 25% of patients with gram-negative bacteremia
- Involves two phases
  - Hyperdynamic, or warm, phase
  - Hypodynamic, or cold, phase

● **Underlying pathophysiology**
- Initially, the body's defenses activate chemical mediators in response to the invading organism
- The release of these mediators results in low systemic vascular resistance and increased cardiac output
- Blood flow is unevenly distributed in the microcirculation, and plasma leaking from capillaries causes functional hypovolemia
- Diffuse increase in capillary permeability occurs
- Eventually, cardiac output decreases
- Poor tissue perfusion and hypotension cause multisystem dysfunction syndrome and death

● **Causes**
- Gram-negative bacteria (70%)
- Gram-positive bacteria

● **Pathophysiologic changes**
- Chills and fever due to infection
- Tachycardia and bounding pulse resulting from sympathetic stimulation
- Restlessness, irritability, and tachypnea due to cerebral hypoxia
- Reduced urine output due to vasoconstriction
- Warm, dry skin resulting form vasodilation
- Hypotension caused by failure of compensatory mechanism
- Cyanosis due to hypoxia
- Unconsciousness and absent reflexes caused by reduced cerebral perfusion, acid-base imbalance, or electrolyte abnormalities
- Rapidly falling blood pressure resulting from decompensation
- Slow, shallow, or Cheyne-Stokes respirations due to respiratory center depression

● **Complications**
- Abnormal liver function
- Death
- DIC
- GI ulcers
- Heart failure
- Renal failure

● **Diagnostic test findings**
- Blood cultures are positive for the causative organism
- CBC shows the presence of anemia and leukopenia, severe or absent neutropenia and, usually, thrombocytopenia

- BUN and creatinine levels are increased and creatinine clearance is decreased
- PT and partial thromboplastin time are abnormal
- Serum LD levels are elevated in patients with metabolic acidosis
- Urine studies show increased specific gravity, increased osmolality, and decreased sodium levels
- ABG analysis shows increased blood pH and PaO_2, decreased $PaCO_2$, and respiratory alkalosis in early stages
- Invasive hemodynamic monitoring findings depend on the stage of shock
  - Cardiac output is increased and systemic vascular resistance is decreased in the warm phase
  - Cardiac output is decreased and systemic vascular resistance is increased in the cold phase

● **Treatment**
- Antibiotic therapy to eradicate the causative organism
- Inotropic and vasopressor drugs, such as dopamine, dobutamine, and norepinephrine (Levophed), to improve perfusion and maintain blood pressure
- Maintenance of patent airway and preparation for intubation and mechanical ventilation to prevent or manage respiratory distress
- Supplemental oxygen to increase oxygenation
- I.V. fluids, crystalloids, colloids, or blood products, as necessary, to maintain intravascular volume
- Monoclonal antibodies to tumor necrosis factor, endotoxin, and interleukin-1 to counteract septic shock mediators (still under investigation)

● **Nursing considerations**
- Remove any I.V., intra-arterial, or urinary drainage catheters and send them to the laboratory to culture for the presence of the causative organism
- Administer appropriate antimicrobial I.V. drugs
- Notify the physician if the patient experiences a progressive drop in blood pressure with a thready pulse and urine output less than 30 ml/hour
- Administer prescribed oxygen
- Provide emotional support to the patient and his family
- Monitor ABG values, pulse oximetry, intake and output, vital signs, peripheral pulses, hemodynamics, cardiac rhythms, and heart and breath sounds

THROMBOPHLEBITIS

● **Definition**
- Development of a blood clot that may cause vessel occlusion or embolization
- An acute condition characterized by inflammation and clot formation
- May occur in deep or superficial veins
- Typically occurs at the valve cusps because venous stasis encourages accumulation and adherence of platelets and fibrin

● **Underlying pathophysiology**
- Alteration in epithelial lining causes platelet aggregation and fibrin entrapment of RBCs, WBCs, and additional platelets
- The thrombus initiates a chemical inflammatory process in the vessel epithelium that leads to fibrosis, which may occlude the vessel lumen or embolize

Key diagnostic test results for septic shock

- Blood cultures: Infective agent
- WBC count: Increased count
- Renal studies: Elevated BUN and creatinine
- Clotting tests: Abnormal

Key treatments for septic shock

- Antibiotic therapy
- Inotropic and vasopressor drugs
- I.V. fluids, crystalloids, colloids, or blood products

Key nursing considerations for septic shock

- Remove all possible sources of infection for culturing.
- Closely monitor hemodynamic parameters.
- Notify physician if patient experiences progressive drop in blood pressure with thready pulse and urine output less than 30 ml/hour.

Key facts about thrombophlebitis

- Development of blood clot
- May cause vessel occlusion or embolization

Key pathophysiologic changes in thrombophlebitis

- Tenderness, redness, and warmth over affected area
- Swelling of affected leg

Key diagnostic test results for thrombophlebitis

- Homans' sign: Positive
- Doppler ultrasonography: Reduced blood flow to a specific area and obstruction to venous flow
- Plethysmography: Decreased circulation distal to affected area

Key treatments for thrombophlebitis

- Anticogulant therapy
- Bed rest
- Elevation of affected extremity

● **Causes**
- May be idiopathic
- Fracture of the spine, pelvis, femur, or tibia
- Hormonal contraceptives such as estrogen
- Neoplasm
- Older age
- Pregnancy and childbirth
- Surgery
- Trauma
- Venous stasis, such as with disease, prolonged bed rest, or inactivity during long airplane or car trips
- Venulitis

● **Pathophysiologic changes**
- Tenderness, redness, and warmth over the affected area due to inflammation
- Swelling of the affected leg from venous congestion

● **Complications**
- Chronic venous insufficiency
- Pulmonary embolism

● **Diagnostic test findings**
- Homans' sign is positive (patient exhibits discomfort in the calf muscles when the foot is forced into dorsiflexion with the knee straight)
- Doppler ultrasonography shows reduced blood flow to a specific area and obstruction to venous flow, particularly in iliofemoral deep vein thrombophlebitis
- Plethysmography shows decreased circulation distal to the affected area and is more sensitive than ultrasonography in detecting deep vein thrombophlebitis
- Phlebography confirms the diagnosis and shows filling defects and diverted blood flow

● **Treatment**
- Application of warm, moist compresses to the affected area
- Application of antiembolism stockings
- Bed rest, with elevation of the affected extremity for a few days
- Drug therapy using anticoagulants, analgesics, and antiplatelet aggregation agents
- Surgery
  - Simple ligation
  - Clipping
  - Vein plication
  - Embolectomy
- Transvenous placement of a vena cava filter to block emboli from passing through the vein

● **Nursing considerations**
- Enforce bed rest initially
  - Elevate the patient's affected arm or leg
  - Avoid compressing the popliteal space
- Apply warm compresses or a covered aquathermia pad
- Give prescribed analgesics

- Mark, measure, and record the circumference of the affected arm or leg daily, and compare this measurement with that of the other arm or leg
- Give prescribed anticoagulants
- Perform or encourage ROM exercises
- Use pneumatic compression devices
- Encourage early ambulation

VARICOSE VEINS

- ### Definition
  - Dilated, tortuous veins, engorged with blood
  - Result from improper venous valve function
  - Primary varicose veins originate in the superficial veins
  - Secondary varicose veins occur in the deep veins

- ### Underlying pathophysiology
  - A weakened valve allows backflow of blood to the previous valve in a vein
  - The valve can't hold the pooling blood
    - It becomes incompetent
    - More blood flows backward
  - The volume of venous blood builds, pressure in the vein increases, and the vein becomes distended
  - The veins are stretched, their walls weaken, and they lose their elasticity
  - The veins enlarge and become lumpy and tortuous
  - As hydrostatic pressure increases, plasma is forced out of the veins and into the surrounding tissues, resulting in edema

- ### Causes
  - Congenital weakness of the valves or venous wall
  - Conditions that produce prolonged venous stasis or increased intra-abdominal pressure
    - Pregnancy
    - Obesity
    - Constipation
    - Wearing tight clothes
  - Occupations that necessitate standing for an extended period
  - Family history of varicose veins
  - Deep vein thrombosis
  - Trauma to the venous system

- ### Pathophysiologic changes
  - Dilated, tortuous, purplish, ropelike veins, particularly in the calves, due to venous pooling
  - Edema of the calves and ankles due to deep vein incompetence
  - Leg heaviness that worsens in the evening and in warm weather caused by venous pooling
  - Dull aching in the legs after prolonged standing or walking, which may be due to tissue breakdown
  - Aching during menses as a result of increased fluid retention

- ### Complications
  - Blood clots secondary to venous stasis

- Venous stasis ulcers
- Chronic venous insufficiency

Diagnostic test findings

- Manual compression test detects a palpable impulse when the vein is firmly occluded at least 8″ (20 cm) above the point of palpation, indicating incompetent valves in the vein
- Trendelenburg's test (retrograde filling test) detects incompetent deep and superficial vein valves
- Photoplethysmography characterizes venous blood flow by noting changes in the skin's circulation
- Doppler ultrasonography detects the presence or absence of venous backflow in deep or superficial veins
- Venous outflow and reflux plethysmography (invasive, not routinely used) detects deep venous occlusion
- Ascending and descending venography demonstrate venous occlusion and patterns of collateral flow

Treatment

- Treatment of the underlying cause
- Antiembolism stockings or elastic bandages to counteract swelling by supporting the veins and improving circulation
- Regular exercise program to promote muscular contraction to force blood through the veins and reduce venous pooling
- Injection of a sclerosing agent into small to medium-sized varicosities
- Surgical stripping and ligation of severe varicose veins
- Phlebectomy (removal of the varicose vein through small incisions in the skin), which may be performed in an outpatient setting
- For the obese patient, weight reduction to reduce increased intra-abdominal pressure
- Elevating the legs above the heart whenever possible to promote venous return
- Instructing the patient to avoid prolonged standing or sitting because these actions enhance venous pooling

Nursing considerations

- Administer analgesics after stripping and ligation or after injection of a sclerosing agent, as ordered, to relieve pain
- Frequently check circulation in toes, and observe elastic bandages for bleeding
  - When ordered, rewrap bandages at least once per shift
  - Wrap from the toe to the thigh, with the leg elevated
- Watch for signs and symptoms of complications
  - Sensory loss in the calves
  - Pain
  - Fever

Key diagnostic test results for varicose veins

- Doppler ultrasonography: Venous backflow
- Venography: Venous occlusion and collateral flow patterns

Key treatments for varicose veins

- Treatment of underlying cause
- Antiembolism stockings
- Elevation of legs above heart level
- Regular exercise

Key nursing considerations for varicose veins

- Monitor circulation in feet.
- Watch for sensory loss in calves, pain, and fever.

NCLEX CHECKS

It's never too soon to begin your licensure examination preparation. Now that you've reviewed this chapter, carefully read each of the following questions and choose the best answer. Then compare your responses to the correct answers.

1. A client with group-A streptococcus is to undergo secondary prevention of rheumatic fever. The nurse is aware that the client should receive antibacterial therapy for how long?

- ☐ **1.** 5 days
- ☐ **2.** 5 weeks
- ☐ **3.** 5 months
- ☐ **4.** 5 years

2. A client with acute chest pain radiating down his left arm is admitted to the emergency department. Serial enzyme and protein tests are ordered.
The nurse will monitor for peak elevations of these tests in what order?

1. Troponin T	
2. CK-MB	
3. LD_1-LD_2	
4. Myoglobin	

3. A nurse is caring for a client with thrombophlebitis. She plans to teach the client that the three conditions that promote thrombus formation are endothelial injury, increased coagulability, and:

- ☐ **1.** increased number of white blood cells.
- ☐ **2.** decreased platelet count.
- ☐ **3.** sluggish blood flow.
- ☐ **4.** rapid pulse rate.

4. A client is admitted to the emergency department with acute coronary syndrome. Testing reveals an acute MI. The nurse knows that she must administer thrombolytic therapy within how many hours of the onset of symptoms?

- ☐ **1.** 3
- ☐ **2.** 5
- ☐ **3.** 8
- ☐ **4.** 12

5. A 6-month-old client has a ventricular heart defect. The nurse will monitor the client for signs and symptoms of:

- ☐ **1.** a right-to-left shunt.
- ☐ **2.** a left-to-right shunt.
- ☐ **3.** an aneurysm.
- ☐ **4.** an embolus.

TOP 5

Items to study for your next test on the cardiovascular system

1. Underlying pathophysiology of key disorders, such as CAD, MI, hypertension, and heart failure
2. Significant pathophysiologic changes associated with cardiovascular disorders, such as chest pain, edema, dyspnea, and abnormal heart sounds
3. Risk factors for developing hypertension, endocarditis, and rheumatic heart disease
4. Treatments for cardiovascular disorders, including surgery and drug therapy for such key disorders as CAD, MI, hypertension, and heart failure
5. Patient-teaching points for cardiovascular disorders

6. Pathophysiologic changes of right-sided heart failure include ascites, nocturia, weight gain, and:

- ☐ **1.** fatigue.
- ☐ **2.** tachycardia.
- ☐ **3.** cool, pale skin.
- ☐ **4.** right upper quadrant pain.

7. A client with coronary artery disease has been admitted to the hospital. The nurse knows that which diagnostic test would show cold spots in the myocardium?

- ☐ **1.** ECG
- ☐ **2.** I.V. ultrasonography
- ☐ **3.** Myocardial perfusion imaging with thallium-201
- ☐ **4.** Stress echocardiography

8. A client is admitted to the facility with complaints of severe shortness of breath, high fever, fatigue, and chest pressure after chemotherapy. The nurse explains that viral or bacterial infections can lead to which type of cardiomyopathy?

- ☐ **1.** Extensive
- ☐ **2.** Dilated
- ☐ **3.** Hypertrophic obstructive
- ☐ **4.** Restrictive

9. A client arrives in the emergency department in shock. After testing, the diagnosis given is "pump failure." The nurse caring for the client knows that "pump failure" is another name for which type of shock?

- ☐ **1.** Septic
- ☐ **2.** Hypovolemic
- ☐ **3.** Hypertensive
- ☐ **4.** Cardiogenic

10. A client diagnosed with cardiac tamponade is to undergo pericardiectomy. This procedure involves:

- ☐ **1.** surgical creation of an opening of the pericardium.
- ☐ **2.** resecting a portion or all of the pericardium.
- ☐ **3.** needle aspiration of the pericardial cavity.
- ☐ **4.** inserting a drainage tube into the pericardium.

ANSWERS AND RATIONALES

1. CORRECT ANSWER: 4
Secondary prevention of rheumatic fever with antibacterial therapy begins after the acute phase of the disease and usually continues for at least 5 years or until age 21, whichever is longer.

2. CORRECT ANSWER:

| **4.** Myoglobin |
| **2.** CK-MB |
| **1.** Troponin T |
| **3.** LD_1-LD_2 |

Serum protein myoglobin peaks 8 to 10 hours after infarction and resolves within 24 hours. CK-MB, an enzyme specific to cardiac muscle, peaks within 24 hours and returns to baseline in approximately 96 hours. Protein troponin T peaks within 48 hours and reverts to normal in 7 to 10 days. LD_1-LD_2 peaks within 72 hours and returns to baseline in 7 to 14 days.

3. CORRECT ANSWER: 3
The presence of Virchow's triad, which includes sluggish blood, endothelial injury, and increased coagulability, promotes thrombus formation. Increased WBC count isn't a factor in this process, although like RBCs, WBCs are caught within the fibrin matrix that accumulates around the increased (not decreased) platelets at the site of a thrombus. Pulse rate isn't a specific indicator for phlebitis.

4. CORRECT ANSWER: 1
Thrombolytic therapy given within 3 hours of onset of symptoms helps restore vessel patency and minimize necrosis. After 3 hours, the effectiveness of thrombolytics in breaking up thrombi decreases, and the risk of adverse reactions such as bleeding increases.

5. CORRECT ANSWER: 2
In a left-to-right shunt, an atrial or ventricular defect allows oxygenated blood to be delivered back to the right side of the heart or to the lungs. This condition leads to hypertrophy of pulmonary vessels and possible right-sided heart failure. In a right-to-left shunt, blood flows from the right side of the heart to the left, or from the pulmonary artery directly into the systemic circulation through a patent ductus arteriosus, adding deoxygenated blood to the systemic circulation. An aneurysm is an abnormal outpouching or dilation of a blood vessel or wall of the heart. An embolus is a substance—commonly a blood clot from a thrombus—that circulates through the bloodstream from one location in the body to another.

6. CORRECT ANSWER: 4
Right-sided heart failure results from ineffective contractile function of the right ventricle, which leads to blood backing up into the right atrium and peripheral circulation, and possible engorgement of other organs. If the liver becomes engorged it could lead to right upper quadrant pain. Tachycardia, fatigue, and cool, pale skin indicate left-sided heart failure.

7. CORRECT ANSWER: 3
Myocardial perfusion imaging may be performed during treadmill exercise to detect ischemic areas of the myocardium. Ischemic areas appear as "cold spots" that normalize during rest, indicating viable tissue. An ECG may reveal the electrical signs of ischemia. Ultrasonography and echocardiography can reveal characteristics of the coronary arteries, such as size, but can't pinpoint specific blockages in the arteries.

8. CORRECT ANSWER: 2

Viral or bacterial infections can lead to dilated cardiomyopathy. Hypertrophic obstructive cardiomyopathy may be caused by a genetic predisposition from an autosomal-dominant trait or hypertension. Restrictive cardiomyopathy may be idiopathic or associated with sarcoidosis or mediastinal radiation from cancer treatment. Extensive isn't a type of cardiomyopathy.

9. CORRECT ANSWER: 4

Cardiogenic shock, a condition in which diminished cardiac output severely impairs tissue perfusion, is also known as *pump failure.* Septic shock is the result of a severe infectious process. Hypovolemia shock occurs when excessive amounts of ECF are lost. "Hypertensive" isn't a type of shock.

10. CORRECT ANSWER: 2

Pericardiectomy, resection of a portion or all of the pericardium, is done to allow full connection with the pleura. A pericardial window is a surgically created opening in the pericardium. Pericardiocentesis involves needle aspiration of the pericardial cavity. A drainage tube is inserted to remove excess fluid if trauma to the chest is the source of the cardiac tamponade.

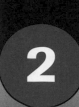

Respiratory system

2

LEARNING OBJECTIVES

After studying this chapter, you should be able to:

● Identify conditions that impede gas exchange.
● Identify signs and symptoms and pathophysiologic changes associated with various respiratory disorders.
● List probable causes of various respiratory disorders.
● Describe medications used to improve respiratory function.
● Write teaching goals for the patient with respiratory dysfunction.
● List nursing interventions for various respiratory disorders.

CHAPTER OVERVIEW

The respiratory system includes the airways, lungs, bony thorax, and respiratory muscles. Its main function is to deliver oxygen to the bloodstream and remove excess carbon dioxide from the body.

Caring for the patient with a respiratory disorder requires an understanding of the pathophysiologic changes that occur and the signs and symptoms such changes produce. This chapter reviews key pathophysiologic concepts related to the respiratory system, and then outlines the underlying pathophysiology, causes, pathophysiologic changes, complications, diagnostic test findings, treatment approaches, and nursing considerations associated with common respiratory disorders.

Key facts about atelectasis

- Occurs when alveolar sacs or entire lung segments expand incompletely
- Produces partial or complete lung collapse

Key facts about bronchiectasis

- Chronic abnormal dilation of bronchi and destruction of bronchial walls
- Has three forms: cylindrical, fusiform, saccular

Key facts about cyanosis

- Bluish discoloration of skin and mucous membranes
- Caused by desaturation of oxygen

Key facts about hypoxemia

- Reduced oxygenation of arterial blood
- Can lead to reduced oxygenation of cells in tissues

PATHOPHYSIOLOGIC CONCEPTS

● **Atelectasis**
- Occurs when alveolar sacs or entire lung segments expand incompletely, producing partial or complete lung collapse
- Removes certain lung regions from gas exchange, allowing unoxygenated blood to pass unchanged through these regions, resulting in hypoxia
- May be chronic or acute
- Commonly occurs in patients undergoing upper abdominal or thoracic surgery

● **Bronchiectasis**
- Chronic abnormal dilation of bronchi and destruction of bronchial walls
    - Can occur throughout the tracheobronchial tree
    - May be confined to a single segment or lobe
- Usually bilateral in nature, involving basilar segments of the lower lobes
- Occurs in three forms
    - Cylindrical
    - Fusiform (varicose)
    - Saccular (cystic)
- Results from conditions associated with repeated damage to bronchial walls and abnormal mucociliary clearance, which causes breakdown of supporting tissue adjacent to airways
    - Debris collects within and occludes bronchi
    - Increasing pressure from retained secretions induces mucosal injury
- Can be accompanied by secondary infection (characterized by inflammation and leukocytic accumulations) caused by sputum stagnating in dilated bronchi

● **Cyanosis**
- Bluish discoloration of the skin and mucous membranes
- Caused by desaturation of oxygen due to sluggish blood flow or reduced hemoglobin levels
- Develops when 5 g of hemoglobin is desaturated of oxygen, even if hemoglobin levels are adequate or reduced

● **Hypoxemia**
- Reduced oxygenation of arterial blood, evidenced by reduced partial pressure of arterial oxygen (PaO_2)
- Has various causes
    - Decreased oxygen content of inspired gas
    - Hypoventilation
    - Diffusion abnormalities
    - Abnormal $\dot{V}/\dot{Q}$ ratios
    - Pulmonary right-to-left shunts
- Variable physiologic mechanism for each cause
- Can lead to reduced oxygenation of cells in tissues
- Can occur anywhere in the body

ACUTE RESPIRATORY DISTRESS SYNDROME

● **Definition**
- Form of pulmonary edema
- Also known as ARDS
- Can quickly lead to acute respiratory failure
- Also known as *shock lung, stiff lung, white lung,* or *wet lung* because of diffuse alveolar damage and acute lung injury
- Difficult to diagnose
- Can cause death within 48 hours if not promptly diagnosed and treated

● **Underlying pathophysiology**
- Diffuse injury to alveolar and pulmonary capillary endothelium reduces normal blood flow to the lungs, allowing platelets to aggregate
- Platelets release substances, such as serotonin, bradykinin and, especially, histamines, that inflame and damage alveolar membrane and later increase capillary permeability
- Increased capillary permeability allows fluid to shift into the interstitial space
- Proteins and more fluid leak out, increasing interstitial osmotic pressure and causing pulmonary edema
- Fluid in the alveoli and decreased blood flow damage surfactant in the alveoli, reducing the cells' ability to produce more surfactant
- Without surfactant, alveoli collapse, impairing gas exchange
- Marked hypoxemia occurs with increased respiratory distress
- Sufficient oxygen can't cross the alveolocapillary membrane
  - Carbon dioxide crosses the membrane more easily and is lost with every exhalation
  - Oxygen and carbon dioxide levels in the blood decrease
- Pulmonary edema worsens
- Inflammation leads to fibrosis, which further impedes gas exchange
- Hypoxemia leads to metabolic acidosis, ultimately resulting in respiratory failure
- Systemically, inflammatory mediators cause generalized endothelial damage and increased capillary permeability
- Multisystem organ dysfunction syndrome (MODS) occurs
- Death may occur (see *Understanding ARDS,* page 62)

● **Causes**
- Anaphylaxis
- Aspiration of gastric contents
- Burns
- Diffuse pneumonia, especially viral pneumonia
- Drug overdose, such as heroin, aspirin, or ethchlorvynol (Placidyl)
- Fat or amniotic fluid emboli
- Idiosyncratic drug reaction to ampicillin (Omnipen) or hydrochlorothiazide (HydroDIURIL)
- Indirect or direct lung trauma
- Inhalation of noxious gases, such as nitrous oxide, ammonia, or chlorine
- Near drowning
- Oxygen toxicity
- Sepsis

Key facts about ARDS

- Develops when injury to alveolar and pulmonary capillary endothelium reduces normal blood flow to the lungs
- Causes platelets to aggregate and release serotonin, bradykinin, and histamines that inflame alveolar membrane and increase capillary permeability
- Leads to increased interstitial osmotic pressure and pulmonary edema because fluid shifts into interstitial spaces
- Impairs gas exchange because reduced blood flow damages surfactant in alveoli
- Progresses to marked hypoxemia with increased respiratory distress
- Results in MODS
- Is difficult to diagnose
- Can cause death within 48 hours if left untreated

Common causes of ARDS

- Diffuse pneumonia
- Fat or amniotic fluid emboli
- Sepsis

Understanding ARDS

In phase 1, injury reduces normal blood flow to the lungs. Platelets aggregate and release histamine (H), serotonin (S), and bradykinin (B).

In phase 2, the released substances inflame and damage the alveolar capillary membrane, increasing capillary permeability. Fluids then shift into the interstitial space.

In phase 3, capillary permeability increases and proteins and fluids leak out, increasing interstitial osmotic pressure and causing pulmonary edema.

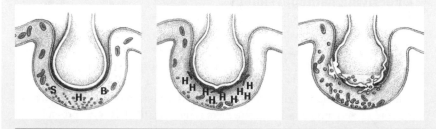

In phase 4, decreased blood flow and fluids in the alveoli damage surfactant and impair the cell's ability to produce more. The alveoli then collapse, impairing gas exchange.

In phase 5, oxygenation is impaired, but carbon dioxide (CO_2) easily crosses the alveolar capillary membrane and is expired. Blood oxygen (O_2) and CO_2 levels are low.

In phase 6, pulmonary edema worsens and inflammation leads to fibrosis. Gas exchange is further impeded.

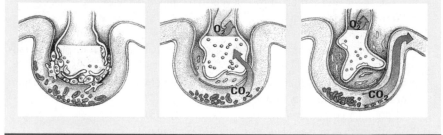

Key pathophysiologic changes in ARDS

- Dyspnea
- Rapid, shallow breathing
- Tachycardia
- Restlessness
- Crackles and rhonchi

● Pathophysiologic changes

- Initially, rapid, shallow breathing and dyspnea due to hypoxemia and its effects on the pneumotaxic center, causing excessive loss of carbon dioxide (respiratory alkalosis)
- Tachycardia related to stimulation of carotid and aortic bodies and the medulla due to decreased carbon dioxide
- Restlessness, apprehension, mental sluggishness, and motor dysfunction due to cerebral vasoconstriction and decreased cerebral blood flow
- Secondary rapid, deep respirations (Kussmaul's respirations) as the body attempts to normalize the alkalosis through the hydrogen-potassium buffer system
- Intercostal and suprasternal retractions resulting from the increased effort required to expand stiff, increasingly fibrotic lungs

- Crackles and rhonchi caused by fluid accumulation in lungs
- Increased blood pressure, possible headache, papilledema, and depressed reflexes as compensatory systems become overwhelmed and carbon dioxide begins to accumulate (respiratory acidosis)
- Coma, minimal respiratory excursion, and hypotension due to failure of compensatory mechanisms (metabolic acidosis)

Complications
- Decreased urine output
- Hypotension
- Metabolic acidosis
- MODS
- Respiratory acidosis
- Ventricular fibrillation
- Ventricular standstill

Diagnostic test findings
- Arterial blood gas (ABG) analysis results vary depending on the progression
  - Results initially reflect respiratory alkalosis
  - As ARDS worsens, respiratory acidosis is evidenced by an increasing partial pressure of arterial carbon dioxide ($PaCO_2$) (greater than 45 mm Hg)
  - Metabolic acidosis is evidenced by decreasing bicarbonate (less than 22 mEq/L) and a declining PaO_2 despite oxygen therapy
- Pulmonary artery catheterization helps identify the cause of pulmonary edema (cardiac versus noncardiac) by measuring pulmonary artery wedge pressure (PAWP), which is usually low to normal
- Serial chest X-rays vary depending on the stage of the disorder
  - Bilateral infiltrates are shown in early stages
  - In later stages, lung fields with a ground-glass appearance and "whiteouts" of both lung fields (with irreversible hypoxemia) may be observed
- Sputum analysis, including Gram stain and culture and sensitivity, identifies causative organisms
- Blood cultures identify infectious organisms
- Toxicology testing screens for drug ingestion
- Serum amylase rules out pancreatitis

Treatment
- Administration of humidified oxygen, ventilatory support with intubation, volume ventilation, and positive end-expiratory pressure (PEEP) to improve oxygenation
- Sedatives, opioids, or neuromuscular blockers during mechanical ventilation to minimize restlessness, oxygen consumption, and carbon dioxide production, and to facilitate ventilation
- Sodium bicarbonate to reverse severe metabolic acidosis
- I.V. fluid administration to maintain blood pressure by treating hypovolemia
- Vasopressors to maintain blood pressure
- Antimicrobial drugs to treat nonviral infections
- Diuretics to reduce interstitial and pulmonary edema
- Correction of electrolyte and acid-base imbalances to maintain cellular integrity (particularly sodium-potassium pump)
- Fluid restriction to prevent increased interstitial and alveolar edema

Key complications of ARDS
- MODS
- Respiratory or metabolic acidosis
- Ventricular fibrillation or standstill

Key diagnostic test results for ARDS
- ABG analysis: Respiratory alkalosis that progresses to acidosis ($PaCO_2$ greater than 45 mm Hg), metabolic acidosis (bicarbonate less than 22 mEq/L), and declining PaO_2
- Serial chest X-rays: Bilateral infiltrates (early stages); lung fields with ground-glass appearance and "whiteouts" of both lung fields (later stages)

Key treatments for ARDS
- Ventilatory support with intubation
- Neuromuscular blockers
- Vasopressors
- Antimicrobial drugs
- Correction of electrolyte and acid-base imbalances

● **Nursing considerations**
- Frequently assess the patient's respiratory status
    - Auscultate for adventitious or diminished breath sounds
    - Check for clear, frothy sputum, which may indicate pulmonary edema
- Observe and document the neurologic status of patients with hypoxemia
- **Maintain a patent airway by suctioning, and using sterile, nontraumatic technique**
- Closely monitor the patient's heart rate and blood pressure
- Watch for arrhythmias
- During pulmonary artery catheterization, know the desired PAWP level
- Monitor serum electrolytes and correct imbalances
- Measure intake and output and weigh the patient daily
- Monitor ABG studies
    - Check for metabolic and respiratory acidosis
    - Check for PaO_2 changes
- Give sedatives, as needed, to reduce restlessness
- **Because positive end-expiratory pressure (PEEP) may decrease cardiac output, check for hypotension, tachycardia, and decreased urine output**
- Suction only as needed to maintain PEEP, or use an in-line suctioning apparatus
- Reposition the patient frequently
- Record increases in secretions and temperature, and document hypotension, all of which may indicate a deteriorating condition
- Monitor peak pressures during ventilation
    - Because of stiff, noncompliant lungs, the patient is at high risk for barotrauma (pneumothorax)
    - Barotrauma is evidenced by increased peak pressures, decreased breath sounds on one side, and restlessness
- Monitor nutrition
    - Record caloric intake
    - Give tube feedings and parenteral nutrition, as ordered
- Maintain joint mobility
- Prevent skin breakdown
- Provide emotional support
    - Tell the patient that recovering from ARDS will take some time

ACUTE RESPIRATORY FAILURE

● **Definition**
- Inadequate ventilation
- Results from the inability of the lungs to adequately maintain arterial oxygenation or eliminate carbon dioxide

● **Underlying pathophysiology**
- If respiratory failure is primarily hypercapnic, it results from inadequate alveolar ventilation
- If respiratory failure is primarily hypoxemic, it results from inadequate exchange of oxygen between the alveoli and capillaries
- Many people experience combined hypercapnic and hypoxemic respiratory failure

Causes

- Atelectasis
- Bronchitis
- Bronchospasm
- Central nervous system (CNS) disease
- CNS depression
  - Head trauma
  - Injudicious use of sedatives, opioids, tranquilizers, or oxygen
- Chronic obstructive pulmonary disease (COPD)
- Cor pulmonale (right ventricular hypertrophy with right-sided heart failure)
- Massive obesity
- Pneumonia
- Pneumothorax
- Pulmonary edema
- Pulmonary emboli
- Ventilatory failure

Pathophysiologic changes

- Increased respiratory rate due to hypoxemia and its effects on pneumotaxic center
- Shallow or deep respirations and cyanosis resulting from decreased oxygen levels in blood
- Crackles on auscultation related to fluid accumulation in lungs
- Restlessness, confusion, loss of concentration, irritability, tremulousness, diminished deep tendon reflexes, papilledema, and coma related to hypoxemia and hypercapnia
- Tachycardia along with increased cardiac output and mildly elevated blood pressure due to adrenal release of catecholamine
- Possible arrhythmias related to myocardial hypoxia
- Increased pressures on the right side of the heart, distended jugular veins, enlarged liver, and peripheral edema resulting from pulmonary capillary vasoconstriction

Complications

- Cardiac arrest
- Metabolic acidosis
- Tissue hypoxia

Diagnostic test findings

- ABG analysis indicates respiratory failure
  - Values deteriorate
  - pH is below 7.35
  - Patients with COPD may have a lower than normal pH compared with previous levels
- Chest X-rays identify pulmonary diseases or conditions, such as emphysema, atelectasis, lesions, pneumothorax, infiltrates, and effusions
- Electrocardiography (ECG) detects ventricular arrhythmias or right ventricular hypertrophy
- Pulse oximetry reveals decreased oxygen saturation (SaO_2)
- White blood cell (WBC) count detects an underlying infection
- Hemoglobin level and hematocrit are abnormally low, which signals blood loss, indicating decreased oxygen-carrying capacity

Common causes of acute respiratory failure

- Bronchitis
- Bronchospasm
- CNS depression
- Pneumonia
- Pulmonary emboli

Key pathophysiologic changes in acute respiratory failure

- Increased respiratory rate
- Crackles
- Restlessness
- Tachycardia
- Arrhythmias

Key diagnostic test results for acute respiratory failure

- ABG analysis: Deteriorating values, pH below 7.35
- Chest X-rays: Pulmonary diseases or conditions
- ECG: Ventricular arrhythmias or right ventricular hypertrophy

- Serum electrolytes reveal hypokalemia from compensatory hyperventilation and hypochloremia, which usually occurs in metabolic alkalosis
- Blood cultures may identify pathogens
- Pulmonary artery catheterization helps to distinguish between pulmonary and cardiovascular causes, and monitors hemodynamic pressures

● Treatment

- Oxygen therapy to promote oxygenation and raise PaO_2
- Mechanical ventilation with an endotracheal (ET) or tracheostomy tube, if needed, to provide adequate oxygenation and reverse acidosis
- If the patient doesn't respond to treatment, high-frequency ventilation to force the airways open, promoting oxygenation and preventing alveoli collapse
- Antibiotics to treat infection
- Bronchodilators to maintain airway patency
- Corticosteroids to decrease inflammation
- Fluid restrictions in cor pulmonale to reduce volume and cardiac workload
- Positive inotropic agents to increase cardiac output
- Vasopressors to maintain blood pressure
- Diuretics to reduce edema and fluid overload
- If patient isn't intubated and mechanically ventilated, deep breathing with pursed lips to help keep airway patent
- Incentive spirometry to increase lung volume

● Nursing considerations

- Maintain a patent airway
- Encourage the patient to cough and to breathe deeply using an incentive spirometer
- Teach the patient to use pursed-lip and diaphragmatic breathing to control dyspnea
- Turn intubated or lethargic patients every 1 to 2 hours
- Use postural drainage and chest physiotherapy to help clear secretions
- For intubated patients, suction the trachea as needed after hyperoxygenation
    - Observe for change in quantity, consistency, and color of sputum
    - Provide humidification to liquefy secretions
- Auscultate for chest sounds
- Monitor ABG levels and report changes immediately
- Monitor and record serum electrolyte levels
- Monitor fluid balance by recording intake and output or daily weight
- Check the cardiac monitor for arrhythmias
- Check ventilator settings and cuff pressures
- Prevent infection by using sterile technique while suctioning
- Check gastric secretions for evidence of bleeding if the patient has a nasogastric tube or complains of epigastric tenderness, nausea, or vomiting
- Monitor hemoglobin level and hematocrit
- Check stool for occult blood
- Administer antacids, histamine-2 receptor antagonists, or sucralfate, as ordered
- **Prevent tracheal erosion, which can result from artificial airway cuff overinflation**
    - Use the minimal leak technique

Key treatments for acute respiratory failure

- Oxygen therapy
- Mechanical ventilation
- Antibiotics
- Bronchodilators
- Corticosteroids

Key nursing considerations for acute respiratory failure

- Maintain patent airway.
- Prevent overinflation of tracheal cuff, if used.
- Closely monitor respiratory status for hypoxia.
- When condition is stable, teach patient respiratory exercises to increase lung capacity.
- Monitor hemodynamic parameters for signs of arrhythmias and heart failure.
- Assess for renal dysfunction, signs of bleeding, and GI irritation.

volume (low-pressure cuff), a foam
n the cuff
ine to prevent oral or vocal cord

n the nostrils and provide good hy-

airway hyperresponsiveness to mul-

intrinsic allergens

to various stimuli, causing episodic
nstrict the airways
s further block the airways
hed to histamine-containing mast
nitiate intrinsic asthma attacks
llen, the IgE antibody combines with

mast cells degranulate and release

n and edema of an asthma attack
flow decreases, trapping gas in the air-
n
egions
s labored breathing

● Causes
- Extrinsic asthma
  - Pollen
  - Animal dander, kapok, or feather pillows
  - House dust or mold
  - Exposure to irritants or noxious fumes
  - Temperature or humidity variations
  - Food additives containing sulfites
- Intrinsic asthma
  - Emotional stress or anxiety
  - Fatigue
  - Endocrine changes
  - Coughing or laughing
  - Genetic factors
  - Exercise

● Pathophysiologic changes
- Sudden dyspnea, wheezing, tightness in the chest, and diminished breath sounds due to bronchial constriction

Key facts about asthma
- Characterized by airflow obstruction and airway hyperresponsiveness
- Initiated by IgE antibodies attached to mast cells, which combine with antigens upon initial exposure to them
- Manifests upon release of mediators after subsequent exposure to antigen, causing bronchoconstriction and edema

Common causes of asthma
- Intrinsic: Internal or genetic
- Exercise
- Stress or anxiety
- Extrinsic: Environmental
- Pollen or mold
- Food additives
- Irritants or noxious fumes

Key pathophysiologic changes in asthma
- Dyspnea
- Diminished breath sounds
- Wheezing

- Initially, nonproductive cough
- Later, coughing with thick, clear, or yellow sputum resulting from excessive mucus production
- Rapid pulse, tachypnea, and use of accessory respiratory muscles due to hypoxemia

● **Complications**
- Hypoxemia
- Respiratory acidosis
- Respiratory failure
- Status asthmaticus

● **Diagnostic test findings**
- Pulmonary function tests (PFTs) provide various findings
  - Signs of airway obstructive disease are present
  - Vital capacity is low-normal or decreased
  - Total lung and residual capacities are increased
  - Pulmonary function may be normal between attacks
- Serum IgE levels may increase from an allergic reaction
- Sputum analysis may indicate the presence of Curschmann's spirals (casts of airways), Charcot-Leyden crystals, and eosinophils
- Complete blood count (CBC) with differential reveals an increased eosinophil count
- Chest X-rays can be used to diagnose or monitor the progress of asthma and may show hyperinflation with areas of atelectasis
- ABG analysis detects hypoxemia and guides treatment
- Skin testing may identify specific allergens
- Bronchial challenge testing evaluates the clinical significance of allergens identified by skin testing
- ECG shows sinus tachycardia during an attack
  - A severe attack may show signs of cor pulmonale (right axis deviation, peaked P wave) that resolve after the attack

● **Treatment**
- Identification and avoidance of precipitating factors (environmental allergens or irritants) to prevent attacks (see *Averting an asthma attack*)
- Desensitization to specific antigens to decrease severity of attacks during future exposure to allergen
- Bronchodilators to decrease bronchoconstriction, reduce bronchial airway edema, and increase pulmonary ventilation
- Corticosteroids to decrease inflammation and edema of airways
- Mast cell stabilizers to block acute obstructive effects of antigen exposure
  - Treatment inhibits degranulation of mast cells, thereby preventing release of chemical mediators responsible for anaphylaxis
- Leukotriene modifiers and leukotriene receptor antagonists to inhibit potent bronchoconstriction and inflammatory effects of cysteinyl leukotrienes
  - May be used as adjunctive therapy to avoid the need for high-dose, inhaled corticosteroids
  - May be used when patient is noncompliant with corticosteroid therapy
- Anticholinergic bronchodilators to block acetylcholine (another chemical mediator)
- Low-flow, humidified oxygen

Key diagnostic test results for asthma

- PFTs: Signs of airway obstructive disease, low-normal or decreased vital capacity, increased total lung and residual capacities
- IgE levels: Elevated in allergic reaction

Key treatments for asthma

- Corticosteroids
- Bronchodilators
- Mast cell stabilizers
- Mechanical ventilation (if necessary)

GO WITH THE FLOW

Averting an asthma attack

This flowchart shows pathophysiologic changes that occur with asthma, and how treatments and interventions alter the physiologic cascade to stop an attack.

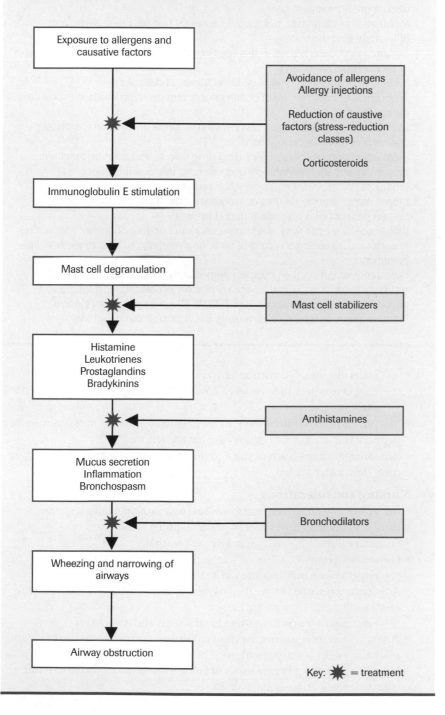

Exposure to allergens and causative factors	

Avoidance of allergens
Allergy injections

Reduction of caustive factors (stress-reduction classes)

Corticosteroids

Immunoglobulin E stimulation

Mast cell degranulation

Mast cell stabilizers

Histamine
Leukotrienes
Prostaglandins
Bradykinins

Antihistamines

Mucus secretion
Inflammation
Bronchospasm

Bronchodilators

Wheezing and narrowing of airways

Airway obstruction

Key: ✴ = treatment

TOP 4

Ways to avert asthma attacks

1. Avoidance of allergens
2. Reduction of causative factors
3. Corticosteroids
4. Allergy injections

TOP 3

Patient teaching topics for asthma patients

1. Explanation of the diagnosis and its causes, effects, and complications
2. Explanation of drug therapy, including therapy specific to exercise-induced asthma
3. Proper use of handheld inhalers and other equipment

TIME-OUT FOR TEACHING

Allergy and asthma sufferers

Be sure to include these points in your teaching plan for patients with allergies or asthma:
- explanation of the diagnosis and its causes, effects, and complications
- discussion of treatment goals
- explanation of diagnostic tests, such as allergy testing, chest X-ray, and pulmonary function testing
- explanation of desensitization therapy (injection of antigens to minimize risk of severe hypersensitivity)
- avoidance of known allergens, noxious fumes, and smoking
- importance of being aware of pollen counts and avoiding outdoor exposure during times of risk
- use of anti-allergy linens and air filters in the home and avoidance of deep-pile carpets to minimize reactions
- explanation of drug therapy, including drug effects and adverse reactions
- proper use of handheld inhalers and extender devices, if required
- proper use of nebulizer equipment, if needed
- proper use of bronchodilators or cromolyn sodium 30 minutes before exercise (in patients with exercise-induced asthma)
- proper use of a peak flow meter to measure the degree of airway obstruction
- importance of keeping a record of peak flow readings to take to medical appointments
- importance of calling the physician immediately if peak flow readings drop suddenly (which may signal severe respiratory problems), or if the patient develops a temperature above 100° F (37.8° C), chest pain, shortness of breath without coughing or exercising, or uncontrollable coughing.

– Treats dyspnea, cyanosis, and hypoxemia
– Should maintain PaO_2 between 65 and 85 mm Hg, as determined by ABG analysis
- Mechanical ventilation if the patient fails to respond to initial ventilatory support and drugs or develops respiratory failure
- Relaxation exercises (such as yoga) to increase circulation and help patient recover from asthma attack

Nursing considerations
- Administer the prescribed treatments and assess the patient's response
- Place the patient in high Fowler's position during an attack
- Encourage pursed-lip and diaphragmatic breathing
- Monitor vital signs
  – Hypertension may indicate asthma-related hypoxemia
- Administer prescribed humidified oxygen by nasal cannula at 2 L/minute to ease breathing and to increase SaO_2
  – Later, adjust oxygen according to vital signs and ABG levels
- Anticipate intubation and mechanical ventilation (if the patient fails to maintain adequate oxygenation)
- Monitor serum theophylline levels (if being used for prophylaxis) to make sure therapeutic range is maintained

Key nursing considerations for asthma

- Assess respiratory status.
- Anticipate intubation and mechanical ventilation (if patient fails to maintain adequate oxygenation).
- Observe for complications of medications.
- Keep room cool for patient comfort.

- Monitor respiratory status
  - Note productive cough
  - Auscultate lungs, noting adventitious or absent breath sounds
  - Suction an intubated patient as needed
- Treat dehydration with I.V. fluids until the patient can tolerate oral fluids
- If conservative treatment fails to improve the airway obstruction, anticipate bronchoscopy or bronchial lavage when a lobe or larger area collapses
- Review ABG levels, pulmonary function test results, and SaO_2 readings
- If the patient is taking systemic corticosteroids, observe for complications
- If the patient is taking corticosteroids by inhaler, watch for signs of candidal infection in the mouth and pharynx
  - Using an extender device and rinsing the mouth afterward may prevent infection
- Observe the patient's anxiety level
  - Measures that reduce hypoxemia and breathlessness should help relieve anxiety.
- Keep the room temperature comfortable
  - Use an air conditioner or a fan in hot, humid weather
- Control exercise-induced asthma
  - Instruct the patient to use a bronchodilator or cromolyn sodium (Intal, Nasalcrom) 30 minutes before exercise
  - Instruct the patient to use pursed-lip breathing while exercising
- Provide patient teaching (see *Allergy and asthma sufferers*)

CHRONIC BRONCHITIS

● Definition
- Form of COPD that involves significant changes in the bronchi
- Involves excessive production of tracheobronchial mucus and chronic cough (cough that lasts at least 3 months each year for 2 consecutive years)
- Characterized by airflow obstruction

● Underlying pathophysiology
- Irritants are inhaled for a prolonged time, which inflames the tracheo-bronchial tree, leading to increased mucus production and a narrowed or blocked airway
- Inflammation continues, causing changes in the cells lining the respiratory tract that result in resistance of the small airways
- Severe ventilation-perfusion imbalance and decreased arterial oxygenation occur
- Several changes follow
  - Hypertrophy and hyperplasia of the bronchial mucous glands
  - Increased goblet cells
  - Ciliary damage
  - Squamous metaplasia of the columnar epithelium
  - Chronic leukocytic and lymphocytic infiltration of bronchial walls (see *Changes in chronic bronchitis,* page 72)

● Causes
- Cigarette smoking
- Genetic predisposition

Key facts about chronic bronchitis

- Develops when irritants are inhaled for a prolonged time
- Inflames the tracheobronchial tree, leading to increased mucus production and a narrowed or blocked airway
- Causes changes in respiratory tract cells causing resistance of small airways

Common causes of chronic bronchitis

- Cigarette smoking
- Respiratory tract infection

Changes in chronic bronchitis

In chronic bronchitis, irritants inflame the tracheobronchial tree over time, leading to increased mucus production and a narrowed or blocked airway. As the inflammation continues, goblet and epithelial cells hypertrophy. Because the natural defense mechanisms are blocked, the airways accumulate debris in the respiratory tract. The illlustrations here show these changes.

CROSS-SECTION OF NORMAL BRONCHIAL TUBE

Epithelial cell
Goblet cell
Cilia

NARROWED BRONCHIAL TUBE IN CHRONIC BRONCHITIS

Epithelial cell
Goblet cell
Cilia

Key pathophysiologic changes in chronic bronchitis

- Copious gray, white, or yellow sputum
- Productive cough
- Dyspnea
- Wheezing and rhonchi

Common complications of chronic bronchitis

- Recurrent respiratory tract infection
- Acute respiratory failure

- Organic or inorganic dusts and noxious gas exposure
- Respiratory tract infection
- Smog

● **Pathophysiologic changes**
- Copious gray, white, or yellow sputum and productive cough due to hypersecretion of goblet cells
- Dyspnea resulting from obstruction of airflow to lower bronchial tree
- Tachypnea, cyanosis, and use of accessory muscles for breathing due to hypoxia
- Wheezing and rhonchi resulting from narrow, mucus-filled respiratory passages
- Prolonged expiratory time resulting from compensatory mechanism to maintain patent airway
- Tachycardia from decreased oxygenation

● **Complications**
- Acute respiratory failure
- Cor pulmonale due to increased right ventricular end-diastolic pressure
- Heart failure, resulting in increased venous pressure, liver engorgement, and dependent edema
- Pulmonary hypertension

- Recurrent respiratory tract infections
- **Diagnostic test findings**
  - Chest X-rays may show hyperinflation and increased bronchovascular markings
  - PFTs reveal various findings
    - Residual volume is increased
    - Vital capacity and forced expiratory flow are decreased
    - Static compliance and diffusing capacity are normal
  - ABG analysis reveals decreased PaO_2 and normal or increased $PaCO_2$
  - Sputum analysis may reveal many microorganisms and neutrophils
  - ECG may show atrial arrhythmias; peaked P waves in leads II, III, and aV_F; and, occasionally, right ventricular hypertrophy
  - CBC reveals a hematocrit level over 50% along with polycythemia due to prolonged hypoxia
- **Treatment**
  - Avoidance of air pollutants (most effective)
  - Smoking cessation and avoidance of second-hand smoke
  - Antibiotics to treat recurring infections
  - Bronchodilators to relieve bronchospasms and facilitate mucociliary clearance
  - Adequate hydration to liquefy secretions
  - Chest physiotherapy to mobilize secretions
  - Ultrasonic or mechanical nebulizers to loosen and mobilize secretions
  - Corticosteroids to combat inflammation
  - Diuretics to reduce edema
  - Oxygen to treat hypoxia
- **Nursing considerations**
  - Provide the patient with smoking-cessation resources or counseling if necessary
  - Assess the patient for changes in baseline respiratory function to detect worsening bronchitis
    - Evaluate sputum quality and quantity
    - Watch for restlessness, increased tachypnea, and altered breath sounds
    - Report changes immediately
  - Perform chest physiotherapy, including postural drainage and chest percussion and vibration for involved lobes, several times daily, as needed
  - Weigh the patient three times weekly, and assess for edema
  - Provide the patient with a high-calorie, protein-rich diet
  - Make sure the patient receives adequate fluids (at least 3 qt [3 L] per day) to loosen secretions
  - Schedule respiratory therapy at least 1 hour before or after meals
  - Provide mouth care after bronchodilator inhalation therapy
  - Advise the patient to avoid crowds and people with known infections
  - Advise the patient to obtain influenza and pneumococcal immunizations
  - Urge the patient to avoid inhaled irritants, such as automobile exhaust fumes, smog, aerosol sprays, and industrial pollutants
  - Warn the patient that exposures to blasts of cold air may precipitate bronchospasm

Key diagnostic test results for chronic bronchitis
- Chest X-rays: Hyperinflation and increased bronchovascular markings
- PFTs: Increased residual volume, decreased vital capacity and forced expiratory flow, normal static compliance and diffusing capacity
- Sputum analysis: Presence of microorganisms and neutrophils

Key treatments for chronic bronchitis
- Avoidance of pollutants
- Nebulizer treatments
- Antibiotics for recurrent infections
- Corticosteroids
- Bronchodilators

Key nursing considerations for chronic bronchitis
- Evaluate patient for signs and symptoms of worsening bronchitis: change in sputum quality or quantity, restlessness, tachypnea, and altered breath sounds.
- Perform chest physiotherapy.
- Advise patient to avoid triggers.

CHRONIC OBSTRUCTIVE PULMONARY DISEASE

- **Definition**
  - Also called *chronic obstructive lung disease* or COPD
  - Results from emphysema, chronic bronchitis, asthma, or a combination of these disorders (bronchitis and emphysema commonly occur together)
  - Doesn't always produce symptoms
  - May cause only minimal disability but worsens with time

- **Underlying pathophysiology**
  - Smoking, one of the major causes of COPD, impairs ciliary action and macrophage function
    - Airways become inflamed
    - Mucus production increases
    - Alveolar septa are destroyed
    - Peribronchiolar fibrosis occurs
    - Early inflammatory changes may reverse if the patient stops smoking before lung disease becomes extensive
  - Mucus plugs and narrowed airways cause air trapping, as in chronic bronchitis and emphysema
  - Alveoli hyperinflate on expiration
  - Air trapping (also called *ball valving*) commonly occurs in asthma and chronic bronchitis (see *Air trapping in COPD*)

- **Causes**
  - Air pollution
  - Allergies
  - Cigarette smoking
  - Familial and hereditary factors such as an alpha$_1$-antitrypsin deficiency

- **Pathophysiologic changes**
  - Fatigue and reduced ability to perform exercises or do strenuous work because of diminished pulmonary reserve
  - Productive cough stimulated by mucus
  - Dyspnea on minimal exertion resulting from decreased oxygenation
  - Thoracic deformities due to overdistention and overinflation of the lungs
  - Dependent edema and possible ascites due to right-sided heart failure

- **Complications**
  - Cor pulmonale
  - Death
  - Overwhelming disability
  - Pulmonary hypertension
  - Severe respiratory failure

- **Diagnostic test findings**
  - ABG analysis determines oxygen need and helps avoid carbon dioxide narcosis by indicating the degree of hypoxia
  - Chest X-rays show air trapping and aeration
  - ECG may show arrhythmias consistent with hypoxemia
  - PFTs show reduced vital capacity and prolonged expiration

Air trapping in COPD

In chronic obstructive pulmonary disease (COPD), mucus plugs and narrowed airways trap air (also called *ball valving*). During inspiration, the airways enlarge and gas enters; on expiration, the airways narrow and air can't escape. This commonly occurs in asthma and chronic bronchitis.

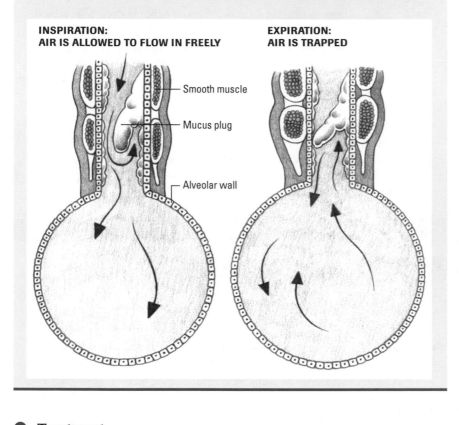

**INSPIRATION:
AIR IS ALLOWED TO FLOW IN FREELY**

**EXPIRATION:
AIR IS TRAPPED**

— Smooth muscle

— Mucus plug

— Alveolar wall

● **Treatment**
  - Bronchodilators to alleviate bronchospasms and enhance mucociliary clearance of secretions
  - Effective coughing to remove secretions
  - Postural drainage to help mobilize secretions
  - Chest physiotherapy to mobilize secretions
  - Low oxygen concentrations as needed (high flow rates can lead to narcosis)
  - Antibiotics to treat respiratory tract infections
  - Smoking cessation
  - Increased fluid intake to thin mucus
  - Use of a humidifier to thin secretions

● **Nursing considerations**
  - Provide smoking cessation counseling or refer the patient to a smoking cessation program
  - Teach the correct use of a metered-dose inhaler
  - Administer antibiotics, as ordered, to treat respiratory infections

**Key treatments
for COPD**

- Bronchodilators
- Effective coughing
- Chest physiotherapy
- Antibiotics
- Smoking cessation
- Increased fluid intake

- Teach the patient to take slow, deep breaths and to exhale through pursed lips to strengthen the respiratory muscles
- Teach the patient how to cough effectively in order to help mobilize secretions
- Teach the family how to perform postural drainage and chest physiotherapy, if needed
- Perform ABG analysis to determine the patient's oxygen needs and to avoid carbon dioxide narcosis
- Teach the patient and his family about safe use of home oxygen therapy, if needed
  - Instruct them not to turn up the flow without physician prescription
  - Explain that excessive oxygen therapy may eliminate the hypoxic respiratory drive, causing confusion and drowsiness, signs of carbon dioxide narcosis
- Emphasize the importance of a balanced diet
  - Because the patient may tire easily when eating, suggest eating frequent, small meals
  - Consider using oxygen, administered by nasal cannula, during meals
- Instruct the patient to allow for daily rest periods
- Instruct the patient to exercise daily as his physician directs

COR PULMONALE

● Definition
- Refers to hypertrophy and dilation of the right ventricle of the heart
- Develops secondary to disease affecting the structure or function of the lungs or their vasculature
- Also called *right-sided heart failure*

● Underlying pathophysiology
- An occluded vessel impairs the heart's ability to generate enough pressure
- Pulmonary hypertension results from the increased blood flow needed to oxygenate the tissues
- Pulmonary hypertension increases the heart's workload
- To compensate, the right ventricle hypertrophies to force blood through the lungs
- In response to hypoxia, the bone marrow produces more red blood cells (RBCs), causing polycythemia
- The blood's viscosity increases, which further aggravates pulmonary hypertension
- Increased blood viscosity increases the right ventricle's workload, causing heart failure (see *Understanding cor pulmonale*)

● Causes
- Bronchial asthma
- COPD (most common cause of chronic cor pulmonale)
- Disorders that affect the pulmonary parenchyma
- External vascular obstruction resulting from a tumor or aneurysm
- Kyphoscoliosis
- Pectus excavatum (funnel chest)
- Primary pulmonary hypertension

Key nursing considerations for COPD

- Teach patient and family about the disease process and its treatment.
- Instruct patient in pursed-lip breathing, effective coughing, and safe use of oxygen therapy, if applicable.

Key facts about cor pulmonale

- Develops when an occluded vessel impairs the heart's ability to generate enough pressure
- Progresses to pulmonary hypertension, which increases cardiac workload
- Results in hypertrophy and dilation of right ventricle

Common causes of cor pulmonale

- Disorders that affect the pulmonary parenchyma
- Primary pulmonary hypertension
- Pulmonary emboli

GO WITH THE FLOW

Understanding cor pulmonale

Various pulmonary restrictive disorders (such as fibrosis or obesity), obstructive disorders (such as bronchitis), and primary vascular disorders (such as recurrent pulmonary emboli) can cause cor pulmonale. However, they all share a common pathway of disease progression.

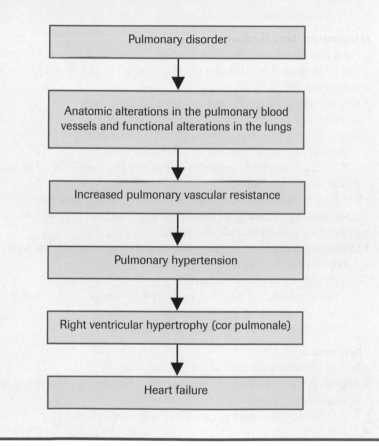

- Pulmonary emboli (most common cause of acute, life-threatening cor pulmonale)
- Vasculitis

Pathophysiologic changes
- Fatigue, weakness, and dyspnea due to hypoxemia
- Tachypnea due to decreased oxygenation to the tissues
- Orthopnea due to pulmonary edema
- Dependent edema and hepatojugular reflux (distention of the jugular vein induced by pressing over the liver)
- Distended jugular veins due to pulmonary hypertension
- Enlarged, tender liver related to polycythemia and decreased cardiac output
- Right upper quadrant discomfort due to liver involvement
- Tachycardia due to decreased cardiac output and increasing hypoxia

Key pathophysiologic changes in cor pulmonale

- Fatigue
- Dyspnea
- Tachypnea
- Orthopnea
- Distended jugular veins

- Weakened pulses due to decreased cardiac output

Complications
- Anasarca (generalized edema)
- Ascites
- Hepatomegaly
- Pleural effusions
- Left-sided heart failure as the heart hypertrophies in an attempt to circulate the blood
- Thromboembolism due to polycythemia

Diagnostic test findings
- Pulmonary artery catheterization shows increased right ventricular pressure and pulmonary artery pressure (PAP) resulting from increased pulmonary vascular resistance
- Echocardiography shows right ventricular enlargement
- Angiography shows right ventricular enlargement
- Chest X-rays reveal large central pulmonary arteries and right ventricular enlargement
- ABG analysis detects decreased PaO_2 (usually less than 70 mm Hg and rarely more than 90 mm Hg)
- ECG shows arrhythmias, such as premature atrial and ventricular contractions, atrial fibrillation, right bundle branch block, and right axis deviation
- PFTs reflect underlying pulmonary disease
- Cardiac catheterization shows increased pulmonary vascular pressures
- Laboratory testing may reveal abnormalities
  - Hematocrit is typically over 50%
  - Aspartate aminotransferase levels may be elevated with hepatic congestion and decreased liver function
  - Serum bilirubin levels may be elevated

Treatment
- Bed rest to reduce myocardial oxygen demands
- Digoxin (Digitek, Lanoxin) to increase the strength of myocardial contractions in chronic cor pulmonale
- Antibiotics to treat underlying respiratory tract infection
- Medications such as pulmonary artery vasodilators (diazoxide [Hyperstat IV], nitroprusside [Nitropress], hydralazine [Apresoline]), angiotensin-converting enzyme (ACE) inhibitors, calcium channel blockers, or prostaglandins
- Continuous administration of low concentrations of oxygen to decrease pulmonary vasoconstriction, polycythemia, and tachypnea
- Mechanical ventilation for acute cor pulmonale
- Low-sodium diet with restricted fluid to reduce edema
- Phlebotomy to decrease excess RBC mass
- Small doses of heparin to decrease the risk of thromboembolism
- Possible tracheotomy if the patient has an upper airway obstruction
- Corticosteroids to treat vasculitis or an underlying autoimmune disorder

Nursing considerations
- Because the patient may lack energy and tire easily when eating, provide small, frequent meals rather than three heavy meals

- Prevent fluid retention
  - Limit the patient's fluid intake to 1 to 2 qt (1 to 2 L)/day
  - Provide a low-sodium diet
- Monitor serum potassium levels closely if the patient is receiving diuretics
- Watch for signs of digoxin toxicity
  - Monitor for cardiac arrhythmias
  - Teach the patient to check his radial pulse before taking digoxin
  - Instruct the patient to notify the physician if he detects changes in pulse rate
- Reposition a bedridden patient frequently to prevent atelectasis
- Provide meticulous respiratory care
  - Periodically measure ABG levels
  - Watch for such signs of respiratory failure
- Teach the patient to detect edema
  - Press the skin over his shins with one finger
  - Hold his finger in place for 1 to 2 seconds
  - Check the site for a finger impression (indicating edema)
- If the patient requires supplemental oxygen therapy at home, refer him to a medical equipment company for assistance
- If the patient has been placed on anticoagulant therapy, emphasize the need to watch for bleeding (epistaxis, hematuria, bruising) and to report signs to the physician
- Tell the patient to watch for and immediately report early signs of infection
- Tell the patient to avoid crowds and persons known to have pulmonary infections, especially during flu season
- Warn the patient to avoid medications that may depress the ventilatory drive, such as sedatives and antihistamines, unless prescribed by his physician

EMPHYSEMA

Definition
- Form of COPD
- Characterized by abnormal, permanent enlargement of the acini accompanied by destruction of alveolar walls
- Involves obstruction due to alveolar wall destruction rather than mucus production
- Limits airflow because of a lack of elastic recoil in the lungs

Underlying pathophysiology
- Recurrent inflammation associated with the release of proteolytic enzymes from lung cells causes abnormal, irreversible enlargement of the air spaces distal to the terminal bronchioles
- This enlargement leads to the destruction of alveolar walls, which results in a breakdown of elasticity

Causes
- Alpha$_1$-antitrypsin deficiency
- Cigarette smoking

Key nursing considerations for cor pulmonale
- Offer small, frequent meals and limit fluids.
- Instruct patient about the therapeutic and adverse effects of prescribed medications.
- Tell patient to avoid exposure to people with infections or influenza.

Key facts about emphysema
- Characterized by permanent enlargement of air spaces distal to the terminal bronchioles
- Leads to destruction of alveolar walls, which results in breakdown of elasticity
- One of the obstructive pulmonary diseases

Key pathophysiologic changes in emphysema

- Tachypnea
- Dyspnea on exertion
- Barrel-shaped chest
- Crackles and wheezing on inspiration
- Prolonged expiration

Key diagnostic test results for emphysema

- Chest X-rays: Flattened diaphragm, reduced vascular markings at lung periphery, overaeration of lungs, vertical heart, enlarged anteroposterior chest diameter, large retrosternal air space
- PFTs: Increased residual volume, total lung capacity, and inspiratory flow; reduced diffusing capacity

Key treatments for emphysema

- Smoking cessation
- Bronchodilators
- Antibiotics
- Adequate hydration
- Oxygen therapy at low settings
- Mucolytics
- Corticosteroids

Key nursing considerations for emphysema

- Offer smoking cessation materials, if applicable.
- Assess for changes in baseline respiratory function.
- Perform chest physiotherapy and offer fluids frequently.
- Provide a high-calorie, protein-rich diet.

Pathophysiologic changes
- Tachypnea and dyspnea on exertion related to decreased oxygenation
- Barrel-shaped chest due to the lungs overdistending and overinflating
- Prolonged expiration and grunting because of accessory muscle use
- Decreased breath sounds and decreased tactile fremitus caused by air-trapping in the alveoli and alveolar wall destruction
- Clubbed fingers and toes related to chronic hypoxic changes
- Decreased chest expansion due to hypoventilation
- Crackles and wheezing on inspiration due to bronchiolar collapse

Complications
- Cor pulmonale
- Respiratory failure
- Recurrent respiratory tract infections

Diagnostic test findings
- Chest X-rays reveal several findings
  - Flattened diaphragm
  - Reduced vascular markings at the lung periphery
  - Overaeration of the lungs
  - Vertical heart
  - Enlarged anteroposterior chest diameter
  - Large retrosternal air space
- PFTs reveal various changes
  - Increased residual volume and total lung capacity
  - Reduced diffusing capacity
  - Increased inspiratory flow
- ABG analysis usually reveals reduced PaO_2 and a normal $PaCO_2$ until late in the disease process
- ECG may show tall, symmetrical P waves in leads II, III, and aV_F
  - A vertical QRS axis and signs of right ventricular hypertrophy are seen late in the disease
- CBC usually reveals increased hemoglobin level and hematocrit late in the disease (when the patient has persistent, severe hypoxia and polycythemia from chronic hypovolemia)

Treatment
- Stopping smoking and avoiding air pollution to preserve the remaining alveoli
- Bronchodilators to reverse bronchospasms and promote mucociliary clearance
- Antibiotics to treat respiratory tract infections
- Pneumococcal 23-valent polysaccharide vaccine (Pneumovax) to prevent pneumococcal pneumonia and influenza vaccine
- Adequate hydration to liquefy and mobilize secretions
- Chest physiotherapy to mobilize secretions
- Oxygen therapy at low settings to correct hypoxia
- Mucolytics to thin secretions and aid in mucus expectoration
- Aerosolized or systemic corticosteroids to decrease inflammation

Nursing considerations
- Provide the patient with smoking-cessation resources or counseling if necessary
- Assess for changes in baseline respiratory function

- Perform chest physiotherapy, as needed, several times daily
- Weigh the patient three times weekly, and assess for edema
- Provide the patient with a high-calorie, protein-rich diet
- Offer small, frequent meals to conserve energy and prevent fatigue
- Make sure the patient receives adequate fluids (at least 3 qt [3 L] per day) to loosen secretions (if not in heart failure)
- Schedule respiratory therapy at least 1 hour before or after meals
- Provide mouth care after bronchodilator inhalation therapy
- Urge the patient to avoid inhaled irritants
- Warn the patient that exposure to blasts of cold air may precipitate bronchospasm

PLEURAL EFFUSION

- **Definition**
  - Excess fluid in the pleural space
  - Can involve various types of fluid
    - Extracellular fluid
    - Pus (as in empyema)
    - Blood (as in hemothorax)
    - Chyle (as in chylothorax)
    - Bilious fluid
  - Classified as transudative (watery) or exudative

- **Underlying pathophysiology**
  - Excessive hydrostatic pressure or decreased osmotic pressure can cause excess fluid to pass across intact capillaries
  - Transudative pleural effusion is a generally clear, ultrafiltrate of plasma containing low concentrations of protein
  - Exudative pleural effusion results when capillaries exhibit increased permeability with or without changes in hydrostatic and colloid osmotic pressures
    - Protein- and leukocyte-rich fluid leak into the pleural space
    - The fluid commonly contains malignant cells or pus from empyema or high levels of fibrinogen that make it opaque to cloudy
  - An infection in the pleural space results from an extension of an infection of nearby structures

- **Causes**
  - Transudative pleural effusions
    - Heart failure
    - Hepatic disease
    - Hypoalbuminemia
    - Renal disease
  - Exudative pleural effusions
    - Bacterial or fungal pneumonitis or empyema
    - Chest trauma
    - Malignancy
    - Subphrenic abscess, pancreatitis
    - Tuberculosis (TB)
    - Carcinoma
    - Idiopathic infection

Key facts about pleural effusion

- Excess fluid in pleural space
- May be transudative or exudative
- Results when capillary permeability increases or excessive hydrostatic pressure or decreased osmotic pressure allows excess fluid to pass across intact capillaries

Causes of transudative pleural effusions

- Heart failure
- Hypoalbuminemia

Causes of exudative pleural effusions

- Bacterial or fungal pneumonitis or empyema
- Idiopathic infection
- Lung abscesses
- Pneumonitis
- Carcinoma

Key pathophysiologic changes in pleural effusion

- Dyspnea
- Pleuritic chest pain
- Fever and malaise

Key diagnostic test results for pleural effusion

- Chest X-ray: Radiopaque fluid in dependent regions
- Thoracentesis: Fluid amylase levels higher than serum levels (if effusion results from esophageal rupture or pancreatitis); presence of acute inflammatory WBCs and microorganisms

Key treatments for pleural effusion

- Thoracentesis
- Chest tube insertion
- Antibiotics
- Oxygen therapy

Key nursing considerations for pleural effusion

- Instruct patient on all procedures ordered to decrease pleural fluid.
- Provide meticulous chest tube care, as needed.
- Closely assess respiratory status and hemodynamic parameters.
- During thoracentesis, monitor closely for complications.

- – Lung abscesses
- – Perforation or esophageal rupture
- – Pneumonitis

● **Pathophysiologic changes**
- Dyspnea due to decreased oxygenation
- Pleuritic chest pain resulting from pleural effusions
- Fever and malaise due to infection

● **Complications**
- Impaired ventilation
- Pericarditis
- Pleurisy
- Septicemia

● **Diagnostic test findings**
- Chest X-ray shows radiopaque fluid in dependent regions
- Thoracentesis, the most useful test, analyses aspirated pleural fluid
  - – If a pleural effusion results from esophageal rupture or pancreatitis, fluid amylase levels are usually higher than the serum levels
  - – Acute inflammatory WBCs and microorganisms are present
- Tuberculin skin test may be positive for TB
- Computed tomography (CT) scanning of the thorax shows small pleural effusions

● **Treatment**
- Thoracentesis to remove fluid, or careful monitoring of the patient's own re-absorption of the fluid
- Chest tube insertion to drain the fluid or to inject a sclerosing agent, such as talc, through the tube to cause adhesions between the parietal and visceral pleura, thereby obliterating the potential space for fluid to recollect
- Decortication (surgical removal of the thick coating over the lung) or rib resection to allow drainage and lung expansion
- Parenteral antibiotics to treat empyema
- Oxygen administration to treat associated hypoxia

● **Nursing considerations**
- Explain thoracentesis to the patient
  - – Instruct the patient to inform the nurse immediately if he feels uncomfortable or has trouble breathing during the procedure
- Carefully monitor the patient during thoracentesis
  - – Monitor vital signs and watch for syncope during the procedure
  - – Monitor the patient for bradycardia, hypotension, pain, pulmonary edema, pneumothorax, and cardiac arrest (may occur if fluid is removed too quickly)
- Encourage the patient to perform deep-breathing exercises to promote lung expansion
  - – Use an incentive spirometer to promote deep breathing
- Provide meticulous chest tube care
  - – In patients with empyema, use aseptic technique for changing dressings around the tube insertion site
  - – Ensure tube patency by watching for fluctuations of fluid in the underwater-seal chamber

– Watch for bubbling in the water-seal chamber
– Record the amount, color, and consistency of tube drainage
- If the patient has open drainage through a rib resection or intercostal tube, use hand and dressing precautions

PNEUMONIA

● Definition
- Acute inflammation of the alveoli and bronchioles
- Sixth-leading cause of death in the United States
- Classified by microbiologic source (bacterial or viral), location (bronchopneumonia or lobular), or type (primary or secondary, typical or atypical)

● Underlying pathophysiology
- Organisms attach to and colonize in the mucus and cells of the nasopharynx (normal process)
- Host defense mechanisms fail to repel organisms from spreading into lower respiratory tract (see *Respiratory defense mechanisms,* page 84)

● Cause
- Aspiration of gastric or oropharyngeal contents
- Protozoan such as *Pneumocystis carinii*
- *Streptococcus pneumoniae* (most common bacterial source) or other bacteria, including *Mycoplasma pneumoniae* and *Legionella pneumophila*
- Viruses, including adenovirus (in young adults), chickenpox (in adults), cytomegalovirus, influenza (most common viral source), and respiratory syncytial virus (in children)

● Pathophysiologic changes
- High temperature as a by-product of phagocytosis and the inflammatory response to antigens (except in elderly patients)
- Productive cough due to increased mucus production and breakdown of alveolar surfaces
    – Initially thin, white, or clear mucus
    – In severe cases, progresses to thick, rust-colored or yellow-green mucus
- Dyspnea and tachypnea related to decreased lung capacity and oxygen saturation
- Crackles, decreased breath sounds, and pleuritic pain resulting from increased fluid in the alveoli and segmental spaces of the lung

● Complications
- Septicemia
- Death

● Diagnostic test findings
- Chest X-ray confirms presence of infiltrates
- Sputum culture and sensitivity testing diagnose the specific organism involve and help determine which drugs will be effective
- WBC count varies depending on the type of pneumonia
    – Elevated in most bacterial sources of infection
    – Normal or low in viral and mycoplasmal pneumonia

Key facts about pneumonia

- Acute inflammation of alveoli and bronchioles
- Infective organisms overwhelm host defenses and spread to lower respiratory tract

Key pathophysiologic changes in pneumonia

- High temperature
- Productive cough
- Decreased breath sounds
- Crackles

Key diagnostic test results for pneumonia

- Chest X-ray: Presence of infiltrates
- Sputum culture and sensitivity testing: Identifies organism involved

---

Respiratory defense mechanisms

MECHANISM	ACTION
Nasopharyngeal defenses	Remove particles from the air; activate surface lysosomes and immunoglobulin A to protect against infection
Glottic and cough reflexes	Prevent aspiration into trachea and bronchi
Mucociliary blanket	Moves secretions, microorganisms, and particles out of the respiratory tract
Pulmonary macrophages	Move microorganisms and foreign particles out of the alveoli

---

- ABG analysis varies depending on the severity of pneumonia and underlying lung diseases
- Pulse oximetry may show a reduced SaO_2 level
- Bronchoscopy or transtracheal aspiration collects material for culture when the patient is unable to cough up a specimen
- Blood cultures may show bacteremia and identify the causative agent

● **Treatment**
- Antibiotics
  - Penicillins and cephalosporins as first choice
  - If bacteria are resistant, clindamycin (Cleocin) or an aminoglycoside, such as gentamicin (Garamycin) or tobramycin (Nebcin)
- Supportive care for viral episodes
  - Acyclovir (Zovirax) I.V. if origin is chickenpox
  - Other antivirals if the patient is immunosuppressed
- Oxygen therapy, if warranted by ABG values or pulse oximetry
- Mucolytics to break up secretions

● **Nursing considerations**
- Encourage fluid intake of 2 qt (2 L)/day to keep secretions thin and the body hydrated
- Monitor temperature, and report recurrences of temperature of 102° F (38.9° C) or greater
- Assist with oxygen therapy and monitoring to maintain SaO_2 of 96% or greater
- Teach the patient and his family about the disease's effects and treatments, and associated precautions
- Instruct the patient and his family about effects of drug treatment and the need to take all doses prescribed
- Instruct the patient to balance rest and activity as his condition improves to prevent relapse of fatigue and malaise

Key treatments for pneumonia

- Antibiotics (if bacterial origin)
- Oxygen therapy
- Mucolytics

Key nursing considerations for pneumonia

- Encourage fluid intake of 2 qt (2 L)/day to keep secretions thin and the body hydrated.
- Teach patient about the disease process and its complications and treatment.
- Instruct patient to balance rest and activity.

PNEUMOTHORAX

● **Definition**
- Accumulation of air or gas in the pleural cavity
- Leads to partial or complete lung collapse
- Has three common types
  - Open
  - Closed
  - Tension

● **Underlying pathophysiology**
- Air accumulates and separates the visceral and parietal pleurae
- Negative pressure is destroyed, and the elastic recoil forces are affected
- The lung recoils by collapsing toward the hilus
- Open pneumothorax
  - Atmospheric air flows directly into the pleural cavity
  - The lung on the affected side collapses
- Closed pneumothorax
  - Air enters the pleural space from within the lung
  - Pleural pressure increases, which prevents lung expansion during normal inspiration
- Tension pneumothorax
  - Air in the pleural space is under higher pressure than air in the adjacent lung
  - Air enters the pleural space from a pleural rupture only on inspiration
  - This air pressure exceeds barometric pressure, causing compression atelectasis
  - Increased pressure may displace the heart and great vessels and cause mediastinal shift (see *Understanding tension pneumothorax,* page 86)

● **Causes**
- Open pneumothorax
  - Chest surgery
  - Insertion of a central venous catheter
  - Penetrating chest injury (gunshot or stab wound)
  - Thoracentesis or closed pleural biopsy
  - Transbronchial biopsy
- Closed pneumothorax
  - Air leakage from ruptured blebs
  - Blunt chest trauma
  - Interstitial lung disease, such as eosinophilic granuloma
  - Rupture resulting from barotrauma caused by high intrathoracic pressures during mechanical ventilation
  - Tubercular or cancerous lesions that erode into the pleural space
- Tension pneumothorax
  - Chest tube occlusion or malfunction
  - Fractured ribs
  - High-level PEEP that causes alveolar blebs to rupture
  - Mechanical ventilation
  - Penetrating chest wound treated with an airtight dressing

Key facts about pneumothorax
- Accumulation of air or gas in pleural cavity

Open
- Results when atmospheric air flows directly into pleural cavity, causing lung on affected side to collapse

Closed
- Occurs when air enters from within lung
- Increases pleural pressure, which prevents lung expansion during inspiration

Tension
- Results from pleural rupture
- Causes air to enter only on inspiration
- Increases air pressure, causing compression atelectasis
- May displace heart and great vessels and cause mediastinal shift

Common causes of pneumothorax
- Chest surgery or penetrating injury
- Emphyseal bleb rupture
- Barotrauma during mechanical ventilation
- Chest tube occlusion
- Fractured ribs
- PEEP

Understanding tension pneumothorax

In tension pneumothorax, air accumulates intrapleurally and can't escape. As intrapleural pressure increases, the ipsilateral lung is affected and also collapses.

On inspiration, the mediastinum shifts toward the unaffected lung, impairing ventilation.

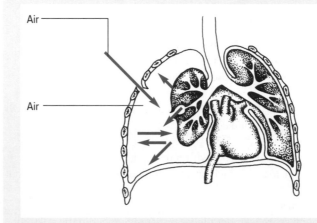

On expiration, the mediastinal shift distorts the vena cava and reduces venous return.

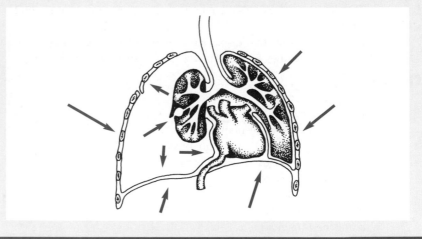

Key pathophysiologic changes in pneumothorax

Open or closed
- Sudden, sharp pleuritic pain
- Asymmetrical chest wall movement
- Absent breath sounds on affected side

Tension
- Hypotension
- Dyspnea
- Anxiety
- Mediastinal shift

Pathophysiologic changes
- Open or closed pneumothorax
  - Sudden, sharp pleuritic pain; asymmetrical chest wall movement; respiratory distress; decreased vocal fremitus; and absent breath sounds on the affected side due to lung collapse
  - Shortness of breath, cyanosis, and tachycardia due to hypoxia
  - Chest rigidity on the affected side due to decreased lung expansion
  - Crackling beneath the skin on palpation (subcutaneous emphysema) due to air leaking into the tissues

- Tension pneumothorax
  - Hypotension; compensatory tachycardia; pallor; and a weak, rapid pulse due to decreased cardiac output from severe hypoxemia
  - Tachypnea, dyspnea, and anxiety due to hypoxia
  - Mediastinal shift due to increasing tension
  - Tracheal deviation to the opposite side resulting from mediastinal shift

● Complications
- Bradycardia
- Cardiac arrest
- Decreased cardiac output
- Hypoxemia
- Shock

● Diagnostic test findings
- Chest X-rays confirm the diagnosis by revealing air in the pleural space and, possibly, a mediastinal shift
- ABG analysis may reveal hypoxemia, possibly with respiratory acidosis and hypercapnia

● Treatment
- Closed pneumothorax with less than 30% lung collapse
  - Bed rest to conserve energy and reduce oxygenation demands
  - Monitoring of blood pressure and pulse for early detection of physiologic compromise
  - Monitoring of respiratory rate to detect early signs of respiratory compromise
  - Oxygen administration to enhance oxygenation and improve hypoxia
  - Aspiration of air with a large-bore needle attached to a syringe to restore negative pressure within the pleural space
- Closed pneumothorax with more than 30% lung collapse
  - Thoracostomy tube connected to underwater-seal and low-pressure suction to try to reexpand the lung by restoring negative intrapleural pressure
  - Possible thoracotomy and pleurectomy for recurrent spontaneous pneumothorax, which causes the lung to adhere to the parietal pleura
- Open pneumothorax
  - Chest tube drainage to reexpand the lung
  - Surgical repair of the lung
- Tension pneumothorax
  - Immediate insertion of a large-bore needle into the pleural space through the second intercostal space to reexpand the lung
  - Insertion of a thoracostomy tube
  - Analgesics to promote comfort and encourage deep breathing and coughing

● Nursing considerations
- Monitor vital signs at least every hour
  - Watch for indications of shock, increasing respiratory distress, or mediastinal shift
  - Watch for falling blood pressure and rising pulse and respiratory rates, which may indicate tension pneumothorax
- Urge the patient to control coughing and gasping during thoracotomy

---

Key diagnostic test results for pneumothorax

- Chest X-rays: Air in pleural space and, possibly, mediastinal shift

Key treatments for pneumothorax

Closed (less than 30% lung collapse)
- Bed rest
- Oxygen therapy
- Aspiration of air

Closed (more than 30% lung collapse)
- Thoracostomy tube

Open
- Chest tube drainage
- Surgical repair of lung

Tension
- Immediate insertion of large-bore needle into pleural space
- Thoracostomy tube

Key nursing considerations for pneumothorax

- Closely monitor breath sounds and vital signs for signs of shock and tension pneumothorax.
- Watch for continuing air leakage from the chest tube.
- Cover dislodged tube site with petroleum gauze.

- After the chest tube is in place, encourage the patient to cough and breathe deeply (at least once per hour) to facilitate lung expansion
- Watch for continuing air leakage (bubbling) from the chest tube, indicating the lung defect has failed to close; this defect may require surgery
- Watch for increasing subcutaneous emphysema by checking around the neck or at the tube insertion site for crackling beneath the skin
- If the patient is on a ventilator, watch for difficulty breathing in time with the ventilator as well as pressure changes on ventilator gauges
- Change dressings around the chest tube insertion site, as necessary
  – Be careful not to reposition or dislodge the tube
  – If the tube dislodges, immediately place petroleum gauze dressing over the opening to prevent rapid lung collapse

PULMONARY EDEMA

- **Definition**
  - Accumulation of fluid in the extravascular spaces of the lungs
  - Common complication of cardiac disorders
  - May be acute or chronic

- **Underlying pathophysiology**
  - Normally, pulmonary capillary hydrostatic pressure and colloid osmotic pressure are balanced
  - Pulmonary edema results from either increased pulmonary capillary hydrostatic pressure or decreased colloid osmotic pressure (see *Understanding pulmonary edema*)
  - If pulmonary capillary hydrostatic pressure increases, several consequences ensue
    – The compromised left ventricle needs higher filling pressures to maintain adequate output
    – These pressures are transmitted to the left atrium, pulmonary veins, and pulmonary capillary bed
    – Fluids and solutes are forced from the intravascular compartment into the lung interstitium
    – With fluid overloading the lung interstitium, some fluid floods peripheral alveoli and impairs gas exchange
  - If colloid osmotic pressure decreases, the following consequences occur
    – The pulling force that contains intravascular fluid is lost, and nothing opposes the hydrostatic forces
    – Fluid flows freely into the interstitium and alveoli, causing pulmonary edema

- **Causes**
  - ARDS
  - Arrhythmias
  - Barbiturate or opioid poisoning
  - Diastolic dysfunction
  - Excess infusion or overly rapid infusion of I.V. fluids
  - Inhalation of irritating gases
  - Left-sided heart failure
  - Mitral stenosis and left atrial myxoma (which impairs left atrial emptying)

Key facts about pulmonary edema

- Involves accumulation of fluid in the extravascular spaces of the lungs
- Results from increased pulmonary capillary hydrostatic pressure or decreased colloid osmotic pressure

Common causes of pulmonary edema

- Left-sided heart failure
- Valvular heart disease
- ARDS

Understanding pulmonary edema

In pulmonary edema, diminished function of the left ventricle causes blood to back up into pulmonary veins and capillaries. The increasing capillary hydrostatic pressure pushes fluid into the interstitial spaces and alveoli. These illustrations show a normal alveolus and an alveolus affected by pulmonary edema.

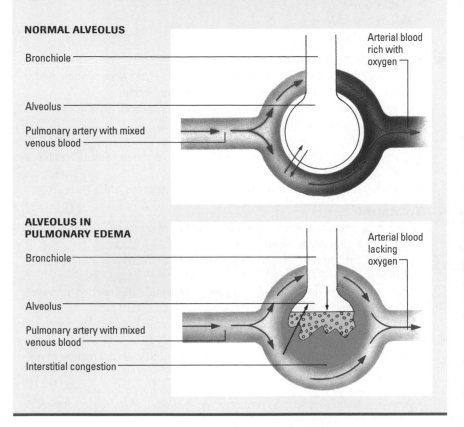

NORMAL ALVEOLUS

Bronchiole

Alveolus

Pulmonary artery with mixed venous blood

Arterial blood rich with oxygen

ALVEOLUS IN PULMONARY EDEMA

Bronchiole

Alveolus

Pulmonary artery with mixed venous blood

Interstitial congestion

Arterial blood lacking oxygen

- Pneumonia
- Valvular heart disease

● Pathophysiologic changes
- Early stages
  - Dyspnea on exertion, mild tachypnea, cough, and tachycardia due to hypoxia
  - Orthopnea due to decreased ability of the diaphragm to expand
  - Increased blood pressure due to increased pulmonary pressures and decreased oxygenation
  - Dependent crackles as air moves through fluid in the lungs
  - Jugular vein distention due to decreased cardiac output and increased pulmonary vascular resistance
- Later stages
  - Labored, rapid respirations; increased tachycardia; cyanosis; and arrhythmias due to hypoxia

Key pathophysiologic changes in pulmonary edema

Early stages
- Dyspnea on exertion
- Orthopnea
- Dependent crackles

Later stages
- Labored, rapid respirations
- Tachycardia
- Cough producing frothy, bloody sputum
- Diaphoresis

Key diagnostic test results for pulmonary edema

- ABG analysis: Hypoxia with variable $PaCO_2$, possible respiratory acidosis
- Chest X-rays: Diffuse haziness of lung fields, cardiomegaly, pleural effusion
- Pulse oximetry: Decreased SaO_2 levels

Key treatments for pulmonary edema

- Oxygen administration
- Assisted ventilation
- Diuretics
- Inotropic agents
- Morphine

Key nursing considerations for pulmonary edema

- Closely assess respiratory status and hemodynamic parameters for deterioration.
- Administer medications as ordered.
- Monitor ABG levels and intake and output.
- Watch for peripheral edema.

- More diffuse crackles and cough producing frothy, bloody sputum as air moves through fluid in the lungs
- Cold, clammy skin due to peripheral vasoconstriction
- Diaphoresis, decreased blood pressure, and a thready pulse due to decreased cardiac output and shock

● Complications
- Cardiac arrest
- Respiratory acidosis
- Respiratory failure

● Diagnostic test findings
- ABG analysis usually reveals hypoxia with variable $PaCO_2$, depending on the patient's degree of fatigue; respiratory acidosis may occur
- Chest X-rays show diffuse haziness of the lung fields and, usually, cardiomegaly and pleural effusion
- Pulse oximetry may reveal decreasing SaO_2 levels
- Pulmonary artery catheterization identifies left-sided heart failure and helps rule out ARDS
- ECG may show previous or current myocardial infarction (MI)

● Treatment
- High concentrations of oxygen administered by nasal cannula to enhance gas exchange and improve oxygenation
- Assisted ventilation to improve oxygen delivery to the tissues and promote acid-base balance
- Diuretics, such as furosemide (Lasix) and bumetanide (Bumex), to increase urination, which helps mobilize extravascular fluid
- Positive inotropic agents, such as digoxin and inamrinone, to enhance contractility in myocardial dysfunction
- Pressor agents to enhance contractility and promote vasoconstriction in peripheral vessels
- Antiarrhythmics for arrhythmias related to decreased cardiac output
- Arterial vasodilators, such as nitroprusside (Nipride), to decrease peripheral vascular resistance, preload, and afterload
- Morphine (Avinza, MSIR, Roxanol) to reduce anxiety and dyspnea and to dilate the systemic venous bed, promoting blood flow from pulmonary circulation to the periphery

● Nursing considerations
- Monitor the patient for early signs of pulmonary edema, especially tachypnea, tachycardia, and abnormal breath sounds
- Check for peripheral edema, which may indicate that fluid is accumulating in pulmonary tissue
- Administer oxygen as ordered
- Administer nitroprusside as ordered
  - Monitor vital signs every 15 to 30 minutes
  - Protect the nitroprusside solution from light by wrapping the bottle or bag with aluminum foil
  - Discard unused solution after 4 hours
- Watch for arrhythmias in the patient receiving cardiac glycosides
- Watch for marked respiratory depression in the patient receiving morphine

- Monitor ABG levels, oral and I.V. fluid intake, urine output and, in the patient with a pulmonary artery catheter, pulmonary end-diastolic pressure, and PAWP
- Check cardiac monitoring frequently and report changes immediately

PULMONARY EMBOLISM

- ● **Definition**
  - Obstruction of the pulmonary arterial bed by a dislodged thrombus, heart valve growths, or a foreign substance
  - Most common pulmonary complication in hospitalized patients
  - Massive emboli may be fatal

- ● **Underlying pathophysiology**
  - Thrombus formation results directly from vascular wall damage, venostasis, or hypercoagulability of the blood
  - Trauma, clot dissolution, sudden muscle spasm, intravascular pressure changes, or a change in peripheral blood flow can cause the thrombus to loosen or fragment
  - The thrombus, now called an *embolus,* floats to the heart's right side and enters the lung through the pulmonary artery
  - The embolus may dissolve, continue to fragment, or grow
  - By occluding the pulmonary artery, the embolus prevents alveoli from producing enough surfactant to maintain alveolar integrity
  - Alveoli collapse and atelectasis develops
  - If the embolus enlarges, it may clog most or all of the pulmonary vessels and cause death

- ● **Causes**
  - Atrial fibrillation
  - Deep vein thrombosis (pelvic, renal, hepatic, great saphenous vein thrombosis), venous stasis, upper extremity thrombosis
  - Hypercoagulable states, congenital or acquired
  - Valvular heart disease
  - Right heart thrombus

- ● **Pathophysiologic changes**
  - Tachypnea, tachycardia, dyspnea, rales, signs of circulatory collapse (weak, thready pulse and hypotension), and respiratory alkalosis resulting from hypoxemia
  - Low-grade fever due to the inflammatory process
  - With a massive embolism, hemoptysis, cyanosis, syncope, and distended jugular veins caused by vasoconstriction and right-sided heart failure

- ● **Complications**
  - Pulmonary infarction
  - Acute respiratory failure
  - Death
  - Acute cor pulmonale

- ● **Diagnostic test findings**
  - Chest X-ray has two purposes
    - It helps rule out other pulmonary diseases

Key facts about pulmonary embolism

- Obstruction of pulmonary arterial bed by dislodged thrombus, heart valve growths, or foreign substance
- Prevents alveoli from producing enough surfactant to maintain alveolar integrity
- Leads to alveoli collapse and atelectasis

TOP 2

Causes of pulmonary embolism

1. Deep vein thrombosis
2. Hypercoagulable states

Key pathophysiologic changes in pulmonary embolism

- Tachypnea
- Tachycardia
- Rales
- Fever

– It can reveal various conditions
  · Areas of atelectasis
  · Elevated diaphragm and pleural effusion
  · Prominent pulmonary artery
  · Occasionally, the characteristic wedge-shaped infiltrate suggestive of pulmonary infarction, or focal oligemia of blood vessels
- Lung scan shows perfusion defects in areas beyond occluded vessels
- Pulmonary angiography is the most definitive test for showing location of emboli
- ECG is inconclusive but helps distinguish pulmonary embolism from MI
- ABG measurements usually show decreased PaO_2 and $PaCO_2$ but these changes don't always occur
- Thoracentesis may rule out pneumonia by detecting whether empyema, an indicator of pneumonia, is present

Treatment
- Oxygen therapy, as needed
- Anticoagulation therapy with heparin (Heparin Sodium Injection) to inhibit new thrombus formation
- Fibrinolytic therapy with urokinase (AbboKinase), streptokinase (Streptase), or alteplase (Activase) to enhance fibrinolysis of the pulmonary emboli and remaining thrombi
- Vasopressors to treat hypotension
- If the patient has septic emboli, administration of antibiotics and evaluation for the infection's source, particularly endocarditis
- Vena cava ligation, plication, or insertion of an umbrella filter to filter blood returning to the heart and lungs

Nursing considerations
- Give oxygen by nasal cannula or mask
- Check ABG levels if the patient develops fresh emboli or worsening dyspnea
- Be prepared to assist with ET intubation with assisted ventilation if breathing is severely compromised
- Monitor coagulation studies daily
  – Effective heparin therapy raises the partial thromboplastin time to more than two times normal
  – Watch closely for signs of abnormal bleeding
- Tell the patient to prevent bleeding by shaving with an electric razor and by brushing his teeth with a soft toothbrush
- After the patient is stable, encourage him to move about frequently, and assist with isometric and range-of-motion exercises
- Check pedal pulses, temperature, and color of the patient's feet to detect venostasis
- Maintain adequate nutrition and fluid balance to promote healing
- Report frequent pleuritic chest pain so that analgesics can be prescribed
- Warn the patient not to cross his legs or sit with his legs in a dependent position for prolonged periods; doing so promotes thrombus formation
- Explain to the patient that an oral anticoagulant (warfarin [Coumadin]) will be taken for 3 to 6 months after a pulmonary embolism
- Advise the patient to watch for signs of bleeding

Key diagnostic test results for pulmonary embolism
- Lung scan: Perfusion defects in areas beyond occluded vessels
- Pulmonary angiography: Presence of emboli in specific areas

Key treatments for pulmonary embolism
- Oxygen therapy
- Anticoagulation therapy
- Fibrinolytic therapy

Key nursing considerations for pulmonary embolism
- Assist with intubation and assisted ventilation.
- Observe for abnormal bleeding during anticoagulant use.
- Instruct patient in long-term use of anticoagulants, safety precautions required, and required follow-up blood testing.
- Monitor for venostasis and assess pain control.

- Tell the patient to take the prescribed medication exactly as ordered, and to avoid taking additional medication (even for headaches or colds)
- Stress the importance of follow-up laboratory tests (prothrombin time) to monitor anticoagulant therapy

PULMONARY HYPERTENSION

Definition
- PAP rises above normal for reasons other than aging or altitude
  - Normal PAP: 15 to 18 mm Hg
  - Pulmonary hypertension: Mean PAP of 25 mm Hg or more
- *Primary,* or idiopathic, pulmonary hypertension
  - Characterized by increased PAP and increased pulmonary vascular resistance
  - Most common in women ages 20 to 40
  - Usually fatal within 3 to 4 years
- *Secondary* pulmonary hypertension
  - Results from existing cardiac or pulmonary disease, or both

Underlying pathophysiology
- Primary pulmonary hypertension
  - The intimal lining of the pulmonary arteries thickens for no apparent reason
  - This thickening narrows the artery and impairs distensibility, increasing vascular resistance
- Secondary pulmonary hypertension
  - Hypoxemia results from conditions involving alveolar hypoventilation, vascular obstruction, or left-to-right shunting

Causes
- Primary pulmonary hypertension
  - Unknown
  - Altered immune mechanisms
  - Hereditary factors
- Secondary pulmonary hypertension
  - Cardiovascular conditions, such as atrial septal defect, heart failure, left atrial myxoma, mitral valve disease, patent ductus arteriosus, vasculitis, and ventricular septal defect
  - Other respiratory, conditions such as COPD, diffuse interstitial pneumonia, hypoxemia, kyphoscoliosis, pulmonary embolism, and sarcoidosis
  - Malignant metastases
  - Obesity
  - Scleroderma and other connective tissue disorders
  - HIV infection
  - Anorexic drug abuse (cocaine, amphetamines)

Pathophysiologic changes
- Increasing dyspnea on exertion, difficulty breathing, shortness of breath, restlessness, agitation, decreased level of consciousness (LOC), and memory loss from left-sided heart failure
- Fatigue, weakness, and syncope from diminished tissue oxygenation
- Pain with breathing due to lactic acid buildup in the tissues

Key facts about pulmonary hypertension

Primary
- Characterized by increased PAP and increased pulmonary vascular resistance resulting from thickening of intimal lining of pulmonary arteries

Secondary
- Results from existing cardiac or pulmonary disease or both

Common causes of pulmonary hypertension

Primary
- Unknown

Secondary
- Congenital heart defects
- Other cardiopulmonary disorders
- Connective tissue disorders

Key pathophysiologic changes in pulmonary hypertension
- Increased dyspnea on exertion
- Weakness
- Fatigue
- Systolic ejection murmur
- Syncope with exertion

- Ascites, jugular vein distention, and peripheral edema due to right ventricular failure
- Decreased diaphragmatic excursion and respiration because of hypoventilation
- Easily palpable right ventricular lift, systolic ejection murmur, and split S_2, S_3, and S_4 due to pulmonary hypertension and altered cardiac output
- Possible displacement of point of maximal impulse beyond the midclavicular line; decreased breath sounds; and loud, tubular breath sounds because of fluid accumulation in the lungs

● **Complications**
- Cardiac arrest
- Heart failure
- Cor pulmonale

● **Diagnostic test findings**
- ABG analysis reveals hypoxemia if severe
- ECG in patients with right ventricular hypertrophy shows right axis deviation and tall or peaked P waves in inferior leads
- Right-heart catheterization reveals pulmonary systolic pressure above 30 mm Hg
  - It may also show an increased PAWP if the underlying cause is left atrial myxoma, mitral stenosis, or left-sided heart failure; otherwise, PAWP is normal
- Pulmonary angiography detects filling defects in pulmonary vasculature such as those that develop with pulmonary emboli
- Pulmonary function studies vary depending on the type of underlying disease
  - Flow rates may be decreased and residual volume may be increased in underlying obstructive disease
  - Total lung capacity may be reduced in underlying restrictive disease
- Radionuclide imaging detects abnormalities in right and left ventricular functioning
- Open lung biopsy may determine the underlying disorder or cause
- Echocardiography can provide several findings
  - It helps estimate pulmonary systolic pressure
  - It helps assess for ventricular wall motion and possible valvular dysfunction
  - It can demonstrate right ventricular enlargement, abnormal septal configuration consistent with right ventricular pressure overload, and reduction in left ventricular cavity size
- Perfusion lung scanning may produce normal or abnormal results, showing multiple patchy and diffuse filling defects that don't suggest pulmonary embolism

● **Treatment**
- Oxygen therapy to correct hypoxemia and resulting increased pulmonary vascular resistance unless patient has a patent formen ovale that provides left-to-right shunting
- Fluid restriction in right-sided heart failure to decrease the heart's workload
- Digoxin to increase cardiac output
- Diuretics to decrease intravascular volume and extravascular fluid accumulation
- Vasodilators to reduce myocardial workload and oxygen consumption
- Calcium channel blockers to reduce myocardial workload and decrease pulmonary vascular resistance
- Bronchodilators to relax smooth muscles and increase airway patency

Key diagnostic test results for pulmonary hypertension

- Right-heart catheterization: Pulmonary systolic pressure above 30 mm Hg
- Echocardiography: Estimated pulmonary systolic pressure and right and left ventricular function

Key treatments for pulmonary hypertension

- Fluid restriction
- Diuretics
- Digoxin
- Anticoagulants
- Vasodilators
- Calcium channel blockers
- Bronchodilators
- Beta-adrenergic blockers

- Beta-adrenergic blockers to improve oxygenation
- Treatment of the underlying cause to correct pulmonary edema
- Heart-lung transplant in severe cases
- Anticoagulant to reduce the risk of thrombus formation in lungs

Nursing considerations
- Administer oxygen therapy as ordered
  - Observe the patient's response
  - Report signs of increasing dyspnea to the physician
- Monitor ABG levels for acidosis and hypoxemia
  - Report changes in LOC immediately
- Record weight daily and carefully measure intake and output
- Check for worsening jugular vein distention, which may indicate fluid overload
- Monitor vital signs, especially blood pressure and heart rate
  - Watch for hypotension and tachycardia
  - If the patient has a pulmonary artery catheter, check PAP and PAWP, as ordered, and report changes
- Before discharge, help the patient adjust to the limitations imposed by this disorder
  - Advise against overexertion and isometric exercise
  - Suggest frequent rest periods between activities
- Explain all medications and diet restrictions to the patient

SEVERE ACUTE RESPIRATORY SYNDROME

Definition
- Life-threatening viral infection
- Also called SARS
- Incubates for a period estimated to range from 2 to 7 days (average 3 to 5 days)
- Not highly contagious when protective measures are used

Underlying pathophysiology
- Coronaviruses cause diseases in pigs, birds, and other animals
- A theory suggests that coronavirus may have mutated, allowing transmission to and infection of humans

Cause
- Transmission of new type of coronavirus known as *SARS-associated coronavirus* (SARS-CoV)
- Risk factors
  - Close contact with an infected person
  - Contact with aerosolized (exhaled) droplets and bodily secretions from infected person
  - Travel to endemic areas

Pathophysiologic changes
- Nonproductive cough, rash, high fever, headache, general discomfort and body aches, and pneumonia due to infectious process
- Shortness of breath and respiratory distress (in later stages) resulting from decreased oxygenation

Key diagnostic test results for SARS

- Serum electrophoresis: Antibodies to coronavirus present
- Gram stain and culture of sputum: Coronavirus present
- SARS-specific polymerase chain reaction test: SARS-CoV RNA present

Key treatments for SARS

- Isolation
- Mechanical ventilation (if severe)
- Antivirals
- Steroids
- Antimicrobials

Key nursing considerations for SARS

- Maintain isolation for patient, as recommended.
- Maintain a patent airway through suctioning if mechanical ventilation is required.
- Monitor vital signs, nutritional status, and respiratory status.

Key facts about TB

- Lung infection characterized by pulmonary infiltrates and formation of granulomas with caseation, fibrosis, and cavitation
- Develops when the bacillus *Mycobacterium tuberculosis* stimulates an inflammatory process followed by a cell-mediated immune response
- Results in formation of granulomas around bacilli
- May lead to active disease in 5% to 15% of those infected
- Is transmitted by airborne droplets

● **Complications**
- Death
- Respiratory difficulties
- Severe thrombocytopenia

● **Diagnostic test findings**
- Serum electrophoresis detects antibodies to coronavirus
- Gram stain and culture of sputum isolate coronavirus
- Platelet count may be low
- Chest X-ray changes (infiltrates) may indicate pneumonia
- SARS-specific polymerase chain reaction test detects SARS-CoV Ribonucleic acid (RNA)

● **Treatment**
- Isolation (for hospitalized patients) to prevent spread of disease
- Strict respiratory and mucosal barrier precautions to prevent spread of the disease
- Quarantine (of exposed individuals) to prevent spread of the disease
- Mechanical ventilation (for severe cases) to treat respiratory failure
- Diet (as tolerated) to provide adequate nutrition
- Global surveillance and reporting of suspected cases to national health authorities to monitor spread of disease
- Antivirals to treat viral infection
- Combination of steroids and antimicrobials to treat inflammation and infection

● **Nursing considerations**
- Maintain isolation for the patient, as recommended
- Practice good hygiene to prevent further transmission
- **Maintain a patent airway through suctioning if mechanical ventilation is required**
- Encourage adequate nutritional intake
- Monitor vital signs, nutritional status, and respiratory status

TUBERCULOSIS

● **Definition**
- Lung infection characterized by pulmonary infiltrates and formation of granulomas with caseation, fibrosis, and cavitation
- May be acute or chronic
- Excellent prognosis with proper treatment and compliance
- Also known as TB

● **Underlying pathophysiology**
- Multiplication of the bacillus *Mycobacterium tuberculosis* causes an inflammatory process
- Cell-mediated immune response follows, usually containing the infection within 4 to 6 weeks
- T-cell response results in the formation of granulomas around the bacilli
  - Bacilli become dormant
  - Immunity to subsequent infection develops

- Bacilli within granulomas may remain viable for many years, indicated by a positive purified protein derivative or other skin test for TB
- Active disease develops in 5% to 15% of those infected
- Transmission occurs in airborne droplets when an infected person coughs or sneezes

Causes
- Exposure to *Mycobacterium tuberculosis*
- Sometimes, exposure to other strains of mycobacterium

Pathophysiologic changes
- Low-grade fever and night sweats; malaise, anorexia and weight loss; adenopathy; productive cough (lasting longer than 3 weeks); hemoptysis, and pleuritic chest pain resulting from inflammatory and immune process

Complications
- Massive pulmonary tissue damage
- Respiratory failure
- Bronchopleural fistulas
- Pneumothorax
- Pleural effusion
- Pneumonia
- Infection of other body organs by small mycobacterium foci
- Liver involvement secondary to drug therapy

Diagnostic test findings
- Tuberculin skin test is positive in active and inactive TB
- Stains and cultures of sputum, cerebrospinal fluid, urine, abscess drainage, or pleural fluid show heat-sensitive, nonmotile, aerobic, acid-fast bacilli
- Chest X-rays show nodular lesions, patchy infiltrates, cavity formation, scar tissue, and calcium deposits
- CT scanning or MRI shows presence and extent of lung damage
- Bronchoscopy shows heat-sensitive, nonmotile, acid-fast bacilli in specimens

Treatment
- Antitubercular drug therapy to treat infection
  - Combination therapy with two or three drugs (rifampin [Rifadin, Rimactane], rifapentine [Priftin], pyrazinamide, ethambutol [Myambutol], streptomycin [Seromycin], or isoniazid [INH, Nydrazid]) taken orally for at least 6 months to treat initial pulmonary infections
  - Drug therapy for 12 months for extrapulmonary infections
  - Drug therapy for up to 2 years for multidrug-resistant pulmonary infections
- Resumption of normal activities (after 2 to 4 weeks, when disease is no longer infectious) to promote independence while taking medication
- Well-balanced, high-calorie diet to maintain or improve nutritional status

Nursing considerations
- Assess for alcohol abuse, liver disease, kidney disease, or acquired immunodeficiency syndrome because many drugs used to treat TB are contraindicated with these conditions
- Administer drug therapy and observe for adverse effects and drug interactions
- Isolate the patient in a quiet, properly ventilated room, and maintain TB precautions

---

Key pathophysiologic changes in TB
- Low-grade fever
- Night sweats
- Malaise
- Productive cough

Key diagnostic test results for TB
- Tuberculin skin test: Positive
- Chest X-rays: Nodular lesions, patchy infiltrates, cavity formation, scar tissue, and calcium deposits

Key treatments for TB
- Antitubercular drug therapy
- Well-balanced, high-calorie diet

Key nursing considerations for TB
- Administer drug therapy and observe for adverse effects and drug interactions.
- Isolate patient in a quiet, properly ventilated room, and maintain TB precautions.
- Provide well-balanced, high-calorie foods.
- Perform chest physiotherapy.

TOP 5

Items to study for your next test on the respiratory system

1. Pathophysiology of high-risk respiratory disorders, such as pneumonia, pulmonary embolism, cor pulmonale, hypertension, and SARS

2. Abnormal breath sounds associated with specific respiratory disorders

3. Common diagnostic tests for respiratory disorders, such as chest X-rays and ABG analysis

4. Significant pathophysiologic changes associated with respiratory disorders, such as dyspnea, tachypnea, and sputum production

5. Treatments, including drug therapy, for key respiratory disorders such as ARDS, asthma, COPD, and pulmonary embolism

- Properly dispose of secretions
- Provide adequate rest periods and diversional activities
- Provide well-balanced, high-calorie foods
- Provide small, frequent meals
- Perform chest physiotherapy
- Monitor vital signs, intake and output, and daily weight
- Provide patient teaching
  - Teach the patient how to perform coughing and deep-breathing exercises
  - Teach the patient about signs and symptoms of recurring TB and when to notify the physician
  - Stress the need for isolation

NCLEX CHECKS

It's never too soon to begin your licensure examination preparation. Now that you've reviewed this chapter, carefully read each of the following questions and choose the best answer. Then compare your responses to the correct answers.

1. A client with a suspected pulmonary embolus is brought to the emergency department. She complains of shortness of breath and chest pain. For which other signs and symptoms of pulmonary embolus should the nurse assess the client? Select all that apply.

☐ **1.** Low-grade fever
☐ **2.** Thick, green sputum
☐ **3.** Bradycardia
☐ **4.** Frothy sputum
☐ **5.** Tachycardia
☐ **6.** Blood-tinged sputum

2. A client is hospitalized with bilateral pleural effusions. The nurse would expect to prepare the client for which diagnostic test to determine the cause of the effusions?

☐ **1.** Thoracentesis
☐ **2.** ABG analysis
☐ **3.** Chest X-ray
☐ **4.** Bronchoscopy

3. A nurse is preparing to instuct a client in the use of antitubercular medications to treat active pulmonary tuberculosis. The nurse should teach the client that treatment will last for how long?

☐ **1.** 6 weeks
☐ **2.** 3 months
☐ **3.** 6 months
☐ **4.** 3 years

4. A client with ARDS has been intubated and placed on a ventilator. The nurse observes increased peak pressures, absent breath sounds in one lobe, and restlessness. The nurse should prepare for emergency testing and treatment for which disorder?

☐ **1.** Cardiac tamponade

☐ **2.** Pulmonary edema

☐ **3.** Heart failure

☐ **4.** Pneumothorax

5. A client is being treated for asthma. The nurse should check the Ig assay report for elevation of which Ig?

☐ **1.** IgA

☐ **2.** IgE

☐ **3.** IgG

☐ **4.** IgM

6. A nurse is caring for a client with chronic bronchitis. The nurse would expect to teach the client that which of the following treatment measures is most effective?

☐ **1.** Corticosteroids

☐ **2.** Nebulizers

☐ **3.** Avoidance of air pollutants

☐ **4.** Antibiotics

7. Which diagnostic test helps determine oxygen needs in a client with COPD?

☐ **1.** ABG analysis

☐ **2.** Chest X-ray

☐ **3.** Pulmonary function studies

☐ **4.** Serum hemoglobin level and hematocrit

8. Pulmonary hypertension is characterized by increased PAP. The mean PAP is usually greater than:

☐ **1.** 15 mm Hg.

☐ **2.** 25 mm Hg.

☐ **3.** 30 mm Hg.

☐ **4.** 35 mm Hg.

9. A nurse is teaching the family of a client with SARS. The family demonstrates understanding of the teaching instructions by stating that the incubation period for SARS is:

☐ **1.** 1 to 3 days.

☐ **2.** 2 to 7 days.

☐ **3.** 5 to 10 days.

☐ **4.** 1 to 3 weeks.

10. A nurse is preparing a staff education program on emphysema. The nurses will be expected to know that the pathophysiologic changes that accompany emphysema include barrel-shaped chest, tachypnea, crackles on inspiration, and:

☐ **1.** peripheral edema.

☐ **2.** decreased tactile fremitus.

☐ **3.** distended jugular veins.

☐ **4.** thick, yellow or green mucus.

ANSWERS AND RATIONALES

1. CORRECT ANSWER: 1, 5, 6

A patient with a pulmonary embolus may present with pleuritic chest pain, dyspnea, low-grade fever, tachycardia, and blood-tinged sputum. Thick, green sputum is more likely in patients with pneumonia. Bradycardia isn't likely to occur in patients with serious respiratory disorders because decreased oxygenation triggers the pneumotaxic center in the brain to increase breathing and heart rates. Frothy sputum is a typical sign of pulmonary edema.

2. CORRECT ANSWER: 1

Thoracentesis, the analysis of aspirated pleural fluid, is the most useful test for determining the cause of pleural effusions. ABG analysis is used to determine the patient's oxygenation level. A chest X-ray may identify the presence of a pleural effusion, but it can't provide information on the source or cause. Bronchoscopy is used to take samples of lung tissue and fluids to evaluate for malignancies and other disorders, but it can't reach the site of a pleural effusion.

3. CORRECT ANSWER: 3

Daily oral doses of antitubercular therapy should continue for 6 months to treat pulmonary infections. Treatment for less than 6 months is insufficient to treat the infection and allows the body to build resistance to the drugs. The maximum time a multidrug-resistant patient would need treatment is 2 years.

4. CORRECT ANSWER: 4

Because of stiff, noncompliant lungs, patients with ARDS are at high risk for pneumothorax, which is characterized by increased peak pressures, absent breath sounds in one lobe, and restlessness. The patient with cardiac tamponade would exhibit muffled heart sounds, not a change in lung sounds in one field, and the central venous pressure would be elevated. Patients with heart failure generally exhibit diminished or adventitious breath sounds and signs of fluid retention. The patient with pulmonary edema has frothy sputum and many adventitious lung sounds.

5. CORRECT ANSWER: 2

IgE antibodies attached to histamine-containing mast cells and receptors on cell membranes initiate intrinsic asthma attacks. When exposed to an antigen such as pollen, the IgE antibody combines with the antigen. On subsequent exposure to the antigen, mast cells degranulate, release mediators, and cause bronchial constriction and edema. IgA, IgG, and IgM antibodies don't initiate intrinsic asthma attacks.

6. CORRECT ANSWER: 3

Avoiding air pollutants, such as dust and noxious gases (including cigarette smoke), is the most effective way to decrease the inflammation of the tracheobronchial tree. Corticosteroids may be administered with a nebulizer in acute exacerbations. Antibiotics are used for secondary lung or upper respiratory tract infections.

7. CORRECT ANSWER: 1

ABG analysis determines oxygen need by indicating the degree of hypoxia. Chest X-ray can show the effects of COPD in the lungs, and pulmonary function studies can reveal breathing capacity, but neither test gives an indication of the amount of oxygen needed to maintain optimum oxygen saturation while minimizing carbon dioxide retention, which ABG analysis does. Blood testing for hemoglobin level and hematocrit can reveal anemia, which may affect the results of ABG analysis.

8. CORRECT ANSWER: 2

Pulmonary hypertension is characterized by a mean PAP of 25 mm Hg or more and increased pulmonary vascular resistance. A PAP of 15 to 18 mm Hg is normal. A mean pulmonary systolic pressure greater than 30 mm Hg confirms the diagnosis.

9. CORRECT ANSWER: 2

The incubation period for SARS is estimated to be in the range of 2 to 7 days. The average incubation is 3 to 5 days.

10. CORRECT ANSWER: 2

A patient with emphysema will have decreased tactile fremitus, decreased breath sounds, a barrel-shaped chest, tachypnea, and crackles on inspiration. Peripheral edema and distended jugular veins are typically found in severe heart failure. Thick, yellow or green mucus is common with bacterial lung infections.

3

Nervous system

LEARNING OBJECTIVES

After studying this chapter, you should be able to:

● Describe conditions related to increased intracranial pressure (ICP).

● Discuss the relationship between signs and symptoms of and the pathophysiologic changes for various nervous system disorders.

● List probable causes of various nervous system disorders.

● Identify nursing interventions for patients with nervous system disorders.

● Describe treatments used to improve increased ICP.

● Identify classes of medications that may improve cerebral edema.

CHAPTER OVERVIEW

The nervous system includes the brain, spinal cord, and peripheral nerves. It receives and interprets stimuli and transmits impulses to other body systems. Because of the nervous system's role in the function of other body systems, it's essential for the nurse to have an understanding of the pathophysiologic changes involved in nervous system disorders and the signs and symptoms such changes produce.

This chapter reviews key pathophysiologic concepts related to the nervous system, and then outlines the underlying pathophysiology, causes, changes, complications, diagnostic test findings, treatment approaches, and nursing considerations associated with common nervous system disorders.

PATHOPHYSIOLOGIC CONCEPTS

● **Altered arousal**
- Can result from various factors
  - Direct destruction of the reticular formation in the brain stem as a result of direct pressure or compression caused by the expansion of other brain structures
  - Destruction of the entire brain stem, including the reticular activating system (RAS) of ascending nerves
    - Can occur directly as a result of tumor invasion, herniation, or increased ICP
    - Can occur indirectly as a result of impaired blood supply
  - Other structural, metabolic, or psychogenic disturbances affecting the RAS
- Occurs in stages
  - Begins with interruption or disruption in the diencephalon (thalamus and hypothalamus)
  - Can manifest as any of the five levels of altered consciousness
    - Confusion
    - Delirium
    - Obtundation
    - Stupor
    - Coma (see *Altered levels of consciousness,* page 104)
- Requires evaluation of five areas of neurologic function to help identify the cause
  - Level of consciousness (LOC)
  - Breathing pattern
  - Pupillary changes
  - Eye movement and reflex responses
  - Motor responses

● **Altered homeostasis**
- Failure of the brain's normal autoregulatory mechanisms
- Can result in increased ICP and cerebral edema
  - Increased ICP
    - Occurs when brain tissue, cerebrospinal fluid (CSF), and cerebral blood (intracranial components) exert pressure against the skull
    - Results in a change in volume of intracranial contents, which triggers reciprocal change in one or more intracranial components to maintain consistent pressure
    - Leads to an attempt by compensatory mechanisms to maintain homeostasis and lower ICP
    - Continues to rise when compensatory mechanisms are overwhelmed and no longer effective (see *What happens when ICP rises,* page 105)
  - Cerebral edema
    - Characterized by increase in intracellular and extracellular fluid volume
    - May result from initial injury to brain tissue
    - May develop in response to cerebral ischemia, hemorrhage, hypoxia, infarct, infection, trauma, or tumor

Key facts about altered arousal

- Results from destruction of the brain stem or its reticular formation or from other structural, metabolic, or psychogenic disturbances
- Can manifest as any of the five levels of altered consciousness

Key facts about altered homeostasis

- Failure of the brain's normal autoregulatory mechanisms
- Can result in increased ICP and cerebral edema

Levels of consciousness

- Confusion
- Delirium
- Obtundation
- Stupor
- Coma

Key facts about altered movement

- Involves neurotransmitters
- Hyperkinesia: Excessive movement
- Hypokinesia: Decreased movement

Key facts about altered muscle tone

- Hypotonia: Severely reduced degree of tension or resistance to movement in a muscle
- Hypertonia: Marked increase in muscle tension and decreased ability to stretch

Altered levels of consciousness

This chart lists the characteristics associated with the five levels of altered consciousness.

LEVEL OF CONSCIOUSNESS	CHARACTERISTICS
Confusion	• Impaired ability to think clearly • Disturbed ability to perceive, respond to, and remember current stimuli • Disorientation • Functional in activities of daily living (ADLs)
Delirium	• Motor restlessness • Increased disorientation • Transient hallucinations • Delusions possible • Requires some assistance with ADLs
Obtundation	• Decreased alertness • Psychomotor retardation • Requires complete assistance with ADLs
Stupor	• Arousable but not alert • Severe disorientation • Little or no spontaneous activity
Coma	• Unarousable • Unresponsive to external stimuli or internal needs • Determination commonly documented using Glasgow Coma Scale score

● **Altered movement**
- Involves certain neurotransmitters (such as dopamine)
- Typically characterized by excessive movement (hyperkinesia) or decreased movement (hypokinesia)
- Marked by paresis
  - Partial loss of motor function and muscle power
  - Commonly described as weakness
  - Can result from dysfunction of various structures
    · Upper motor neurons (in cerebral cortex, subcortical white matter, internal capsule, brain stem, or spinal cord)
    · Lower motor neurons (in brain stem and anterior horn of spinal cord); may also result from problems with neuronal axons of the peripheral nerves as they travel to skeletal muscle
    · Motor units affecting muscle fibers or neuromuscular junction

● **Altered muscle tone**
- Classified as two major types
  - Hypotonia (severely reduced degree of tension or resistance to movement in a muscle)
  - Hypertonia (marked increase in muscle tension and decreased ability of a muscle to stretch)

GO WITH THE FLOW

What happens when ICP rises

Intracranial pressure (ICP) is the pressure exerted within the intact skull by the intracranial volume—about 10% blood, 10% cerebrospinal fluid (CSF), and 80% brain tissue. The rigid skull has little space for expansion of these substances.

The brain compensates for increases in ICP by regulating the volume of the three substances in the following ways:

● limiting blood flow to the head
● displacing CSF into the spinal canal
● increasing absorption or decreasing production of CSF—withdrawing water from brain tissue and excreting it through the kidneys.

When compensatory mechanisms become overworked, small changes in volume lead to large changes in pressure. The following chart will help you understand increased ICP's pathophysiology.

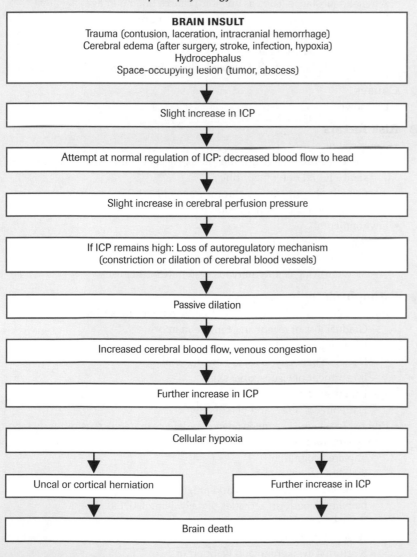

BRAIN INSULT
Trauma (contusion, laceration, intracranial hemorrhage)
Cerebral edema (after surgery, stroke, infection, hypoxia)
Hydrocephalus
Space-occupying lesion (tumor, abscess)

↓

Slight increase in ICP

↓

Attempt at normal regulation of ICP: decreased blood flow to head

↓

Slight increase in cerebral perfusion pressure

↓

If ICP remains high: Loss of autoregulatory mechanism
(constriction or dilation of cerebral blood vessels)

↓

Passive dilation

↓

Increased cerebral blood flow, venous congestion

↓

Further increase in ICP

↓

Cellular hypoxia

↓   ↓

Uncal or cortical herniation   Further increase in ICP

↓   ↓

Brain death

Ways the brain compensates for increased ICP

● Limits blood flow to the head
● Displaces CSF into the spinal canal
● Increases absorption or decreases production of CSF

Key facts about Alzheimer's disease

- Disorder of the cerebral cortex
- Involves three distinguishing features of brain tissue: granulovacuolar degeneration, neurofibrillary tangles, and amyloid plaques

TOP 4

Risk factors for Alzheimer's disease

1. Advancing age
2. Neurotransmitter deficiencies
3. Repeated head trauma
4. Lipoprotein E-epsilon 4 genotype

Key pathophysiologic changes in Alzheimer's disease

Initial stage
- Gradual loss of recent and remote memory
- Impairment of visuospatial skills
- Language deficits

Progressive stage
- Impaired cognition
- Difficulty with abstraction and judgment
- Inability to perform ADLs
- Personality changes

ALZHEIMER'S DISEASE

● **Definition**
- Disorder of the cerebral cortex (especially frontal lobe and hippocampus)
- Degenerative effect of amyloid plaques and neurofibrillary tangles of proteins in the affected areas
- Accounts for more than one-half of all cases of dementia
- Progressive, with poor prognosis

● **Underlying pathophysiology**
- Exact pathophysiology is unknown, but several theories exist
  - A genetic abnormality may occur on chromosomes 14, 19, and 21
  - Loss of neurotransmitter stimulation may occur
  - Encoding amyloid precursor protein may mutate
  - Alteration in apolipoprotein E may occur
- A genetic substance (such as amyloid) causes brain damage
- Brain tissue develops three distinguishing features
  - Granulovacuolar degeneration
  - Neurofibrillary tangles
  - Amyloid plaques (see *Abnormal cellular structures in Alzheimer's disease*)

● **Causes**
- Unknown

● **Risk factors**
- Neurochemical
  - Deficiencies in the neurotransmitters acetylcholine, somatostatin, substance P, and norepinephrine
  - Genetic abnormality on chromosomes 14, 19, 21
  - Lipoprotein E-epsilon 4 genotype
- Environmental
  - Repeated head trauma
  - Exposure to aluminum or manganese
  - Slow-growing central nervous system (CNS) viruses

● **Pathophysiologic changes**
- Initial stage — changes related to defects in neurotransmitter metabolism
  - Gradual loss of recent and remote memory
  - Disorientation to time and date
  - Decrease in ability to learn new material
  - Impairment of visuospatial skills
  - Language deficits
  - Flattening of affect and personality
- Progressive stage — changes related to defects in neurotransmitter metabolism or structural loss of brain
  - Impaired cognition
  - Inability to concentrate
  - Difficulty with abstraction and judgment
  - Inability to perform activities of daily living (ADLs)
  - Restlessness and agitation
  - Personality changes
  - Nocturnal awakening and wandering

Abnormal cellular structures in Alzheimer's disease

The brain tissue of patients with Alzheimer's disease exhibits three distinct and characteristic features: granulovacuolar degeneration, neurofibrillary tangles, and amyloid plaques.

GRANULOVACUOLAR DEGENERATION

Granulovacuolar of degeneration occurs inside the neurons of the hippocampus. An abnormally high number of fluid-filled spaces (vacuoles) enlarge the cell's body, possibly causing the cell to die.

NEUROFIBRILLARY TANGLES

Neurofibrillary tangles are bundles of filaments inside the neuron that abnormally twist around one another. They are found in the brain areas associated with memory and learning (hippocampus), fear and aggression (amygdala), and thinking (cerebral cortex). These tangles may play a role in the memory loss and personality changes that commonly occur in Alzheimer's disease.

AMYLOID PLAQUES

Also called *senile plaques*, amyloid plaques are found outside neurons in the extracellular space of the cerebral cortex and hippocampus. They contain a core of beta amyloid protein surrounded by abnormal nerve endings (neurites).

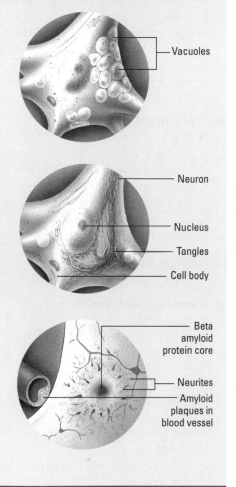

Vacuoles

Neuron

Nucleus

Tangles

Cell body

Beta amyloid protein core

Neurites

Amyloid plaques in blood vessel

- Severe deterioration in memory, language, and motor function
- Loss of coordination
- Inability to write or speak
- Acute confusion, agitation, compulsive behavior, fearfulness
- Disorientation and emotional lability
- Urinary and fecal incontinence

● **Complications**
• Injury secondary to violent behavior or wandering
• Pneumonia and other infections
• Malnutrition
• Dehydration

Key diagnostic test results for Alzheimer's disease

- CT scan: Excessive and progressive brain atrophy
- Autopsy: Confirms diagnosis

Key treatments for Alzheimer's disease

- Cholinesterase inhibitors
- Glutamate regulator
- Antianxiety drugs
- Antidepressants
- Antipsychotics

Key nursing considerations for Alzheimer's disease

- Provide patient with safe environment.
- Maintain daily routine.
- Ensure adequate nutrition.
- Help agitated or fearful patient focus on another activity.

Key facts about ALS

- Progressively debilitating and fatal motor system disease
- Involves upper and lower motor neuron degeneration
- Causes affected motor units to no longer be innervated

- Aspiration
- Death

● **Diagnostic test findings**
- Diagnosis is made by exclusion; tests are performed to rule out other diseases
- Positive diagnosis is made on autopsy
- Positron emission tomography shows metabolic activity of the cerebral cortex
- Computed tomography (CT) scan reveals excessive and progressive brain atrophy
- Magnetic resonance imaging (MRI) rules out intracranial lesions
- Cerebral blood flow studies show abnormalities in blood flow to the brain
- CSF analysis uncovers chronic neurologic infection
- EEG detects slowing of the brain waves in late stages of the disease
- Neuropsychologic tests reveal impaired cognitive ability and reasoning

● **Treatment**
- Cognitive symptoms
    - Cholinesterase inhibitors: donepezil (Aricept), rivastigmine (Exelon), galantamine (Reminyl), tacrine (Cognex)
    - Glutamate regulator: memantine (Namenda)
    - Experimental agents to slow progression: CX516 (Ampalex), atorvastatin (Lipitor), dimethylaminoethanol (Deanol), nefiracetam (Translon)
- Behavioral symptoms
    - Antianxiety drugs
    - Antidepressants
    - Antipsychotics

● **Nursing considerations**
- Provide the patient with a safe environment; this may involve admission to a facility outside of the home
- Assist the patient with exercise, as ordered, to help maintain mobility
- Maintain an established daily routine to decrease confusion and disorientation
- Ensure adequate nutrition by basing food choices on the patient's current abilities, including ability to chew and swallow or use utensils
- Intervene with an agitated or fearful patient by helping him focus on another activity
- Refer the patient and his family to appropriate community resources and support services
- Establish an effective communication system with the patient and his family to help them adjust to the patient's altered abilities
- Offer emotional support to the patient and his family

AMYOTROPHIC LATERAL SCLEROSIS

● **Definition**
- Progressively debilitating and fatal motor system disease
- Commonly called *Lou Gehrig disease* and ALS
- Doesn't affect sensory system, regulatory mechanisms of control and coordination of movement, or the intellect
- Onset usually between ages 40 and 60

Underlying pathophysiology
- Upper and lower motor neuron degeneration occurs without inflammation
- Excitatory neurotransmitter accumulates to toxic levels at the synapses
- Affected motor units are no longer innervated
- Progressive degeneration of axon causes loss of myelin

Causes
- Unknown
- Genetic defect occurring on chromosome 21 (in 5% to 10% of those affected)
- Possible contributing mechanisms
  - Autoimmune disorders
  - Metabolic interference in nucleic acid production by the nerve fibers
  - Nutritional deficiency related to a disturbance in enzyme metabolism
  - Slow-acting virus

Pathophysiologic changes
- Fasciculations, accompanied by spasticity, atrophy, and weakness, due to degeneration of the upper and lower motor neurons, and loss of functioning motor units
- Impaired speech, difficulty chewing and swallowing, choking, and excessive drooling from degeneration of cranial nerves V, IX, X, and XII
- Difficulty breathing resulting from brain stem involvement and muscle weakness
- Emotional lability due to progressive bulbar palsy

Complications
- Aspiration
- Fractures from falls
- Respiratory failure
- Respiratory infections

Diagnostic test findings
- Diagnosis is made by exclusion; tests are performed to rule out other diseases
- Electromyography reveals abnormalities of electrical activity in involved muscles
- Muscle biopsy uncovers atrophic fibers interspersed among normal fibers
- Nerve conduction studies are normal
- CT scan and EEG are normal, thus ruling out multiple sclerosis, spinal cord neoplasm, polyarteritis, syringomyelia, myasthenia gravis, progressive muscular dystrophy, and progressive stroke

Treatment
- Treatment is supportive
- Drug therapy
  - Diazepam (Valium), dantrolene (Dantrium), or baclofen (Lioresal) for decreasing spasticity
  - Quinidine (Quinaglute Dura-Tabs) to relieve painful muscle cramps
  - Riluzole (Rilutek) to modulate glutamate activity and slow disease progression
- Respiratory, speech, and physical therapy to maintain function as much as possible
- Psychological support to help the patient cope with this progressive, fatal illness

---

Key pathophysiologic changes in ALS
- Fasciculations
- Weakness
- Spasticity
- Difficulty chewing and swallowing
- Difficulty breathing

Key diagnostic test results for ALS
- Electromyography: Electrical activity abnormalities in involved muscles
- Muscle biopsy: Atrophic fibers

Key treatments for ALS
- Diazepam, dantrolene, or baclofen
- Riluzole
- Respiratory therapy
- Physical therapy

- Thyrotropin-releasing hormone to temporarily improve motor function (successful only in some patients)

Nursing considerations
- Implement a rehabilitation program designed to maintain the patient's independence for as long as possible
- Help the patient obtain assistive devices, such as a walker or a wheelchair
- Arrange for a visiting nurse to oversee the patient's status, provide support, and teach the family about the illness
- Assist with bathing, personal hygiene, and transfers from wheelchair to bed
- Help establish a regular bowel and bladder routine
- Teach the patient and family how to perform suction to help handle an increased accumulation of secretions and dysphagia
- Provide good skin care when the patient is bedridden
  - Turn him often
  - Use pressure-reducing devices such as an alternating air mattress
- If the patient has trouble swallowing, give him soft, solid foods and position him upright during meals
- Gastrostomy or nasogastric (NG) tube feedings may be necessary if the patient can no longer swallow
- Teach the patient and his family how to administer gastrostomy feedings
- Encourage the patient and his family to discuss directives regarding health care decisions before the patient becomes unable to communicate his wishes
- Refer the patient to a hospice program or a local ALS support group

ARTERIOVENOUS MALFORMATIONS

Definition
- Tangled masses of thin-walled, dilated blood vessels with interlinking fistulas, lacking capillary beds that appear between arteries (when a deficient muscularis layer is present) and veins
- Lack of development or injury to the capillary bed in the brain
- Commonly involve more than one malformation
  - Develop primarily in the posterior portion of the cerebral hemispheres
  - One-half superficially located, one-half buried deeply
- Range in size from a few millimeters to large malformations extending from the cerebral cortex to the ventricles

Underlying pathophysiology
- Arteriovenous malformations (AVMs) lack the typical structural characteristics of the blood vessels
  - Vessels of the AVM are very thin
  - One or more arteries feed into the AVM, causing it to appear dilated and torturous
- High-pressured arterial flow moves into the venous system through the fistulas to increase venous pressure, engorging and dilating the venous structures
- Abnormal channels between the arterial and venous system mix oxygenated and unoxygenated blood, preventing adequate perfusion of brain tissue

---

Key nursing considerations for ALS

- Implement rehabilitation program.
- Help establish regular bowel and bladder routine.
- Teach patient and family how to perform suction.
- If patient has trouble swallowing, offer soft, solid foods and position him upright during meals.
- Refer patient to hospice program or ALS support group.

Key facts about AVMs

- Involve tangled masses of thin-walled, dilated blood vessels and abnormal channels between arteries and veins
- Cause oxygenated and unoxygenated blood to mix
- Prevent adequate perfusion of brain tissue
- May cause hemorrhage into brain

- If the AVM is large enough, the shunting can deprive the surrounding tissue of adequate blood flow
- Thin-walled vessels may ooze small amounts of blood or rupture, causing hemorrhage into the brain or subarachnoid space

● **Causes**
- Congenital
- Penetrating injuries such as trauma

● **Pathophysiologic changes**
- Chronic mild to severe throbbing headache (sometimes felt to throb in time with the pulse) resulting from vessel engorgement
- Confusion caused by AVM dilation, vessel engorgement, and increased ICP
- Seizures secondary to compression of the surrounding tissues by the engorged vessels and impaired oxygenation
- Systolic bruit over carotid artery, mastoid process, or orbit, indicating turbulent blood flow
- Focal neurologic deficits (depending on the location) resulting from compression of normal brain tissue and diminished perfusion to surrounding brain cells
- Sudden severe headache, seizures, confusion, lethargy, and meningeal irritation from bleeding into the brain tissue or subarachnoid space
- Hydrocephalus from AVM extension into the cerebral ventricular lining

● **Complications**
- Aneurysm development and subsequent rupture
- Intracerebral, subarachnoid, or subdural hemorrhage, depending on the location of the AVM
- Hydrocephalus

● **Diagnostic test findings**
- Cerebral arteriogram confirms presence of AVMs and evaluates blood flow
- Doppler ultrasonography of the cerebrovascular system reveals abnormal, turbulent blood flow

● **Treatment**
- Aneurysm precautions to prevent possible rupture
- Surgery, such as block dissection, laser, or ligation, to repair the fistulas and remove the damaged arteries
- If surgery isn't possible, embolization or radiation therapy to close the fistulas and damaged arteries and thus reduce the blood flow to the AVM

● **Nursing considerations**
- Monitor vital signs frequently
- Control hypertension, seizure activity, and other activity that could elevate the patient's blood pressure
  - Administer drug therapy as ordered
  - Perform ongoing neurologic assessments
  - Maintain a quiet, therapeutic environment
- If the AVM has ruptured, work to control increased ICP and intracranial hemorrhage

Key pathophysiologic changes in AVMs
- Chronic mild to severe throbbing headache
- Confusion
- Seizures

Key diagnostic test results for AVMs
- Cerebral arteriogram: Presence of AVMs

Key treatments for AVMs
- Aneurysm precautions
- Surgery
- Embolization or radiation therapy

Key nursing considerations for AVMs
- Monitor vital signs and neurologic status.
- Maintain blood pressure control.
- If AVM has ruptured, work to control increased ICP and intracranial hemorrhage.

BELL'S PALSY

Key facts about Bell's palsy

- Inflammatory reaction around cranial nerve VII
- Inhibits neural stimulation of the muscle by motor fibers of the facial nerve
- Produces unilateral or bilateral facial weakness or paralysis

Key pathophysiologic changes in Bell's palsy

- Unilateral facial weakness
- Drooping mouth and drooling
- Impaired ability to close the eye on the weak side
- Bell's phenomenon

Key diagnostic test results for Bell's palsy

- Electromyography: Distinguishes temporary conduction defects from pathologic interruption of nerve fibers

● Definition
- Disease of cranial nerve VII (the facial nerve) that produces unilateral or bilateral facial weakness or paralysis
- Involves rapid onset of symptoms
- Resolves spontaneously in 80% to 90% of patients, with complete recovery in 1 to 8 weeks
- Recovery may be delayed in the elderly
- If recovery is partial, contractures may develop on the paralyzed side of the face

● Underlying pathophysiology
- An inflammatory reaction occurs around cranial nerve VII, usually at the internal auditory meatus, where the nerve leaves bony tissue
- The inflammatory reaction produces a conduction block that inhibits appropriate neural stimulation to the muscle by the motor fibers of the facial nerve, resulting in the characteristic unilateral or bilateral facial weakness (see *Neurologic dysfunction in Bell's palsy*)

● Causes
- Hemorrhage
- Herpes simplex or herpes zoster
- Infection
- Local trauma
- Meningitis
- Tumor
- Viral disease

● Pathophysiologic changes
- Unilateral facial weakness
- Drooping mouth and drooling saliva
- Taste perception distortion or loss of taste
- Smooth forehead appearance
- Impaired ability to close the eye on the weak side
- Upward rolling of the eyes when attempting to close them (Bell's phenomenon)
- Excessive tearing
- Ringing in the ear

● Complications
- Corneal abrasion
- Infection (masked by steroid use)
- Poor functional recovery

● Diagnostic test findings
- Diagnosis is based on clinical presentation
- MRI rules out tumor
- Electromyography 10 days after the onset of symptoms helps predict the level of expected recovery by distinguishing temporary conduction defects from a pathologic interruption of nerve fibers

Neurologic dysfunction in Bell's palsy

This illustration shows how motor conduction of the facial nerve (cranial nerve VII) is blocked in Bell's palsy, causing a unilateral facial weakness.

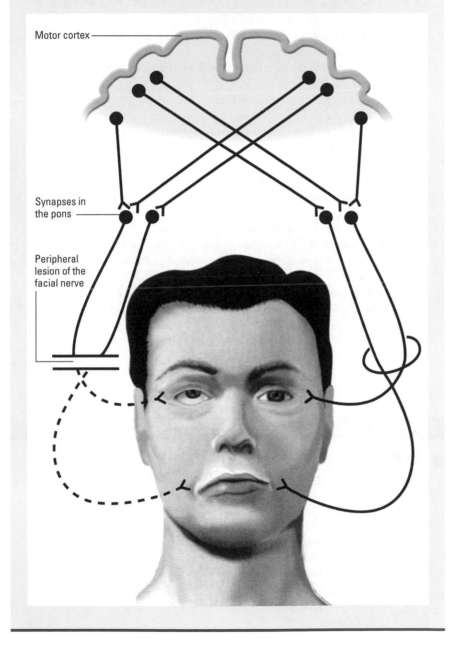

Motor cortex

Synapses in the pons

Peripheral lesion of the facial nerve

Treatment
- Analgesics to relieve pain
- Steroids to reduce facial nerve edema and improve nerve conduction and blood flow

Key treatments for Bell's palsy
- Analgesics
- Steroids

- Possible electrotherapy after the 14th day of steroid therapy to help prevent atrophy of facial muscles
- Surgery for persistent paralysis

● **Nursing considerations**
- Watch for adverse effects of steroid use, GI distress, and fluid retention
- Antacids usually provide relief for GI distress
- Use prednisone cautiously in patients with diabetes; monitor serum glucose levels frequently in these patients
- Apply moist heat to the affected side of the face to reduce pain, taking care not to burn the skin
- Help the patient maintain muscle tone
    - Massage the patient's face with a gentle upward motion two to three times daily for 5 to 10 minutes, or have him massage his face himself.
    - When he's ready for active exercises, teach him to exercise by grimacing in front of a mirror
- Advise the patient to protect his face, especially his eye
    - Have him cover his eye with an eye patch, especially when he's outdoors or sleeping
    - Tell the patient to keep warm and avoid exposure to dust and wind
    - When exposure is unavoidable, instruct him to cover his face
- To prevent excessive weight loss, help the patient cope with difficulty in eating and drinking
    - Instruct him to chew on the unaffected side of his mouth
    - Provide a soft, nutritionally balanced diet, eliminating hot foods and fluids
    - Apply a facial sling to improve lip alignment
- Provide frequent and complete mouth care, being particularly careful to remove residual food that collects between the cheeks and gums
- Offer psychological support

GUILLAIN-BARRÉ SYNDROME

● **Definition**
- Acute, rapidly progressive, and potentially fatal form of acquired inflammatory disease that results in demyelination of the peripheral nerves
- Occurs in three phases
    - Acute phase
        - Begins with the onset of the first definitive symptom and ends 1 to 3 weeks later
        - Ascending motor paralysis produces a symmetrical flaccid paralysis
    - Plateau phase
        - Lasts several days to 2 weeks
        - No changes occur
    - Recovery phase
        - Extends over 4 to 6 months but may last up to 2 to 3 years if the disease is severe
        - Involves remyelinization and regrowth of axonal processes

Understanding sensorimotor nerve degeneration

Guillain-Barré syndrome attacks the peripheral nerves so that they can't transmit messages to the brain correctly. Here's what goes wrong.

The myelin sheath degenerates for unknown reasons. This sheath covers the nerve axons and conducts electrical impulses along the nerve pathways. Degeneration brings inflammation, swelling, and patchy demyelination. As this disorder destroys myelin, the nodes of Ranvier (at the junction of the myelin sheaths) widen. This widening delays and impairs impulse transmission along the dorsal and anterior nerve roots.

Because the dorsal nerve roots handle sensory function, the patient may experience tingling and numbness. Similarly, because the anterior nerve roots are responsible for motor function, impairment causes varying weakness, immobility, and paralysis.

Underlying pathophysiology

- Segmental demyelination of the peripheral nerves prevents normal transmission of electrical impulses along the sensorimotor nerve roots
- Inflammation and degenerative changes occur in the posterior (sensory) and the anterior (motor) nerve roots
- Signs of sensory and motor losses occur simultaneously (see *Understanding sensorimotor nerve degeneration*)
- Autonomic nerve transmission may be impaired

Causes

- Unknown
- Possible precipitating factors
  - Cell-mediated immune response to viral or bacterial infection (commonly GI or respiratory)
  - Recent history of *Campylobacter jejuni* infection (precedes the syndrome in 60% of patients)
  - Surgery
  - Rabies or swine influenza vaccination
  - Hodgkin's disease or other malignant disease
  - Systemic lupus erythematosus

Pathophysiologic changes

- Symmetrical muscle weakness (ascending type) from impaired anterior nerve root transmission
  - Major neurologic sign
  - Appears first in the legs
  - Extends to the arms and facial nerves within 24 to 72 hours
- Muscle weakness (descending type), developing in the arms first or in the arms and legs simultaneously, from impaired anterior nerve root transmission
- Paresthesia, sometimes preceding muscle weakness but vanishing quickly, from impairment of the dorsal nerve root transmission
- Diplegia, possibly with ophthalmoplegia (ocular paralysis), caused by impaired motor nerve root transmission and involvement of cranial nerves III, IV, and VI

TOP 2

Precipitating factors in Guillain-Barré syndrome

1. Recent history of *Campylobacter jejuni* infection
2. Cell-mediated immune response to infection

Key pathophysiologic changes in Guillain-Barré syndrome

- Ascending or descending symmetrical muscle weakness
- Cranial nerve involvement
- Pain

- Pain caused by inflamed nerve roots and paralysis with resultant immobility
- Dysphagia or dysarthria and, less commonly, weakness of the muscles supplied by cranial nerve XI (spinal accessory nerve)
- Hypotonia and areflexia resulting from reflex arc interruption

● **Complications**
- Aspiration
- Hypertension and orthostatic hypotension
- Joint contractures
- Loss of bladder and bowel sphincter control
- Mechanical respiratory failure
- Muscle wasting
- Pressure ulcers
- Respiratory tract infections
- Sepsis
- Moderate to severe residual muscle weakness or paralysis
- Thrombophlebitis or pulmonary emboli

● **Diagnostic test findings**
- CSF analysis by lumbar puncture provides various findings
  - Protein levels are elevated without cellular abnormality and peak in 4 to 6 weeks
  - White blood cell (WBC) count remains normal
  - In severe disease, CSF pressure may rise above normal
- Complete blood count reveals leukocytosis with immature WBCs (such as band cells) early in the illness, and then quickly returns to normal
- Electromyography may show repeated firing of the same motor unit, instead of widespread sectional stimulation
- Nerve conduction velocities slow soon after paralysis develops
- Serum immunoglobulin levels are elevated
- Pulmonary function tests (PFTs) show decreased expiratory vital capacity and decreased oxygen saturation as muscles of expiration weaken

● **Treatment**
- Endotracheal (ET) intubation or tracheotomy if respiratory muscle involvement causes difficulty in clearing secretions
- Ventilatory support if required
- Trial dose (7 days) of a steroid to reduce inflammatory response
  - Used if the disease is relentlessly progressive
  - Discontinued if drug doesn't produce noticeable improvement
- Plasmapheresis during the initial phase to reduce the number of circulating antibodies in the plasma
  - Decreases the recovery time
  - No benefit if started 2 weeks after onset
- High-dose I.V. immunoglobulin therapy (possibly) to reduce inflammatory effects and decrease antibody formation
- Continuous cardiac monitoring to watch for possible arrhythmias from autonomic dysfunction
- Propranolol to treat tachycardia and hypertension
- Atropine to treat bradycardia
- Volume replacement in cases of severe hypotension

Key diagnostic test results for Guillain-Barré syndrome

- CSF analysis: Elevated protein levels, normal WBC count, CSF pressure above normal (in severe disease)
- Electromyography: repeated firing of same motor unit
- PFTs: Results of impaired neuromuscular function

Key treatments for Guillain-Barré syndrome

- ET intubation or tracheotomy
- Ventilatory support
- Steroids
- Plasmapheresis
- Cardiac medications to treat arrhythmias

Nursing considerations
- Monitor the patient for worsening of symptoms
- Watch for ascending sensory loss, which precedes motor loss
- Monitor vital signs and LOC
- Assess respiratory function and provide treatment as necessary
  - Auscultate for breath sounds
  - If respiratory muscles are weak, take serial vital capacity recordings
  - Obtain arterial blood gas measurements and watch for signs of respiratory failure
  - Turn and position the patient
  - Encourage coughing and deep breathing
  - **Begin respiratory support at the first sign of dyspnea or with decreasing partial pressure of arterial oxygen**
  - If respiratory failure is imminent, establish an emergency airway with an ET tube
- Give meticulous skin care to prevent skin breakdown and contractures
  - Reposition the patient every 2 hours
  - Use foam, gel, or alternating pressure pads at points of contact
- Perform passive range-of-motion (ROM) exercises within the patient's pain limits
- When the patient's condition stabilizes, assist with gentle stretching and active exercises
- Prevent aspiration
  - **Test the gag reflex, and elevate the head of the bed before giving the patient anything to eat**
  - If the gag reflex is absent, give NG tube feedings until this reflex returns
  - A gastrostomy tube may be necessary to provide adequate nourishment
- Monitor the patient's blood pressure and pulse when tilting him to a vertical position
- Take steps to prevent thrombophlebitis
  - Apply antiembolism stockings
  - Inspect the legs regularly
  - Give prophylactic anticoagulants as ordered
- Provide appropriate care if the patient has facial paralysis
  - Perform eye and mouth care every 4 hours
  - Protect the corneas with isotonic eye drops and conical eye shields
- Measure and record intake and output every 8 hours
  - Offer the bedpan every 3 to 4 hours
  - Encourage adequate fluid intake (2 qt [2 L]/day), unless contraindicated
- Provide assistance, as needed, if urine retention develops
  - The patient may need manual pressure on the bladder (Credé's maneuver) before urination
  - If Credé's maneuver isn't effective, begin intermittent catheterization, as ordered
- Prevent or relieve constipation
  - Offer prune juice and a high-bulk diet
  - If necessary, give daily or alternate-day suppositories (glycerin or bisacodyl [Dulcolax]) or enemas, as ordered
- Before discharge, teach the patient how to perform transfers and how to walk short distances with a walker or a cane

- Provide patient teaching to the patient and his family
  - Show the family how to help the patient eat
  - Teach how to avoid skin breakdown
  - Stress the need for a regular bowel and bladder routine

HEADACHE

Definition
- Common neurologic disorder
- Usually a benign symptom
- Classified as migraine, cluster, paroxysmal hemicrania, or tension headache
- May be primary or secondary
  - Primary—no organic or structural cause
  - Secondary—indicative of an underlying structural or organic disease, such as aneurysm, meningitis, or tumor

Underlying pathophysiology
- Intracranial and extracranial arteries constrict and dilate
- Pain may emanate from the pain-sensitive structures of the skin, scalp, muscles, arteries, and veins; cranial nerves V, VII, IX, and X; or cervical nerves 1, 2, and 3
- Intracranial mechanisms include traction or displacement of arteries, venous sinuses, or venous tributaries and inflammation of or direct pressure on cranial nerves with afferent pain fibers
- With migraines, various biochemical abnormalities are thought to occur
  - Local leakage of neurokinin, a vasodilator polypeptide, through the dilated arteries
  - Decrease in the plasma level of serotonin

Causes
- Diseases of the scalp, teeth, extracranial arteries, or external or middle ear
- Emotional stress or fatigue
- Environmental stimuli, such as noise, crowds, or bright lights
- Glaucoma
- Head trauma or tumor
- Hypertension
- Increased ICP
- Inflammation of the eyes or mucosa of the nasal or paranasal sinuses
- Intracranial bleeding, abscess, or aneurysm
- Menstruation
- Systemic disease
- Vasodilators, such as nitrates, alcohol, and histamine

Pathophysiologic changes
- With migraine headaches, unilateral, pulsating pain, which later becomes more generalized
- Dull, persistent ache; tender spots on the head, face, and neck; feeling of tightness around the head with a characteristic "hat-band" distribution caused by muscle contraction and traction-inflammatory vascular headaches
- Photophobia caused by pressure on the optic nerve

Key facts about headache
- Pain caused by constriction and dilation of intracranial and extracranial arteries
- May be primary or secondary
- Classified as migraine, cluster, paroxysmal hemicrania, or tension headache

Key pathophysiologic changes in headache
- Unilateral, pulsating pain
- Dull, persistent ache
- Tender spots on head, face, and neck
- Feeling of tightness around head

- Neurologic deficits, such as paresthesia and muscle weakness, resulting from associated intracranial bleeding
- Pain that disrupts sleep, exertional headaches, and headaches accompanied by neurologic symptoms indicating a tumor or other intracranial pathology

Complications
- Status migraines
- Drug dependency
- Disruption of lifestyle

Diagnostic test findings
- Skull X-rays may show skull fracture (with trauma)
- CT scan may show a tumor, subarachnoid hemorrhage, or other intracranial disorders and possibly disorders of sinuses
- MRI may show presence of a tumor
- Lumbar puncture may show increased ICP, suggesting a tumor, edema, or hemorrhage
- EEG may show alterations in the brain's electrical activity, suggesting intracranial lesions, head injury, meningitis, or encephalitis

Treatment
- Analgesics, ranging from aspirin to codeine or meperidine (Demerol), may provide symptomatic relief
- Identification and elimination of causative factors
- Possible psychotherapy if headaches are caused by emotional stress
- Muscle relaxants for chronic tension headaches
- Drug therapy for migraine headaches
  - Drugs such as propranolol (Inderal), atenolol (Tenormin), clonidine (Catapres), or amitriptyline (Elavil) to prevent migraine headaches
  - Sumatriptan (Imitrex) and other serotonin receptor agonists for acute migraine attacks or cluster headaches (drugs of choice)
  - Ergotamine (Ergomar) or similar ergotamine derivatives, alone or with caffeine
    - Work best when taken early in the course of an attack
    - Use of rectal suppositories if nausea and vomiting make oral administration difficult

Nursing considerations
- Obtain a complete history
  - Duration and location of the headache
  - Time of day it usually begins
  - Nature of the pain
  - Associated symptoms such as blurred vision
  - Medications taken
  - History of prolonged fasting
  - Precipitating factors, such as tension, menstruation, loud noises, menopause, or alcohol
- Help the patient avoid exacerbating factors
- Advise the patient to lie down in a dark, quiet room during an attack and place ice packs on the forehead or a cold cloth over the eyes
- Instruct the patient to take the prescribed medication at the onset of migraine symptoms

- Tell the patient to prevent dehydration by drinking plenty of fluids after nausea and vomiting subside
- Avoid repeated use of opioids if possible

HUNTINGTON'S DISEASE

Definition

- Hereditary disorder in which degeneration of the cerebral cortex and basal ganglia causes chronic progressive chorea (involuntary and irregular movements) and cognitive deterioration that ends in dementia
- Onset generally between ages 25 and 55
- Usually results in death 10 to 15 years after onset due to suicide, heart failure, or pneumonia

Underlying pathophysiology

- Levels of neurotransmitter substances — primarily gamma-aminobutyric acid (GABA) and dopamine — are disturbed
- In the basal ganglia, frontal cortex, and cerebellum, GABA neurons are destroyed and replaced by glial cells
- The consequent deficiency of GABA (an inhibitory neurotransmitter) results in a relative excess of dopamine and abnormal neurotransmission along the affected pathways
- Degeneration in the cerebral cortex and basal ganglia leads to chronic progressive chorea and mental deterioration that ends in dementia

Causes

- Unknown
- Transmitted as an autosomal dominant trait with high penetrance, which either sex can transmit and inherit

Pathophysiologic changes

- Progressively severe choreic movements due to the relative excess of dopamine
- Bradykinesia (slow movement), commonly accompanied by rigidity, due to impaired neurotransmission
- Impairment of voluntary and involuntary movement due to the combination of chorea, bradykinesia, and patient's normal muscle strength
- Dementia without significant impairment of immediate memory resulting from dysfunction of the subcortex (an early indication of the disease)
- Problems with recent memory due to retrieval rather than encoding problems
- Deficits of executive function (planning, organizing, regulating, and programming) due to frontal lobe involvement
- Depression and possible mania (earliest symptom) related to altered levels of dopamine and GABA

Complications

- Aspiration
- Choking
- Heart failure
- Infections
- Pneumonia

● **Diagnostic test findings**
- Genetic testing reveals the autosomal dominant marker G8 on chromosome 4
- Positron emission tomography reveals brain atrophy and areas of functional loss
- CT scan and MRI show brain atrophy in the caudate nuclei and putamen (the outer, darker gray layer of the caudate nuclei) and ventricular enlargement

● **Treatment**
- Palliative care to manage symptoms
- Haloperidol (Haldol) or diazepam (Valium) to modify choreic movements and control behavioral manifestations
- Psychotherapy and psychotropic drugs to decrease anxiety and stress and manage psychiatric symptoms
- Transfer to a long-term care facility or 24-hour home health services to manage progressive mental deterioration and self-care deficits

● **Nursing considerations**
- Provide physical support by attending to the patient's basic needs, such as hygiene, skin care, bowel and bladder care, and nutrition
- Offer emotional support to the patient and his family
  - Teach them about the disease
  - Listen to their concerns and special problems
  - Allow the patient extra time to express himself to help decrease frustration
  - Teach the family to participate in the patient's care
- **Control the patient's environment to protect him from suicide or other self-inflicted injury**
- If the patient has difficulty walking, provide a walker to help him maintain his balance
- Make sure that affected families receive genetic counseling
- Refer the patient and his family to the Huntington's Disease Association

INTRACRANIAL ANEURYSM

● **Definition**
- Dilation, bulging, or ballooning of part of a vein or artery wall within the brain
- Also called *cerebral aneurysm*
- Has various forms
  - Berry
    - Saclike outpouching in the media of a cerebral artery
    - Most common
  - Fusiform
  - Mycotic
  - Traumatic
- Usually arises at an arterial junction in the Circle of Willis, the circular anastomosis forming the major cerebral arteries at the base of the brain, the vertebrobasilar arteries, or within the carotid system
- May rupture and cause subarachnoid hemorrhage (rupture occurs in 1 out of 100 people with aneurysm)

Key diagnostic test results for Huntington's disease

- Genetic testing: Autosomal dominant marker G8 on chromosome 4
- Positron emission tomography: Brain atrophy, areas of functional loss

Key treatments for Huntington's disease

- Palliative care
- Haloperidol or diazepam
- Psychotherapy
- Psychotropic drugs

Key nursing considerations for Huntington's disease

- Provide physical and emotional support.
- Control environment to protect patient from suicide or other self-inflicted injury.
- Refer patient and family to Huntington's Disease Association.

Key facts about intracranial aneurysm

- Dilation, bulging, or ballooning of vein or artery wall within brain
- Can lead to rupture because blood flow exerts pressure on weakened vessel walls
- Can cause subarachnoid hemorrhage

Key pathophysiologic changes in intracranial aneurysm

- Sudden severe headache
- Nausea
- Projectile vomiting
- Altered LOC
- Nuchal rigidity
- Hemiparesis

Key diagnostic test results for intracranial aneurysm

- Cerebral angiography: Altered cerebral blood flow, vessel lumen dilation, differences in arterial filling
- CT scan: Subarachnoid or ventricular bleeding, displaced midline structures

Key treatments for intracranial aneurysm

- Surgical repair
- Embolization
- Bed rest in a quiet, darkened room
- Sedation
- Aminocaproic acid

● **Underlying pathophysiology**
- Blood flow exerts pressure against a congenitally weak arterial wall, stretching it like an overblown balloon and making it likely to rupture
- Rupture is followed by a subarachnoid hemorrhage, in which blood spills into the space normally occupied by CSF
- Blood spills into brain tissue, where a clot can cause potentially fatal increased ICP and brain tissue damage

● **Causes**
- Atherosclerosis
- Binge alcohol use
- Cigarrette use
- Cocaine use
- Congenital defect
- Degenerative process
- Combination of congenital defect and degenerative process
- Infection
- Inflammation
- Trauma

● **Pathophysiologic changes**
- Subarachnoid hemorrhage caused by rupture of the intracranial aneurysm (see *Classifying subarachnoid hemorrhage*)
- Sudden severe headache caused by increased pressure from bleeding into a closed space
- Nausea and projectile vomiting related to increased ICP
- Altered LOC, depending on the severity and location of bleeding, due to increased ICP caused by increased cerebral blood volume
- Meningeal irritation, resulting in nuchal rigidity, back and leg pain, fever, restlessness, irritability, occasional seizures, photophobia, and blurred vision, secondary to bleeding into the subarachnoid space
- Hemiparesis, hemisensory defects, dysphagia, and visual defects from bleeding into the brain tissues
- Diplopia, ptosis, dilated pupil, and inability to rotate the eye caused by compression on the oculomotor nerve (if the aneurysm is near the internal carotid artery)

● **Complications**
- Death from increased ICP and brain herniation
- Rebleeding
- Vasospasm

● **Diagnostic test findings**
- Cerebral angiography shows altered cerebral blood flow, vessel lumen dilation, and differences in arterial filling
- CT scan reveals subarachnoid or ventricular bleeding and displaced midline structures
- MRI shows a void in cerebral blood flow
- Skull X-rays show the calcified wall of the aneurysm and areas of bone erosion

● **Treatment**
- Surgical repair by clipping, ligation, or wrapping (before or after rupture)

Classifying subarachnoid hemorrhage

The severity of symptoms accompanying subarachnoid hemorrhage varies from patient to patient, depending on the site and the amount of bleeding.

GRADE	CHARACTERISTICS
I (minimal bleeding)	Alert and oriented, neurologically intact; may have slight headache and nuchal tension
II (mild bleeding)	Alert and oriented, with mild to severe headache, nuchal rigidity, possible photophobia, and third cranial nerve involvement (sign of meningeal irritation)
III (moderate bleeding)	Lethargic, confused or drowsy, with continued nuchal rigidity, and possible mild focal deficit such as hemiparesis
IV (severe bleeding)	Stuporous, with nuchal rigidity and possible moderate to severe focal deficits (hemiplegia, early decerebrate rigidity, and vegetative disturbances such as dysphagia)
V (moribund or fatal bleeding)	In deep coma, with severe neurologic deficits, such as decerebrate rigidity, when nonfatal

TOP 4

Precautions to prevent rebleeding in ruptured aneurysm

1. Promoting bed rest
2. Avoiding strenuous activity
3. Preventing elevated blood pressure
4. Administering aminocaproic acid

- Microcoil thrombus or balloon embolization
- Bed rest in a quiet, darkened room with minimal stimulation
- Avoidance of coffee, other stimulants, and aspirin to reduce the risk of blood pressure elevation
- Codeine or another analgesic, as needed, to maintain rest and minimize risk of pressure changes
- Antihypertensives if the patient is hypertensive
- Sedation to prevent agitation leading to hypertension
- Calcium channel blockers to decrease spasm and subsequent rebleeding
- Corticosteroids to manage headache in subarachnoid hemorrhage
- Anticonvulsants to prevent or treat seizures secondary to pressure and tissue irritation from bleeding
- Aminocaproic acid (Amicar), an inhibitor of fibrinolysis, to minimize the risk of rebleeding by delaying blood clot lysis

● **Nursing considerations**
- After hemorrhage, establish and maintain a patent airway
- Position the patient to promote pulmonary drainage and prevent upper airway obstruction
- If the patient is intubated, administer 100% oxygen before suctioning to remove secretions
  – Doing so prevents hypoxia and vasodilation resulting from carbon dioxide accumulation
  – Suction no longer than 20 seconds to avoid increased ICP
- Impose aneurysm precautions to minimize the risk of rebleed and to avoid increased ICP

Key nursing considerations for intracranial aneurysm

- After hemorrhage, establish and maintain patent airway.
- Position patient to promote pulmonary drainage and prevent upper airway obstruction.
- If patient is intubated, administer 100% oxygen before suctioning.
- Don't suction longer than 20 seconds.
- Impose aneurysm precautions.
- Monitor for indicators of enlarging aneurysm, rebleeding, intracranial clot, vasospasm, or change in respiratory status.
- Watch for intermittent signs of increasing ICP.

  - Bed rest in a quiet, darkened room with the head of the bed flat or less than 30 degrees, as ordered
  - Limiting of visitors
  - Avoidance of strenuous physical activity and straining with bowel movements
  - Restricted fluid intake
- Turn the patient often
- Encourage occasional deep breathing and leg movement
- Assist with active ROM exercises; if the patient is paralyzed, perform regular passive ROM exercises
- Monitor ABG levels, LOC, and vital signs often
- Measure intake and output
- **Monitor the patient for indicators of an enlarging aneurysm, rebleeding, intracranial clot, vasospasm, or change in respiratory status**
  - Unilateral enlarged pupil
  - Onset or worsening of hemiparesis or motor deficit
  - Increased blood pressure and slowed pulse
  - Worsening of headache or sudden onset of a headache
  - Renewed or worsened nuchal rigidity
  - Renewed or persistent vomiting
- **Watch for intermittent signs that can indicate increasing ICP, such as restlessness, extremity weakness, and speech alterations**
- Give fluids, as ordered, and monitor I.V. infusions to avoid increased ICP
- If the patient has facial weakness, assess the gag reflex and assist him during meals
  - Place food in the unaffected side of his mouth
  - If the patient can't swallow, insert an NG tube, as ordered
  - Give all tube feedings slowly
- If the patient can eat, provide a high-fiber diet to prevent straining at stool, which can increase ICP
- Obtain an order for a stool softener or a mild laxative, and administer as ordered
- If the patient is receiving steroids, check the stools for blood
- With palsy involving the third or seventh cranial nerve, administer artificial tears or ointment to the affected eye and tape the eye shut at night to prevent corneal damage
- To minimize stress, encourage relaxation techniques
- Administer antihypertensives as ordered
  - Carefully monitor blood pressure
  - Immediately report any significant change
- Administer aminocaproic acid (Amicar) I.V., orally, or as ordered at least every 2 hours to maintain therapeutic blood levels, and monitor the patient for adverse reactions, such as nausea, diarrhea, and phlebitis
- Prevent deep vein thrombosis by applying antiembolism stockings or sequential compression sleeves
- If the patient can't speak, establish a simple means of communication, or use cards or a notepad

Key indicators of enlarging aneurysm or rebleeding

- Unilateral enlarged pupil
- Onset or worsening of hemiparesis or motor deficit
- Worsening of headache or sudden onset of headache
- Renewed or persistent vomiting

LYME DISEASE

● **Definition**
- Multisystem disorder caused by *Borrelia burgdorferi* (a spirochete transmitted through a deer tick bite)
- Primarily occurs in areas inhabited by deer
- Typically manifests in three stages
  - Early localized stage (distinctive red rash accompanied by flulike symptoms)
  - Early disseminated stage (neurologic and cardiac abnormalities)
  - Late stage (arthritis, chronic neurologic problems), which may occur up to 2 years after the tick bite

● **Underlying pathophysiology**
- A tick injects spirochete-laden saliva into the bloodstream or deposits fecal matter on the skin
- After incubating for 3 to 32 days, spirochetes migrate outward, causing the characteristic red macular or papular rash (bull's-eye rash)
- Spirochetes disseminate to other skin sites or organs through bloodstream or lymph
- Spirochetes can survive in the joints for years, or they can trigger an inflammatory response in the host and die

● **Causes**
- Infestation of spirochete *B. burgdorferi* resulting from deer tick bite

● **Pathophysiologic changes**
- Distinctive red bull's-eye rash, flulike symptoms (fever, chills, myalgia, headache, malaise), and regional lymphadenopathy resulting from local infection of *B. burgdorferi* spirochete
- Neurologic abnormalities (peripheral and cranial neuropathy), cardiac abnormalities (carditis, conduction disturbances, first-degree heart block), and eye abnormalities (conjunctivitis) due to dissemination of spirochetes into bloodstream
- Inflammation, joint swelling, and arthritis caused by presence of organisms in the synovium

● **Complications**
- Arrhythmias
- Heart block
- Meningitis
- Myocarditis
- Pericarditis

● **Diagnostic test findings**
- Assays for anti-*B. burgdorferi* (Anti-B) show evidence of previous or current infection
- Enzyme-linked immunosorbent assay (ELISA), enzyme immunoassay, or indirect immunofluorescence microscopy reveal presence of antibodies
  - Immunoglobulin (Ig) M levels peak 3 to 6 weeks after infection
  - IgG antibodies are detected several weeks after infection and may continue to develop for months and persist for years

Key facts about Lyme disease
- Caused by a spirochete transmitted through a deer tick bite
  - Incubates for 3 to 32 days
  - Disseminates to other skin sites or organs through bloodstream or lymph
  - Can survive in joints for years

Key pathophysiologic changes in Lyme disease
- Red bull's-eye rash
- Flulike symptoms
- Joint swelling
- Arthritis
- Peripheral and cranial neuropathy

Key diagnostic test results for Lyme disease
- ELISA, enzyme immunoassay, or indirect immunofluorescence microscopy: Presence of antibodies
- Western blot assay: Positive for *B. burgdorferi*

- Western blot assay is positive, showing serologic evidence of past or current infection with *B. burgdorferi*
- Polymerase chain reaction (PCR) is used when joints and CSF are involved

Treatment
- Antibiotics to treat infection
- Anti-inflammatory agents to treat joint inflammation and pain
- Close observation for ptosis, strabismus, and diplopia, which indicate increased ICP and cranial nerve involvement
- Electrocardiography to detect arrhythmias or conduction abnormalities

Nursing considerations
- Report infections to the Centers for Disease Control and Prevention (CDC)
- Plan care to allow for adequate rest
- Administer antibiotics and other drugs prescribed for specific symptoms
- Assist with ROM and strengthening exercises
- Encourage verbalization and provide support
- Teach the patient ways of preventing Lyme disease, such as avoiding tick-infested areas, covering the skin with clothing, and using insect repellents

MENINGITIS

Definition
- Inflammation of the brain and spinal cord meninges
- Usually a result of bacterial infection
- May result from a virus, fungus, parasite, or other toxin
- Two primary types
    - Acute pyrogenic, which is commonly caused by *Streptococcus pneumoniae*, *Haemophilus influenzae*, *Neisseria meningitidis*, or *Escherichia coli*
    - Acute lymphatic, which is usually viral in origin
- Classified as acute, subacute, or chronic
- May involve all three meningeal membranes—the dura mater, arachnoid, and pia mater
- Complications are rare
- Factors contributing to good prognosis
    - Early recognition of the disease
    - Response of infecting organism to treatment
- If untreated, mortality is 70% to 100%
- Poorer prognosis for infants and elderly patients

Underlying pathophysiology
- Inflammation of the pia-arachnoid and subarachnoid space progresses to congestion of adjacent tissues and nerve cell destruction
- ICP increases because of exudates
- These changes lead to engorged blood vessels, disrupted cerebral blood supply, possible thrombosis, or rupture and cerebral infarction

Causes
- Bacterial pneumonia, sinusitis, or other bacterial infection
- Brain abscess
- Empyema
- Encephalitis

Key treatments for Lyme disease

- Antibiotics
- Anti-inflammatory agents

Key nursing considerations for Lyme disease

- Report infections to CDC.
- Allow for adequate rest.
- Administer antibiotics and other drugs.

Key facts about meningitis

- Inflammation of brain and spinal cord meninges
- Progresses to congestion of adjacent tissues and nerve cell destruction
- Associated with increased ICP
- May lead to thrombosis or rupture and cerebral infarction

- Endocarditis
- Fungal infection
- Lumbar puncture
- Myelitis
- Osteomyelitis
- Aseptic meningitis
- Otitis media
- Penetrating head wound
- Skull fracture
- Tuberculosis
- Ventricular shunting
- Viral infection

Pathophysiologic changes

- Fever, chills, malaise, petechial rash, and tachycardia resulting from infection and inflammation
- Headache, vomiting and, rarely, papilledema (inflammation and edema of the optic nerve) due to increased ICP
- Nuchal rigidity, positive Brudzinski's and Kernig's signs, exaggerated and symmetrical deep tendon reflexes, and opisthotonos (a spasm in which the back and extremities arch backward so that the body rests on the head and heels) due to meningeal irritation
- Sinus arrhythmias due to irritation of the nerves of the autonomic nervous system
- Irritability because of increasing ICP
- Photophobia, diplopia, and other vision problems resulting from cranial nerve irritation
- Delirium, deep stupor, and coma caused by increased ICP and cerebral edema

Complications

- Amputation of one or more extremities
- Brain abscess
- Cerebral infarction
- Coma
- Cranial nerve deficits including optic neuritis and deafness
- Death
- Encephalitis
- Endocarditis
- Hydrocephalus
- Increased ICP
- Paresis or paralysis
- Seizures
- Syndrome of inappropriate antidiuretic hormone secretion
- Additional complications in children
  - Epilepsy
  - Mental retardation
  - Subdural effusions
  - Unilateral or bilateral sensory hearing loss

Diagnostic test findings

- Lumbar puncture findings vary depending on the type of meningitis (see *Lumbar puncture,* page 128)

(see *Lumbar puncture,* page 128)

Key pathophysiologic changes in meningitis

- Fever and malaise
- Petechial rash
- Headache
- Vomiting
- Nuchal rigidity

Key complications of meningitis in children

- Seizure disorder
- Mental retardation
- Hearing loss

Key diagnostic test results for meningitis

- Lumbar puncture: Elevated CSF pressure, cloudy or milky white CSF, high protein level, positive Gram stain and culture in bacterial meningitis; elevated CSF pressure, lymphocytes, and protein level in viral meningitis
- Blood, urine, and nose cultures: Presence of offending organism

TOP 4

Teaching points about lumbar puncture

1. Purpose of procedure
2. Proper position for procedure
3. Need for remaining still throughout procedure
4. Length of time to lay flat after procedure

TIME-OUT FOR TEACHING

Lumbar puncture

Lumbar puncture is a common test for patients with meningitis. Teaching your patient what to expect can help minimize complications and adverse effects. Be sure to include these points in your teaching:

- Lumbar puncture involves inserting a hollow needle into the subarachnoid space surrounding the spinal cord to remove spinal fluid for analysis. This test also measures spinal column pressure.
- The procedure takes about 15 minutes.
- The patient lies on his side with his chin and knees tucked in, or sits with his head bent toward his knees.
- The patient is encouraged to void before the procedure.
- Before inserting the needle, the puncture site is cleaned with an antiseptic that may feel cold to the skin. Then, a local anesthetic is administered with a tiny needle. This drug may cause temporary stinging before the numbness occurs. The patient should report any other sensations, such as tingling or sharp pain.
- The patient needs to remain still throughout the procedure to avoid dislodging the needle. He may be asked to breathe deeply or straighten his legs. He may feel pressure applied briefly to his jugular vein at this time.
- After the test, the patient must lie flat (keep his head at or below hip level) for 4 to 24 hours and drink plenty of fluids to prevent a headache.

- Bacterial meningitis
  - CSF pressure is elevated due to obstructed CSF outflow at the arachnoid villi
  - CSF is cloudy or milky white
  - Protein level is high
  - Gram stain and culture are positive
  - Glucose concentration is decreased
- Viral meningitis
  - CSF pressure is elevated
  - Lymphocytes are elevated
  - Protein level is slightly elevated
  - Glucose concentration is normal
- Cultures of blood, urine, and nose and throat secretions reveal the offending organism (if cause is bacterial)
- Chest X-ray may reveal pneumonitis or lung abscess, tubercular lesions, or granulomas secondary to a fungal infection
- Sinus and skull X-rays may identify cranial osteomyelitis or paranasal sinusitis as the underlying infectious process, or a skull fracture, which can serve as an entrance for the causative microorganism
- WBC count is elevated
- CT scan may reveal hydrocephalus or rule out cerebral hematoma, hemorrhage, or tumor as the underlying cause

Treatment

- Appropriate I.V. antibiotics for at least 2 weeks, followed by oral antibiotics selected by culture and sensitivity testing
- Digoxin (Lanoxin) to control arrhythmias
- Mannitol (Osmitrol) to decrease cerebral edema
- **Anticonvulsant (usually given I.V.) or a sedative to reduce restlessness and prevent or control seizure activity**
- Aspirin or acetaminophen (Tylenol) to relieve headache and fever
- Bed rest to prevent increases in ICP
- Fluid therapy (given cautiously if cerebral edema and increased ICP are present) to prevent dehydration
- Appropriate therapy for any coexisting conditions, such as endocarditis or pneumonia
- Possible prophylactic antibiotics after ventricular shunting procedures, skull fracture, or penetrating head wounds to prevent infection (controversial)
- Ventilatory support if needed

Nursing considerations

- Maintain standard precautions during care
- Use droplet precautions in addition to standard precautions for meningitis caused by *H. influenzae* and *N. meningitidis* until 24 hours after the start of effective therapy
- **Assess neurologic function often**
  - Observe LOC
  - Monitor the patient for signs of increased ICP (vomiting, seizures, and a change in motor function and vital signs)
  - Monitor the patient for signs of cranial nerve involvement (ptosis, strabismus, and diplopia)
- Monitor fluid balance
  - Measure central venous pressure, and intake and output accurately
- Watch for adverse effects of I.V. antibiotics and other drugs
- Position the patient carefully to prevent joint stiffness and neck pain
  - Turn him often, according to positioning schedule
  - Assist with ROM exercises
- Maintain adequate nutrition and elimination
  - It may be necessary to provide frequent small meals or to supplement meals with NG tube or parenteral feedings
  - To prevent constipation and straining at stool, give the patient a mild laxative or stool softener, as ordered
- Provide mouth care regularly
- Maintain a quiet environment
- Darkening the room may decrease photophobia
- Teach patients with chronic sinusitis or other chronic infections the importance of proper medical treatment
- **Follow strict sterile technique when treating patients with head wounds or skull fractures**
- Give prophylactic antibiotics to persons in close physical contact with the patient before and during illness
- Provide meningitis vaccine to college-age persons as a preventative measure
- Monitor respiratory status for complications

MULTIPLE SCLEROSIS

Key facts about MS

- Involves sporadic patches of axon demyelination and nerve fiber loss throughout the CNS
- Results in varied neurologic dysfunction
- Characterized by exacerbations and remissions

Conditions that can precede onset or exacerbation of MS

- Emotional stress
- Fatigue
- Pregnancy
- Acute respiratory infections

Key pathophysiologic changes in MS

- Sensory impairment, such as burning and pins and needles
- Weakness
- Diplopia, blurred vision, and nystagmus
- Gait ataxia
- Fatigue

Definition
- Also known as MS
- Involves demyelination of the white matter of the brain, spinal cord, and optic nerve and damage to nerve fibers and their targets, which affects the CNS
- Is a major cause of chronic disability in individuals between ages 20 and 50
- Generally characterized by exacerbations and remissions (relapsing-remitting type)
- Allows 70% of patients to lead active, productive lives with prolonged remissions
- May progress rapidly (primary progressive, secondary progressive, and progressive-relapsing types)
  - Can disable the patient by early adulthood or cause death within months of onset

Underlying pathophysiology
- Widely disseminated and varied neurologic dysfunction induced by sporadic patches of axon demyelination and nerve fiber loss throughout the CNS (see *How myelin breaks down*)

Causes
- Unknown
- Possible autoimmune response to slow-acting or latent viral infection
- Environmental factors
- Genetic factors
- Conditions that appear to precede onset or exacerbation
  - Emotional stress
  - Fatigue (physical or emotional)
  - Pregnancy
  - Acute respiratory infections

Pathophysiologic changes
- Sensory impairment, such as burning, pins and needles, and electrical sensations; fatigue related to conduction deficits and impaired impulse transmission along the nerve fiber due to demyelination
- Optic neuritis, diplopia, ophthalmoplegia, blurred vision, and nystagmus resulting from impaired cranial nerve function and conduction deficits to the optic nerve
- Weakness, paralysis ranging from monoplegia to quadriplegia, spasticity, hyperreflexia, intention tremor, and gait ataxia from impaired motor reflex
- Incontinence, urinary frequency and urgency, and frequent infections from impaired transmission involving sphincter innervation
- Involuntary evacuation or constipation from altered impulse transmission to internal sphincter
- Poorly articulated or measured and slow speech and dysphagia from impaired transmission to the cranial nerves and sensory cortex
- Cognitive symptoms, including depression, euphoria, inattentiveness, apathy, forgetfulness, and memory loss, due to primary damage in the cerebrum

Complications
- Constipation

How myelin breaks down

Myelin speeds electrical impulses to the brain for interpretation. This lipoprotein complex formed of glial cells or oligodendrocytes protects the neuron's axon much like the insulation on an electrical wire. Its high electrical resistance and low capacitance allow the myelin to conduct nerve impulses from one node of Ranvier to the next.

Myelin is susceptible to injury; for example, by hypoxemia, toxic chemicals, vascular insufficiencies, or autoimmune responses. The sheath becomes inflamed, and the membrane layers break down into smaller components that become well-circumscribed plaques (filled with microglial elements, macroglia, and lymphocytes). This process is called *demyelination*.

The damaged myelin sheath can't conduct normally. The partial loss or dispersion of the action potential causes neurologic dysfunction.

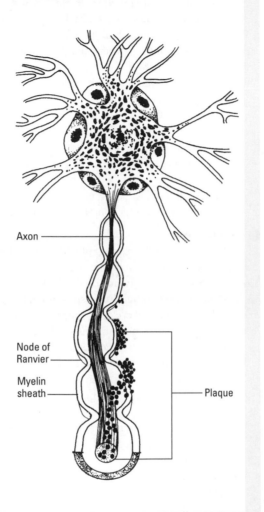

ABNORMAL NEURON

Axon

Node of Ranvier

Myelin sheath

Plaque

Key facts about myelin

- Speeds electrical impulses to the brain for interpretation
- Is susceptible to injury

- Depression
- Injuries from falls
- Joint contractures
- Pneumonia
- Pressure ulcers
- Rectal distention
- Seizures
- Sexual dysfunction
- Spasticity
- Speech and swallowing disorders
- Urinary tract infection

Key diagnostic test results for MS

- MRI: Multifocal white matter lesions
- Lumbar puncture: Normal total CSF protein, elevated IgG, possible elevated CSF WBC count
- Evoked potential studies: Slowed conduction of nerve impulses

Key treatments for MS

- Immune system therapy
- Stretching and ROM exercises
- Baclofen and tizanidine
- Frequent rest periods
- Treatment of associated bowel and bladder problems
- Adaptive devices
- Physical therapy
- Speech therapy
- Vision therapy or adaptive lenses

● **Diagnostic test findings**
- Diagnosis requires evidence of two or more neurologic dysfunctions
- MRI reveals multifocal white matter lesions
- EEG demonstrates abnormalities in brain waves in one-third of patients
- Lumbar puncture provides several findings
  - Total CSF protein is normal
  - IgG (gamma globulin) is elevated
    - IgG reflects hyperactivity of the immune system due to chronic demyelination
    - An elevated CSF IgG level is significant only when serum IgG level is normal
  - CSF WBC count may be elevated
- CSF electrophoresis detects bands of IgG in most patients, even when the percentage of IgG in CSF is normal
  - Presence of kappa light chains provides additional support to the diagnosis
- Evoked potential studies (visual, brain stem, auditory, and somatosensory) reveal slowed conduction of nerve impulses in most patients

● **Treatment**
- I.V. methylprednisolone (Solu-Medrol) followed by oral therapy
  - Reduces edema of the myelin sheath
  - Speeds recovery from acute attacks
- Possible use of other drugs, such as azathioprine (Imuran) or methotrexate (Rheumatrex) and cyclophosphamide (Cytoxan)
- Immune system therapy consisting of interferon (Actimmune) and glatiramer (Copaxone; a combination of four amino acids) to reduce frequency and severity of relapses and possibly slow CNS damage
- Stretching and ROM exercises, coupled with correct positioning, to relieve the spasticity resulting from opposing muscle groups relaxing and contracting at the same time
- Baclofen (Lioresal) and tizanidine (Zanaflex) to treat spasticity
- Botulinum toxin injections, intrathecal injections, nerve blocks, and surgery for severe spasticity
- Frequent rest periods, aerobic exercise, and cooling techniques (such as air conditioning, breezes, water sprays) to minimize fatigue
- Amantidine (Symmetrel), pemoline (Cylert), methylphenidate (Ritalin), or antidepressants to manage fatigue
- Treatment of associated bladder problems (failure to store urine, empty the bladder, or both) as appropriate
  - Drinking cranberry juice
  - Insertion of an indwelling urinary catheter and suprapubic tubes
  - Intermittent self-catheterization and postvoid catheterization programs
  - Anticholinergic medications
- Treatment of bowel problems (constipation and involuntary evacuation) as appropriate
  - Increasing fiber intake
  - Using bulking agents
  - Using bowel-training strategies, such as daily suppositories and rectal stimulation

- Management of sensory symptoms, such as pain, numbness, burning, and tingling sensations, with low-dose tricyclic antidepressants, phenytoin (Dilantin), or carbamazepine (Tegretol)
- Adaptive devices and physical therapy to assist with motor dysfunction, such as problems with balance, strength, and muscle coordination
- Possible use of beta-adrenergic blockers, sedatives, or diuretics to alleviate tremors
- Speech therapy to help manage dysarthria
- Antihistamines, vision therapy, or exercises to minimize vertigo
- Vision therapy or adaptive lenses to manage visual problems

● **Nursing considerations**
- Assist with physical therapy
- Increase patient comfort with massages and relaxing baths
- Educate the patient and his family about the disease
- Emphasize the need to avoid stress, infections, and fatigue and to maintain independence by developing new ways of performing daily activities
- Stress the importance of eating a nutritious, well-balanced diet that contains sufficient roughage and adequate fluids to prevent constipation
- Evaluate the need for bowel and bladder training during hospitalization
- Watch for adverse drug effects, such as muscle weakness and decreased muscle tone caused by skeletal muscle relaxers
- Promote emotional stability
  - Help the patient establish a daily routine to maintain optimal functioning
  - Encourage regular rest periods to prevent fatigue
  - Encourage daily physical exercise
- Inform the patient that exacerbations are unpredictable, necessitating physical and emotional adjustments in lifestyle
- Refer the patient to the National Multiple Sclerosis Society

MYASTHENIA GRAVIS

● **Definition**
- Autoimmune disease caused by antibody-mediated loss of acetylcholine receptors in the neuromuscular junction
- Commonly affects muscles innervated by the cranial nerves (face, lips, tongue, neck, and throat), but can affect any muscle group
- Involves sporadic but progressive weakness and abnormal fatigability of striated (skeletal) muscles
- Exacerbated by exercise and repeated movement
- Follows an unpredictable course of periodic exacerbations and remissions
- Onset generally between ages 20 and 30
- Is three times more common in women than in men
- Occurs along with thymic abnormalities in 75% of patients

● **Underlying pathophysiology**
- Transmission of nerve impulses at the neuromuscular junction fails
- Antireceptor antibodies block, weaken, or reduce the number of acetylcholine receptors available at each neuromuscular junction, thereby impairing the muscle depolarization necessary for movement (see *Impaired transmission in myasthenia gravis,* page 134)

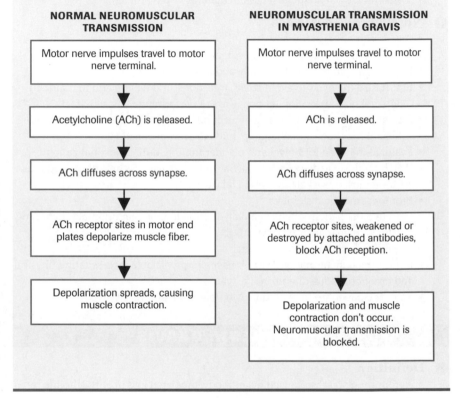

GO WITH THE FLOW

Impaired transmission in myasthenia gravis

In myasthenia gravis, transmission of nerve impulses at the neuromuscular junction fails. These flowcharts compare the sequence of normal neuromuscular transmission with the impaired transmission that occurs in myasthenia gravis.

NORMAL NEUROMUSCULAR TRANSMISSION

Motor nerve impulses travel to motor nerve terminal.

↓

Acetylcholine (ACh) is released.

↓

ACh diffuses across synapse.

↓

ACh receptor sites in motor end plates depolarize muscle fiber.

↓

Depolarization spreads, causing muscle contraction.

NEUROMUSCULAR TRANSMISSION IN MYASTHENIA GRAVIS

Motor nerve impulses travel to motor nerve terminal.

↓

ACh is released.

↓

ACh diffuses across synapse.

↓

ACh receptor sites, weakened or destroyed by attached antibodies, block ACh reception.

↓

Depolarization and muscle contraction don't occur. Neuromuscular transmission is blocked.

Key pathophysiologic changes in myasthenia gravis

- Weak eye closure
- Ptosis
- Diplopia
- Progressive muscle weakness and loss of function
- Blank, expressionless facial appearance
- Weakened respiratory muscles
- Difficulty chewing, swallowing, or talking

Cause
- Autoimmune response leading to ineffective acetylcholine (ACh) release and inadequate muscle fiber response to ACh

Pathophysiologic changes
- Weak eye closure, ptosis, and diplopia resulting from impaired neuromuscular transmission to the cranial nerves supplying the eye muscles (may be the only symptom)
- Progressive muscle weakness, fatigue, and accompanying loss of function (depending on muscle group affected) due to impaired neuromuscular transmission
  - In the early stages, may present as easy fatigability of certain muscles with no other findings
  - In later stages, may be severe enough to cause paralysis

- Blank and expressionless facial appearance and nasal vocal tones secondary to impaired transmission of cranial nerves innervating the facial muscles
- Frequent nasal regurgitation of fluids and difficulty chewing and swallowing due to cranial nerve involvement
- Weakened neck muscles, with head tilting back to see or possible bobbing, due to impaired neuromuscular transmission
- Weakened respiratory muscles and decreased tidal volume and vital capacity resulting from impaired neuromuscular transmission to the diaphragm due to loss of ACh receptors in the appropriate junctions
    - Lead to breathing difficulties
    - Predispose the patient to pneumonia and other respiratory tract infections
    - Can lead to myasthenic crisis (mucles of respiration fail and ventilatory support is required)

Complications
- Aspiration
- Myasthenic crisis
- Pneumonia
- Respiratory distress

Diagnostic test findings
- Tensilon test (anticholinesterase test) confirms diagnosis by revealing temporarily improved muscle function within 30 to 60 seconds after I.V. injection of edrophonium (Tensilon) or neostigmine (Prostigmin), lasting up to 30 minutes
- Single-fiber electromyography with neural stimulation a specific muscle fiber shows progressive decrease in muscle fiber contraction (repetitive nerve stimulation of muscle groups is less accurate)
- Immunoassay tests demonstrate the presence of ACh receptor antibodies circulating in the blood
- Chest X-ray reveals thymoma in approximately 15% of patients

Treatment
- Anticholinesterase drugs, such as neostigmine and pyridostigmine (Regonol)
    - Counteract fatigue and muscle weakness and allow for about 80% of normal muscle function
    - Less effective as disease worsens
- Immunosuppressive therapy with corticosteroids, azathioprine (Imuran), cyclosporine (Neoral), and cyclophosphamide used in a progressive fashion to decrease the immune response toward acetylcholine receptors at the neuromuscular junction
- IgG during acute relapses, or plasmapheresis in severe exacerbations to suppress the immune system (effect is temporary)
- Thymectomy to remove thymomas and possibly induce remission in some cases of adult-onset myasthenia
- Tracheotomy, positive pressure ventilation, and vigorous suctioning to remove secretions and treat acute exacerbations that cause severe respiratory distress

Nursing considerations
- Establish neurologic and respiratory baselines
    - Monitor tidal volume and vital capacity regularly

Key diagnostic test results for myasthenia gravis
- Tensilon test: Temporarily improved muscle function within 30 to 60 seconds after I.V. injection of edrophonium or neostigmine, lasting up to 30 minutes
- Single-fiber electromyography: Progressive decrease in muscle fiber contraction

Key treatments for myasthenia gravis
- Anticholinesterase drugs
- Immunosuppressive therapy with corticosteroids, azathioprine, cyclosporine, and cyclophosphamide
- IgG during acute relapses
- Plasmapheresis in severe exacerbations

– The patient may need a ventilator and frequent suctioning to remove accumulating secretions
- Be alert for signs of an impending crisis
  – Increased muscle weakness
  – Respiratory distress
  – Difficulty in talking or chewing
- Anticipate immediate hospitalization and vigorous respiratory support for patients in myasthenic crisis
- Discontinue anticholinesterase drugs in myasthenic crisis until respiratory function improves
- Adhere closely to the ordered drug administration schedule to prevent relapses
- Be prepared to give atropine for anticholinesterase overdose or toxicity
- Plan exercise, meals, patient care, and activities to make the most of energy peaks; for example, give medication 20 to 30 minutes before meals to facilitate chewing or swallowing
- Allow the patient to participate in his care
- If the patient has difficulty swallowing, give soft, solid foods instead of liquids to lessen the risk of choking
- After a severe exacerbation, try to increase social activity as soon as possible
- Teach the patient how to recognize the adverse effects and signs and symptoms of toxicity of anticholinesterase drugs and corticosteroids
- Warn the patient to avoid strenuous exercise, stress, infection, and needless exposure to the sun or cold
- For patients with diplopia, suggest wearing an eye patch or glasses with one frosted lens
- Avoid aminoglycoside antibiotics, which can exacerbate myasthenia gravis
- Refer the patient to the Myasthenia Gravis Foundation

PARKINSON'S DISEASE

Definition
- Slowly progressive degenerative disorder of basal ganglia function that results in variable combinations of tremor, rigidity, and bradykinesia
- Onset usually after age 40
- More common in men than women

Underlying pathophysiology
- Dopaminergic neurons degenerate, causing loss of available dopamine
- Dopamine deficiency prevents affected brain cells from performing their normal inhibitory function
- Excess excitatory ACh occurs at the synapses
- Nondopaminergic receptors are also involved
- Motor neurons are depressed

Causes
- Exact cause unknown
- Possible causes

  – Dopamine deficiency, which prevents affected brain cells from performing their normal inhibitory function in the CNS
  – Exposure to toxins, such as manganese dust or carbon monoxide
  – Repeated trauma to the brain (such as in boxing injuries)
  – Stroke
  – Brain tumors

● **Pathophysiologic changes**
  • Muscle rigidity, akinesia, and an insidious tremor beginning in the fingers (unilateral pill-roll tremor) secondary to loss of inhibitory dopamine activity at the synapse
    – Increases during stress or anxiety
    – Decreases with purposeful movement and sleep
  • Muscle rigidity with resistance to passive muscle stretching, which may be uniform (lead-pipe rigidity) or jerky (cogwheel rigidity); high-pitched, monotone voice; masklike facial expression; and loss of posture control secondary to depletion of dopamine
  • Akinesia resulting from impaired dopamine action
    – Causes difficulty walking
    – Alters gait
      · Lacks normal parallel motion
      · May be retropulsive or propulsive
  • Drooling secondary to impaired regulation of motor function
  • Dysarthria, dysphagia, or both; excessive sweating; decreased motility of GI and genitourinary smooth muscle from impaired autonomic transmission
  • Orthostatic hypotension resulting from impaired vascular smooth muscle response
  • Oily skin secondary to inappropriate regulation of androgen production by the hypothalamic-pituitary axis
  • Endogenous depression, dementia from impaired dopamine metabolism, and neurotransmitter dysfunction

● **Complications**
  • Aspiration
  • Injury from falls
  • Pressure ulcers
  • Urinary tract infections

● **Diagnostic test findings**
  • Diagnosis primarily made by clinical history and neurologic examination
  • Diagnostic testing performed to rule out other disorders
  • CT scan or MRI rules out such other disorders as intracranial tumors
  • Positron emission tomography scan and single-photon emission CT can be diagnostic but are not readily available or affordable

● **Treatment**
  • Levodopa (Larodopa) to replace dopamine
    – Most effective during early stages
    – Given in increasing doses until symptoms are relieved or adverse effects appear

---

Key pathophysiologic changes in Parkinson's disease

● Muscle rigidity
● Akinesia that alters gait
● Drooling
● Dysarthria, dysphagia, or both
● Excessive sweating
● Decreased motility of GI and genitourinary smooth muscle

Key diagnostic test results for Parkinson's disease

● None readily available except to rule out other disorders
● CT scan or MRI: Rules out other disorders

Key treatments for Parkinson's disease

● Levodopa
● Anticholinergics and antihistamines
● Amantadine or selegiline
● Stereotactic neurosurgery

TOP 3

Teaching topics for patients with Parkinson's disease

1. Disease process and its progressive stages
2. Adverse effects of drug therapy
3. Safety measures to prevent injury

TIME-OUT FOR TEACHING

Topics for patients with Parkinson's disease

Be sure to include these points in your teaching plan for patients with Parkinson's disease:
- disease process and its progressive stages
- adverse effects of drug therapy
- ways to prevent falls, pressure ulcers, and contractures
- dietary restrictions imposed by use of levodopa
- household safety measures to prevent accidents
- referral to the National Parkinson Foundation and the United Parkinson Foundation
- referral to resources for home assistance or financial aid as needed.

  – Usually given in combination with carbidopa (Sinemet) to halt peripheral dopamine synthesis
- Alternative drug therapy, including anticholinergics and antihistamines, amantadine (Symmetrel), or selegiline (Eldepryl), to conserve dopamine and enhance the therapeutic effect of levodopa when levodopa is no longer effective
- Stereotactic neurosurgery to prevent involuntary movement
  – Most effective in young, otherwise healthy patients with unilateral tremor or muscle rigidity
- Deep brain stimulation to decrease tremors and allow normal function
  – An alternative for patients for whom conventional treatment fails
  – Involves implantation of neurostimulator and electrodes that stimulate the globus pallidus subthalmic nucleus
- Fetal cell transplantation (experimental), in which fetal brain tissue is injected into the patient's brain to possibly allow the brain to process dopamine, thereby halting or reducing the disease progression
- Active and passive ROM exercises, maintenance of routine daily activities, walking, baths, and massage to help relax muscles

Nursing considerations
- Monitor drug treatment and adjust dosage, if necessary, to minimize adverse effects.
- After surgery, watch for signs and symptoms of hemorrhage and increased ICP by frequently checking LOC and vital signs
- Encourage the patient to achieve partial control of his body by sitting on a chair and using its arms to steady himself
- Advise the patient to change position slowly and dangle his legs before getting out of bed
- Help the patient overcome problems related to eating and elimination
  – Help establish a regular bowel routine by encouraging him to drink at least 2 qt (about 2 L) of liquids daily and eat high-fiber foods

Key nursing considerations for Parkinson's disease

- Monitor drug treatment and adjust dosage, if necessary.
- After surgery, watch for signs and symptoms of hemorrhage and increased ICP.
- Advise patient to change position slowly and dangle legs before getting out of bed.
- Help patient overcome problems related to eating and elimination.

– The patient may need an elevated toilet seat to assist his movement from a standing to a sitting position
• Give the patient and his family emotional support and provide patient teaching (see *Topics for patients with Parkinson's disease*)

SEIZURE DISORDER

● **Definition**
• Sudden explosive and disorderly discharge of cerebral neurons
• Characterized by a sudden, transient alteration in brain function
• Primary seizure disorder (epilepsy)
  – Idiopathic
  – No apparent structural changes in the brain
• Secondary epilepsy
  – Has a known cause, such as trauma or stroke
  – Characterized by structural changes or metabolic alterations of the neuronal membranes that cause increased automaticity
• Types of seizures
  – Partial seizures
    • Caused by electrical abnormality in the brain
    • Arise from a localized part of the brain
    • Simple partial seizures
      - Remain local
      - Affect autonomic, sensory, and psychiatric areas without altering consciousness
    • Complex partial seizures
      - Cascade further into adjacent nerve cells
      - Alter consciousness
      - Patient maintains ability to follow simple commands during the episode
  – Generalized seizures
    • Caused by electrical abnormality in the brain
    • Tonic-clonic seizures
      - Convulsive
      - Involve loss of consciousness
      - Last 2 to 5 minutes
    • Absence seizures
      - Involve brief change in LOC
      - No associated motor involvement
    • Myoclonic seizures
      - Don't affect consciousness
      - Involve brief muscle jerking
  – Status epilepticus
    • Prolonged seizure state
    • Can occur in any type of seizure
    • Most life-threatening in tonic-clonic seizures
    • May lead to unconsciousness, loss of sphincter control, and apnea
  – Unclassified seizures
    • Involve seizure episodes with features that don't match any of the above criteria

Key facts about seizure disorder
● Sudden explosive and disorderly discharge of cerebral neurons
● Occurs when cerebral neurons function as an epileptogenic focus, which fires more readily than normal and spreads electric current to surrounding cells
● Stimulates cells to fire and the impulse cascades to one side of the brain, both sides of the brain, or the cortical, subcortical, and brain stem areas

Main seizure types
● Partial seizures
● Generalized seizures
● Status epilepticus
● Unclassified seizure

Underlying pathophysiology
- Some neurons in the brain may depolarize easily or be hyperexcitable
  - These neurons function as an epileptogenic focus
  - The epileptogenic focus fires more readily than normal when stimulated
  - In these neurons, the membrane potential (the potential energy maintained within the membrane surrounding the nerve cell) at rest is less negative or inhibitory connections are missing, possibly as a result of decreased GABA activity or localized shifts in electrolytes
- On stimulation, the epileptogenic focus fires locally or throughout the cerebrum and spreads electric current to surrounding cells
- Cells fire in turn and the impulse cascades to one side of the brain (a partial seizure), both sides of the brain (a generalized seizure), or the cortical, subcortical, and brain stem areas

Causes
- Idiopathic (in about two-thirds of all seizure disorders)
- Anoxia
- Birth trauma (inadequate oxygen supply to the brain, blood incompatibility, or hemorrhage)
- Brain tumors
- Drug or alcohol abuse or rapid withdrawal from abused drugs
- Febrile illness (especially common in young children)
- Genetic predisposition
- Head injury or trauma
- Infectious diseases (meningitis, encephalitis, or brain abscess)
- Ingestion of toxins (mercury, lead, or carbon monoxide)
- Inherited disorders or degenerative disease, such as phenylketonuria or tuberous sclerosis
- Metabolic disorders, such as hypoglycemia and hypoparathyroidism
- Myoclonic syndromes
- Perinatal infection
- Stroke (hemorrhage, thrombosis, or embolism)

Pathophysiologic changes
- Recurring seizures, possibly of more than one type (hallmark of epilepsy)
- Visual, olfactory, or auditory hallucinations; sweating or flushing; dream states, anger, or fear reactions resulting from simple partial seizures
- Altered consciousness, such as amnesia for events around the time of the seizure, resulting from complex partial seizures
- Movement and muscle involvement resulting from tonic-clonic or myoclonic seizures
- Brief changes in LOC without motor involvement due to absence seizures

Complications
- Hypoxia or anoxia from airway occlusion
- Traumatic injury
- Brain damage
- Depression and anxiety

Diagnostic test findings
- CT scan or MRI reveals abnormalities
- EEG reveals paroxysmal abnormalities and provides evidence of the continuing tendency to have seizures

– In tonic-clonic seizures, high, fast voltage spikes are present in all leads
– In absence seizures, rounded spike wave complexes are present
– A negative EEG doesn't rule out epilepsy because the abnormalities occur intermittently
- Skull X-ray may show evidence of fractures or shifting of the pineal gland, bony erosion, or separated sutures
- Serum chemistry blood studies may reveal hypoglycemia, electrolyte imbalances, and elevated liver enzyme and alcohol levels

● **Treatment**
- Drug therapy specific to the type of seizure
  – Phenytoin (Dilantin), carbamazepine (Tegretol), phenobarbital (Barbita, Luminal), gabapentin (Neurontin), and primidone (Mysoline) for generalized tonic clonic seizures and complex partial seizures
  – I.V. fosphenytoin (Cerebyx), an alternative to phenytoin that can be administered rapidly without the adverse cardiovascular effects that occur with phenytoin
  – Valproic acid (Depakene), clonazepam (Klonopin), and ethosuximide (Zarontin) for absence seizures
  – Gabapentin and felbamate (Felbatol) — used alone or in combination — for partial seizures when other drugs are ineffective
- If drug therapy is ineffective, surgery to remove a demonstrated focal lesion, or to remove the underlying cause, such as a tumor, abscess, or vascular problem
- Vagus nerve stimulator implant to help reduce the incidence of focal seizure
- I.V. diazepam (Valium), lorazepam (Ativan), phenytoin, or phenobarbital for status epilepticus
- Administration of dextrose (when seizures are secondary to hypoglycemia) or thiamine (in chronic alcoholism or withdrawal)

● **Nursing considerations**
- Assure the patient and his family that epilepsy is controllable for most patients who follow a prescribed regimen of medication and that most patients maintain a normal lifestyle
- Teach them about drug therapy and the need for compliance with the prescribed drug schedule
- Instruct the patient to report adverse effects of drug therapy immediately
  – Drowsiness, lethargy, hyperactivity, confusion, and vision and sleep disturbances indicate the need for dosage adjustment
  – Phenytoin therapy may lead to hyperplasia of the gums
- When administering phenytoin I.V., use a large vein
  – Monitor vital signs frequently
  – Avoid I.M. administration and mixing with dextrose solutions
- Emphasize the importance of having certain anticonvulsant drug blood levels checked at regular intervals, even if the seizures are under control
- Warn the patient against drinking alcoholic beverages
- Make appropriate referrals
  – Epilepsy Foundation of America for general information
  – State motor vehicle department for information about driving restrictions
- **Take proper precautions during a seizure**
  – Avoid restraining the patient

Key treatments for seizure disorder
● Drug therapy specific to type of seizure
● Surgery (if drug therapy isn't effective)
● I.V. therapy for status epilepticus

Key nursing considerations for seizure disorder
● Teach patient and family about the disease, safety precautions, and prescribed treatment.
● Focus on patient safety and breathing during seizure activity.
● Refer patient to support groups.

- Help the patient to a lying position
- Loosen any tight clothing
- Place something flat and soft, such as a pillow, jacket, or hand, under his head
- Clear the area of hard objects
- Don't force anything into the patient's mouth; doing so could lacerate the mouth and lips or displace teeth, precipitating respiratory distress
- If vomiting occurs, turn the head to provide an open airway
• After the seizure subsides
- Reorient the patient to time and place
- Inform him that he had a seizure

STROKE

● **Definition**
  • Sudden impairment of cerebral circulation in one or more blood vessels
  • Can be ischemic (a thrombus or embolus blocks circulation) or hemorrhagic (a blood vessel ruptures)
  • Varies in symptoms depending on artery affected, severity of damage, and extent of collateral circulation
  • Signs appear on opposite side of the body from where stroke occurred
  • Affects structures on same side of the body if cranial nerves are damaged

● **Underlying pathophysiology**
  • Thrombotic or embolic stroke
    - Arteries become blocked, leading autoregulatory mechanisms to maintain cerebral circulation until collateral circulation develops to deliver blood to the affected area
    - If the compensatory mechanisms become overworked, or if cerebral blood flow remains impaired for more than a few minutes, oxygen deprivation leads to infarction of brain tissue
    - Brain cells cease to function because they can't store glucose or glycogen or engage in anaerobic metabolism
    - Ischemia results in cerebral infarction
    - Tissue injury triggers an inflammatory response that in turn increases ICP
  • Hemorrhagic stroke
    - Impaired cerebral perfusion from hemorrhage causes infarction, and the blood itself acts as a space-occupying mass, exerting pressure on the brain tissues
    - Increased ICP forces CSF out, thus restoring the balance
    - If the hemorrhage is small, the patient may survive with only minimal neurologic deficits
    - If the bleeding is heavy, ICP increases rapidly and perfusion stops; even if the pressure returns to normal, many brain cells die
  • Specific manifestations of stroke are determined by the cerebral artery affected, the brain tissue supplied by that vessel, and the adequacy of the collateral circulation

Key facts about stroke

• Sudden impairment of cerebral circulation in one or more blood vessels

Thrombotic or embolic stroke
• Results when arteries become blocked and blood flow becomes impaired
• Leads to infarction of brain tissue
• Comprises 80% of strokes

Hemorrhagic stroke
• Occurs when impaired cerebral perfusion from hemorrhage causes infarction
• Comprises 20% of strokes

Causes
- Occluded blood flow caused by thrombosis of the cerebral arteries supplying the brain or the intracranial vessels (see *Understanding stroke,* page 144)
- Embolism from thrombus outside the brain, such as in the heart, aorta, or common carotid artery
- Hemorrhage from an intracranial artery or vein, such as from hypertension, ruptured aneurysm, AVMs, trauma, hemorrhagic disorder, or septic embolism

Risk factors
- Alcohol or cocaine
- Cardiac disease including atrial fibrillation and valvular disease
- Cigarette smoking
- Diabetes
- Familial hyperlipidemia
- Family history of stroke
- History of transient ischemic attacks
- Hypercholesterolemia
- Hypertension
- Increased alcohol intake
- Obesity, sedentary lifestyle
- Sickle cell disease
- Use of hormonal contraceptives

Pathophysiologic changes
- Aphasia, dysphasia; visual field deficits; and hemiparesis of affected side (more severe in face, arms) resulting from thrombosis or hemorrhage of middle cerebral artery
- Weakness, paralysis, numbness; sensory changes; altered LOC; bruits over carotid artery; and headache caused by thrombosis or hemorrhage of carotid artery
- Weakness, paralysis; numbness around lips and mouth; visual field deficits, diplopia, nystagmus; poor coordination, dizziness; dysphagia, slurred speech; amnesia; and ataxia resulting from thrombosis or hemorrhage of vertebro-basilary artery
- Confusion; weakness, numbness; urinary incontinence; impaired motor and sensory functions; and personality changes caused by thrombosis or hemorrhage of anterior cerebral artery
- Visual field deficits; sensory impairment; dyslexia; cortical blindness; and coma resulting from thrombosis or hemorrhage of posterior cerebral artery

Complications
- Altered LOC
- Aspiration
- Cerebral edema
- Cognitive impairment
- Contractures
- Fluid imbalances
- Infections such as pneumonia
- Paralysis
- Pulmonary embolism
- Sensory impairment

TOP 5
Risk factors for stroke
1. Advanced age
2. Hypertension
3. Smoking
4. Cardiac disease
5. Hypercholesterolemia

Key pathophysiologic changes in stroke
- Hemiparesis
- Visual field deficits
- Aphasia
- Dysphasia
- Confusion
- Personality changes

Understanding stroke

Strokes are typically classified as ischemic or hemorrhagic, depending on the underlying cause. In either type of stroke, the patient's brain is deprived of oxygen and nutrients.

ISCHEMIC STROKE

Ischemic stroke results from a blockage or reduction of blood flow to an area of the brain. The blockage may result from atherosclerosis or blood clot formation

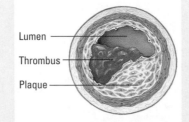

Lumen

Thrombus

Plaque

HEMORRHAGIC STROKE

Hemorrhagic stroke is caused by bleeding within and around the brain. Bleeding that fills the spaces between the brain and the skull (called *subarachnoid hemorrhage*) is caused by ruptured aneurysms, arteriovenous malformation, and head trauma. Bleeding within the brain tissue itself (known as *intracerebral hemorrhage*) is primarily caused by hypertension.

COMMON SITES OF PLAQUE FORMATION

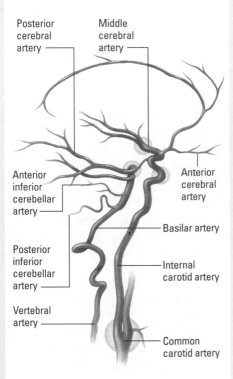

Posterior cerebral artery

Middle cerebral artery

Anterior inferior cerebellar artery

Posterior inferior cerebellar artery

Vertebral artery

Anterior cerebral artery

Basilar artery

Internal carotid artery

Common carotid artery

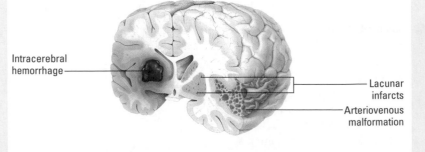

Intracerebral hemorrhage

Lacunar infarcts

Arteriovenous malformation

- Unstable blood pressure (from loss of vasomotor control)
- Death

● **Diagnostic test findings**
- CT scan identifies an ischemic stroke within the first 72 hours of symptom onset or evidence of a hemorrhagic stroke (lesions larger than 1 cm) immediately
- MRI assists in identifying areas of ischemia or infarction and cerebral swelling
- Cerebral angiography reveals an occlusion, such as stenosis or acute thrombus, or hemorrhage, that disrupts or displaces the cerebral circulation
- Digital subtraction angiography shows evidence of occlusion of cerebral vessels, lesions, or vascular abnormalities
- Carotid duplex scan identifies the degree of stenosis
- Brain scan shows ischemic areas but may not be conclusive for up to 2 weeks after a stroke
- Single photon emission CT and positron emission tomography scans identify areas of altered metabolism surrounding lesions
- Transesophageal echocardiogram reveals cardiac disorders, such as atrial thrombi, atrial septal defect, or patent foramen ovale, as causes of thrombotic stroke
- Lumbar puncture (performed if there are no signs of increased ICP) reveals bloody CSF in cases of hemorrhagic stroke
- Ophthalmoscopy may identify signs of hypertension and atherosclerotic changes in retinal arteries
- EEG helps identify damaged areas of the brain

● **Treatment**
- ICP management with monitoring and hyperventilation to reduce arterial carbon dioxide levels and ICP
- Osmotic diuretics (mannitol), and corticosteroids (dexamethasone), to reduce inflammation and cerebral edema
- Stool softeners to prevent straining, which increases ICP
- Anticonvulsants to treat or prevent seizures
- Surgery for large cerebellar infarction to remove infarcted tissue and decompress remaining live tissue
- Aneurysm repair to prevent further hemorrhage
- Percutaneous transluminal angioplasty or stent insertion to open occluded vessels
- For ischemic stroke
  - Thrombolytic therapy (tissue plasminogen activator, alteplase [Activase]) within the first 3 hours after the onset of symptoms to dissolve the clot, remove occlusion, and restore blood flow, thus minimizing cerebral damage
  - Anticoagulant therapy (heparin, warfarin) to maintain vessel patency and prevent further clot formation in cases of high-grade carotid stenosis or in newly diagnosed cardiovascular disease
- For hemorrhagic stroke
  - Analgesics, such as acetaminophen, to relieve headache

● **Nursing considerations**
- Maintain a patent airway and oxygenation
- If the patient is unconscious, he could aspirate saliva

Key nursing considerations for stroke

- Maintain patent airway and oxygenation.
- Keep patient in lateral position, as needed.
- Insert artificial airway and start mechanical ventilation or supplemental oxygen, if necessary.
- Monitor for signs and symptoms of increased ICP and nuchal rigidity or flaccidity.
- Check for gag reflex before feeding.
- If patient vomits, position him on his side to prevent aspiration.
- Position patient and align extremities correctly.
- Assist patient with exercises.
- Establish and maintain patient communication.
- Assist with rehabilitation.

- Keep him in a lateral position to allow secretions to drain naturally or suction secretions, as needed
- Insert an artificial airway, and start mechanical ventilation or supplemental oxygen, if necessary
- Check vital signs and neurologic status
  - Monitor blood pressure, LOC, pupillary changes, motor function, sensory function, speech, skin color, and temperature
  - Monitor the patient for signs and symptoms of increased ICP and nuchal rigidity or flaccidity
  - Report significant changes to the physician
- Watch for signs and symptoms of pulmonary emboli, such as chest pains, shortness of breath, dusky color, tachycardia, fever, and changed sensorium
- If the patient is unresponsive, monitor his blood gases often
- Maintain fluid and electrolyte balance
  - Administer I.V. fluids, as ordered; never give too much too fast because this can increase ICP
  - Offer the urinal or bedpan every 2 hours
- Ensure adequate nutrition
  - Check for gag reflex before offering small oral feedings of semisolid foods
  - Place the food tray within the patient's visual field because loss of peripheral vision is common
  - If oral feedings aren't possible, insert an NG tube
- Be alert for signs that the patient is straining at elimination because this increases ICP
  - Modify diet
  - Administer stool softeners, as ordered, and give laxatives, if necessary
- If the patient vomits (usually during the first few days), keep him positioned on his side to prevent aspiration
- Provide careful mouth care
- Provide meticulous eye care
  - Instill eyedrops as ordered
  - Patch the patient's affected eye if he can't close the lid
- Position the patient and align his extremities correctly
  - Use high-topped sneakers to prevent footdrop
  - Use contracture and convoluted foam, flotation, or pulsating mattress or sheepskin to prevent pressure ulcers
- Turn the patient at least every 2 hours to prevent pneumonia
- Elevate the affected hand to control dependent edema, and place it in a functional position
- Assist the patient with exercise
  - Perform ROM exercises for the affected and unaffected sides
  - Teach and encourage the patient to use his unaffected side to exercise his affected side
- Give medications, as ordered, and watch for and report adverse effects
- Establish and maintain communication with the patient; if he's aphasic, set up a simple method of communicating basic needs
- Provide psychological support
  - Set realistic short-term goals
  - Involve the patient's family in his care when possible

 – Explain his deficits and strengths
- Assist with rehabilitation
  – The amount of teaching needed depends on the extent of neurologic deficit
  – If necessary, reteach the patient to comb his hair, dress, and wash
  – With the aid of a physical therapist and an occupational therapist, obtain assistive devices, such as walking frames, hand bars by the toilet, and ramps, as needed
  – Be aware that the patient may experience unilateral neglect, in which he fails to recognize that he has a paralyzed side
    · Teach him to inspect the paralyzed side of his body for injury
    · Show him how to protect his body from harm
  – If indicated, encourage the patient to begin speech therapy as soon as possible and follow through with the speech pathologist's suggestions
- Instruct the patient or his family to report premonitory signs of a stroke, such as severe headache, drowsiness, confusion, and dizziness
- Emphasize the importance of regular follow-up visits
- If aspirin has been prescribed to minimize the risk of ischemic stroke, tell the patient to watch for possible GI bleeding

WEST NILE ENCEPHALITIS

● **Definition**
- Vector-borne infectious disease that primarily causes encephalitis (inflammation) of the brain
- Mortality is 3% to 15% (higher among elderly population)

● **Underlying pathophysiology**
- Virus has an incubation period of 5 to 15 days after exposure
- Mosquitoes become infected by feeding on birds contaminated with the virus
- The virus is transmitted to a human by the bite of an infected mosquito (mostly the *Culex* species)
- Encephalitis of the brain results

● **Cause**
- West Nile virus, a flavivirus commonly found in birds, mosquitoes, humans, and other vertebrates

● **Pathophysiologic changes**
- Mild infection (most common); flulike symptoms (headache and body aches); swollen lymph glands; and rash resulting from transmission of the virus into the bloodstream
- Severe infection characterized by headache, high fever, neck stiffness, stupor, disorientation, coma, tremors, occasional seizures, paralysis caused by inflammation of brain and spinal cord (occurs as virus travels to neurologic system)

● **Complications**
- Neurologic impairment
- Seizures
- Death

● Diagnostic test findings

- WBC count is normal or increased
- MAC-ELISA detects the IgM for the virus
- CSF analysis reveals elevated WBC count and protein levels
- MRI may show inflammation
- Plaque reduction neutralization test (PRNT) differentiates the specific type of flavivirus when the MAC-ELISA test is false-positive

● Treatment

- Hospitalization for severe infection
- I.V. fluids to maintain adequate hydration
- Airway management to maintain open airway
- Ventilator support to provide adequate oxygenation and ventilation
- Medications such as antipyretics

● Nursing considerations

- Maintain adequate hydration with I.V. fluids
- Provide respiratory support measures when needed
- Follow standard precautions when handling blood or other body fluids
- Report suspected cases of West Nile encephalitis to the state department of health
- Provide rest periods when the patient is fatigued
- Monitor fluid and electrolyte status, neurologic status, and vital signs
- Discuss with the patient precautions to control propagation of mosquitoes at home

NCLEX CHECKS

It's never too soon to begin your licensure examination preparation. Now that you've reviewed this chapter, carefully read each of the following questions and choose the best answer. Then compare your responses with the correct answers.

1. Behavioral problems in a client with Alzheimer's disease can be worsened by:
- ☐ **1.** effective communication.
- ☐ **2.** reorientation.
- ☐ **3.** excess stimulation.
- ☐ **4.** exercise.

2. A client presents to the emergency department with hyperreflexia, difficulty swallowing, and emotional lability. These signs and symptoms most likely indicate which nervous system disorder?
- ☐ **1.** ALS
- ☐ **2.** Myasthenia gravis
- ☐ **3.** MS
- ☐ **4.** Alzheimer's disease

3. A client is being evaluated for Bell's palsy. The nurse teaches the client that Bell's palsy is a disease of which cranial nerve?
- ☐ **1.** II
- ☐ **2.** III
- ☐ **3.** V
- ☐ **4.** VII

4. A client with a subarachnoid hemorrhage has been admitted to the unit. His neurologic assessment indicates right-sided weakness and stupor with nuchal rigidity. What grade would you assign this aneurysm?

- ☐ **1.** II
- ☐ **2.** III
- ☐ **3.** IV
- ☐ **4.** V

5. To minimize the risk of rebleed in a client with an intracranial aneurysm, a nurse should place the head of the bed no higher than:

- ☐ **1.** 45 degrees.
- ☐ **2.** 30 degrees.
- ☐ **3.** 15 degrees.
- ☐ **4.** 10 degrees.

6. A client is hospitalized for observation following a head injury. On the second day, he's found having continuous tonic-clonic seizures. The physician orders an immediate injection of 15 mg/kg phenytoin I.V. The client's weight on admission was 176 lb. In grams, what total dose of phenytoin should be administered by slow I.V. infusion?

_____

7. A nurse is reviewing laboratory test results for a client with Lyme disease. The nurse would expect which of the following diagnostic test to show elevated Ig levels?

- ☐ **1.** Assays for Anti-B
- ☐ **2.** Western blot assay
- ☐ **3.** PCR
- ☐ **4.** ELISA

8. A client is being treated for Parkinson's disease. The nurse should monitor the client for which skin abnormality?

- ☐ **1.** Acne
- ☐ **2.** Psoriasis
- ☐ **3.** Oily skin
- ☐ **4.** Dry skin

9. A client reports that he's having episodes in which he becomes hot and flushed, sees lights flashing, and feels extremely fearful for a few seconds. About what type of seizure should the nurse expect to teach the client?

- ☐ **1.** Complex partial
- ☐ **2.** Simple partial
- ☐ **3.** Generalized
- ☐ **4.** Status epilepticus

TOP 6

Items to study for your next test on the nervous system

1. Pathophysiology of common disorders of the nervous system, such as multiple sclerosis, Parkinson's disease, seizure disorder, and stroke
2. Causes of and treatments for increased ICP
3. Preparation and postprocedure care for lumbar puncture
4. Classes of medications that improve cerebral edema
5. Primary nursing considerations for patients with nervous system emergencies, such as intracranial hemorrhage, myasthenic crisis, status epilepticus, and ischemic stroke
6. The five levels of altered consciousness

10. A client comes to the emergency department with unilateral weakness and aphasia. The nurse anticipates preparing the client for testing and, potentially, thrombolytic therapy if symptoms occur within how many hours of onset?

- ☐ **1.** 3
- ☐ **2.** 4
- ☐ **3.** 8
- ☐ **4.** 12

ANSWERS AND RATIONALES

1. CORRECT ANSWER: 3

Excess stimulation and changes in established routine can worsen behavioral problems in the patient with Alzheimer's disease because changes in neurotransmitter metabolism can lead to emotional lability. Effective communication, reorientation, and exercise are all appropriate nursing interventions for the patient with Alzheimer's disease.

2. CORRECT ANSWER: 1

ALS is a motor neuron disease that causes muscle atrophy and bulbar palsy. Hyperreflexia is caused by degeneration of upper and lower motor neurons. Difficulty swallowing is related to degeneration of cranial nerves V, IX, X, and XII. Emotional lability is a result of progressive bulbar palsy. Myasthenia gravis can also present with difficulty swallowing, but this disease is related to an intermittent muscular weakness and doesn't involve emotional lability. MS is characterized by visual or sensory changes, fatigue, and weakness that persists or remits. Memory and cognitive decline are symptoms of Alzheimer's disease.

3. CORRECT ANSWER: 4

In Bell's palsy, cranial nerve VII (the facial nerve) develops an inflammatory reaction that produces unilateral or bilateral facial weakness or paralysis. Cranial nerve II is the optic nerve controlling sight. Cranial nerve III is the oculomotor nerve involved primarily with eye movement. Cranial nerve V is the trigeminal nerve that primarily affects facial sensation.

4. CORRECT ANSWER: 3

The severity of a subarachnoid hemorrhage is graded according to the patient's signs and symptoms on a scale from I to V. Grade IV is characterized by severe bleeding, stupor, nuchal rigidity and, possibly, mild to severe hemiparesis.

5. CORRECT ANSWER: 2

Aneurysm precautions, which include bed rest in a quiet, darkened room with the head of the bed flat or less than 30 degrees, are imposed to minimize the risk of rebleed and to avoid increased ICP.

6. CORRECT ANSWER: 1.2

First, calculate the patient's weight in kilograms by using the conversion factor 1 kg = 2.2 lb:

$$\frac{1 \text{ kg}}{2.2 \text{ lb}} = \frac{x \text{ kg}}{176 \text{ lb}}$$

Cross-multiply and divide both sides by 2.2:

$$2.2x = 176$$
$$x = 80$$

Next, determine how many milligrams of phenytoin would be given:

$$15 \text{ mg} \times 80 \text{ kg} = 1{,}200 \text{ mg}$$

Finally, convert milligrams to grams:

$$1{,}200 \text{ mg} \div 1{,}000 = 1.2 \text{ g}.$$

7. CORRECT ANSWER: 4

ELISA shows IgM levels, which peak 3 to 6 weeks after infection, and IgG antibodies, which can be detected several weeks after infection and may continue to develop for several months to years. Assay for anti-B is a screening test for hepatitis. The Western blot assay is used to confirm HIV infection. The PCR test is used specifically for Lyme disease with joint and CSF involvement.

8. CORRECT ANSWER: 3

Oily skin may develop in patients with Parkinson's disease secondary to inappropriate regulation of androgen production by the hypothalamic-pituitary axis. Acne, dry skin, and psoriasis are unrelated to nervous system disorders.

9. CORRECT ANSWER: 2

Simple partial seizures affect autonomic, sensory, and psychiatric areas without altering consciousness. They result in visual, olfactory, or auditory hallucinations; sweating or flushing; and dream states, anger, or fear reactions. Complex partial seizures cascade further into adjacent nerve cells, resulting in altered consciousness. Status epilepticus occurs when neurons all over the brain depolarize together, causing prolonged involuntary motor activity that may lead to unconsciousness, loss of sphincter control, and apnea. Generalized seizures are similar to those seen in status epilepticus, but of a short duration as one burst of energy is discharged over the cerebrum.

10. CORRECT ANSWER: 1

Thrombolytic therapy must be used within the first 3 hours after the onset of symptoms to dissolve the clot, remove occlusion, and restore blood flow, thus minimizing cerebral damage.

Musculoskeletal system

LEARNING OBJECTIVES

After studying this chapter, you should be able to:

● Discuss the pathophysiology of altered bone conditions.

● Describe the relationship between presenting signs and symptoms of and the pathophysiologic changes for various musculoskeletal disorders.

● Identify causes for various musculoskeletal disorders.

● Identify classes of medications used to treat musculoskeletal disorders.

● Describe nursing considerations for various musculoskeletal disorders.

● List teaching goals for the patient with a musculoskeletal disorder.

CHAPTER OVERVIEW

The musculoskeletal system is a complex system of bones, joints, muscles, ligaments, tendons, and other tissues that protects vital organs and gives the body form and shape. It also stores calcium and other minerals in the bony matrix and provides sites for hematopoiesis in the marrow. In addition, the musculoskeletal system makes movement possible.

To care for a patient with a musculoskeletal disorder, you'll need an understanding of the signs and symptoms of these disorders and the pathophysiologic changes that occur. This chapter outlines key pathophysiologic concepts relating to the musculoskeletal system as well as to common musculoskeletal system disorders, including their underlying pathophysiology, associated changes, complications, diagnostic test findings, treatments, and nursing considerations.

PATHOPHYSIOLOGIC CONCEPTS

- **Altered bone density**
  - Normally, resorption and formation of bone occur in tandem to maintain bone mass in a steady state
  - Occurs when resorption exceeds formation
  - Common causes
    - Decreased estrogen levels in menopause, which may lead to diminished osteoblastic activity and loss of bone mass (called *osteoporosis*)
    - Vitamin D deficiency and inadequate calcium absorption in children, which prevents normal bone calcification

- **Altered bone growth**
  - Insufficient blood supply to growing bones, resulting in avascular necrosis of epiphyseal growth plates (in children and adolescents)
  - Lack of blood to femoral head, leading to septic necrosis and bone softening and resorption
  - Revascularization, which initiates new bone formation in femoral head or tibial tubercle, causing femoral head malformation

- **Altered bone strength**
  - Weakened bone due to loss of inorganic salts that constitute the chemical structure of bone
  - Occurs in cancellous (porous) bone more quickly than in cortical bone because cancellous bone is more sensitive to metabolic influences of conditions that produce rapid bone loss

- **Muscle atrophy**
  - Decrease in the size of muscle tissues or cells
  - Decrease in the size and thickness of myofibrils (the filaments within each muscle cell that align to form bands of muscle fibers with neighboring cells)
  - Conditions promoting atrophy
    - After prolonged inactivity due to bed rest or trauma
      - Associated with muscle deconditioning
      - Muscle deconditioning may be apparent in a matter of days
    - When local nerve damage makes movement impossible
    - When illness removes needed nutrients from muscles

CARPAL TUNNEL SYNDROME

- **Definition**
  - Form of repetitive stress injury
  - Most common nerve entrapment syndrome
  - Involves compression of the median nerve as it passes through the canal (tunnel) formed by the carpal bones and transverse carpal ligaments

- **Underlying pathophysiology**
  - Inflammation or fibrosis of the tendon sheaths that pass through the carpal tunnel usually causes edema and compression of the median nerve (see *The carpal tunnel*, page 154)

Key facts about altered bone density

- Occurs when resorption exceeds formation
- Commonly caused by decreased estrogen levels, vitamin D deficiency, or inadequate calcium intake

Key facts about altered bone growth

- Insufficient blood supply to growing bones

Key facts about altered bone strength

- Weakened bone due to loss of inorganic salts
- Occurs in cancellous bone more quickly than in cortical bone

Key facts about muscle atrophy

- Decrease in the size of muscle tissues or cells
- Decrease in the size and thickness of myofibrils
- Promoted by prolonged inactivity, local nerve damage, or illness

Key facts about carpal tunnel syndrome

- Form of repetitive stress injury
- Results from inflammation or fibrosis of the tendon sheaths that pass through the carpal tunnel
- Causes edema and compression of median nerve

The carpal tunnel

The carpal tunnel is clearly visible in this palmar view and cross section of a right hand. Note the blood vessels and median nerve flexor tendons of the fingers passing through the tunnel on their way from the forearm to the hand.

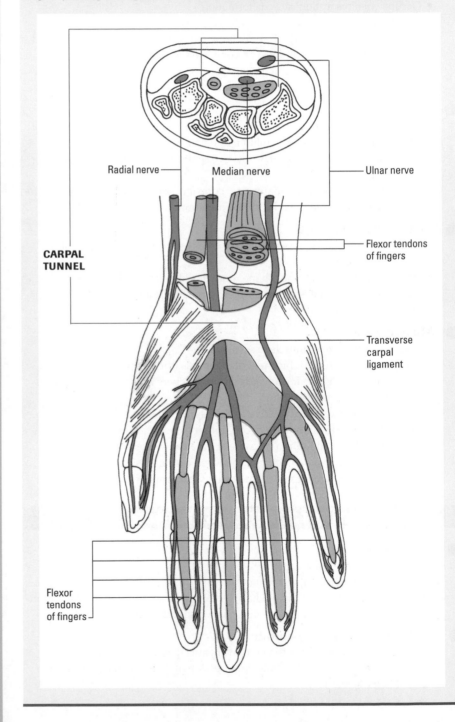

Radial nerve

Median nerve

Ulnar nerve

CARPAL
TUNNEL

Flexor tendons
of fingers

Transverse
carpal
ligament

Flexor
tendons
of fingers

- Sensory and motor changes in the median distribution of the hands occurs, initially impairing sensory transmission to the thumb, index finger, second finger, and inner aspect of the third finger

Causes
- Congenital predisposition
- Development of cyst or tumor within canal
- Fluid retention during pregnancy or menopause
- Hypothyroidism
- Mechanical problems in wrist joint
- Obesity
- Overactive pituitary gland
- Rheumatoid arthritis
- Trauma or injury to wrist
- Work-related stress

Pathophysiologic changes
- Weakness, pain, burning, numbness, or tingling of thumb, forefinger, middle finger, and one-half of fourth finger in one or both hands; atrophic nails; dry, shiny skin; and inability to clench the hand into a fist resulting from nerve compression
- Worsening of symptoms at night and in morning due to vasodilation and venous stasis

Complications
- Decreased wrist function
- Permanent nerve damage, with loss of movement and sensation

Diagnostic test findings
- Tinel's sign (tingling over the median nerve on light percussion) is positive
- Phalen's maneuver reproduces symptoms of carpal tunnel syndrome
- Compression test provokes paresthesia along the distribution of the median nerve

Treatment
- Splinting of the wrist in neutral extension for 1 to 2 weeks to rest the hand
- Nonsteroidal anti-inflammatory drugs (NSAIDs) to relieve symptoms
- Injection of hydrocortisone and lidocaine (Xylocaine) to provide significant but temporary relief of symptoms
- Surgery to relieve compression on the nerve
    - Resection of the entire transverse carpal tunnel ligament
    - Endoscopic surgical techniques
- Occupational therapy or job retraining (if a definite link has been established) to prevent recurrence of symptoms

Nursing considerations
- Administer mild analgesics as needed
- Encourage the patient to use his hands appropriately as much as possible, but with rest periods between activities
- Teach the patient how to apply a splint if necessary
    - Tell him not to make it too tight
    - Show him how to remove the splint to perform daily gentle range-of-motion (ROM) exercises

---

Key pathophysiologic changes in carpal tunnel syndrome

- Pain, burning, numbness, or tingling of thumb, forefinger, middle finger, and one-half of fourth finger in one or both hands
- Worsening of symptoms at night and in morning

Key diagnostic test results for carpal tunnel syndrome

- Tinel's sign: Positive
- Phalen's maneuver: Reproduces symptoms of carpal tunnel syndrome

Key treatments for carpal tunnel syndrome

- Splinting of wrist
- NSAIDs
- Hydrocortisone and lidocaine injection
- Surgery

Key nursing considerations for carpal tunnel syndrome
- After surgery, monitor vital signs and regularly check color, sensation, and motion of affected hand.
- Encourage patient to use hands as much as possible, resting between activities.

Key facts about gout
- Metabolic disease that causes painful arthritic joints
- Marked by urate deposits in the connective tissue, which trigger an acute inflammatory response
- May lead to hypertension or urate renal calculi

Key pathophysiologic changes in gout
- Joint pain due to inflammation
- Redness and swelling in joints caused by uric acid formation
- Tophi in great toe, ankle, and pinna of ear caused by urate deposits

- After surgery
  - Monitor vital signs and regularly check the color, sensation, and motion of the affected hand
  - Advise the patient who's about to be discharged to perform hand exercises
  - If the patient's arm is in a sling, tell him to remove the sling several times per day to perform exercises for his elbow and shoulder

GOUT

Definition
- Metabolic disease marked by urate deposits that cause painful arthritic joints
- Urate deposits found mostly in the foot (especially the great toe), ankle, and midfoot, but may affect any joint
- Follows an intermittent course; patient may be asymptomatic for years

Underlying pathophysiology
- Uric acid becomes supersaturated in the blood and body fluids
- Uric acid then crystallizes and forms a precipitate of urate salts that accumulates in connective tissue throughout the body
- Crystal deposits (called *tophi*) trigger an acute inflammatory response when neutrophils begin to ingest them
- Neutrophils release lysosomes that damage tissues and perpetuate the inflammation
- With gout that produces no symptoms
  - Serum urate levels increase but don't crystallize
  - Progression may cause hypertension or urate renal calculi

Causes
- Exact cause unknown
- Possible causes
  - Genetic defect in purine metabolism causing hyperuricemia
  - Retention of uric acid
  - Combination of the above
- Causes of secondary gout (develops during the course of another disease)
  - Alcoholism
  - Diabetes mellitus
  - Hypertension
  - Obesity
  - Renal disease
  - Sickle cell anemia

Pathophysiologic changes
- Joint pain due to uric acid deposits and inflammation
- Redness and swelling in joints due to uric acid deposits and irritation
- Tophi in the great toe, ankle, and pinna of ear due to urate deposits
- Elevated skin temperature resulting from inflammation

Complications
- Renal calculi
- Atherosclerotic disease

- Cardiovascular lesions
- Stroke
- Coronary thrombosis

● Diagnostic test findings
- Needle aspiration of synovial fluid shows needlelike monosodium urate crystals
- Serum uric acid levels are elevated with a gout attack
- White blood cell (WBC) count is elevated in acute attack
- Urine uric acid level is elevated in 20% of patients
- X-ray of the articular cartilage and subchondral bone shows evidence of chronic gout

● Treatment
- For acute gout
  - Immobilization and protection of the inflamed, painful joints
  - Local application of heat to stimulate circulation in the area and clear cellular debris from the inflammation
  - Local application of cold to decrease pain
  - Increased fluid intake (to 3 qt [3 L]/day if not contraindicated) to prevent renal calculi formation
  - Colchicine (oral or I.V.) every hour for 8 hours
    - Inhibits phagocytosis of uric acid crystals by neutrophils
    - Given until the pain subsides or nausea, vomiting, cramping, or diarrhea develops
  - NSAIDs to reduce pain and inflammation
- For chronic gout
  - Maintenance dosages of allopurinol (Aloprim) to suppress uric acid formation or control uric acid levels, preventing further attacks (used cautiously in patients with renal failure)
  - Cholchicine to prevent recurrent acute attacks until uric acid level returns to normal
  - Uricosuric agents and sulfinpyrazone (Anturane) to promote uric acid excretion and inhibit uric acid accumulation
  - Avoiding purine-rich foods (shellfish, liver, sardines, anchovies, cod, and kidneys) that increase urate levels

● Nursing considerations
- Encourage bed rest, but use a foot cradle to keep bed covers off extremely sensitive, inflamed joints
- Give pain medication as needed, especially during acute attacks
- Apply hot or cold packs to inflamed joints according to what the patient finds most effective
- Urge the patient to drink plenty of fluids to prevent formation of renal calculi
- Watch for gout attacks 24 to 96 hours after surgery
- Before and after surgery, administer colchicine, as ordered, to help prevent attacks
- Make sure the patient understands the importance of checking serum uric acid levels periodically and avoiding high-purine foods
- Teach the patient to report any adverse effects from medications immediately

Key diagnostic test results for gout

- Needle aspiration of synovial fluid: Presence of needlelike monosodium urate crystals
- Serum uric acid levels: Elevated
- X-ray of the articular cartilage and subchondral bone: Evidence of chronic gout

Key treatments for gout

Acute gout
- Immobilization and protection of joints
- Heat or cold application
- Colchicine
- NSAIDs

Chronic gout
- Allopurinol
- Colchicine
- Avoiding purine-rich foods

Key nursing considerations for gout

- Give pain medication as needed, especially during acute attacks.
- Urge patient to drink plenty of fluids to prevent renal calculi.
- Before and after surgery, administer colchicine, as ordered.
- Make sure patient understands importance of checking serum uric acid levels periodically and avoiding high-purine foods.

Key facts
about herniated
intervertebral disk

- Occurs when physical stress tears or ruptures the anulus fibrosus
- Causes nucleus pulposus to be forced through the disk's damaged anulus fibrosus
- Creates pressure on nerve roots, causing pain

Key pathophysiologic
changes in herniated
intervertebral disk

- Severe low back pain and sciatic pain
- Weakness and atrophy of leg muscles
- Numbness and tingling in nerve roots

Key diagnostic test
results for herniated
intervertebral disk

- Straight-leg raising test: Positive if patient has sciatic pain
- Myelogram, CT scan, and MRI: Spinal canal compression

HERNIATED INTERVERTEBRAL DISK

- **Definition**
  - Occurs when all or part of the nucleus pulposus (the soft, gelatinous, central portion of an intervertebral disk) is forced through the disk's weakened or torn outer ring (anulus fibrosus)
  - Occurs in the lumbar and lumbosacral regions (L5 and S1) in about 90% of cases

- **Underlying pathophysiology**
  - An intervertebral disk has two parts
    - Nucleus pulposus—the soft center
    - Anulus fibrosus—the tough, fibrous surrounding ring
  - Physical stress, usually a twisting motion, can tear or rupture the anulus fibrosus so that the nucleus pulposus herniates into the spinal canal
  - Vertebrae move closer together and the ruptured disk material exerts pressure on the nerve roots, causing pain and, possibly, sensory and motor loss
  - Herniation occurs in three stages
    - Protrusion—the nucleus pulposus presses against the anulus fibrosus
    - Extrusion—the nucleus pulposus bulges forcibly through the anulus fibrosus, pushing against the nerve root
    - Sequestration—the anulus fibrosus gives way as the disk's core bursts and presses against the nerve root
  - Minor trauma may lead to herniation if the patient has intervertebral joint degeneration (see *How a herniated disk develops*)

- **Causes**
  - Severe trauma or strain
  - Intervertebral joint degeneration

- **Pathophysiologic changes**
  - In lumbosacral disk disease, severe low back pain and sciatic pain resulting from compression of nerve roots supplying buttocks, legs, and feet
  - Muscle spasms due to pressure and irritation of sciatic nerve root
  - Weakness and atrophy of leg muscles (in later stages) resulting from inactivity
  - Pain, numbness, and tingling in affected spinal nerve roots caused by nerve irritation and inflammation from toxic reaction to release of proteoglycans that make the nucleus pulposus

- **Complications**
  - Neurologic deficits
  - Bowel and bladder problems

- **Diagnostic test findings**
  - Straight-leg raising test is positive only if the patient has posterior leg (sciatic) pain, not back pain
  - Lasègue's test reveals resistance and pain as well as loss of ankle or knee-jerk reflex, indicating spinal root compression
  - Spinal X-rays rule out other abnormalities but may not diagnose a herniated disk because a marked disk prolapse may not be apparent
  - Myelogram, computed tomography (CT) scan, and magnetic resonance imaging (MRI) reveal spinal canal compression by herniated disk material

How a herniated disk develops

These illustrations show how herniation of an intervertebral disk develops.

NORMAL VERTEBRA AND INTERVERTEBRAL DISK

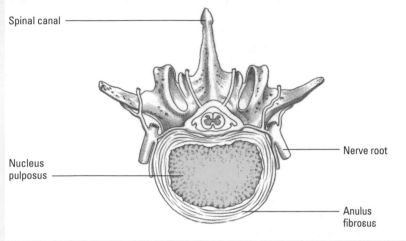

Spinal canal

Nucleus pulposus

Nerve root

Anulus fibrosus

Physical stress, from severe trauma or strain, or intervertebral joint degeneration may cause herniation. Herniation occurs in three stages: protrusion, extrusion, and sequestration.

PROTRUSION

EXTRUSION AND SEQUESTRATION

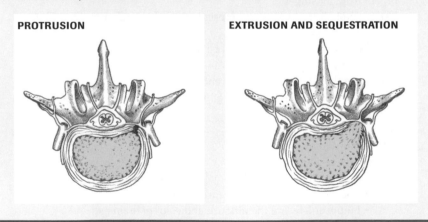

● **Treatment**
- Heat application to decrease muscle spasm and provide pain relief
- Exercise program to strengthen associated muscles and prevent further deterioration
- Corticosteroids or NSAIDs to reduce inflammation and edema at the site of injury
- Muscle relaxants to minimize muscle spasm from nerve root irritation
- Analgesics or epidural injections at the level of the protrusion to relieve pain

- Minimally invasive procedures, such as laser-assisted internal disc compression, coblation, automated percutaneous lumbar disc decompression, endoscopic disc excision, and chemonucleolysis with chymopapain (Chymodiactin when available) to repair small disc tears or ruptures
- Microsurgical laminoforaminotomy and disc excision (most commonly performed surgical treatment for ruptured discs and various related spinal conditions or multiple levels of abnormality)
- Surgery, including laminectomy to remove the extruded disk, spinal fusion to overcome segmental instability, or both to stabilize the spine when other treatment measures have failed

● **Nursing considerations**
- Before myelography
  - Ask about allergies to iodides, iodine-containing substances, or seafood
  - Such allergies may indicate sensitivity to the test's radiopaque dye
- After myelography
  - Urge the patient to remain in bed with his head elevated (especially if metrizamide was used)
  - Encourage the patient to drink plenty of fluids
  - Monitor intake and output
  - Watch for seizures and allergic reaction
- During conservative treatment, watch for deterioration in neurologic status (especially during the first 24 hours after admission), which may indicate an urgent need for surgery
- Use antiembolism stockings, as prescribed, and encourage the patient to move his legs, as allowed
- Work closely with a physical therapist to ensure a consistent regimen of leg and back stretching and strengthening exercises
- Encourage fluid intake to prevent renal stasis
- Encourage coughing and deep breathing to avoid pulmonary complications
- Provide good skin care
- Assess for bowel function
- After laminectomy or spinal fusion
  - Enforce bed rest as ordered
  - Check the tubing of blood drainage system frequently
    - Look for kinks; ensure a secure vacuum
    - Empty and record the amount and color of drainage
    - Report colorless or excessive drainage immediately
  - Observe neurovascular status of legs (color, motion, temperature, and sensation)
  - Monitor vital signs and check for bowel sounds and abdominal distention
  - Use the logrolling technique to turn the patient
  - Administer analgesics, as ordered, especially 30 minutes before initial attempts at sitting or walking
- Teach the patient who has undergone spinal fusion how to wear a brace and to use proper body mechanics
- Assist with straight-leg-raising and toe-pointing exercises, as ordered

---

Key nursing considerations for herniated intervertebral disk

- Ask about allergies to iodides, iodine-containing substances, or seafood.
- During conservative treatment, watch for deterioration in neurologic status.
- Ensure a consistent regimen of leg and back stretching and strengthening exercises.
- Advise patient to sleep on his side.
- If patient requires chemonucleolysis, make sure he isn't allergic to meat tenderizers.

After laminectomy or spinal fusion
- Enforce bed rest as ordered.
- Observe neurovascular status of legs.
- Administer analgesics, as ordered.

- Advise the patient to lie down when tired and to sleep on his side (never on his abdomen) on a moderately firm to extra-firm mattress
- Urge the patient to maintain proper weight to prevent lordosis caused by obesity
- **If the patient requires chemonucleolysis, make sure that he isn't allergic to meat tenderizers**
  - Chymopapain is a substance similar to meat tenderizers
  - **Such an allergy contraindicates the use of this enzyme, which can produce severe anaphylaxis in a sensitive patient**
- After chemonucleolysis, enforce bed rest, as ordered
  - Administer analgesics and apply heat, as needed
  - Urge the patient to cough and deep breathe
  - Teach him special exercises, and advise him to continue these exercises after discharge
- Teach the patient about adverse effects of prescribed medications
  - Muscle relaxants cause drowsiness
  - Advise the patient to avoid activities that require alertness

MUSCULAR DYSTROPHY

● Definition
- Group of congenital disorders characterized by progressive symmetrical wasting of skeletal muscles without neural or sensory defects
- Includes four main types
  - Duchenne's, or pseudohypertrophic (50% of all cases)
  - Becker's, or benign pseudohypertrophic
  - Landouzy-Dejerine, or facioscapulohumeral
  - Erb's (limb-girdle)

● Underlying pathophysiology
- Abnormally permeable cell membranes allow leakage of various muscle enzymes, particularly creatine kinase
- Phagocytosis of the muscle cells by inflammatory cells causes scarring and loss of muscle function
- As the disease progresses, skeletal muscle is almost totally replaced by fat and connective tissue
- Skeleton eventually becomes deformed, causing progressive immobility
- Cardiac and smooth muscles of the GI tract typically become fibrotic

● Causes
- Various genetic mechanisms typically involving an enzymatic or metabolic defect
- X-linked recessive disorders
- Autosomal dominant disorder (Landouzy-Dejerine)
- Autosomal recessive disorder (Erb's)

● Pathophysiologic changes
- Duchenne's
  - Waddling gait, toe-walking, and lumbar lordosis due to muscle weakness
  - Enlarged, firm calf muscles because of connective tissue and fat replacing muscle tissue

Key pathophysiologic changes in muscular dystrophy

Duchenne's and Becker's
- Waddling gait
- Toe-walking
- Lumbar lordosis

Landouzy-Dejerine
- Masklike expression
- Winging of the scapulae
- Inability to raise arms above the head

Erb's
- Winging of the scapulae
- Lordosis with abdominal protrusion
- Poor balance

Key diagnostic test results for muscular dystrophy

- Electromyography: Short, weak bursts of electrical activity in affected muscles
- Muscle biopsy: Confirms diagnosis

Key treatments for muscular dystrophy

- Coughing and deep-breathing exercises
- Physical therapy
- Surgery to promote or maintain mobility
- Low-calorie, high-protein, high-fiber diet
- Adequate fluid intake

– Tachycardia, electrocardiogram abnormalities, and pulmonary complications resulting from weakening of cardiac and respiratory muscles
- Becker's
  – Changes similar to those seen in Duchenne's but with a slower progression
- Landouzy-Dejerine
  – Pendulous lip, absence of the nasolabial fold, and inability to pucker mouth or whistle due to weakness of the voluntary facial muscles
  – Diffuse facial flattening that leads to a masklike expression caused by weakening of the facial muscles
  – Winging of the scapulae and inability to raise arms above the head resulting from weakened muscles of the shoulders and arms
- Erb's
  – Winging of the scapulae, lordosis with abdominal protrusion, waddling gait, poor balance, and inability to raise the arms caused by muscle weakness

Complications
- Arrhythmias
- Cardiac hypertrophy
- Contractures
- Crippling disability
- Dysphagia
- Pneumonia

Diagnostic test findings
- Electromyography shows short, weak bursts of electrical activity in affected muscles
- Muscle biopsy confirms the diagnosis
- Laboratory tests reveal elevated urine creatinine, serum creatine kinase, lactate dehydrogenase, alanine aminotransferase, and aspartate aminotransferase levels

Treatment
- Coughing and deep-breathing exercises and diaphragmatic breathing
- Teaching parents to recognize early signs of respiratory complications
- Orthopedic appliances, exercise, physical therapy, and surgery to correct contractures
- Genetic counseling regarding risk of transmitting the disease from family members who are carriers
- Adequate fluid intake, increased dietary bulk, and stool softener to prevent constipation due to inactivity
- Low-calorie, high-protein, high-fiber diet to prevent obesity due to physical inactivity
- Surgery to promote or maintain motility, such as tendon releases for contractures and spinal fusions for scoliosis
- Splints, braces, and surgery to correct contractures
- Trapeze bars, overhead slings, and a wheelchair to help preserve mobility
- Footboard or high-topped sneakers and a foot cradle to increase comfort and prevent footdrop

Nursing considerations

- Encourage and assist with active and passive ROM exercises to preserve joint mobility and prevent muscle atrophy
- Advise the patient to avoid long periods of bed rest and inactivity
- Provide emotional support to help the patient cope with continual changes in body image
- Refer the patient and his family to the Muscular Dystrophy Association
- Refer family members for genetic counseling

OSTEOARTHRITIS

Definition

- Chronic condition causing the deterioration of joint cartilage and the formation of reactive new bone at the margins of subchondral areas of the joints
- Usually affects weight-bearing joints, such as knees, feet, hips, and lumbar vertebrae

Underlying pathophysiology

- Synovial joint cartilage deteriorates as a result of damage to chondrocytes (cells responsible for binding cartilage)
- Cartilage softens with age, narrowing the joint space
- Mechanical injury also erodes articular cartilage
- Bone underneath the cartilage is unprotected and scleroses
- Cartilage flakes irritate the synovial lining, which becomes fibrotic, limiting joint movements
- Synovial fluid may be forced into bone defects, causing cysts
- New bone (osteophyte, or bone spur) forms at joint margins as the articular cartilage erodes, causing gross alteration of the bony contours and enlargement of the joint

Causes

- Primary osteoarthritis (a normal part of aging)
  - Metabolic factors (endocrine disorders such as hyperthyroidism) and genetic factors (decreased collagen synthesis)
  - Chemical factors (drugs such as steroids that stimulate the collagen-digesting enzymes in synovial membrane)
  - Mechanical factors (repeated stress on joint)
- Secondary osteoarthritis (follows an identifiable predisposing event that leads to degenerative changes)
  - Trauma (most common cause)
  - Congenital deformity
  - Obesity

Pathophysiologic changes

- Deep, aching joint pain that's usually relieved by rest (most common symptom) and stiffness in the morning and after exercise that's usually relieved by rest resulting from degradation of cartilage, inflammation, and bone stress (particularly after exercise or weight-bearing activities)

TOP 6

Ways to cope with arthritis

1. Daily stretching
2. Regular exercise
3. Rest when needed
4. Healthy weight
5. Good posture
6. Use of good body mechanics

Key diagnostic test results for osteoarthritis

- Synovial fluid analysis: Rules out inflammatory arthritis
- X-rays: Narrowing of joint space and margins, sclerosis of subchondral space, joint deformity, or articular damage

---

TIME-OUT FOR TEACHING

Tips for coping with arthritis

You can help your patient live a healthier and happier life by offering these tips for coping with arthritis:

- **Stretch.** Daily stretching exercises within the full range of motion will maintain flexibility of the joints and decrease pain and stiffness. Stretch again after prolonged periods of immobility.
- **Exercise regularly.** The health care provider will help determine what exercises are safest. Perform these exercises consistently. Be sure to include some strengthening exercises; doing so will enable the muscles to help support the joints and spine.
- **Rest when needed.** Learn to listen to the body. Give it a short rest after strenuous activities or if coping with pain. A good night's sleep is also helpful.
- **Watch the weight.** The heavier a person is, the more stress and strain is put on the joints and spine. Follow a varied diet and use portion control to ensure a healthy weight.
- **Straighten up.** Keep walking tall with good spinal posture and a balanced center of gravity to allow the joints to remain in their more natural and comfortable position for all activities.
- **Think mechanically.** Use good body mechanics for lifting, holding, and carrying objects. Ask for help when objects are too heavy or awkward to handle. The more the joints and spine are protected, the less chance pain and complications will occur.

- Crepitus or "grating" of the joint during motion due to cartilage damage
- Heberden's nodes (bony enlargement of distal interphalangeal joints) and Bouchard's nodes (bony enlargement of proximal interphalangeal joints) due to repeated inflammation
- Altered gait (from contractures) caused by overcompensation of muscles supporting the joints
- Decreased ROM due to pain and stiffness
- Deformity related to bone stress and altered bone growth
- Localized headaches as a result of cervical spine arthritis

● Complications
- Decreased joint ROM
- Irreversible joint changes and node formation
- Loss of independence in activities of daily living (ADLs)
- Pain (debilitating in later stages)
- Subluxation of the joint

● Diagnostic test findings
- Synovial fluid analysis rules out inflammatory arthritis
- X-rays of the affected joint may show a narrowing of the joint space and margins, sclerosis of the subchondral space, joint deformity, or articular damage
- Radionuclide bone scan is used to rule out inflammatory arthritis

- MRI shows affected joint, adjacent bones, and disease progression
- Arthroscopy shows internal joint structures and identifies soft-tissue swelling

Treatment
- Weight loss to reduce extra stress on weight-bearing joints
- Exercise to keep joints flexible and improve muscle strength
- Medications (corticosteroids, NSAIDs, cyclooxygenase-2 inhibitors) to control pain
- Glucocorticoid injections for inflamed joints unresponsive to NSAIDs
- Heat or cold therapy for temporary pain relief
- Joint protection to prevent strain or stress on painful joints
- Surgery (arthroplasty, osteoplasty, osteotomy) to relieve chronic pain in damaged joints

Nursing considerations
- Teach self-care skills to promote joint health (see *Tips for coping with arthritis*)
- Assist with physical therapy, and encourage the patient to perform gentle isometric ROM exercises
- If the patient needs surgery, provide appropriate preoperative and postoperative care
- Provide emotional support and reassurance to help the patient cope with limited mobility

OSTEOGENESIS IMPERFECTA

Definition
- Genetic disease in which bones are thin, poorly developed, and fracture easily
- Congenital form (rare)
  - Involves fractures that are present at birth
  - Usually fatal within first days or weeks of life
- Late-appearing form
  - Occurs after the first year of life
  - Manifests as recurring fractures

Underlying pathophysiology
- Genes that determine the structure of collagen mutate
- Possible mutations in other genes may cause variations in the assembly and maintenance of bone and other connective tissue
- Collectively or alone, these mutated genes lead to pathologic fractures and impaired healing

Causes
- Genetic disease, typically autosomal dominant (characterized by a defect in the synthesis of connective tissue)
- Autosomal recessive gene defect that produces osteogenesis imperfecta in homozygotes (osteoporosis in some)

Pathophysiologic changes
- Frequent fractures and poor healing due to falls as toddler begins to walk
- Short stature due to multiple fractures caused by minor physical stress

Key diagnostic test results for osteogenesis imperfecta

- Prenatal ultrasound (second trimester): Bowing of long bones, fractures, limb shortening, and decreased skull echogenicity
- Skull, long bone, and pelvis X-rays: Thin bones, fractures with deformities, beaded ribs, and osteopenia
- DEXA scan: Mean bone density approximately three-fourths normal level

Key treatments for osteogenesis imperfecta

- Prevention of fractures
- Internal fixation of fractures

Key nursing considerations for osteogenesis imperfecta

- Teach parent and child how to recognize fractures and correctly splint them.
- Teach parents how to protect the child during diapering, dressing, and other ADLs.
- Stress importance of good nutrition.
- Administer analgesics, as ordered.
- Monitor dental and hearing needs.

- Deformed cranial structures and limbs as a result of multiple fractures
- Thin skin, bluish sclera, and thin collagen fibers of the sclera, which allow the choroid layer to be seen, caused by mutation of connective tissue
- Abnormal tooth and enamel development due to improper deposition of dentin

Complications
- Deafness
- Cerebral hemorrhage caused by birth trauma
- Hyperplastic callus formation
- Repeated respiratory tract infections
- Spinal cord compression
- Stillbirth or death within the first year of life (autosomal-recessive disorder)

Diagnostic test findings
- Serum alkaline phosphatase levels are elevated during periods of rapid bone formation and cellular injury
- Skin culture shows reduced number of fibroblasts
- Echocardiography may show mitral insufficiency or floppy mitral valve
- Prenatal ultrasound during second trimester reveals bowing of long bones, fractures, limb shortening, and decreased skull echogenicity
- Skull, long bone, and pelvis X-rays reveal thin bones, fractures with deformities, beaded ribs, and osteopenia
- Dual-energy X-ray absorptiometry (DEXA) scan shows a mean bone density that is 77% of normal level in the lumbar spine and 71% of normal level in the femoral neck

Treatment
- Prevention of fractures
- Internal fixation of fractures to ensure stabilization and prevent deformities

Nursing considerations
- Teach the parent and child how to recognize fractures and correctly splint them
- Teach the parents how to protect the child during diapering, dressing, and other ADLs
- Advise the parents to encourage their child to develop fine motor skills and interests that don't require strenuous physical activity
- Teach the child to assume responsibility for precautions during physical activities to help foster his independence
- Stress the importance of good nutrition to heal bones
- Refer the parents and child for genetic counseling to assess the risk of passing on the condition
- Administer analgesics, as ordered, to relieve pain from frequent fractures
- Monitor dental and hearing needs
- Stress the need for regular dental care and immunizations

OSTEOMYELITIS

- **Definition**
  - Bone infection characterized by progressive inflammatory destruction after formation of new bone
  - May be chronic or acute
  - Commonly results from a combination of local trauma causing a hematoma and an acute infection originating elsewhere in the body

- **Underlying pathophysiology**
  - Organisms settle in a hematoma or weakened area
  - Organisms travel through the bloodstream to the metaphysis, the section of a long bone that's continuous with the epiphyseal plates, where blood flows into sinusoids (see *Understanding osteomyelitis*, page 168)

- **Causes**
  - *Staphylococcus aureus* (most common infective organism)
  - *Escherichia coli*
  - Fungi or viruses
  - *Pasteurella multocida*
  - Pneumococcus
  - *Proteus vulgaris*
  - *Pseudomonas aeruginosa*
  - *Streptococcus pyogenes*

- **Pathophysiologic changes**
  - Rapid onset of sudden pain in the affected bone; tenderness, heat, swelling, erythema, and guarding of affected region of the limb; and restricted movement resulting from inflammation
  - Dehydration (in young patients) resulting from inflammation and infection
  - Irritability and poor feeding (in infants) caused by infection and pain
  - Fever and tachycardia resulting from inflammation

- **Complications**
  - Chronic infection
  - Skeletal deformities
  - Joint deformities
  - Disturbed bone growth in children
  - Differing leg lengths
  - Impaired mobility

- **Diagnostic test findings**
  - WBC count is elevated
  - Erythrocyte sedimentation rate is increased
  - Blood culture identifies pathogens
  - X-rays show bone involvement
  - Bone scans may detect early infection
  - CT scan and MRI can show extent of infection

Key facts about osteomyelitis

- Bone infection
- Occurs when organisms settle in a hematoma or weakened area and travel through the bloodstream to the metaphysis
- Most commonly involves *S. aureus*

Key pathophysiologic changes in osteomyelitis

- Rapid onset of pain in affected bone
- Fever
- Guarding of affected region

Key diagnostic test results for osteomyelitis

- WBC count: Elevated
- Erythrocyte sedimentation rate: Increased
- X-rays: Bone involvement

GO WITH THE FLOW

Understanding osteomyelitis

Bones are essentially isolated from the body's natural defense system after an organism gets through the periosteum. Bones are limited in their ability to replace necrotic tissue caused by infection, which may lead to chronic osteomyelitis.

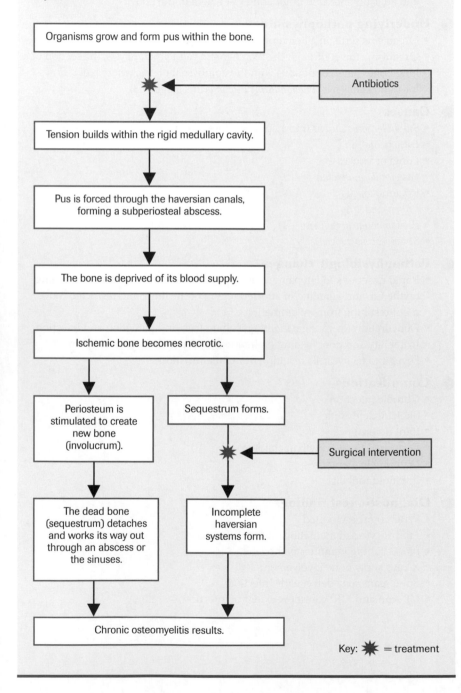

Treatments

- Large doses of I.V. antibiotics (usually a penicillinase-resistant penicillin, such as nafcillin or oxacillin)
- Early surgical drainage to relieve pressure and abscess formation
- Immobilization of the affected body part by cast, traction, or bed rest to prevent failure to heal or recurrence
- Supportive measures, such as analgesics for pain and I.V. fluids to maintain hydration
- Incision and drainage, followed by a culture of the drainage (if an abscess or sinus tract forms)
- Intracavitary instillation of antibiotics through closed-system continuous irrigation with low intermittent suction
- Packed, wet, antibiotic-soaked dressings
- Hyperbaric oxygen to stimulate normal immune mechanisms

Nursing considerations

- Use strict sterile technique when changing dressings and irrigating wounds
- If the patient is in skeletal traction for compound fractures, cover insertion points of pin tracks with small, dry dressings
- Administer I.V. fluids to maintain adequate hydration, as necessary
- Provide a diet high in protein and vitamin C
- Assess vital signs, the wound's appearance, and whether the patient experiences new pain, which may indicate secondary infection
- Support the affected limb with firm pillows while keeping the limb level with the body
- Provide good skin care
  - Turn the patient gently every 2 hours
  - Observe for signs of pressure ulcer formation
- Provide good cast care
  - Support the cast with pillows
  - Petal the cast to smooth rough edges
  - Check circulation and drainage
  - Mark wet spots on cast and report any enlargements
- Provide emotional support and appropriate diversions

OSTEOPOROSIS

Definition

- Metabolic bone disorder in which the rate of bone resorption accelerates while the rate of bone formation slows, causing a loss of bone mass
- Occurs when affected bones lose calcium and phosphate salts
- Causes bones to become porous, brittle, and abnormally vulnerable to fractures
- May be classified as primary disease (commonly called *postmenopausal osteoporosis*) or secondary to other causes

Underlying pathophysiology

- The remodeling of bone resorption and formation is interrupted

How osteoporosis develops

A metabolic bone disorder, osteoporosis develops as the rate of bone resorption accelerates while the rate of bone formation slows, causing a loss of bone mass. Bone weakens as local cells reabsorb bone tissue. Trabecular bone at the core becomes less dense, and cortical bone on the perimeter loses thickness. Bones affected by this disease lose calcium and phosphate salts and become porous, brittle, and abnormally vulnerable to fractures.

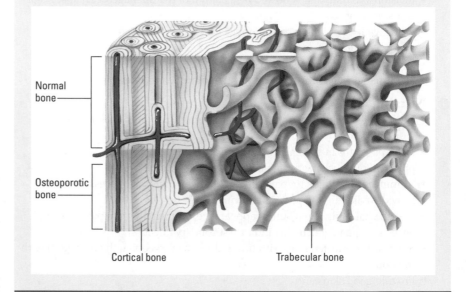

Normal bone

Osteoporotic bone

Cortical bone   Trabecular bone

- New bone formation falls behind resorption
- When bone is resorbed faster than it forms, the bone becomes less dense (see *How osteoporosis develops*)

● **Causes**
- Unknown (in primary disease)
- Alcoholism
- Bone immobilization
- Hyperthyroidism
- Liver disease
- Malnutrition, particularly diet low in calcium
- Osteogenesis imperfecta
- Prolonged therapy with steroids or heparin
- Rheumatoid arthritis

● **Pathophysiologic changes**
- Loss of height, spinal deformities, spontaneous wedge fractures, pathologic fractures of neck and femur, Colles' fractures of distal radius (common after minor fall), vertebral collapse, and hip fractures resulting from weakened bones
- Pain caused by fractures

Key pathophysiologic changes in osteoporosis

- Loss of height
- Spinal deformities
- Pain caused by fractures

- **Complications**
  - Spontaneous fractures
  - Shock, hemorrhage, or fat embolism

- **Diagnostic test findings**
  - Parathyroid hormone level is elevated
  - X-rays show characteristic degeneration in the lower thoracolumbar vertebrae
  - CT scan assesses spinal bone loss
  - Bone biopsy shows thin, porous, but otherwise normal bone
  - Dual or single photon absorptiometry shows loss of bone mass

- **Treatment**
  - Physical therapy emphasizing gentle exercises and activity and regular, moderate weight-bearing exercise
    - Slows bone loss
    - Possibly reverses demineralization
    - Provides mechanical stress, which stimulates bone formation
  - Supportive devices such as a back brace
  - Surgery, if indicated, for pathologic fractures
  - Hormone replacement therapy with estrogen to slow bone loss and prevent occurrence of fractures (controversial)
  - Analgesics and local heat to relieve pain
  - Calcium and vitamin D supplements to support normal bone metabolism
  - Calcitonin (Calcimar) to reduce bone resorption and slow the decline in bone mass
  - Bisphosphonates to increase bone density and restore bone loss
  - Fluoride to stimulate bone formation
    - Requires strict dosage precautions
    - Can cause gastric distress
  - Vitamin C, calcium, and protein to support skeletal metabolism through a balanced diet rich in nutrients
  - Early mobilization after surgery or trauma
  - Decreased alcohol and tobacco consumption
  - Careful observation for signs of malabsorption (fatty stools, chronic diarrhea)

- **Nursing considerations**
  - Check the patient's skin daily
    - Look for redness, warmth, and new sites of pain
    - These signs and symptoms may indicate fractures
  - Encourage activity
    - Help the patient walk several times daily
    - As appropriate, perform ROM exercises or encourage the patient to perform active exercises
  - Impose safety precautions
    - Move the patient gently and carefully at all times
    - Explain to the patient's family how easily an osteoporotic patient's bones can fracture
  - Teach the patient and his family about the patient's prescribed drug regimen and how to recognize and report adverse effects
  - Instruct the patient to report new pain sites immediately
  - Teach the patient good body mechanics

Key diagnostic test results for osteoporosis
- X-rays: Degeneration in lower thoracolumbar vertebrae
- Photon absorptiometry: Loss of bone mass

Key treatments for osteoporosis
- Calcium and vitamin D supplements
- Regular, moderate weight-bearing exercise

Key nursing considerations for osteoporosis
- Encourage activity.
- Teach patient and family about prescribed drug regimen and how to recognize and report adverse effects.
- Instruct patient to immediately report new pain.
- Teach good body mechanics.

– Stoop before lifting anything
– Avoid twisting movements and prolonged bending

PAGET'S DISEASE

● **Definition**
  • Slow, progressive metabolic bone disease characterized by accelerated patterns of bone remodeling
  • Affects one or several skeletal areas (spine, pelvis, femur, and skull)
  • Can be fatal, particularly when associated with heart failure, bone sarcoma, or giant-cell tumors

● **Underlying pathophysiology**
  • Initial phase of excessive bone resorption (osteoclastic phase) is followed by a reactive phase of excessive abnormal bone formation (osteoblastic phase)
  • Collagen fibers in the new bone are disorganized, and glycoprotein levels in the matrix decrease
  • Partially resorbed trabeculae thicken and enlarge because of excessive bone formation, and the bone becomes soft and weak

● **Causes**
  • Exact cause is unknown
  • Possible causes (theories)
    – Autoimmune disease
    – Benign or malignant bone tumors
    – Estrogen deficiency
    – Slow or dormant viral infection
    – Vitamin D deficiency during childhood

● **Pathophysiologic changes**
  • Severe and persistent pain intensifying with weight bearing, possibly with impaired movement, due to impingement of abnormal bone on the spinal cord or sensory nerve root and the constant inflammation accompanying cell breakdown
  • Characteristic cranial enlargement over frontal and occipital areas (hat size may increase) and possibly headaches, sensory abnormalities, and impaired motor function resulting from skull involvement
  • Kyphosis accompanied by a barrel-shaped chest due to compression fractures of vertebrae
  • Asymmetrical bowing of the tibia and femur (commonly reducing height) resulting from weakened and softened bones
  • Waddling gait caused by softening of pelvic bones
  • Blindness and hearing loss with tinnitus and vertigo caused by bony impingement on cranial nerves

● **Complications**
  • Blindness and hearing loss
  • Fractures
  • Gout
  • Heart failure

Key facts about Paget's disease

• Slow, progressive metabolic bone disease
• Involves osteoclastic phase followed by osteoblastic phase
• Causes partially resorbed trabeculae to thicken
• Results in soft and weak bones

Key pathophysiologic changes in Paget's disease

• Severe and persistent pain intensifying with weight bearing
• Cranial enlargement over frontal and occipital areas
• Kyphosis and barrel-shaped chest
• Asymmetrical bowing of tibia and femur

- Hypercalcemia
- Hypertension
- Osteoarthritis
- Paraplegia
- Renal calculi
- Sarcoma

Diagnostic test findings

- Red blood cell count shows anemia
- Serum alkaline phosphatase level is elevated
- Serum calcium level is normal or elevated
- 24-hour urine hydroxyproline level is elevated
- X-ray studies show bone expansion and increased bone density
- Bone scans clearly show early pagetic lesions
- Bone biopsy shows a characteristic mosaic pattern of bone tissue

Treatment

- Bisphosphonates (alendronate [Fosamax] and etidronate [Didronel]) to inhibit osteoclast-mediated bone resorption
- Calcitonin, a hormone, and etidronate to retard bone resorption and reduce serum alkaline phosphate and urine hydroxyproline secretion
- Mithramycin (Mithracin), a cytotoxic antibiotic, to decrease serum calcium, urine hydroxyproline, and serum alkaline phosphatase levels
  - Produces remission of symptoms within 2 weeks and biochemical improvement in 1 to 2 months
  - May destroy platelets or compromise renal function
- Surgery to reduce or prevent pathologic fractures, correct secondary deformities, and relieve neurologic impairment
- Drug therapy with calcitonin and etidronate or mithramycin before surgery to decrease the risk of excessive bleeding from hypervascular bone
- Joint replacement
- Aspirin, indomethacin (Indocin), or ibuprofen (Motrin) to control pain

Nursing considerations

- Assess pain level daily
  - Watch for new areas of pain or restricted movements, which may indicate new fracture sites
- Watch for sensory or motor disturbances, such as difficulty in hearing, seeing, or walking
- Monitor serum calcium and alkaline phosphatase levels
- If the patient is confined to prolonged bed rest, provide good skin care to prevent pressure ulcers
  - Reposition the patient frequently
  - Use a flotation mattress
  - Provide high-topped sneakers to prevent footdrop
- Monitor intake and output
- Encourage adequate fluid intake to minimize renal calculi formation
- Demonstrate how to inject calcitonin properly and rotate injection sites, or how to use the nasal inhalation form

- Teach the patient about prescribed medications, and instruct him to report adverse effects
- Teach the patient how to pace activities and, if necessary, how to use assistive devices
- Encourage him to follow a recommended exercise program
- Suggest a moderately firm to firm mattress to minimize spinal deformities
- Emphasize the importance of regular check-ups, including those for the eyes and ears
- Refer the patient and his family to the Paget Foundation

RHABDOMYOLYSIS

● **Definition**
  - Breakdown of muscle tissue
  - May cause myoglobinuria
  - Usually follows major muscle trauma, especially a muscle crush injury
  - Good prognosis if contributing causes are alleviated or disease is controlled before damage becomes irreversible
  - Can cause renal failure if left untreated

● **Underlying pathophysiology**
  - Muscle trauma compresses tissues, causing ischemia and necrosis
  - Ensuing local edema further increases compartment pressure and tamponade
  - Pressure from swelling causes blood vessels to collapse, leading to tissue hypoxia, muscle infarction, neural damage in the area of the fracture, and release of myoglobin, potassium, and creatine kinase from the necrotic muscle fibers into the circulation
  - Myoglobin can become trapped in renal capillaries or tubules, leading to acute renal failure

● **Causes**
  - Excessive muscle activity (such as status epilepticus, electroconvulsive therapy, severe dystonia)
  - Familial tendency
  - Infection
  - Medications (antihistamines, salicylates, fibric acid derivatives, HMG-CoA reductase inhibitors, neuroleptics, anesthetics, paralytic agents, corticosteroids, tricyclic antidepressants, selective serotonin reuptake inhibitors)
  - Severe muscle trauma (such as blunt injury, extensive burns, electric shock, near drowning)
  - Sporadic strenuous exertion (such as running a marathon)

● **Pathophysiologic changes**
  - Tenderness, swelling, and muscle weakness resulting from muscle trauma and pressure
  - Dark, reddish brown urine caused by myoglobin release

● **Complications**
  - Amputation
  - Renal failure

Key facts about rhabdomyolysis

- Occurs when muscle trauma compresses tissues, causing ischemia and necrosis
- Leads to tissue hypoxia, muscle infarction, and release of myoglobin, from necrotic muscle fibers
- Can cause acute renal failure

Key pathophysiologic changes in rhabdomyolysis

- Tenderness, swelling, and muscle weakness
- Dark, reddish brown urine

Diagnostic test findings
- Urine myoglobin level exceeds 0.5 mg/dl (evident with only 200 g of muscle damage)
- Creatine kinase level is elevated due to muscle damage
- Serum potassium, phosphate, creatinine, and creatine levels are elevated
- Serum calcium levels show hypocalcemia in early stages, hypercalcemia in later stages
- Intracompartmental pressure measurements are elevated
- CT scan, MRI, and bone scintigraphy detect muscle necrosis

Treatment
- Treatment of the underlying disorder
- Hydration with I.V. crystalloid to increase intravascular volume and glomerular filtration rate
- Urine alkalinization and osmotic or loop diuretics to prevent renal failure
- Analgesics for pain
- If compartment syndrome develops and venous pressure is greater than 25 mm Hg, immediate fasciotomy and debridement to relieve pressure and prevent tissue death
- Exercise modification (prolonged low-intensity training rather than short bursts of intense exercise) to prevent muscle injury and disease

Nursing considerations
- Administer I.V. fluids and diuretics, as ordered, to reduce nephrotoxicity
- Monitor intake and output
- Recommend exercise modification to prevent recurrence of rhabdomyolysis

TENDINITIS AND BURSITIS

Definition
- Tendinitis
  - Painful inflammation of tendons (the dense, fibrous connective tissue that attaches muscle to bone) and tendon-muscle attachments to bone (see *Anatomy of tendons and bursae*, page 176)
  - Usually occurs in the rotator cuff, hip, Achilles tendon, or hamstring
- Bursitis
  - Painful inflammation of one or more bursae (small sacs of connective tissue lined with a synovial membrane and synovial fluid)
  - Usually occurs in the subdeltoid, olecranon, trochanteric, calcaneal, or prepatellar area

Underlying pathophysiology
- Tendinitis
  - Inflammation causes localized pain around the affected area
  - Joint movement is restricted
  - Swelling results from fluid accumulation
  - Calcium deposits form in and around the tendon
  - Further swelling and immobility result

Anatomy of tendons and bursae

Tendons, like stiff rubber bands, hold the muscles in place and enable them to move the bones. Bursae are located at friction points around joints and between tendons, cartilage, or bone. Bursae keep these body parts lubricated so they move freely.

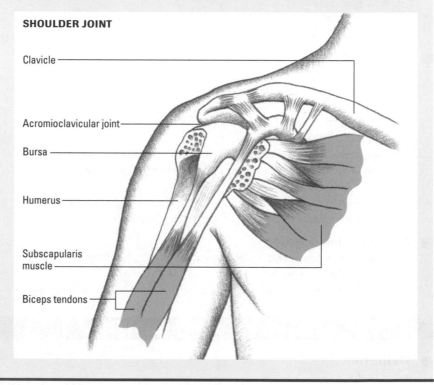

SHOULDER JOINT

- Clavicle
- Acromioclavicular joint
- Bursa
- Humerus
- Subscapularis muscle
- Biceps tendons

- Bursitis
  - Bursae sacs hold lubricating synovial fluid
  - Inflammation leads to excessive production of fluid in the sacs
  - Bursae become distended and press on sensory nerve endings, causing pain

● **Causes**
  - Tendinitis
    - Abnormal body development
    - Hypermobility
    - Musculoskeletal disorders (rheumatic diseases, congenital defects)
    - Overuse
    - Postural misalignment
  - Bursitis
    - Inflammatory joint disease (rheumatoid arthritis, gout)
    - Recurring trauma that stresses or presses joint
    - Wound infection or bacterial invasion of skin over bursa (septic bursitis)

Key causes of tendinitis and bursitis

- Overuse
- Recurring trauma

Pathophysiologic changes

- Tendinitis
  - Restricted movement resulting from inflammation of affected tendon
  - Localized pain that's most severe at night and interferes with sleep due to inflammation
  - Swelling at affected site caused by fluid accumulation
- Bursitis
  - Sudden or gradual pain, limited movement, and irritation resulting from fluid accumulation in the bursae

Complications

- Scar tissue and subsequent disability, if left untreated
- Acute calcific bursitis if calcium erodes into adjacent tissue
- Extreme pain and restricted movement

Diagnostic test findings

- Arthrocentesis may identify causative microorganisms and other causes of inflammation
- CT scan and MRI identify tears, inflammation, or tumor
- X-rays in tendinitis may show bony fragments, osteophyte sclerosis, or calcium deposits
- X-rays in calcific bursitis may show calcium deposits in the joint
- Arthrography results are usually normal in tendinitis, with minor irregularities on the tendon under the surface

Treatment

- Resting the joint by immobilization with a sling, splint, or cast
- Systemic analgesics to relieve pain
- Application of cold or heat, ultrasound, or local injection of an anesthetic and corticosteroid to reduce inflammation
- Oral NSAIDs, such as ibuprofen, naproxen, indomethacin, or oxaprozin, until the patient is free from pain and can perform ROM exercises easily
- Short-term analgesics, including propoxyphene, codeine, acetaminophen with codeine and, occasionally, oxycodone, to relieve pain when NSAIDs alone are ineffective
- Fluid removal by aspiration and heat therapy
- For calcific tendinitis, ice packs, physical therapy, ultrasonography, or hydrotherapy to maintain or regain ROM
- Rarely, surgical removal of calcium deposits
- Changes in lifestyle to prevent recurring joint irritation

Nursing considerations

- Assess the severity of pain and the ROM to determine effectiveness of the treatment
- **Before injecting corticosteroids or local anesthetics, ask the patient about his drug allergies**
- Tell the patient to take anti-inflammatory agents with milk to minimize GI distress and to immediately report any signs of distress
- Advise the patient to perform stretching and strengthening exercises as prescribed and avoid activities that aggravate the joint

---

Key pathophysiologic changes in tendinitis and bursitis

Tendinitis
- Restricted movement
- Pain, especially at night

Bursitis
- Sudden or gradual pain
- Limited movement
- Irritation

Key diagnostic test results for tendinitis and bursitis

- Arthrocentesis: Causative microorganisms and other causes of inflammation
- X-rays: Bony fragments, osteophyte sclerosis, or calcium deposits in tendinitis; calcium deposits in joint in calcific bursitis

Key treatments for tendinitis and bursitis

- Joint immobilization
- Analgesics
- Cold or heat application
- NSAIDs
- Injection of an anesthetic and corticosteroids

Key nursing considerations for tendinitis and bursitis

- Ask patient about drug allergies.
- Tell patient to take anti-inflammatory agents with milk and to immediately report signs of distress.
- Advise patient to perform stretching and strengthening exercises and physical therapy regimen.

• Remind the patient to wear a triangular sling during the first few days of an attack of subdeltoid tendinitis or bursitis to support the arm and protect the shoulder, particularly at night
• Advise the patient to maintain joint mobility and prevent muscle atrophy by performing exercises or physical therapy when he's free from pain

NCLEX CHECKS

It's never too soon to begin your licensure examination preparation. Now that you've reviewed this chapter, carefully read each of the following questions and choose the best answer. Then compare your responses with the correct answers.

1. The nurse is teaching a class on musculoskeletal disorders. A student in the class shows understanding by stating that altered bone density is caused by:
☐ **1.** increased uric acid production.
☐ **2.** insufficient blood supply.
☐ **3.** loss of inorganic calcium salts.
☐ **4.** decreased estrogen production.

2. A client with which type of muscular dystrophy would be unable to pucker his mouth?
☐ **1.** Duchenne's
☐ **2.** Becker's
☐ **3.** Landouzy-Dejerdine
☐ **4.** Erb's

3. A client who is diagnosed with osteoarthritis complains that several of her finger joints are inflamed and painful. Identify the joint on which the nurse would expect to find a Bouchard's node.

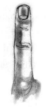

4. A client reports chronic neck pain and stiffness that improve after he takes a warm shower and stretches. Neck X-rays confirm the presence of osteoarthritis. The nurse instructs the client that which factor can cause primary osteoarthritis?
☐ **1.** Trauma
☐ **2.** Congenital deformity
☐ **3.** Hyperthyroidism
☐ **4.** Obesity

5. A client has been referred to physical therapy to learn exercises that she can safely perform to help manage her osteoporosis. The nurse explains to the patient that the primary benefit of weight-bearing exercise in osteoporosis is:
☐ **1.** to stimulate bone formation.
☐ **2.** to improve posture.
☐ **3.** to improve the patient's emotional status and feeling of well-being.
☐ **4.** to stimulate appetite.

TOP 6

Items to study for your next test on the musculoskeletal system

1. Pathophysiology of altered bone and muscle conditions
2. Key pathophysiologic changes in herniated intervertebral disk, osteoarthritis, osteoporosis, and osteogenesis imperfecta
3. Classes of medications that reduce inflammation and pain
4. The similarities and differences between tendinitis and bursitis and carpal tunnel syndrome
5. Tests used to diagnose rhabdomyolysis, osteomyelitis, and Paget's disease
6. Five nursing considerations common to all musculoskeletal disorders

6. In Paget's disease, the phase of excessive abnormal bone formation is known as the:

- ☐ **1.** osteoclastic phase.
- ☐ **2.** osteoblastic phase.
- ☐ **3.** osteophytic phase.
- ☐ **4.** osteomalacia phase.

7. A client is admitted with rhabdomyolysis following a crush injury. The nurse monitors his myoglobin levels because elevated levels could lead to:

- ☐ **1.** heart failure.
- ☐ **2.** renal failure.
- ☐ **3.** shock.
- ☐ **4.** stroke.

8. A nurse monitors the laboratory cultures and sensitivity reports for a client who has osteomyelitis. The nurse is aware that the most common infective organism in osteomyelitis is:

- ☐ **1.** *Streptococcus pyogenes.*
- ☐ **2.** *Escherichia coli.*
- ☐ **3.** *Staphylococcus aureus.*
- ☐ **4.** *Pseudomonas aeruginosa.*

9. Which stage of a herniated intervertebral disk involves the nucleus pulposus pressing against the anulus fibrosus?

- ☐ **1.** Protrusion
- ☐ **2.** Extrusion
- ☐ **3.** Sequestration
- ☐ **4.** Herniation

10. A client is diagnosed with acute gout. Tophi are visible on X-ray, and the client has a red, hot, and swollen left great toe. What other sign would the nurse expect to see?

- ☐ **1.** Below normal uric acid level
- ☐ **2.** Decreased hemoglobin
- ☐ **3.** Elevated WBC count
- ☐ **4.** Below normal blood pressure

ANSWERS AND RATIONALES

1. CORRECT ANSWER: 4
Decreased estrogen production during menopause leads to diminished osteoblastic activity and loss of bone mass. Increased uric acid production can lead to gout. An insufficient blood supply indicates altered bone growth. Loss of inorganic calcium salts relates to altered bone strength.

2. CORRECT ANSWER: 3
Landouzy-Dejerdine muscular dystrophy, also known as *facioscapulohumeral dystrophy*, is a slowly progressive form of muscular dystrophy. It weakens the muscles of the face, shoulders, and upper arms and eventually spreads to all voluntary muscles,

---

producing an inability to pucker or whistle. The other forms of muscular dystrophy don't affect the facial muscles.

3. CORRECT ANSWER:

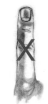

Bouchard's nodes are bony enlargements of the proximal interphalangeal joints due to repeated inflammation from osteoarthritis.

4. CORRECT ANSWER: 3

Metabolic factors, including endocrine disorders such as hyperthyroidism and diabetes mellitus, are causes of primary osteoarthritis. Other causes of primary osteoarthritis are genetic factors, chemical factors, such as steroids, and mechanical factors, such as repeated stress on a joint. Trauma, congenital deformity, and obesity are all causes of secondary osteoarthritis.

5. CORRECT ANSWER: 1

The primary benefit of weight-bearing exercise for the patient with osteoporosis is that the mechanical stress of such exercise stimulates bone formation. Secondary benefits of weight-bearing exercises may be improved posture and sense of emotional well-being. Whether the patient's appetite is stimulated isn't a primary benefit of weight-bearing exercises for osteoporosis.

6. CORRECT ANSWER: 2

Paget's disease is a metabolic bone disease characterized by accelerated patterns of bone remodeling. An initial phase of bone resorption (the osteoclastic phase) is followed by a reactive phase of excessive abnormal bone formation, known as the *osteoblastic phase*. Osteophyte formation occurs in osteoarthritis. Osteomalacia is a disease caused by vitamin D deficiency.

7. CORRECT ANSWER: 2

Muscle trauma leads to tissue damage and release of myoglobin into the bloodstream. The myoglobin can become trapped in renal capillaries or tubules, leading to acute renal failure. Elevated myoglobin levels don't cause heart failure, shock, or stroke.

8. CORRECT ANSWER: 3

The most common infective organism in osteomyelitis is *S. aureus*. Organisms find a culture site in a hematoma or in a weakened area and travel through the bloodstream to the bone.

9. CORRECT ANSWER: 1

Herniation occurs in three stages. The first stage, during which the nucleus pulposus presses against the anulus fibrosus, is protrusion. During the extrusion stage, the nucleus pulposus bulges forcibly through the anulus fibrosus, pushing against the nerve root. During the sequestration stage, the anulus fibrosus gives way as the disk's core bursts and presses against the nerve root.

10. CORRECT ANSWER: 3

In gout, an elevated WBC count occurs as neutrophils rally to ingest the urate crystals. Uric acid levels would be increased. Hypertension, not hypotension, may occur in severe cases. Hemoglobin isn't affected by gout.

5

Gastrointestinal system

LEARNING OBJECTIVES

After studying this chapter, you should be able to:

● Describe the relationship between presenting signs and symptoms and the pathophysiologic changes associated with various GI disorders.

● List probable causes of various GI disorders.

● Identify interventions for a patient with a GI disorder.

● Write teaching goals for a patient with a GI disorder.

● Identify classes of medications that may improve or control GI dysfunction.

CHAPTER OVERVIEW

The GI system ingests and digests food and eliminates waste products. Structures of the GI system include the GI tract, which extends from the mouth to the anus and contains the pharynx, esophagus, stomach, small intestine, and large intestine. Accessory organs of the GI system include the liver, pancreas, gallbladder, and bile ducts.

Because GI disorders directly affect nutrition, understanding pathophysiologic changes can help protect a patient's overall nutritional status. This chapter reviews key pathophysiologic concepts related to the GI system, and then outlines the underlying pathophysiology, causes, changes, complications, diagnostic test findings, treatment approaches, and nursing considerations associated with common GI disorders.

PATHOPHYSIOLOGIC CONCEPTS

● **Anorexia**
- Loss of appetite or lack of desire for food despite the normal stimulation of hunger in the hypothalamus by falling blood glucose levels
- Causes
  - Slow gastric emptying or gastric stasis
  - High levels of neurotransmitters (such as serotonin)
  - Excess cortisol levels, which suppress hypothalamic control of hunger, contributing to satiety

● **Diarrhea**
- Increase in fluidity of feces and frequency of defecation
- Three types
  - Osmotic diarrhea
    - Nonabsorbable substance or increased numbers of osmotic particles in intestine increase osmotic pressure and draw excess water into intestine
    - Weight and volume of stool increases
  - Secretory diarrhea
    - Pathogen or tumor irritates muscle and mucosal layers of intestine
    - Consequent increase in motility and secretions (water, electrolytes, mucus) results in diarrhea
  - Motility diarrhea
    - Inflammation, neuropathy, or obstruction causes reflex increase in intestinal motility
    - Patient may expel the irritant or clear the obstruction

● **Jaundice**
- Yellow pigmentation of skin and sclera
- Results when production of bilirubin exceeds metabolism and excretion and bilirubin accumulates in blood
- Occurs when bilirubin levels exceed 2 mg/dl

● **Nausea**
- Urge to vomit
- May occur independently of vomiting, or may precede or accompany it
- Marked by increased salivation, diminished functional activities of the stomach, and altered small intestinal motility
- May be stimulated by the vomiting center in the medulla and signals from the hypothalamus

● **Vomiting**
- Forceful oral expulsion of gastric contents
- Occurs when chemoreceptor trigger zone in medulla is stimulated
  - Abdominal muscles and diaphragm contract
  - Reverse peristalsis begins, causing intestinal material to flow back into stomach, distending it
  - Stomach pushes diaphragm into thoracic cavity, raising intrathoracic pressure
  - Pressure forces upper esophageal sphincter open, glottis closes, and soft palate blocks nasopharynx

Key facts about anorexia
- Loss of appetite despite normal stimulation of hunger
- Causes gastric stasis, high neurotransmitter levels, and excess cortisol levels

Key facts about diarrhea
- Increase in fluidity of feces and frequency of defecation
- Classified as osmotic, secretory, or motility

Key facts about jaundice
- Yellow pigmentation of skin and sclera caused by excess bilirubin production
- Occurs when bilirubin levels exceed 2 mg/dl

Key facts about nausea
- Urge to vomit
- May precede, accompany, or occur independently of vomiting

Key facts about vomiting
- Forceful oral expulsion of gastric contents
- Results when chemoreceptor trigger zone in medulla is stimulated

– Pressure forces material up through the sphincter and out through the mouth

Key facts about cholecystitis

- Inflammation of gallbladder wall
- Usually associated with a gall-stone impacted in the cystic duct
- May be acute or chronic

Key pathophysiologic changes in cholecystitis

- Acute abdominal pain in right upper quadrant
- Colic
- Nausea and vomiting

Key diagnostic test results for cholecystitis

- Ultrasonography: Presence of gallstones (distinguishes be-tween obstructive and nonob-structive jaundice)
- Percutaneous transhepatic cholangiography: Calculi (sup-ports diagnosis of obstructive jaundice)
- Laboratory studies: Elevated serum alkaline phosphate, lac-tate dehydrogenase, AST, and total bilirubin

CHOLECYSTITIS

Definition
- Acute or chronic inflammation causing painful distention of the gallbladder
- Usually associated with a gallstone impacted in the cystic duct
- Acute form most common among middle-aged women
- Chronic form most common among elderly people

Underlying pathophysiology
- Inflammation of the gallbladder wall usually develops after a gallstone lodges in the cystic duct (see *Understanding gallstone formation*)

Causes
- Gallstones (most common cause)
- Abnormal metabolism of cholesterol and bile salts
- Poor or absent blood flow to the gallbladder

Pathophysiologic changes
- Acute abdominal pain in the right upper quadrant that may radiate to the back, between the shoulders, or to the front of the chest secondary to inflam-mation and irritation of nerve fibers
- Colic due to the passage of gallstones along the bile duct
- Nausea and vomiting triggered by the inflammatory response
- Chills related to fever
- Low-grade fever secondary to inflammation
- Jaundice from obstruction of the common bile duct by calculi

Complications
- Carcinoma
- Cholangitis
- Empyema
- Fistula formation
- Gallstone ileus
- Gangrene
- Hepatitis
- Pancreatitis
- Perforation and abscess formation

Diagnostic test findings
- X-ray reveals gallstones (if they contain enough calcium to be radiopaque) and helps detect porcelain gallbladder (hard, brittle gallbladder due to calcium deposited in wall), limy bile, and gallstone ileus
- Ultrasonography detects gallstones as small as 2 mm and distinguishes be-tween obstructive and nonobstructive jaundice
- Technetium-labeled scan reveals cystic duct obstruction and acute or chronic cholecystitis if ultrasound doesn't visualize the gallbladder
- Percutaneous transhepatic cholangiography supports the diagnosis of ob-structive jaundice and reveals calculi in the ducts

Understanding gallstone formation

Abnormal metabolism of cholesterol and bile salts plays an important role in gallstone formation. The liver makes bile continuously. The gallbladder concentrates and stores it until the duodenum signals that bile is needed to help digest fat. Changes in the composition of bile may allow gallstones to form. Changes to the absorptive ability of the gallbladder lining may also contribute to gallstone formation.

ABNORMAL BILE

Certain conditions, such as age, obesity, and estrogen imbalance, cause the liver to secrete bile that's abnormally high in cholesterol or lacking the proper concentration of bile salts.

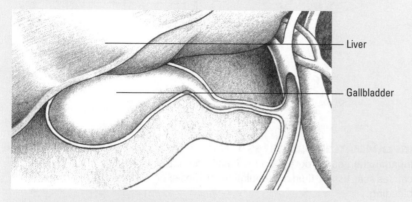

Liver

Gallbladder

INSIDE THE GALLBLADDER

When the gallbladder concentrates this abnormal bile, inflammation may occur. Excessive reabsorption of water and bile salts makes the bile less soluble. Cholesterol, calcium, and bilirubin precipitate into gallstones.

Fat entering the duodenum causes the intestinal mucosa to secrete the hormone cholecystokinin, which stimulates the gallbladder to contract and empty. If a stone lodges in the cystic duct, the gallbladder contracts but can't empty.

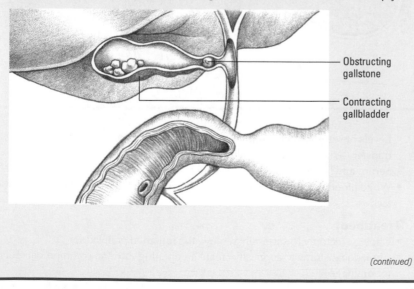

Obstructing gallstone

Contracting gallbladder

Factors causing abnormal metabolism of cholesterol and bile salts

- Age
- Obesity
- Estrogen imbalance

(continued)

Understanding gallstone formation *(continued)*

JAUNDICE, IRRITATION, INFLAMMATION

If a stone lodges in the common bile duct, the bile can't flow into the duodenum. Bilirubin is absorbed into the blood and causes jaundice.

Biliary narrowing and swelling of the tissue around the stone can also cause irritation and inflammation of the common bile duct.

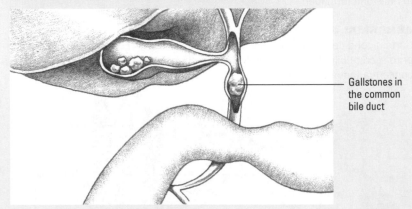

Gallstones in the common bile duct

INFLAMMATION PROGRESSION

Inflammation can progress up the biliary tree into any of the bile ducts. This causes scar tissue, fluid accumulation, cirrhosis, portal hypertension, and bleeding.

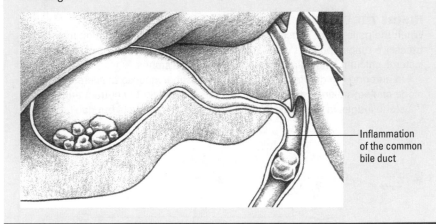

Inflammation of the common bile duct

- Levels of serum alkaline phosphate, lactate dehydrogenase, aspartate aminotransferase (AST), and total bilirubin are high
- Serum amylase level is slightly elevated
- White blood cell (WBC) counts are slightly elevated during a cholecystitis attack

● **Treatment**
  - Cholecystectomy to surgically remove the inflamed gallbladder
  - Choledochostomy to surgically create an opening into the common bile duct for drainage

- Percutaneous transhepatic cholecystostomy
- Endoscopic retrograde cholangiopancreatography (ERCP) to remove gall-stones
- Lithotripsy to break up gallstones and relieve obstruction
- Oral chenodeoxycholic acid (Chenodiol) or ursodeoxycholic acid (Actigall) to dissolve calculi
- Low-fat diet to prevent attacks
- Vitamin K to relieve itching, jaundice, and bleeding tendencies caused by vitamin K deficiencies
- Antibiotics to treat infection during an acute attack
- Nasogastric (NG) tube insertion during an acute attack for abdominal decompression

● **Nursing considerations**
- Before surgery
  - Teach the patient to deep-breathe, cough, expectorate, and perform leg exercises that are necessary after surgery
  - Teach splinting, repositioning, and ambulation techniques
- After surgery
  - Monitor the patient's vital signs for signs of bleeding, infection, or atelectasis
  - Evaluate the incision site for bleeding
    - Serosanguineous drainage is common during the first 24 to 48 hours if the patient has a wound drain
  - If a T-tube drain is placed in the duct and attached to a drainage bag, make sure that the drainage tube has no kinks and is well secured
  - Measure and record T-tube drainage daily (200 to 300 ml is normal)
  - Teach patients who will be discharged with a T tube how to perform dressing changes and routine skin care
  - Monitor intake and output
    - Allow the patient nothing by mouth for 24 to 48 hours or until bowel sounds return and nausea and vomiting stop
    - Postoperative nausea may indicate a full bladder
    - If the patient doesn't void within 8 hours or if the amount voided is inadequate, check for bladder distention
  - Encourage deep breathing and leg exercises every hour
  - Have the patient ambulate after surgery
  - Provide elastic stockings to prevent stasis and clot formation
- Evaluate the location, duration, and character of pain and administer adequate medication to relieve it
- At discharge
  - Advise the patient against heavy lifting or straining for 6 weeks
  - Urge him to walk daily
  - Instruct the patient to notify the surgeon if he has pain for more than 24 hours, anorexia, nausea or vomiting, fever, or tenderness in the abdominal area, or if he notices any jaundice, because these signs may indicate a biliary tract injury from the cholecystectomy, requiring immediate attention
- Patients who have had a laparoscopic cholecystectomy may be discharged the same day or within 24 hours after surgery

Key treatments for cholecystitis
- Surgery
- ERCP
- Lithotripsy
- Drug therapy with chenodeoxycholic acid or ursodeoxycholic acid

Key nursing considerations for cholecystitis
- Before surgery, teach about deep-breathing and coughing, leg exercises, and splinting.
- After surgery, monitor for bleeding, infection, and atelectasis.
- Monitor vital signs and intake and output.

– These patients should have minimal pain, be able to tolerate a regular diet within 24 hours after surgery, and be able to return to normal activity within 1 week

CIRRHOSIS

Key facts about cirrhosis

- Occurs when hepatic cells undergo destruction and fibrotic regeneration
- Alters liver structure and normal vasculature
- Results in buildup of toxins, which impairs blood and lymph
- Leads to hepatic insufficiency

Primary types of cirrhosis

- Biliary
- Idiopathic
- Laënnec's
- Postnecrotic

TOP 2

Causes of cirrhosis

1. Hepatitis C
2. Alcoholic liver disease

● **Definition**
  - Chronic disease characterized by diffuse destruction and fibrotic regeneration of hepatic cells
  - Damages liver tissue and normal vasculature
  - Ultimately causes hepatic insufficiency
  - Most common types
    - Biliary cirrhosis
    - Idiopathic cirrhosis
    - Laënnec's cirrhosis
    - Postnecrotic cirrhosis
  - High mortality; many patients die within 5 years of onset

● **Underlying pathophysiology**
  - Hepatic cells undergo diffuse destruction and fibrotic regeneration
  - Necrotic tissue becomes fibrotic as cells die
  - Liver structure and normal vasculature are altered by the cellular loss and resultant fibrosis
  - Blood and normal vasculature are altered by the change in the liver's capacity to filter toxins and essential nutrients
  - Blood and lymph are impaired by buildup of toxins
  - Hepatic insufficiency occurs

● **Causes**
  - Biliary cirrhosis
    - Prolonged biliary tract obstruction or inflammation
  - Idiopathic cirrhosis
    - No known cause
    - Contributing factors
      - Sarcoidosis
      - Chronic inflammatory bowel disease
  - Laënnec's cirrhosis
    - Chronic alcoholism
    - Malnutrition
  - Postnecrotic cirrhosis
    - Viral hepatitis
    - Exposure to liver toxins, such as arsenic, carbon tetrachloride, and phosphorus

● **Pathophysiologic changes**
  - Early stages
    - Anorexia resulting from distaste for certain foods
    - Nausea and vomiting resulting from inflammatory response and systemic effects of liver inflammation
    - Diarrhea caused by malabsorption
    - Dull abdominal ache due to liver inflammation

TIME-OUT FOR TEACHING

Esophageal varices

If your patient is at risk for portal hypertension, teach him about the danger of ruptured esophageal varices. Explain that esophageal varices are stretched veins whose walls are very thin. Like fragile balloons, they may break without warning, causing profuse bleeding that may be fatal without prompt intervention.

Explain that esophageal varices result from portal hypertension — increased pressure in the portal vein from obstruction in the portal circulation. As blood to the liver backs up, it begins to flow through collateral channels such as the esophageal veins. The excessive pressure causes these thin-walled veins to become varicose. If the pressure continues, they may rupture. The resulting hemorrhage can lead to hypovolemic shock.

Urge the patient to call the physician immediately if he detects signs of GI bleeding, such as dark, tarry stools or vomit that contains blood or looks like coffee grounds.

Teach him about procedures to treat esophageal varices. Electrocoagulation cauterizes the varices. Sclerotherapy, performed after the initial bleeding is controlled, involves injecting a sclerosing agent directly into the esophageal varices. Surgery is the only treatment for portal hypertension.

- Late stages
  - Pleural effusion and limited thoracic expansion due to abdominal ascites, leading to inefficient gas exchange
  - Hepatomegaly due to fibrotic changes
  - Anorexia resulting from gastric stasis
  - Jaundice related to impaired hepatic function
  - Ascites and edema of the legs from portal hypertension and decreased plasma proteins
  - Esophageal varices resulting from portal hypertension (see *Esophageal varices*)

Complications
- Ascites
- Bleeding esophageal varices, acute GI bleeding
- Coagulopathy
- Hepatic encephalopathy
- Jaundice
- Liver failure
- Portal hypertension
- Renal failure
- Respiratory compromise

Diagnostic test findings
- Liver biopsy reveals tissue destruction and fibrosis
- Abdominal X-rays show an enlarged liver, cysts, or gas within the biliary tract or liver; liver calcification; and massive fluid accumulation (ascites)
- Computed tomography (CT) and liver scans show liver size, abnormal masses, hepatic blood flow, and obstruction

Key pathophysiologic changes in cirrhosis

Early stages
- Anorexia
- Nausea and vomiting
- Diarrhea

Late stages
- Jaundice
- Ascites
- Esophageal varices

Key diagnostic test results for cirrhosis

- Liver biopsy: Tissue destruction and fibrosis
- CT and liver scans: Liver size, presence of abnormal masses or obstruction, hepatic blood flow
- Blood studies: Elevated liver enzyme, total serum bilirubin, and indirect bilirubin levels; decreased total serum albumin and protein levels; prolonged PT; decreased hemoglobin level, hematocrit, and serum electrolytes

Key treatments for cirrhosis

- Vitamins and nutritional supplements
- Antacids
- Gastric lavage
- Paracentesis

TOP 4

Areas to monitor for bleeding

1. Skin
2. Gums
3. Stools
4. Vomitus

Key nursing considerations for cirrhosis

- Monitor patient for bleeding.
- Check for signs of hepatic encephalopathy.
- Observe for signs of hypovolemic shock.

- Esophagogastroduodenoscopy (EGD) reveals bleeding esophageal varices, stomach irritation or ulceration, or duodenal bleeding and irritation
- Blood studies reveal various abnormalities
  - Liver enzyme levels are elevated
  - Total serum bilirubin and indirect bilirubin levels are elevated
  - Total serum albumin and protein levels are decreased
  - Prothrombin time (PT) is prolonged
  - Hemoglobin level, hematocrit, and serum electrolytes are decreased
  - Vitamins A, C, and K are deficient
- Urine studies show increased bilirubin and urobilirubinogen level
- Fecal studies show decreased fecal urobilirubinogen level

● Treatment

- Vitamins and nutritional supplements to help heal damaged liver cells and improve nutritional status
- Antacids to reduce gastric distress and decrease the potential for GI bleeding
- Potassium-sparing diuretics to reduce fluid accumulation
- Vasopressin (Pitressin) to treat esophageal varices
- Esophagogastric intubation with multilumen tubes to control bleeding from esophageal varices or other hemorrhage sites by using balloons to exert pressure on the bleeding site
- Gastric lavage along with antacids and histamine antagonists if the bleeding is secondary to a gastric ulcer
- Esophageal balloon tamponade to compress bleeding vessels and stop blood loss from esophageal varices
- Paracentesis to relieve abdominal pressure and remove ascitic fluid
- Surgical shunt placement to divert ascites into venous circulation, leading to weight loss, decreased abdominal girth, increased sodium excretion from the kidneys, and improved urine output
- Sclerosing agents injected into oozing vessels to induce clotting and sclerosis

● Nursing considerations

- Monitor the patient for bleeding
  - Check skin, gums, stools, and vomitus regularly
  - Apply pressure to injection sites to prevent bleeding
  - Warn the patient against taking nonsteroidal anti-inflammatory drugs (NSAIDs), straining at stool, and blowing his nose or sneezing too vigorously
  - Suggest using an electric razor and soft toothbrush
- Observe closely for signs of behavioral or personality changes
  - **Report increasing stupor, lethargy, hallucinations, or neuromuscular dysfunction**
  - **Watch for asterixis, a sign of developing hepatic encephalopathy**
- Weigh the patient and measure abdominal girth at least daily
- Inspect the ankles and sacrum for dependent edema
- Accurately record intake and output
- **Carefully evaluate the patient before, during, and after paracentesis; this drastic loss of fluid may induce shock**
- Prevent skin breakdown
  - Avoid using soap when you bathe the patient; use lubricating lotion or moisturizing agents

– Handle the patient gently
– Turn and reposition the patient often to keep his skin intact
- Refer the patient to Alcoholics Anonymous, if necessary

CROHN'S DISEASE

⬤ **Definition**
- Inflammation of any part of the GI tract, extending through all layers of the intestinal wall
  – Usually involves the proximal portion of the colon
  – May involve the terminal ileum (less common)
- May also involve inflamed or enlarged regional lymph nodes and mesentery due to fighting secondary infection

⬤ **Underlying pathophysiology**
- Inflammation spreads slowly and progressively
- Enlarged lymph nodes block lymph flow in the submucosa
- Lymphatic obstruction leads to edema, mucosal ulceration and fissures, abscesses and, sometimes, granulomas
- Oval, elevated patches of closely packed lymph follicles — called *Peyer's patches* — develop in the lining of the small intestine
- Subsequent fibrosis thickens the bowel wall and causes stenosis, or narrowing of the lumen
- Serous membrane becomes inflamed, inflamed bowel loops adhere to other diseased or normal loops, and diseased bowel segments become interspersed with healthy ones
- Diseased parts of the bowel become thicker, narrower, and shorter

⬤ **Causes**
- Exact cause unknown
- Contributing factors
  – Allergies
  – Genetic predisposition
  – Immune disorders
  – Infection
  – Lymphatic obstruction

⬤ **Pathophysiologic changes**
- Steady, colicky pain in the right lower quadrant due to acute inflammation and nerve fiber irritation
- Cramping and tenderness due to acute inflammation
- Palpable mass in the right lower quadrant
- Diarrhea due to bile salt malabsorption, loss of healthy intestinal surface area, and bacterial growth
- Weight loss secondary to diarrhea and malabsorption
- Steatorrhea secondary to fat malabsorption
- Bloody stools secondary to bleeding resulting from inflammation and ulceration

⬤ **Complications**
- Anal fistula
- Fistulas to the bladder or vagina or to the skin in an old scar area

---

Key facts about Crohn's disease
- Slow and progressive inflammation through all layers of intestinal wall
- Involves lymphatic obstruction, which leads to edema, mucosal ulceration, and fissures
- Leads to fibrosis, which causes stenosis of bowel lumen

Common factors contributing to Crohn's disease
- Genetic predisposition
- Immune disorders
- Lymphatic obstruction

Key pathophysiologic changes in Crohn's disease
- Colicky, right-lower-quadrant pain
- Diarrhea
- Bloody stools

Key diagnostic test results for Crohn's disease

- Small bowel X-ray: Irregular mucosa, ulceration, and stiffening
- Barium enema: String sign, possible fissures, and narrowing of bowel
- Sigmoidoscopy and colonoscopy: Patchy areas of inflammation, with cobblestone-like mucosal surface

Key treatments for Crohn's disease

- Corticosteroids
- Sulfasalazine
- Immunosuppressants
- Antidiarrheals
- Opioid analgesics

Key nursing considerations for Crohn's disease

- Monitor fluid and electrolyte status, hemoglobin level, hematocrit, and vital signs.
- Monitor for abdominal pain and bleeding.
- Stress importance of diet therapy.
- Refer patient to a support group.

- Fluid imbalances
- Intestinal obstruction
- Nutrient deficiencies from poor digestion and malabsorption of bile salts and vitamin B_{12}
- Perineal abscess

● **Diagnostic test findings**
- Fecal occult test reveals minute amounts of blood in stools
- Small bowel X-ray shows irregular mucosa, ulceration, and stiffening
- Barium enema reveals the string sign (segments of stricture separated by normal bowel) and possibly fissures and narrowing of the bowel
- Sigmoidoscopy and colonoscopy reveal patchy areas of inflammation, with a cobblestone-like mucosal surface
    - This finding helps to rule out ulcerative colitis
    - With colon involvement, ulcers may be seen
- Biopsy reveals granulomas in up to one-half of all specimens
- Blood tests reveal various findings
    - WBC count and erythrocyte sedimentation rate (ESR) are increased
    - Potassium, calcium, magnesium, and hemoglobin levels are decreased

● **Treatment**
- Corticosteroids to reduce inflammation and, subsequently, diarrhea, pain, and bleeding
- Sulfasalazine (Azulfidine) to reduce inflammation
- Immunosuppressants to suppress the response to antigens
- Metronidazole (Flagyl) to treat perianal complications
- Antidiarrheals to combat diarrhea (not used with patients with significant bowel obstruction)
- Opioid analgesics to control pain and diarrhea
- Stress reduction and reduced physical activity to rest the bowel and allow it to heal
- Vitamin supplements to compensate for the bowel's inability to absorb vitamins
- Elimination of fruits, vegetables, high fiber foods, dairy products, spicy and fatty foods, foods that irritate the mucosa, carbonated or caffeinated beverages, and other foods or liquids that stimulate excessive intestinal activity
- Surgery, if necessary, to repair bowel perforation and correct massive hemorrhage, fistulas, or acute intestinal obstruction
- Colectomy with ileostomy in patients with extensive disease of the large intestine and rectum

● **Nursing considerations**
- Record fluid intake and output, and weigh the patient daily
- Watch for dehydration and maintain fluid and electrolyte balance
- Stay alert for signs of intestinal bleeding (bloody stools); check stools daily for occult blood
- If the patient is receiving steroids
    - Watch for adverse effects such as GI bleeding
    - Steroids can mask signs of infection
- Check hemoglobin level and hematocrit regularly
- Give iron supplements and blood transfusions, as ordered
- Give analgesics as ordered

- Provide good patient hygiene and meticulous mouth care if the patient is restricted to nothing by mouth
- After each bowel movement, give good perineal skin care
- Monitor the patient for complications
  - Fever and pain or pneumaturia may signal a bladder fistula
  - Abdominal pain and distention and fever may indicate intestinal obstruction
  - Watch for stools from the vagina and an enterovaginal fistula
- Before ileostomy, arrange for a visit by an enterostomal therapist
- After surgery
  - Frequently check the patient's I.V. line and NG tube for proper functioning
  - Monitor the patient's vital signs and fluid intake and output
  - Watch for wound infection
- Provide meticulous stoma care
  - Teach stoma care to the patient and his family
  - Offer reassurance and emotional support
- Stress the need for a severely restricted diet and bed rest, which may be challenging, particularly for the young patient
- Refer the patient to a support group such as the Crohn's and Colitis Foundation of America

DIVERTICULAR DISEASE

● Definition
- Characterized by bulging pouches (diverticula) in the GI wall that push the mucosal lining through the surrounding muscle
- Two clinical forms
  - Diverticulosis — diverticula are present but may cause only mild or no symptoms; may progress to diverticulitis
  - Diverticulitis — diverticula are inflamed and may cause potentially fatal obstruction, infection, or hemorrhage

● Underlying pathophysiology
- Results from high intraluminal pressure on an area of weakness in the GI wall, where blood vessels enter
- Retained undigested food and bacteria accumulate in the diverticular sac, cutting off the blood supply to the thin walls of the sac, making the walls more susceptible to attack by colonic bacteria
- Inflammation follows and may lead to perforation, abscess, peritonitis, obstruction, or hemorrhage
- Occasionally, the inflamed colon segment may adhere to the bladder or other organs and cause a fistula

● Causes
- Defects in colon wall strength
- Diminished colonic motility and increased intraluminal pressure
- Low-fiber diet

● Pathophysiologic changes
- Mild diverticulitis

Key facts about diverticular disease

- Characterized by diverticula in the GI wall that push the mucosal lining through surrounding muscle
- Leads to inflammation caused by accumulated food and bacteria in diverticular sac
- Has two types: diverticulosis (mild or no symptoms) and diverticulitis (potentially fatal)

– Moderate left-lower-abdominal pain secondary to inflammation of diverticula
– Low-grade fever from trapping of bacteria-rich stool in the diverticula
– Leukocytosis from infection secondary to trapping of bacteria-rich stool in the diverticula
- Severe diverticulitis
  – Abdominal rigidity resulting from rupture of the diverticula, abscesses, and peritonitis
  – Left lower quadrant pain secondary to rupture of the diverticula and subsequent inflammation and infection
  – High fever, chills, hypotension from sepsis, and shock from the release of fecal material from the rupture site
  – Microscopic or massive hemorrhage resulting from rupture of diverticulum near a vessel
- Chronic diverticulitis
  – Constipation, ribbonlike stools, intermittent diarrhea, and abdominal distention resulting from intestinal obstruction
  – Abdominal rigidity and pain, diminishing or absent bowel sounds, nausea, and vomiting secondary to intestinal obstruction

Complications
- Bowel obstruction
- Fistula formation (vesicosigmoid is common)
- Hemorrhage
- Peritonitis

Diagnostic test findings
- Upper GI series confirms or rules out diverticulosis of the esophagus and upper bowel
- Barium enema reveals filling of diverticula, which confirms diagnosis
- Biopsy reveals evidence of benign disease, ruling out cancer
- Blood studies show an elevated ESR in diverticulitis

Treatment
- Liquid or bland diet, stool softeners, and occasional doses of mineral oil for symptomatic diverticulosis to relieve symptoms, minimize irritation, and lessen the risk of progression to diverticulitis
- High-residue diet for treatment of diverticulosis after pain has subsided to help decrease intra-abdominal pressure during defecation
- Exercise to increase the rate of stool passage
- Antibiotics to treat infection of the diverticula
- Analgesics, such as meperidine (Demerol) or morphine, to control pain and to relax smooth muscle
- Antispasmodics to control muscle spasms
- Colon resection with removal of involved segment to correct cases refractory to medical treatment
- Temporary colostomy, if necessary, to drain abscesses and rest the colon in diverticulitis accompanied by perforation, peritonitis, obstruction, or fistula
- Blood transfusions, if necessary, to treat blood loss from hemorrhage and fluid replacement, as needed

Nursing considerations

- Make sure that the patient understands the importance of dietary fiber and the harmful effects of constipation and straining during defecation; encourage increased intake of foods high in indigestible fiber
- Advise the patient to relieve constipation with stool softeners or bulk-forming cathartics
  - Instruct the patient to take bulk-forming cathartics with plenty of water
  - If swallowed dry, bulk-forming cathartics may absorb enough moisture in the mouth and throat to swell and obstruct the esophagus or trachea
- In mild disease
  - Administer medications as ordered
  - Explain diagnostic tests and preparations for such tests
  - Observe stools carefully
  - Monitor the patient's vital signs and intake and output
- If the patient is hospitalized
  - Administer medications as ordered
  - Observe his stools carefully for frequency, color, and consistency
  - Keep accurate pulse and temperature charts because they may signal developing inflammation or complications
- If diverticular bleeding occurs, the patient may require angiography and catheter placement for vasopressin infusion
  - Inspect the insertion site frequently for bleeding
  - Check pedal pulses often
  - Keep the patient from flexing his legs at the groin
- Watch for vasopressin-induced fluid retention and severe hyponatremia
- After surgery
  - Watch for signs of infection and bleeding
  - Encourage coughing and deep breathing to prevent atelectasis
  - Record intake and output accurately
  - Keep the NG tube patent
  - Teach ostomy care as needed
  - Arrange for a visit by an enterostomal therapist

GASTROESOPHAGEAL REFLUX DISEASE

Definition

- Backflow of gastric contents, duodenal contents, or both past the lower esophageal sphincter (LES) into the esophagus without associated belching or vomiting
- Causes acute epigastric pain
  - Usually occurs after a meal
  - May radiate to the chest or arms
- Also known as GERD

Underlying pathophysiology

- Reflux occurs when LES pressure is deficient or pressure in the stomach exceeds LES pressure
- The LES relaxes, and gastric contents regurgitate into the esophagus

How heartburn occurs

Hormonal fluctuations, mechanical stress, and the effects of certain foods and drugs can decrease lower esophageal sphincter (LES) pressure. When LES pressure falls and intra-adominal or intragastric pressure rises, the normally contracted LES relaxes inappropriately and allows reflux of gastric acid or bile secretions into the lower esophagus. There, the reflux irritates and inflames the esophageal mucosa, causing pyrosis.

Persistent inflammation can cause LES pressure to decrease even more and may trigger a recurrent cycle of reflux and pyrosis.

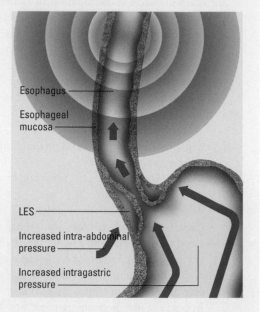

Esophagus

Esophageal mucosa

LES

Increased intra-abdominal pressure

Increased intragastric pressure

Causes of GERD

- Food, alcohol, or cigarettes that lower LES pressure
- Increased abdominal pressure
- Hiatal hernia
- Weakened esophageal sphincter

Key pathophysiologic changes in GERD

- Burning pain in epigastric area
- Pain after meals or when lying down

- The degree of mucosal injury is based on the amount and concentration of refluxed gastric acid, proteolytic enzymes, and bile acids (see *How heartburn occurs*)

Causes

- Food, alcohol, or cigarettes that lower LES pressure
- Hiatal hernia
- Increased abdominal pressure, such as with obesity or pregnancy
- Medications, such as morphine, diazepam (Valium), calcium channel blockers, meperidine, and anticholinergics
- NG intubation for more than 4 days
- Weakened esophageal sphincter

Pathophysiologic changes

- Burning pain in the epigastric area, possibly radiating to the arms and chest, resulting from the reflux of gastric contents into the esophagus causing irritation and esophageal spasm
- Pain, usually after a meal or when lying down, secondary to increased abdominal pressure causing reflux
- Feeling of fluid accumulation in the throat without a sour or bitter taste due to hypersecretion of saliva

Complications

- Chronic pulmonary disease from aspiration of gastric contents in the throat
- Esophageal stricture
- Esophageal ulceration
- Reflux esophagitis

- **Diagnostic test findings**
  - Esophageal acidity test evaluates the competence of the LES and provides an objective measure of reflux
  - Acid perfusion test confirms esophagitis and distinguishes it from cardiac disorders
  - Esophagoscopy allows visual examination of the lining of the esophagus to reveal the extent of the disease and confirm pathologic changes in mucosa
  - Barium swallow identifies hiatal hernia as the cause
  - Upper GI series detects hiatal hernia or motility problems
  - Esophageal manometry evaluates resting pressure of the LES and determines sphincter competence

- **Treatment**
  - Diet therapy to reduce abdominal pressure and reduce the incidence of reflux
    - Frequent, small meals
    - Avoidance of eating before going to bed
  - Positioning to reduce abdominal pressure and prevent reflux
    - Sitting up during and after meals
    - Sleeping with head of bed elevated
  - Increased fluid intake to wash gastric contents out of the esophagus
  - Antacids to neutralize acidic content of the stomach and minimize irritation
  - Histamine-2 (H_2) receptor antagonists to inhibit gastric acid secretion
  - Proton pump inhibitors to reduce gastric acidity
  - Cholinergic agents to increase LES pressure
  - Smoking cessation to improve LES pressure (nicotine lowers LES pressure)
  - Surgery (if hiatal hernia is the cause, or if the patient has refractory symptoms)

- **Nursing considerations**
  - Teach the patient about the causes of reflux and symptoms to report
  - Tell the patient how to avoid reflux with an antireflux regimen
    - Instruct the patient to avoid circumstances that increase intra-abdominal pressure, such as bending, coughing, vigorous exercise, tight clothing, constipation, and obesity
    - Instruct the patient to avoid substances that reduce sphincter control (cigarettes, alcohol, fatty foods, and caffeine)
    - Advise the patient to sit upright, particularly after meals, and to eat small, frequent meals
    - Tell the patient to avoid highly seasoned food, acidic juices, alcoholic drinks, bedtime snacks, and foods high in fat or carbohydrates, which reduce LES pressure
    - Instruct the patient to eat meals at least 2 hours before lying down
    - Tell the patient to take antacids, as ordered, usually 1 and 3 hours after meals and at bedtime
  - Teach the patient correct preparation for diagnostic testing, such as not eating for 6 to 8 hours before a barium swallow or endoscopy
  - After surgery involving a thoracic approach
    - Carefully watch and record chest tube drainage and respiratory status
    - If needed, give chest physiotherapy and oxygen
    - Position the patient with an NG tube in semi-Fowler's position to help prevent reflux
    - Offer reassurance and emotional support

Key diagnostic test results for GERD
- Esophagoscopy: Extent of disease; pathologic changes in mucosa
- Barium swallow: Hiatal hernia

Key treatments for GERD
- Diet therapy
- Proper positioning after meals and during sleep
- Antacids
- H_2-receptor antagonists
- Proton pump inhibitors

Key nursing considerations for GERD
- Teach patient to avoid foods that cause reflux.
- Instruct patient to eat meals at least 2 hours before lying down.
- Instruct patient about use of antacids.

Key facts about nonviral hepatitis

- Inflammation of liver
- Leads to hepatic cellular necrosis and scarring

Key pathophysiologic changes in nonviral hepatitis

- Jaundice
- Dark urine
- Clay-colored stool

Key diagnostic test results for nonviral hepatitis

- Liver enzyme levels: Elevated
- Total and direct bilirubin levels: Elevated
- ALP level: Elevated

Key treatments for nonviral hepatitis

- Lavage, catharsis, or hyperventilation
- Acetylcysteine

Key nursing considerations for nonviral hepatitis

- Teach patient about drug use and proper handling of cleaning agents and solvents.

HEPATITIS (NONVIRAL)

- **Definition**
  - Inflammation of the liver
  - Usually results from exposure to certain chemicals or drugs
  - May develop into fulminating hepatitis or cirrhosis, but most patients recover

- **Underlying pathophysiology**
  - Toxic hepatitis
    - After exposure to hepatotoxins, hepatic cellular necrosis, scarring, Kupffer cell hyperplasia, and infiltration by mononuclear phagocytes occur with varying severity
    - Alcohol, anoxia, and preexisting liver disease exacerbate the effects of some toxins
  - Drug-induced (idiosyncratic) hepatitis
    - This type may begin with a hypersensitivity reaction unique to the individual, which appears to affect all exposed people indiscriminately
    - Symptoms of hepatic dysfunction may appear at any time during or after drug exposure, but it usually manifests after 2 to 5 weeks of therapy

- **Causes**
  - Hepatotoxic chemicals
  - Hepatotoxic drugs

- **Pathophysiologic changes**
  - Anorexia, nausea, and vomiting due to systemic effects of liver inflammation
  - Jaundice from decreased bilirubin metabolism, leading to hyperbilirubinemia
  - Dark urine resulting from elevated urobilinogen
  - Hepatomegaly due to inflammation
  - Possible abdominal pain caused by liver inflammation
  - Clay-colored stool secondary to decreased bile in the GI tract resulting from liver necrosis
  - Pruritus secondary to jaundice and hyperbilirubinemia

- **Complications**
  - Cirrhosis
  - Hepatic failure

- **Diagnostic test findings**
  - Liver enzyme levels are elevated
  - Total and direct bilirubin levels are elevated
  - Alkaline phosphatase (ALP) level is elevated
  - WBC and eosinophil counts are elevated
  - Liver biopsy identifies underlying pathology, especially infiltration with WBCs

- **Treatment**
  - Lavage, catharsis, or hyperventilation, depending on the route of exposure, to remove the causative agent
  - Acetylcysteine (Mucomyst) as an antidote for acetaminophen poisoning
  - Corticosteroids to relieve symptoms of drug-induced nonviral hepatitis

- **Nursing considerations**
  - Instruct the patient about the proper use of drugs and the proper handling of cleaning agents and solvents

HEPATITIS (VIRAL)

● Definition

- Infection of the liver, resulting in hepatic cell destruction, necrosis, and autolysis
- In most patients, hepatic cells eventually regenerate with little or no residual damage
- Five major forms recognized
  - Type A
    - Infectious or short-incubation hepatitis
    - Commonly spread via the fecal-oral route by the ingestion of fecal contaminants
  - Type B
    - Serum or long-incubation hepatitis
    - Spread through contact with contaminated blood, secretions, and stools
  - Type C
    - Blood-borne disease
    - Associated with shared needles, blood transfusions
  - Type D (delta hepatitis)
    - Linked to chronic hepatitis B infection
    - Can be severe and lead to fulminant hepatitis
    - In the United States, occurs only in people who are frequently exposed to blood and blood products, such as I.V. drug users and patients with hemophilia
    - Depends on the double-shelled type B virus to replicate; for this reason, type D infection can't outlast a type B infection
  - Type E
    - Formerly grouped with types C and D under the name *non-A, non-B hepatitis*
    - Occurs primarily among patients who have recently returned from an endemic area (see *Viral hepatitis from A to E,* pages 200 and 201)
- If chronic and persistent, may prolong recovery up to 8 months

● Underlying pathophysiology

- Virus causes hepatocyte injury and death by directly killing the cells or by activating inflammatory and immune reactions
- Inflammatory and immune reactions injure or destroy hepatocytes by lysing the infected or neighboring cells
- Direct antibody attack against the viral antigens causes further destruction of the infected cells
- Edema and swelling of the interstitium lead to collapse of capillaries and decreased blood flow, tissue hypoxia, and scarring and fibrosis

● Causes

- Infection with the causative viruses (hepatitis A, B, C, D, or E)

● Pathophysiologic changes

- Prodromal stage
  - Systemic effects of liver inflammation
    - Easy fatigue and generalized malaise

Key facts about viral hepatitis

- Infection of liver
- Results from a virus that causes hepatocyte injury and death
- Leads to immune reactions against viral antigens and further destruction of hepatic cells
- Classified as type A, B, C, D, or E

Key pathophysiologic changes in viral hepatitis

Prodromal stage
- Malaise
- Fatigue
- Nausea and vomiting
- Right-upper-quadrant tenderness
- Dark urine and clay-colored stools

Clinical stage
- Itching
- Jaundice
- Abdominal pain or tenderness

Recovery stage
- Return of appetite

Hepatitis severity by type

- A: Mild
- B: Commonly severe
- C: Moderate
- D: Can be severe and lead to fulminant hepatitis
- E: Highly virulent with progression to fulminant hepatitis

Viral hepatitis from A to E

This chart compares the features of each (characterized) type of viral hepatitis. Other types are emerging.

FEATURE	HEPATITIS A	HEPATITIS B
Incubation	15 to 45 days	30 to 180 days
Onset	Acute	Insidious
Age-group most affected	Children, young adults	Any age
Transmission	Fecal-oral, sexual (especially oral-anal contact), nonpercutaneous (sexual, maternal–neonatal), percutaneous (rare)	Blood-borne; parenteral route, sexual, maternal–neonatal; virus is shed in all body fluids
Severity	Mild	Commonly severe
Prognosis	Generally good	Worsens with age and debility
Progression to chronicity	None	Occasional

- Anorexia and mild weight loss
- Arthralgia and myalgia
- Nausea and vomiting resulting from GI effects of liver inflammation
  - Changes in the senses of taste and smell related to liver inflammation
  - Fever secondary to inflammatory process
  - Right upper quadrant tenderness resulting from liver inflammation and irritation of area nerve fibers
  - Dark colored urine resulting from urobilinogen
  - Clay-colored stools due to decreased bile in the GI tract
- Clinical stage
  - Worsening of all symptoms of prodromal stage
  - Itching and jaundice due to increased bilirubin in the blood
  - Abdominal pain or tenderness resulting from continued liver inflammation
- Recovery stage
  - Subsiding of symptoms
  - Return of appetite

Complications
- Cirrhosis
- Hepatic failure and death
- Primary hepatocellular carcinoma

HEPATITIS C	HEPATITIS D	HEPATITIS E
15 to 160 days	14 to 64 days	14 to 60 days
Insidious	Acute and chronic	Acute
More common in adults	Any age	Ages 20 to 40
Blood-borne; parenteral route	Parenteral route; most people infected with hepatitis D are also infected with hepatitis B	Primarily fecal-oral
Moderate	Can be severe and lead to fulminant hepatitis	Highly virulent with common progression to fulminant hepatitis and hepatic failure, especially in pregnant patients
Moderate	Fair, worsens in chronic cases; can lead to chronic hepatitis D and chronic liver disease	Good unless pregnant
10% to 50% of cases	Occasional	None

● **Diagnostic test findings**
  • Hepatitis profile study identifies antibodies specific to the causative virus, establishing the type of hepatitis
  • Serum AST and alanine aminotransferase (ALT) levels are increased in the prodromal stage
  • Serum ALP level is slightly increased
  • Serum bilirubin level may remain high in late disease, especially in severe cases
  • PT is prolonged (greater than 3 seconds longer than normal indicates severe liver damage)
  • WBC counts reveal transient neutropenia and lymphopenia followed by lymphocytosis
  • Liver biopsy confirms suspicion of chronic hepatitis

● **Treatment**
  • Rest to minimize energy demands
  • Avoidance of alcohol or other drugs to prevent further liver damage
  • Diet therapy with small, high-calorie meals to combat anorexia
  • Parenteral nutrition if patient can't eat due to persistent vomiting
  • Vaccination against hepatitis A and B to provide immunity before transmission occurs

Key diagnostic test results for viral hepatitis
● Hepatitis profile study: Antibodies specific to causative virus
● Serum studies: Increased AST and ALT levels in prodromal stage, slightly increased ALP level

Key treatments for viral hepatitis
● Rest
● Diet therapy
● Avoidance of alcohol

Key nursing considerations for viral hepatitis

- Use standard precautions.
- Encourage fluid and foods.
- Schedule rest periods.
- Watch for signs of complications, such as hepatic coma.

- **Nursing considerations**
  - Use standard precautions for all patients
  - Use enteric precautions when caring for patients with type A or E hepatitis
  - Inform visitors about isolation precautions
  - Schedule treatments and tests so that the patient can rest between bouts of activity
  - Encourage the patient to eat
    - Don't overload his meal tray or overmedicate him
    - Doing so will diminish his appetite
  - Encourage intake of fluids (at least 135 oz [4,000 ml] per day)
    - Encourage the anorectic patient to drink fruit juices
    - Offer chipped ice and effervescent soft drinks to maintain hydration without inducing vomiting
  - Administer supplemental vitamins and commercial feedings as ordered
  - If symptoms are severe and the patient can't tolerate oral intake, provide I.V. therapy and parenteral nutrition, as ordered
  - Record the patient's weight daily, and keep intake and output records
    - Observe stools for color, consistency, and amount
    - Record the frequency of bowel movements
  - Watch for signs of fluid shift, such as weight gain and orthostasis
  - Watch for signs of hepatic coma, dehydration, pneumonia, vascular problems, and pressure ulcers
  - Fulminant hepatitis
    - Maintain electrolyte balance and a patent airway
    - Prevent infections
    - Control bleeding
    - Correct hypoglycemia and other complications while awaiting liver regeneration and repair
  - Before discharge
    - Emphasize the importance of having regular medical check-ups for at least 1 year
    - Warn the patient against drinking alcohol or taking over-the-counter drugs during this period
    - Teach the patient to recognize the signs of recurrence

INTESTINAL POLYPS

Key facts about intestinal polyps

- Small, tumorlike growths that project from mucous membrane surface
- Result from unrestrained cell growth in upper epithelium
- Classified as adenomatous or nonadenomatous

- **Definition**
  - Small, tumorlike growths that project from a mucous membrane surface
  - May develop in the colon or rectum, where they protrude into the GI tract
  - May be described by their appearance
    - Pedunculated — attached by a stalk to the intestinal wall
    - Sessile — attached to the intestinal wall with a broad base and no stalk
  - Classified according to tissue type involved
    - Adenomatous polyps (benign tumors that originate from glandular tissues in the epithelial layer of the intestine), such as tubular adenoma, tubulovillous adenoma, and villous adenoma
    - Nonadenomatous polyps, such as hyperplastic polyps, which result from overgrowth of cells

Underlying pathophysiology
- Unrestrained cell growth in the upper epithelium leads to masses of tissue that rise above the mucosal membrane and protrude into the GI tract

Causes
- Unknown

Risk factors
- Age
- Heredity
- High-fat, low-fiber diet

Pathophysiologic changes
- Because intestinal polyps don't generally cause symptoms, they're usually discovered incidentally during a digital examination or rectosigmoidoscopy
- Rectal bleeding is a common sign
  - High rectal polyps leave a streak of blood on the stool
  - Low rectal polyps bleed freely

Complications
- Anemia
- Bowel obstruction
- Colorectal cancer (villous adenomas and familial polyps)
- Intussusception
- Rectal bleeding

Diagnostic test findings
- Sigmoidoscopy or colonoscopy and rectal biopsy identifies rectal polyps, confirming diagnosis
- Barium enema can help identify polyps that are located high in the colon
- Supportive laboratory findings
  - Occult blood is in the stools
  - Hemoglobin level and hematocrit (with anemia) are low
  - Serum electrolyte imbalances may be present in patients with villous adenomas

Treatment
- Surgical procedures
  - Polypectomy, commonly by fulguration (destruction by high-frequency electricity) during endoscopy
  - Abdominoperineal resection, low anterior resection, ileostomy, colostomy
  - Biopsy

Nursing considerations
- During diagnostic evaluation
  - Check sodium, potassium, and chloride levels daily in the patient with fluid imbalance
  - Adjust fluid and electrolytes, as necessary
  - Weigh the patient daily, and record the amount of diarrhea
  - Watch for signs of dehydration (decreased urine and increased blood urea nitrogen [BUN] levels)
  - Tell the patient to watch for and report evidence of rectal bleeding
- After biopsy and fulguration

Key pathophysiologic change with intestinal polyps
- Rectal bleeding

Key diagnostic test results for intestinal polyps
- Sigmoidoscopy or colonoscopy and rectal biopsy: Presence of polyps
- Barium enema: Identification of polyps located high in the colon

Key treatments for intestinal polyps
- Polypectomy
- Abdominoperineal resection
- Low anterior resection

Key nursing considerations for intestinal polyps

- During diagnostic tests, monitor fluid, electrolyte, and BUN levels.
- Tell patient to watch for and report rectal bleeding.
- Prevent postoperative embolism with ambulation, antiembolism stockings, and ROM exercises.
- Monitor postoperative patients for signs of perforation or hemorrhage.

Key facts about IBS

- Involves chronic abdominal pain
- Alternates between constipation and diarrhea
- May result from motor disturbances of the entire colon, leading to strong contractions of intestinal smooth muscle

Key causes of IBS

- Psychological stress
- Ingestion of irritants
- Hormonal changes

      – Check for signs of perforation and hemorrhage, such as sudden hypotension, decrease in the hemoglobin level or hematocrit, shock, abdominal pain, and passage of red blood through the rectum
      – Have the patient walk as soon as possible after the procedure
      – Watch for and record the first bowel movement, which may not occur for 2 to 3 days
      – If the patient has benign polyps, stress the need for routine follow-up studies to check for new polypoid growth
      – Prepare the patient with precancerous or familial lesions for abdominoperineal resection
        • Provide emotional support and preoperative instruction
- After ileostomy or subtotal colectomy with ileoproctostomy
      – Properly care for abdominal dressings, I.V. lines, and indwelling urinary catheter
      – Record intake and output
      – Check the patient's vital signs for hypotension and surgical complications
      – Administer pain medication, as ordered
      – Prevent embolism development
        • Have the patient walk as soon as possible
        • Apply antiembolism stockings
        • Encourage range-of-motion (ROM) exercises
      – Provide enterostomal therapy and teach stoma care

IRRITABLE BOWEL SYNDROME

Definition
- Chronic abdominal pain, alternating constipation and diarrhea, excess flatus, sense of incomplete evacuation, and abdominal distention
- Common, stress-related disorder
- Predominant in women
- Benign condition; has no anatomical or physiologic abnormality or inflammatory component
- Also known as IBS

Underlying pathophysiology
- Appears to reflect motor disturbances of the entire colon in response to stimuli
- Muscles of the small bowel are sensitive to certain factors
    – Some muscles are sensitive to motor abnormalities and distention
    – Others are sensitive to certain foods and drugs or hypersensitive to the hormones gastrin and cholecystokinin
- Pain seems to be caused by abnormally strong contractions of the intestinal smooth muscle as it reacts to distention, irritants, or stress

Causes
- Abuse of laxatives
- Hormonal changes (menstruation)
- Ingestion of irritants, such as coffee, fatty foods, raw fruit, or vegetables
- Lactose intolerance
- Psychological stress (most common)

Pathophysiologic changes

- Crampy lower abdominal pain secondary to muscle contraction
- Pain that intensifies 1 to 2 hours after a meal from irritation of nerve fibers by causative stimulus
- Constipation alternating with diarrhea, with one condition being dominant, secondary to motor disturbances from causative stimulus
- Mucus passed through the rectum resulting from altered secretion in intestinal lumen caused by motor abnormalities
- Abdominal distention and bloating caused by flatus and constipation

Complications

- None known

Diagnostic test findings

- Stool samples for ova, parasites, bacteria, and blood rule out infection
- Lactose intolerance test to determine if lactose intolerance is a factor in the disease
- Barium enema may reveal colon spasm and tubular appearance of descending colon without evidence of cancers and diverticulosis
- Sigmoidoscopy or colonoscopy may reveal spastic contractions without evidence of colon cancer or inflammatory bowel disease
- Rectal biopsy rules out malignancy

Treatment

- Stress relief measures, including counseling or mild anti-anxiety agents
- Identification and avoidance of food irritants
- Heat application to the abdomen
- Bulking agents to reduce episodes of diarrhea and minimize effect of non-propulsive colonic contractions
- Antispasmodics (propantheline [Pro-Banthine] or diphenoxylate and atropine sulfate [Lomotil]) for pain
- Loperamide (Imodium) possibly to reduce urgency and fecal soiling in patients with persistent diarrhea
- Bowel training (if the cause is chronic laxative abuse) to regain muscle control

Nursing considerations

- Tell the patient to avoid irritating foods
- Encourage the patient to develop regular bowel habits
- Help the patient deal with stress
- Warn the patient about the adverse effects of sedatives and antispasmodics, including altered bowel habits
- Encourage the patient to have regular check-ups because pancreatitis is associated with a higher than normal incidence of diverticulitis and colon cancer
- For patients older than age 40, emphasize the need for an annual sigmoidoscopy and rectal examination

PANCREATITIS

Definition

- Inflammation of the pancreas
- May be acute or chronic
- May be due to edema, necrosis, or hemorrhage

Key pathophysiologic changes in IBS

- Crampy lower abdominal pain
- Constipation alternating with diarrhea
- Abdominal distention and bloating

Key diagnostic test results for IBS

- Barium enema: Colon spasm and tubular appearance of descending colon
- Sigmoidoscopy or colonoscopy: Spastic contractions

Key treatments for IBS

- Stress management
- Avoidance of food irritants
- Antispasmodics
- Antidiarrheals

Key nursing considerations for IBS

- Encourage patient to develop regular bowel habits.
- Encourage patient to have regular check-ups.

TOP 2

Causes of pancreatitis

1. Alcoholism
2. Biliary tract disease

- Good prognosis if associated with biliary tract disease
- Poor prognosis if associated with alcoholism
- Mortality as high as 60% when associated with necrosis and hemorrhage

● **Underlying pathophysiology**
- Acute pancreatitis occurs in two forms
  - Edematous pancreatitis causes fluid accumulation and swelling
  - Necrotizing pancreatitis causes cell death and tissue damage
- Inflammation that occurs with both types is caused by premature activation of enzymes, which causes tissue damage
- Enzymes back up and spill out into the pancreatic tissue resulting in autodigestion of the pancreas
- In chronic pancreatitis, persistent inflammation produces irreversible changes in the structure and function of the pancreas
  - It sometimes follows an episode of acute pancreatitis
  - Protein precipitates block the pancreatic duct and eventually harden or calcify, leading to fibrosis and atrophy of the glands
  - Growths called pseudocysts contain pancreatic enzymes and tissue debris
  - An abscess results if *pseudocysts* become infected
  - It damages the islets of Langerhans, and the damage may cause diabetes mellitus
- Sudden severe pancreatitis causes massive hemorrhage and total destruction of the pancreas, manifested as diabetic acidosis, shock, or coma

● **Causes**
- Abnormal organ structure
- Alcoholism
- Biliary tract disease
- Blunt or surgical trauma
- Drugs, such as glucocorticoids, sulfonamides, thiazides, hormonal contraceptives, and NSAIDs
- Endoscopic examination of the bile ducts and pancreas
- Kidney failure or transplantation
- Metabolic or endocrine disorders, such as high cholesterol levels or overactive thyroid
- Pancreatic cysts or tumors
- Penetrating peptic ulcers

● **Pathophysiologic changes**
- Midepigastric abdominal pain, which may radiate to the back, caused by several factors
  - Escape of inflammatory exudate and enzymes into the back of the peritoneum
  - Edema and distention of the pancreatic capsule
  - Obstruction of the biliary tract
- Mottled skin from hemorrhagic necrosis of the pancreas
- Tachycardia secondary to dehydration and possible hypovolemia
- Low-grade fever resulting from the inflammatory response
- Cold, sweaty extremities secondary to cardiovascular collapse
- Restlessness related to pain associated with acute pancreatitis
- Extreme malaise (in chronic pancreatitis) related to malabsorption or diabetes

- In severe attack
  - Persistent vomiting from hypermotility or paralytic ileus secondary to pancreatitis or peritonitis
  - Abdominal distention from bowel hypermotility and the accumulation of fluids in the abdominal cavity
  - Diminished bowel activity suggesting altered motility secondary to peritonitis
  - Crackles at lung bases secondary to heart failure
  - Left pleural effusion from circulating pancreatic enzymes

Complications
- Biliary and duodenal obstruction
- Diabetes mellitus
- Massive hemorrhage and shock
- Portal and splenic vein thrombosis
- Pseudocysts
- Respiratory failure

Diagnostic test findings
- Elevated serum amylase and lipase confirm diagnosis
- Blood and urine glucose tests reveal transient glucose in urine and hyperglycemia
  - In chronic pancreatitis, serum glucose levels may be transiently elevated
- WBC count is elevated
- Serum bilirubin levels are elevated in acute and chronic pancreatitis
- Blood calcium levels may be decreased
- Stool analysis reveals elevated lipid and trypsin levels in chronic pancreatitis
- Abdominal and chest X-rays
  - Detect pleural effusions
  - Differentiate pancreatitis from diseases that cause similar symptoms
  - May detect pancreatic calculi
- CT scan and ultrasonography show an enlarged pancreas with cysts and pseudocysts
- ERCP has two functions
  - Identifies ductal system abnormalities, such as calcification or strictures
  - Helps differentiate pancreatitis from other disorders such as pancreatic cancer

Treatment
- I.V. replacement of fluids, protein, and electrolytes to treat shock
- Fluid volume replacement to help correct metabolic acidosis
- Blood transfusions to replace blood loss from hemorrhage
- Withholding food and fluids to rest the pancreas and reduce pancreatic enzyme secretion
- NG tube suctioning to decrease stomach distention and suppress pancreatic secretions
- Antiemetics to alleviate nausea and vomiting
- Meperidine to relieve abdominal pain
- Antacids to neutralize gastric secretions
- Histamine antagonists to decrease hydrochloric acid production
- Antibiotics to fight bacterial infections
- Anticholinergics to reduce vagal stimulation, decrease GI motility, and inhibit pancreatic enzyme secretion

Key diagnostic test results for pancreatitis
- Serum amylase and lipase levels: Elevated
- WBC count: Elevated
- ERCP: Ductal system abnormalities; differentiates pancreatitis from other disorders

Key treatments for pancreatitis
- I.V. replacement of fluids, protein, and electrolytes (if patient is in shock)
- Blood transfusions
- Meperidine
- Anticholinergics
- Withholding of food and fluids

- Insulin to correct hyperglycemia
- Surgical drainage to treat a pancreatic abscess or pseudocyst or to reestablish drainage of the pancreas
- Laparotomy (if biliary tract obstruction causes acute pancreatitis) to remove obstruction

Nursing considerations
- Monitor the patient's vital signs and hemodynamics closely
  - Give plasma or albumin, if ordered, to maintain blood pressure
  - Record fluid intake and output
  - Check urine output hourly, and monitor electrolyte levels
  - Assess for crackles, rhonchi, or decreased breath sounds
- Maintain constant NG suctioning for bowel decompression, and give nothing by mouth
- Perform good mouth and nose care
- Watch for calcium deficiency
  - Signs and symptoms include tetany, cramps, carpopedal spasm, and seizures
  - If you suspect hypocalcemia, keep airway and suction apparatus handy and pad side rails
- Administer analgesics as needed to relieve the patient's pain and anxiety
- Warn the patient that he may experience dry mouth and facial flushing because anticholinergics reduce salivary and sweat gland secretions
- **Remember that narrow-angle glaucoma contraindicates the use of atropine or its derivatives**
- Watch for adverse reactions to antibiotics
  - Nephrotoxicity may occur with aminoglycosides
  - Pseudomembranous enterocolitis may occur with clindamycin
  - Blood dyscrasias may occur with chloramphenicol
- Don't confuse thirst due to hyperglycemia with dry mouth due to NG intubation and anticholinergics
- Watch for complications due to total parenteral nutrition (TPN), such as sepsis, hypokalemia, overhydration, and metabolic acidosis
- Use strict aseptic technique when caring for the catheter insertion site

PEPTIC ULCERS

Definition
- Circumscribed lesions in the mucosal membrane extending below the epithelium
- Can develop in the lower esophagus, stomach, pylorus, duodenum, or jejunum
- May be acute or chronic
  - If chronic, they have scar tissue at their base (see *Understanding peptic ulcers*)
- Gastric ulcers are most common in middle-aged and elderly men, especially in chronic users of NSAIDs, alcohol, or tobacco

Underlying pathophysiology
- Peptic ulcers resulting from *Helicobacter pylori*
  - *H. pylori* releases a toxin that destroys the gastric and duodenal mucosa

---

Key nursing considerations for pancreatitis
- Monitor for signs of calcium deficiency (tetany, cramps, carpopedal spasm, seizures).
- Maintain NG suctioning.
- Give nothing by mouth.
- In patient with narrow-angle glaucoma, don't give atropine or its derivatives.

Key facts about peptic ulcers
- Involve lesions in the mucosal membrane extending below the epithelium
- Can develop in the lower esophagus, stomach, pylorus, duodenum, or jejunum
- Result when *H. pylori* releases a toxin that destroys the gastric and duodenal mucosa
- May result from inhibition of prostaglandin synthesis

Understanding peptic ulcers

A GI lesion isn't necessarily an ulcer. Lesions that don't extend below the mucosal lining (epithelium) are called *erosions*. Lesions of acute and chronic ulcers can extend through the epithelium and perforate the stomach wall. Chronic ulcers also have scar tissue at the base.

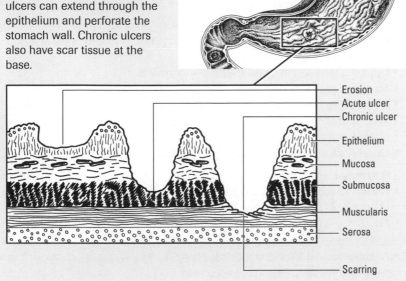

- Erosion
- Acute ulcer
- Chronic ulcer
- Epithelium
- Mucosa
- Submucosa
- Muscularis
- Serosa
- Scarring

Key types of gastric lesions

- Erosions
- Acute ulcers
- Chronic ulcers

- The epithelium's resistance to acid digestion is reduced, causing gastritis and ulcer disease
- Acid isn't the dominant cause of bacterial infection but contributes to the consequences
- Peptic ulcers resulting from other causes
  - Ulceration stems from inhibition of prostaglandin synthesis (such as by NSAIDs), increased gastric acid and pepsin secretion, reduced gastric mucosal blood flow, or decreased cytoprotective mucus production

Causes
- *H. pylori* infection
- Pathologic hypersecretory disorders
- Use of NSAIDs

Pathophysiologic changes
- Gastric ulcer
  - Pain that worsens with eating due to stretching of the mucosa by food
  - Nausea and anorexia secondary to mucosal stretching
- Duodenal ulcer
  - Epigastric pain that's gnawing, dull, aching, or "hungerlike" due to excessive acid production
  - Pain that's relieved by food or antacids, but usually recurring 2 to 4 hours later secondary to food acting as a buffer for acid

Key pathophysiologic changes with peptic ulcers

- Pain with eating (gastric ulcer)
- Pain relieved with food or antacids (duodenal ulcer)

● **Complications**
- Gastric outlet obstruction
- Gastric perforation
- Hemorrhage
- Shock

● **Diagnostic test findings**
- Barium swallow or upper GI and small bowel series may reveal the presence of the ulcer
  - This is the first test performed on a patient when symptoms aren't severe
- EGD confirms the presence of an ulcer and permits cytologic studies and biopsy to rule out *H. pylori* or cancer
- Upper GI tract X-rays reveal mucosal abnormalities
- Stool analysis may reveal occult blood
- Serologic testing may disclose clinical signs of infection such as an elevated WBC count
- Gastric secretory studies show hyperchlorhydria
- Urea breath test results show *H. pylori* activity

● **Treatment**
- Antimicrobial agents (tetracycline, bismuth subsalicylate, and metronidazole) to eradicate *H. pylori* infection (see *Treating peptic ulcers,* pages 212 and 213)
- Misoprostol (Cytotec), a prostaglandin analog, to inhibit gastric acid secretion and increase carbonate and mucus production, to protect the stomach lining
- Antacids to neutralize acidic gastric contents by elevating the gastric pH, thus protecting the mucosa and relieving pain
- Anticholinergic drugs to inhibit the effect of the vagal nerve on acid-secreting cells
- H$_2$-receptor antagonists to reduce acid secretion
- Sucralfate (Carafate), a mucosal protectant, to form an acid-impermeable membrane that adheres to the mucous membrane and accelerates mucus production
- Proton gastric acid pump inhibitor, omeprazole (Prilosec), to decrease gastric acid secretion
- Dietary therapy
  - Small frequent meals
  - Avoidance of eating before bedtime to neutralize gastric contents
  - Avoidance of caffeine and alcohol to inhibit gastric acid secretion
- Insertion of an NG tube (in instances of GI bleeding)
  - Allows gastric decompression and rest
  - Permits iced saline lavage, which may contain norepinephrine
- Gastroscopy to allow visualization of the bleeding site and coagulation by laser or cautery to control bleeding
- Surgery to repair perforation or to treat unresponsiveness to conservative treatment or suspected malignancy

● **Nursing considerations**
- Administer prescribed medications
- Watch for adverse reactions to H$_2$-receptor antagonists and omeprazole, such as dizziness, fatigue, rash, and mild diarrhea

TIME-OUT FOR TEACHING

Topics for patients with peptic ulcers

Be sure to include these points when teaching your patient about treatment for a peptic ulcer:

- adverse reactions to histamine-2 receptor antagonists and proton pump inhibitors (such as dizziness, fatigue, rash, and mild diarrhea)
- use of antacids containing low amounts of sodium if the patient has cardiac disease or follows a sodium-restricted diet
- importance of avoiding steroids and nonsteroidal anti-inflammatory drugs because these medications irritate the gastric mucosa
- importance of stopping smoking
- importance of avoiding stressful situations, excessive intake of coffee, and ingestion of alcoholic beverages during exacerbations of peptic ulcer disease
- potential adverse effects of antibiotic therapy, such as superinfection and diarrhea, and when to notify the physician if such effects occur
- potential adverse effects of bismuth subsalicylate such as constipation
- description of follow-up testing that the physician will order to confirm eradication of *Helicobacter pylori* infection, if such infection is the cause.

- Teach the patient proper self-care techniques (see *Topics for patients with peptic ulcers*)
- After gastric surgery
  - Keep the NG tube patent
    - If the tube isn't functioning, don't reposition it; you might damage the suture line or anastomosis
    - Notify the surgeon promptly
  - Monitor intake and output, including NG tube drainage
    - Check for bowel sounds
    - Allow the patient nothing by mouth until peristalsis resumes and the NG tube is removed or clamped
  - Replace fluids and electrolytes
  - Assess for signs of dehydration, sodium deficiency, and metabolic alkalosis, which may occur secondary to gastric suction
  - **Monitor for possible complications**
    - **Hemorrhage or shock**
    - Iron, folate, or vitamin B_{12} deficiency anemia from malabsorption (pernicious anemia) due to lack of intrinsic factor
    - Dumping syndrome (a rapid gastric emptying produced by a bolus of food, causing distention of the duodenum or jejunum)
  - Take steps to avoid dumping syndrome
    - Advise the patient to lie down after meals
    - Tell the patient to drink fluids between meals rather than with meals
    - Tell the patient to avoid eating large amounts of carbohydrates, and to eat four to six small, high-protein, low-carbohydrate meals during the day

Key nursing considerations for peptic ulcers

- Watch for adverse reactions to prescribed medications.

After gastric surgery
- Monitor intake and output, bowels sounds, and electrolytes.
- Watch for signs of hemorrhage, shock, dumping syndrome, and vitamin or mineral deficiency.

(Text continues on page 214.)

GO WITH THE FLOW

Treating peptic ulcers

Peptic ulcers can result from factors that increase gastric acid production or from factors that impair mucosal barrier protection. This flowchart highlights the actions of the major treatments used for peptic ulcer and where they interfere with the pathophysiologic chain of events.

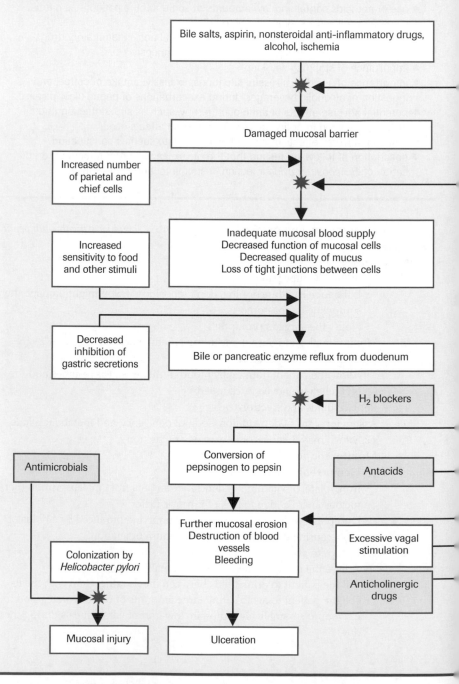

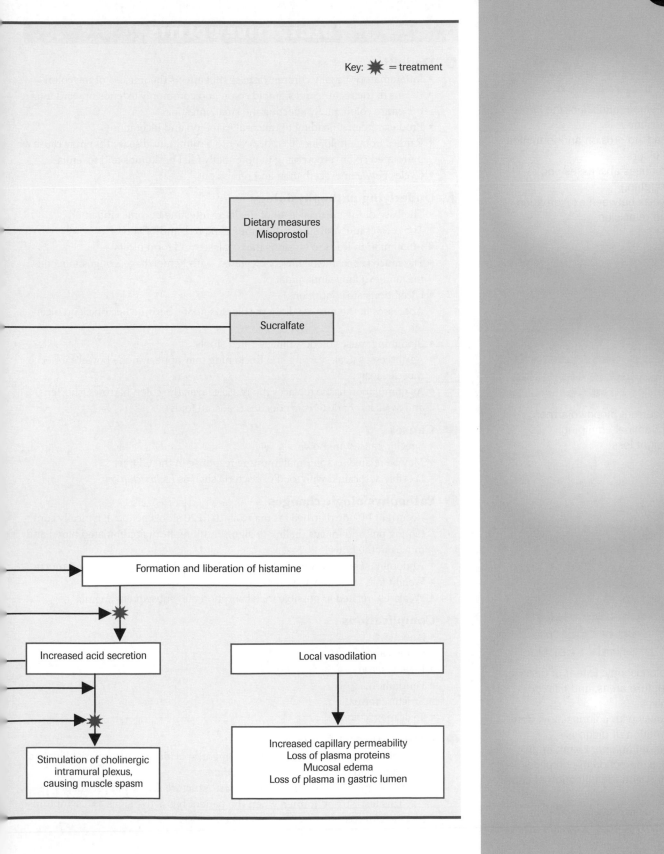

Key: ✸ = treatment

Dietary measures
Misoprostol

Sucralfate

Formation and liberation of histamine

Increased acid secretion

Local vasodilation

Stimulation of cholinergic
intramural plexus,
causing muscle spasm

Increased capillary permeability
Loss of plasma proteins
Mucosal edema
Loss of plasma in gastric lumen

ULCERATIVE COLITIS

Key facts about ulcerative colitis

- Inflamed mucosa of the large intestines
- Leads to erosion and formation of ulcers
- Produces abscesses and sloughing
- Cycles between exacerbation and remission

Key pathophysiologic changes in ulcerative colitis

- Recurrent bloody diarrhea
- Abdominal cramping
- Weight loss

Key diagnostic test results for ulcerative colitis

- Colonoscopy: Extent of disease, stricture areas, and pseudo-polyps
- Biopsy with colonoscopy: Confirmation of diagnosis
- Barium enema: Extent of disease, detection of complications, and identification of cancer

Definition

- Inflammatory, usually chronic, disease that affects the mucosa of the colon
- Begins in the rectum and sigmoid colon and commonly extends upward into the entire colon, rarely affecting the small intestine
- Produces edema (leading to mucosal friability) and ulcerations
- Ranges from a mild, localized disorder to a fulminant disease that may cause a perforated colon, progressing to potentially fatal peritonitis and toxemia
- Cycles between exacerbation and remission

Underlying pathophysiology

- The base of the mucosal layer of the large intestine becomes inflamed
- The colon's mucosal surface becomes dark, red, and velvety
- Inflammation leads to erosions that coalesce and form ulcers
- The mucosa becomes diffusely ulcerated, with hemorrhage, congestion, edema, and exudative inflammation
- Ulcerations are continuous
- Abscesses in the mucosa drain purulent exudate, become necrotic, and ulcerate
- Sloughing causes bloody, mucus-filled stools
- As abscesses heal, scarring and thickening may appear in the bowel's inner muscle layer
- As granulation tissue replaces the muscle layer, the colon narrows, shortens, and loses its characteristic pouches (haustral folds)

Causes

- Specific causes unknown
- May be related to abnormal immune response in the GI tract
- Possibly associated with food or bacteria such as *Escherichia coli*

Pathophysiologic changes

- Recurrent bloody diarrhea (as many as 10 to 20 stools per day), typically containing pus and mucus (hallmark sign), resulting from accumulated blood and mucus in the bowel
- Abdominal cramping and rectal urgency from accumulated blood and mucus
- Weight loss secondary to malabsorption
- Weakness related to possible malabsorption and subsequent anemia

Complications

- Anemia
- Colon cancer
- Liver disease
- Perforation
- Stricture formation
- Toxic megacolon

Diagnostic test findings

- Sigmoidoscopy confirms rectal involvement, specifically mucosal friability and flattening and thick, inflammatory exudate
- Colonoscopy reveals extent of the disease, stricture areas, and pseudopolyps
  – This test isn't performed when the patient has active signs and symptoms
- Biopsy with colonoscopy confirms the diagnosis

- Barium enema reveals the extent of the disease, detects complications, and identifies cancer
  - This test isn't performed when the patient has active signs and symptoms
- Stool specimen analysis reveals blood, pus, and mucus but no disease-causing organisms
- Serology reveals various findings
  - Serum potassium, magnesium, and albumin levels are decreased
  - WBC count is decreased
  - Hemoglobin level is decreased
  - PT is prolonged
- Elevated ESR correlates with the severity of the attack

Treatment
- Corticotropin and adrenal corticosteroids to control inflammation
- Sulfasalazine for its anti-inflammatory and antimicrobial effects
- Antidiarrheals to relieve frequent, troublesome diarrhea in patients whose ulcerative colitis is otherwise under control
- Iron supplements to correct anemia
- TPN and nothing by mouth for patients with severe disease to rest the intestinal tract, decrease stool volume, and restore nitrogen balance
- Fortified liquids to supplement nutrition in patients with moderate symptoms
- I.V. hydration to replace fluid loss from diarrhea
- Surgery to correct massive dilation of the colon and to treat patients with symptoms that are unbearable or unresponsive to drugs and supportive measures
- Proctocolectomy with ileostomy
  - Diverts stool
  - Allows rectal anastomosis to heal
  - Removes potentially malignant epithelia of the rectum and colon

Nursing considerations
- Accurately record intake and output, particularly the frequency and volume of stools
- Watch for signs of dehydration and electrolyte imbalances, especially signs and symptoms of hypokalemia (muscle weakness and paresthesia) and hypernatremia (tachycardia, flushed skin, fever, and dry tongue)
- Monitor the patient's hemoglobin level and hematocrit, and give blood transfusions, as ordered
- Provide good mouth care for the patient who's on nothing-by-mouth status
- After each bowel movement, thoroughly clean the skin around the rectum
- Provide an air mattress or sheepskin to help prevent skin breakdown
- Administer medications as ordered
  - Watch for adverse effects of prolonged corticosteroid therapy (moon face, hirsutism, edema, and gastric irritation)
  - Be aware that corticosteroid therapy may mask infection
- If the patient needs TPN
  - Change dressings as ordered
  - Assess for inflammation at the insertion site
  - Check capillary blood glucose levels every 4 to 6 hours
- If the patient is prone to bleeding
  - Take precautionary measures

Key treatments for ulcerative colitis
- I.V. hydration
- TPN
- Sulfasalazine
- Antidiarrheals
- Corticosteroids

Key nursing considerations for ulcerative colitis
- Monitor fluid and electrolyte status.
- Provide good mouth care for patients on nothing-by-mouth status.
- Watch for adverse effects of corticosteroid therapy.
- For patients receiving TPN, assess for inflammation at insertion site.
- Observe for signs of complications, such as perforated colon and peritonitis.

– Watch closely for signs of complications
  · Perforated colon and peritonitis (fever, severe abdominal pain, abdominal rigidity and tenderness, and cool, clammy skin)
  · Toxic megacolon (abdominal distention and decreased bowel sounds)
• For patients requiring surgery
  – Carefully prepare the patient for surgery
    · Inform the patient about ileostomy
    · Perform bowel preparation, as ordered
  – After surgery
    · Provide meticulous supportive care
    · Continue teaching correct stoma care
    · Keep the NG tube patent
    · After removal of the NG tube, provide a clear-liquid diet, and gradually advance to a low-residue diet, as tolerated
  – After a proctocolectomy and ileostomy
    · Teach good stoma care
    · Wash the skin around the stoma with soapy water and dry it thoroughly
    · Apply karaya gum around the stoma's base to avoid irritation, and make a watertight seal
    · Attach the pouch over the karaya ring
    · Cut an opening in the ring to fit over the stoma, and secure the pouch to the skin
    · Empty the pouch when it's one-third full.
  – After a pouch ileostomy
    · Uncork the catheter every hour to allow contents to drain
    · After 10 to 14 days, gradually increase the time the catheter is left corked until it can be opened every 3 hours, and then remove the catheter and reinsert it every 3 to 4 hours for drainage
    · Teach the patient how to insert the catheter and how to take care of the stoma
  – Encourage the patient to have regular physical examinations

TOP 5

Items to study for your next test on the GI system

1. Types of GI surgeries
2. Five types of hepatitis
3. Diet therapies for patients with GI disorders
4. Common GI disorders, including cholecystitis, cirrhosis, peptic ulcer, and ulcerative colitis
5. Types of GI medications, such as antacids, diarrheals, and corticosteroids

NCLEX CHECKS

It's never too soon to begin your licensure examination preparation. Now that you've reviewed this chapter, carefully read each of the following questions and choose the best answer. Then compare your responses to the correct answers.

1. The most common cause of cholecystitis is:
☐ **1.** poor or absent blood flow to the gallbladder.
☐ **2.** abnormal metabolism of cholesterol and bile salts.
☐ **3.** a high-fat diet.
☐ **4.** gallstones.

2. The nurse is measuring and recording T-tube drainage of a patient with cholecystitis. The normal daily amount is:
☐ **1.** 50 to 100 ml.
☐ **2.** 100 to 200 ml.
☐ **3.** 200 to 300 ml.
☐ **4.** 300 to 400 ml.

3. The nurse is caring for a patient with cirrhosis and a history of alcohol abuse. Which type of cirrhosis is caused by chronic alcoholism?
- [ ] **1.** Postnecrotic
- [ ] **2.** Laënnec's
- [ ] **3.** Biliary
- [ ] **4.** Idiopathic

4. A 28-year-old patient is admitted with Crohn's disease. Which of the following treatments should the nurse expect to be part of the care plan? Select all that apply.
- [ ] **1.** Lactulose therapy
- [ ] **2.** High-fiber diet
- [ ] **3.** High-protein milkshakes
- [ ] **4.** Corticosteroid therapy
- [ ] **5.** Antidiarrheal medications

5. The three parts of an antireflux regimen that the nurse should teach the patient with GERD are diet, medication, and:
- [ ] **1.** positional therapy.
- [ ] **2.** exercise.
- [ ] **3.** stress reduction therapy.
- [ ] **4.** increased fluid intake.

6. The type of viral hepatitis that's linked to chronic hepatitis B is:
- [ ] **1.** A.
- [ ] **2.** C.
- [ ] **3.** D.
- [ ] **4.** E.

7. A patient develops dumping syndrome after gastric surgery for a peptic ulcer. Which measure helps prevent dumping syndrome?
- [ ] **1.** Sitting up after meals
- [ ] **2.** Drinking fluids between meals rather than with meals
- [ ] **3.** Eating large amounts of carbohydrates
- [ ] **4.** Eating four to six small low-protein meals during the day

8. Ulcerative colitis usually begins in which part of the colon?
- [ ] **1.** Small intestine
- [ ] **2.** Rectum
- [ ] **3.** Transverse colon
- [ ] **4.** Descending colon

9. A patient presents with midepigastric abdominal pain that radiates to the back. This pathologic change most likely indicates:
- [ ] **1.** hepatitis.
- [ ] **2.** irritable bowel syndrome.
- [ ] **3.** Crohn's disease.
- [ ] **4.** pancreatitis.

10. A patient reports passing ribbonlike stools. This finding suggests which type of diverticular disease?

- ☐ **1.** Diverticulosis
- ☐ **2.** Mild diverticulitis
- ☐ **3.** Chronic diverticulitis
- ☐ **4.** Severe diverticulitis

ANSWERS AND RATIONALES

1. CORRECT ANSWER: 4

Cholecystitis (inflammation of the gallbladder) is most commonly caused by gallstones that lodge in the cystic duct. A high-fat diet, poor or absent blood flow to the gallbladder, and abnormal metabolism of bile salts and cholesterol are predisposing factors to cholecystitis, but none of these factors is considered the most common cause.

2. CORRECT ANSWER: 3

The normal daily amount of drainage from a T tube is 200 to 300 ml. Lower amounts of drainage may indicate an obstruction of the tube or decreased bile production in the liver.

3. CORRECT ANSWER: 2

Chronic alcoholism can lead to Laënnec's cirrhosis. Postnecrotic cirrhosis is a complication of viral hepatitis or results from exposure to liver toxins. Biliary cirrhosis is caused by a prolonged biliary tract obstruction or inflammation. Idiopathic cirrhosis has no known cause but may be associated with sarcoidosis or chronic inflammatory bowel disease.

4. CORRECT ANSWER: 4, 5

In patients with Crohn's disease, corticosteroids reduce the signs and symptoms of diarrhea, pain, and bleeding by decreasing inflammation. Antidiarrheals combat diarrhea by decreasing peristalsis. Dietary changes, such as eliminating fruits, vegetables, high-fiber foods, dairy products, spicy and fatty foods, foods that irritate the mucosa, carbonated or caffeinated beverages, and other foods or liquids that stimulate excessive intestinal activity, are prescribed for patients with Crohn's disease to decrease bowel activity. Lactulose would be contraindicated in a patient with Crohn's disease.

5. CORRECT ANSWER: 1

Positional therapy for patients with GERD involves teaching the patient to sit up during and after meals and to sleep with the head of the bed elevated. These actions reduce abdominal pressure and prevent reflux. Increasing fluid intake would help wash down gastric contents, but this isn't a preventive measure. Vigorous exercise can worsen reflux if it's performed too soon after a meal. There's no documented relationship between stress and GERD.

6. CORRECT ANSWER: 3

The type D virus depends on the double-shelled type B virus to replicate. For this reason, type D infection can't outlast a type B infection. Hepatitis A, C, and E aren't linked to hepatitis B.

7.   CORRECT ANSWER: 2

Dumping syndrome (rapid gastric emptying) causes distention of the duodenum or jejunum. Drinking fluids between meals rather than with meals helps to avoid distention. Patients should also lie down after meals, avoid eating large amounts of carbohydrates, and eat frequent small meals that are high in protein.

8.   CORRECT ANSWER: 2

Ulcerative colitis, a chronic disease that affects the mucosa of the colon, usually begins in the rectum and sigmoid colon and commonly extends into the entire colon. It rarely affects the small intestine.

9.   CORRECT ANSWER: 4

Midepigastric abdominal pain that may radiate to the back is a pathophysiologic change associated with pancreatitis. The symptom results from the escape of inflammatory exudate and enzymes into the back of the peritoneum, edema and distention of the pancreatic capsule, and obstruction of the biliary tract.

10.   CORRECT ANSWER: 3

Ribbonlike stools along with constipation and intermittent diarrhea are present in chronic diverticulitis. Diverticulosis is the presence of diverticuli on examination but without associated symptoms. Mild diverticulitis involves inflammation of the diverticuli and evidence of the body fighting the potential infection. Severe diverticulitis is characterized by hemorrhaging as the infected polyps rupture and severe abdominal pain due to blood loss in the abdominal cavity or peritonitis.

6

Hematologic system

LEARNING OBJECTIVES

After studying this chapter, you should be able to:

- Describe the relationship between presenting signs and symptoms and the pathophysiologic changes for various hematologic disorders.
- Identify conditions that lead to an excess of or a deficiency of various types of cells in the body.
- List probable causes for various hematologic disorders.
- Identify treatments for various hematologic disorders.
- Write teaching goals for a patient with a hematologic disorder.
- List classes of medications used to treat hematologic disorders.

CHAPTER OVERVIEW

Blood is one of the most complex tissues in the body. It consists of plasma (liquid protein) and the formed elements within it (blood cells). Plasma carries antibodies and nutrients to the tissues and removes waste material. The red blood cells (RBCs), or erythrocytes, carry oxygen to tissues and remove carbon dioxide as waste. The white blood cells (WBCs), or leukocytes, are involved in inflammatory and immune responses. Platelets, or thrombocytes, and plasma coagulation factors form the basis of the clotting process.

Hematopoiesis is the process of blood formation. This process occurs primarily in the red bone marrow. Red bone marrow is located in the ends of the bones, whereas yellow bone marrow appears in the center of the bone and forms the bone's hard structure.

This chapter first reviews key pathophysiologic concepts related to the hematologic system, and then outlines the underlying pathophysiology, causes, changes, complications, diagnostic test findings, treatment approaches, and nursing considerations associated with common hematologic disorders.

PATHOPHYSIOLOGIC CONCEPTS

- ● **RBC deficiency (anemia)**
  - Inhibited RBC production
    - Marked by increased tissue demand for oxygen (hypoxia)
    - Triggers release of erythropoietin (the hormone that activates RBC production in bone marrow)
  - Early destruction of RBCs in association with various factors
    - Drugs or toxins
    - Ionizing radiation
    - Congenital or acquired defects
    - Metabolic abnormalities or deficiency of vitamins or minerals
    - Excessive chronic or acute blood loss
    - Chronic illnesses

- ● **RBC excess (polycythemia)**
  - Abnormal increase in RBC production
    - Marked by chronic tissue hypoxia
    - Triggers increased erythropoietin release and excessive RBC production
  - Decreased plasma volume causing relative excess of RBCs (commonly related to dehydration, stress)

- ● **WBC deficiency (leukopenia)**
  - Suppressed production of WBCs, in bone marrow (see *WBC types and functions,* page 222)
  - May be congenital or acquired because of drugs, radiation, prolonged stress, systemic disease, or viral infection
  - Can affect any or all types of WBCs but most commonly affects neutrophils (predominant type of granular leukocyte, or granulocyte), typically resulting in neutropenia
  - Alters body's defense mechanism, increasing risk of infection

- ● **WBC excess (leukocytosis)**
  - Is initiated by inflammatory response or infection
  - Triggers cellular response of phagocytic cells (WBCs that engulf and digest foreign bodies in the bloodstream) to site of injury or infection
  - Results when mobilization of the body's defense mechanism leads to increased WBC production
  - If pathogenic, commonly associated with cancer and bone marrow depression

Key facts about anemia

- ● RBC deficiency
- ● Results from inhibited RBC production or early destruction of RBCs

Key facts about polycythemia

- ● RBC excess
- ● Results from increased RBC production or decreased plasma volume

Key facts about leukopenia

- ● WBC deficiency
- ● Results from suppressed WBC production
- ● May be congenital or acquired
- ● Alters body's defense mechanism

Key facts about leukocytosis

- ● WBC excess
- ● Results when the body increases WBC production

Types of WBCs

Granular
- Neutrophils
- Eosinophils
- Basophils

Agranular
- Lymphocytes
- Monocytes
- Plasma cells

WBC types and functions

White blood cells (WBCs), or leukocytes, protect the body against harmful bacteria and infection. WBCs are classified as granular leukocytes (basophils, neutrophils, and eosinophils) or agranular leukocytes (lymphocytes, monocytes, and plasma cells). WBCs are usually produced in bone marrow; lymphocytes and plasma cells are produced in lymphoid tissue as well. Neutrophils have a circulating half-life of less than 6 hours, whereas some lymphocytes may survive for weeks or months. Normally, WBCs number between 5,000 and 10,000 µl. There are six types of WBCs.

GRANULAR

- Neutrophils—The predominant form of granulocyte, they make up about 60% of WBCs and help devour invading organisms by phagocytosis.
- Eosinophils—Minor granulocytes, they may defend against parasites and lung and skin infections and act in allergic reactions. They account for 1% to 5% of the total WBC count.
- Basophils—Minor granulocytes, they may release heparin and histamine into the blood and participate in delayed hypersensitivity reactions. They account for 0% to 1% of the total WBC count.

AGRANULAR

- Lymphocytes—They occur as B cells and T cells. B cells form lymphoid follicles, produce humoral antibodies, and help T-cell mediated delayed hypersensitivity reactions and the rejection of foreign cells or cell products. Lymphocytes account for 20% to 40% of the total WBC count.
- Monocytes—Along with neutrophils, they help devour invading organisms by phagocytosis. Monocytes help process antigens for lymphocytes and form macrophages in the tissues. They account for 1% to 6% of the total WBC count.
- Plasma cells—They develop from lymphoblasts, reside in the tissue, and produce antibodies.

APLASTIC ANEMIA

Key facts about aplastic anemia

- Results from injury to or destruction of stem cells, which inhibits blood cell production
- May create an unfavorable environment for cell growth
- Has two forms: hypoplastic anemia and Fanconi's syndrome

● **Definition**
- Refers to pancytopenia (anemia, leukopenia, and thrombocytopenia) resulting from the decreased functional capacity of a hypoplastic, fatty red bone marrow
- Results from injury to or destruction of stem cells in bone marrow or the bone marrow matrix
- Produces severe anemia, fatal bleeding, or infection, especially when caused by chloramphenicol (Chloromycetin) use or infectious hepatitis or if idiopathic
- If severe, has an 80% to 90% death rate
- Two identified forms of congenital aplastic anemia
    - Hypoplastic, or Blackfan-Diamond, anemia (develops between ages 2 and 3 months)
    - Fanconi's syndrome (develops between birth and age 10)

Underlying pathophysiology
- Damaged or destroyed stem cells inhibit blood cell production
- Less commonly, damaged bone marrow microvasculature creates an unfavorable environment for cell growth and maturation

Causes
- Autoimmune reactions (unconfirmed)
- Severe disease (especially hepatitis)
- Preleukemic and neoplastic infiltration of bone marrow
- Drugs (antibiotics, anticonvulsants) or toxic agents (such as benzene or chloramphenicol)
- Radiation (in about half of aplastic anemia cases)

Pathophysiologic changes
- Progressive weakness and fatigue, shortness of breath, headache, pallor, and ultimately tachycardia and heart failure due to hypoxia and increased venous return
- Ecchymosis, petechiae (small purplish hemorrhagic spots on skin), and hemorrhage, especially from the mucous membranes (nose, gums, rectum, vagina) or into the retina or central nervous system (CNS), due to thrombocytopenia
- Infection (fever, oral and rectal ulcers, sore throat) without characteristic inflammation due to neutropenia (neutrophil deficiency)

Complications
- Life-threatening hemorrhage from the mucous membranes

Diagnostic test findings
- RBC studies reveal 1 million/μl or fewer RBCs of normal color and size (normochromic and normocytic)
    - RBCs may be macrocytic (larger than normal) and anisocytotic (excessive variation in size)
    - Absolute reticulocyte count is very low
- Serum iron level is elevated (unless bleeding occurs), but total iron-binding capacity is normal or slightly reduced
- Platelet, neutrophil, and lymphocyte counts are decreased
- Coagulation test results, such as bleeding time, are abnormal, reflecting decreased platelet count
- Bone marrow biopsy reveals various findings
    - A useful specimen will show diminished number of cells, particularly normoblasts (precursor RBCs), megakaryocytes (platelet precursors), and neutrophils as well as varied amounts of fat, fibrous tissue, or gelatinous replacement material in the red bone marrow
    - Several sites may show no cells ("dry tap") because of the reduced number of cells

Treatment
- Packed RBC or platelet transfusion
- Histocompatibility locus antigen-matched leukocyte transfusions (experimental)
- Bone marrow transplantation (treatment of choice for anemia due to severe aplasia and for patients who need constant RBC transfusions)

Key pathophysiologic changes in aplastic anemia
- Weakness
- Fatigue
- Ecchymosis
- Petechiae
- Hemorrhage from mucous membranes

Key diagnostic test results for aplastic anemia
- RBC studies: 1 million/μl or fewer RBCs of normal color and size
- Coagulation tests: Abnormal, reflecting decreased platelet count
- Bone marrow biopsy: Diminished number of cells, particularly normoblasts, megakaryocytes, and neutrophils, or no cells

- For patients with leukopenia, special measures to prevent infection, such as avoiding exposure to communicable diseases and diligent hand washing
- Specific antibiotics for infection (not given prophylactically because they encourage resistant strains of organisms)
- Respiratory support with oxygen in addition to blood transfusions (for patients with low hemoglobin levels)
- Drug therapy as appropriate
    - Corticosteroids to stimulate erythropoiesis
    - Marrow-stimulating agents such as androgens (controversial)
    - Antithymocyte globulin (experimental)
    - Immunosuppressive agents (if the patient doesn't respond to other therapy)
    - Colony-stimulating factors to encourage growth of specific cellular components

Nursing considerations

- If the platelet count is less than 20,000/µl, monitor for and prevent bleeding
    - Avoid I.M. injections
    - Suggest the use of an electric razor and a soft toothbrush
    - Use humidifying oxygen to prevent drying of mucous membranes
    - Avoid using enemas and taking rectal temperatures
    - Promote regular bowel movements through the use of a stool softener and a proper diet
    - Apply pressure to venipuncture sites until bleeding stops
    - Detect bleeding early by checking for blood in urine and stool and assessing skin for petechiae
    - Take safety precautions to prevent falls that could lead to prolonged bleeding or hemorrhage
- Help prevent infection
    - Wash your hands thoroughly before entering the patient's room
    - Make sure that the patient is receiving a nutritious diet (high in vitamins and proteins) to improve his resistance
    - Encourage meticulous mouth and perianal care
- **Watch for life-threatening hemorrhage, infection, adverse effects of drug therapy, or blood transfusion reaction**
- Teach the patient to recognize signs of infection and to report them immediately
- If the patient has a low hemoglobin level, which causes fatigue, schedule frequent rest periods
- Administer oxygen therapy as needed
- If blood transfusions are necessary, assess for a transfusion reaction by checking the patient's temperature and watching for the development of other signs and symptoms, such as rash, hives, itching, back pain, restlessness, and chills
- Reassure and support the patient and his family
    - Explain the disease and its treatment, particularly if the patient has recurring acute episodes
    - Explain the purpose of all prescribed drugs and discuss possible adverse effects, including which ones he should report promptly (see *Answering patients' questions about aplastic anemia*)

TIME-OUT FOR TEACHING

Answering patients' questions about aplastic anemia

When teaching your patient about aplastic anemia, keep these answers to commonly asked questions in mind.

WHY DO I NEED SO MANY RED BLOOD CELL AND PLATELET TRANSFUSIONS?
Transfusions help to replenish the blood cells that your bone marrow suppresses or fails to produce. Blood cells are living cells with a limited life span. Red blood cells usually live for 120 days, whereas platelets live only for 8 to 10 days. Normally, bone marrow produces replacements for the cells that die.

WHY CAN'T I HAVE A TRANSFUSION OF WHITE BLOOD CELLS?
White blood cells have a short life span. They don't survive long enough

to be helpful when given by transfusion.

WHY CAN'T I JUST TAKE ANTIBIOTICS TO PREVENT INFECTIONS?
Taking antibiotics to prevent infection may encourage the growth of resistant strains of bacteria. Remember, infections sometimes come from germs existing in your own body. Preventive treatment with antibiotics will kill this normal flora and encourage the growth of bacteria resistant to treatment. You're safer practicing standard hygiene (such as washing your hands before eating) and avoiding crowds and people that you know are sick.

TOP 3

Ways to prevent infection

1. Wash your hands.
2. Provide the patient with a nutritious diet.
3. Encourage meticulous mouth and perianal care.

- To prevent aplastic anemia, monitor blood studies carefully in the patient receiving anemia-inducing drugs
- Support efforts to educate the public about the hazards of toxic agents
- Tell parents to keep toxic agents out of the reach of children

FOLIC ACID DEFICIENCY ANEMIA

● **Definition**
- Common, slowly progressive, megaloblastic anemia
- Usually occurs in infants, adolescents, pregnant and lactating females, alcoholics, the elderly, and people with malignant or intestinal diseases

● **Underlying pathophysiology**
- Folic acid (pteroylglutamic acid, folacin) is found in most body tissues
  - It acts as a coenzyme in metabolic processes involving one carbon transfer
  - It's essential for RBC formation and maturation and for deoxyribonucleic acid synthesis
- When body stores of folic acid are low or if diet is insufficient, folic acid deficiency will develop within 4 months
- Deficiency of folic acid inhibits cell growth, particularly of RBCs, leading to production of scant, enlarged RBCs

Key facts about folic acid deficiency anemia

- Is slowly progressive
- Results from deficiency of folic acid, which is needed for RBC formation
- Results in inhibited cell growth and development of megaloblasts, which have a shortened life span

TOP 3

Causes of folic acid deficiency anemia

1. Poor diet (age, alcohol use, poverty)
2. Increased folic acid requirements, such as during pregnancy or childhood
3. Limited capacity to store folic acid (infants)

Key pathophysiologic changes in folic acid deficiency anemia

- Fatigue
- Shortness of breath
- Pallor
- Nausea

Key diagnostic test results for folic acid deficiency anemia

- Schilling test: Macrocytosis, decreased reticulocyte count, abnormal platelets, serum folate level less than 4 mg/ml

Key treatments for folic acid deficiency anemia

- Folic acid supplements
- Well-balanced diet

- Enlarged RBCs, or megaloblasts, have a shortened life span of weeks rather than months, resulting in anemia

● **Causes**
- Alcohol abuse (alcohol may suppress metabolic effects of folate)
- Bacteria competing for available folic acid
- Excessive cooking, which can destroy a high percentage of folic acid in foods
- Impaired absorption (due to intestinal dysfunction from bowel resection and such disorders as celiac disease, tropical sprue, and regional jejunitis)
- Increased folic acid requirements during certain growth stages or situations
  - Pregnancy
  - Rapid growth in infancy (common because of recent increase in survival of premature infants)
  - Childhood and adolescence (because of general use of folate-poor cow's milk)
  - Neoplastic disease or certain skin diseases (such as chronic exfoliative dermatitis)
- Limited capacity to store folic acid (in infants)
- Poor diet
- Prolonged drug therapy with anticonvulsants and estrogens, including hormonal contraceptives

● **Pathophysiologic changes**
- Progressive fatigue, shortness of breath, palpitations, weakness, and pallor resulting from hypoxemia
- Nausea and anorexia caused by decreased GI blood flow
- Headache, fainting, irritability, and forgetfulness due to decreased blood flow to the brain

● **Complications**
- Neural tube defects in infants if mother is deficient during pregnancy

● **Diagnostic test findings**
- The Schilling test and a therapeutic trial of vitamin B$_{12}$ injections distinguish between folic acid deficiency anemia and pernicious anemia
  - Significant findings include macrocytosis, decreased reticulocyte count, abnormal platelets, and serum folate level less than 4 mg/ml

● **Treatment**
- Elimination of contributing cause
- Folic acid supplements given orally (usually 1 to 5 mg/day) or parenterally (to patients who are severely ill, have malabsorption, or can't take oral medication)
- Well-balanced diet to ensure adequate intake of folic acid

● **Nursing considerations**
- Teach the patient to meet daily folic acid requirements by including a food from each food group in every meal
- If the patient has a severe deficiency, explain that diet only reinforces folic acid supplementation and isn't therapeutic by itself
- Urge compliance with the prescribed course of therapy
- Advise the patient to continue taking the supplements even after he begins to feel better

- Encourage the avoidance of alcohol, nonherbal teas, antacids, and phosphates, which impair the absorption of B vitamins and iron
- If the patient has a combined vitamin B_{12} and folic acid deficiency, folic acid replenishment alone may aggravate neurologic dysfunction
- If the patient has glossitis
  - Emphasize the importance of good oral hygiene
  - Suggest regular use of mild or diluted mouthwash and a soft toothbrush
- Watch fluid and electrolyte balance, particularly in the patient who has severe diarrhea and is receiving parenteral fluid replacement therapy
- Because anemia causes severe fatigue, schedule regular rest periods until the patient can resume normal activity
- Try to prevent folic acid deficiency anemia
  - Emphasize the importance of a well-balanced diet high in folic acid
  - Identify alcoholics with poor dietary habits, and try to arrange for appropriate counseling
  - Tell mothers who aren't breast-feeding to use commercially prepared formulas

IRON DEFICIENCY ANEMIA

Definition
- Disorder of oxygen transport in which hemoglobin synthesis is deficient
- Occurs most commonly in premenopausal women, infants (particularly premature or low-birth-weight infants), children, and adolescents (especially girls)

Underlying pathophysiology
- Occurs when the iron supply is inadequate for optimal RBC formation, resulting in smaller (microcytic) cells with less color (hypochromic) on staining
- Body stores of iron, including plasma iron, become depleted
- The serum transferrin concentration, which binds with and transports iron, decreases
- Insufficient iron stores lead to a depleted RBC mass with subnormal hemoglobin concentration and, in turn, subnormal oxygen-carrying capacity of the blood

Causes
- Blood loss resulting from drug-induced GI bleeding (such as with anticoagulants, aspirin, and steroids), heavy menses, hemorrhage from trauma, peptic ulcers, cancer, increased laboratory blood sampling in chronically ill patients, sequestration in patients on dialysis, or varices
- Inadequate dietary intake of iron (less than 1 to 2 mg/day), as in prolonged nonsupplemented breast-feeding or bottle-feeding of infants, or during periods of stress, such as rapid growth, in children and adolescents
- Intravascular hemolysis-induced hemoglobinuria or paroxysmal nocturnal hemoglobinuria
- Iron malabsorption
- Mechanical trauma to RBCs caused by a prosthetic heart valve or vena cava filters
- Pregnancy
- Possibly related to lead poisoning in children

Key pathophysiologic changes in iron deficiency anemia

- Dyspnea on exertion
- Fatigue
- Pallor
- Koilonychia
- Sore, dry skin in corners of mouth

Key diagnostic test results for iron deficiency anemia

- Hemoglobin level: Decreased (less than 12 g/dl in males; less than 10 g/dl in females)
- Hematocrit: Decreased (less than 47 in males; less than 42 in females)
- Serum iron: Decreased with a high binding capacity level
- Serum ferritin: Decreased

Key treatments for iron deficiency anemia

- Identification of underlying cause
- Oral or parenteral iron supplementation

TOP 3

Signs of allergic reaction to I.V. iron

1. Dizziness
2. Headache
3. Thrombophlebitis around I.V. site

● **Pathophysiologic changes**
- Dyspnea on exertion, fatigue, listlessness, pallor, inability to concentrate, irritability, headache, and a susceptibility to infection due to decreased oxygen-carrying capacity of the blood caused by decreased hemoglobin level
- Increased cardiac output and tachycardia due to decreased oxygen perfusion
- Coarsely ridged, spoon-shaped, brittle, thin nails (koilonychia) resulting from decreased capillary circulation
- Sore, red, and burning tongue due to papillae atrophy
- Sore, dry skin in the corners of the mouth caused by epithelial changes

● **Complications**
- Bleeding
- Infection
- Oral or I.M. iron supplement overdose
- Pica (compulsive eating of nonfood materials, such as starch or dirt)
- Pneumonia

● **Diagnostic test findings**
- Hemoglobin level is decreased (less than 12 g/dl in males; less than 10 g/dl in females)
- Hematocrit is decreased (less than 47 in males; less than 42 in females)
- Serum iron is decreased with a high binding capacity level
- Serum ferritin level is decreased
- RBC count is decreased with microcytic and hypochromic cells
  - In early stages, RBC count may be normal, except in infants and children
- Mean corpuscular hemoglobin level is decreased in severe anemia
- Bone marrow studies reveal depleted or absent iron stores (by specific staining) and hyperplasia of normal precursor cells
- GI studies, such as guaiac stool tests, barium swallow and enema, endoscopy, and sigmoidoscopy, determine whether bleeding is causing the iron deficiency

● **Treatment**
- Determine appropriate treatment by identifying the underlying cause of anemia
- Oral iron preparation (treatment of choice) or a combination of iron and ascorbic acid (enhances iron absorption)
- Parenteral iron
  - Used if patient is noncompliant with oral dose, needs more iron than can be given orally, or has a malabsorption problem that prevents adequate iron absorption
  - Used when a maximum rate of hemoglobin regeneration is needed

● **Nursing considerations**
- Monitor the patient's compliance with the prescribed iron supplement therapy (see *Iron deficiency anemia*)
- If the patient receives I.V. iron, monitor the infusion rate carefully, and observe for an allergic reaction
  - Watch for dizziness and headache and for thrombophlebitis around the I.V. site
  - Stop the infusion and begin supportive treatment immediately if the patient shows signs of an adverse reaction
- Because total-dose I.V. infusion of supplemental iron is painless and requires fewer injections, it's usually preferred to I.M. administration

TIME-OUT FOR TEACHING

Iron deficiency anemia

Include these points in your teaching plan for patients with iron deficiency anemia to improve their understanding of and compliance with the treatment plan:

- body's need for iron to build healthy red blood cells, which carry oxygen to all parts of the body
- route of iron supplement administration (I.V., I.M., or oral), dosing, and reason for administration
- dangers of lead poisoning, especially in children, if iron deficiency causes pica, and how to keep a home free from dangerous lead paints
- importance of continuing therapy, even when the patient starts to feel better
- drug interactions, such as absorption interference when iron preparations are taken with milk or antacids and increased iron absorption if vitamin C is consumed
- importance of drinking liquid preparations with a straw to avoid staining teeth
- basics of a nutritionally balanced diet
- importance of avoiding infection and when to report signs of infection
- importance of taking supplements with a meal (except dairy products) to decrease gastric distress
- adverse effects to report to the prescriber, such as nausea, vomiting, diarrhea, constipation (especially in elderly or immobile patients), fever, or severe stomach pain
- need for regular check-ups and repeat blood testing for iron and anemia.

Key nursing considerations for iron deficiency anemia

- Monitor compliance with prescribed iron supplement therapy.
- Advise patient to have regular check-ups and blood studies.

— I.V. test dose is given first to minimize the risk of an allergic reaction
- Use the Z-track injection method when administering iron I.M. to prevent skin discoloration, scarring, and irritating iron deposits in the skin
- Because an iron deficiency may recur, advise the patient to have regular check-ups and blood studies

PERNICIOUS ANEMIA

● **Definition**
- Most common type of megaloblastic anemia
- Involves a vitamin B_{12} deficiency
- Characterized by decreased gastric production of hydrochloric acid and a deficiency of intrinsic factor, especially essential for vitamin B_{12} absorption
- Fatal if not treated
- May result in some permanent neurologic deficits — even with treatment

● **Underlying pathophysiology**
- An inherited autoimmune response may cause gastric mucosal atrophy and resultant decreased production of hydrochloric acid and intrinsic factor, a substance normally secreted by parietal cells of the gastric mucosa
- Intrinsic factor deficiency impairs vitamin B_{12} absorption
- Vitamin B_{12} deficiency inhibits cell growth, particularly of RBCs, leading to production of scant, deformed RBCs with poor oxygen-carrying capacity
- Neurologic damage occurs because vitamin B_{12} deficiency impairs myelin formation

Key facts about pernicious anemia

- Involves a vitamin B_{12} deficiency
- Develops when decreased production of intrinsic factor decreases vitamin B_{12} absorption
- Impairs cell growth and myelin formation, causing neurologic damage

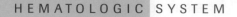

Key pathophysiologic changes in pernicious anemia

- Weakness
- Numbness and tingling in extremities
- Sore tongue
- Pale lips and gums
- Lack of coordination
- Altered vision
- Palpitations

Key diagnostic test results for pernicious anemia

- Hemoglobin level: Decreased (4 to 5 g/µl)
- Mean corpuscular volume: Greater than 120 µl
- Serum vitamin B_{12}: Less than 0.1 µg/ml
- Schilling test for excretion of radiolabeled vitamin B_{12}: Lower-than-normal excretion of radioactive vitamin B_{12} in urine in 24-hour period

● Causes
- Gastric bypass
- Genetic predisposition (suggested by familial incidence)
- Immunologically related diseases, such as thyroiditis, myxedema, and Graves' disease
- Older age (progressive loss of vitamin B_{12} absorption)
- Partial gastrectomy (iatrogenic induction)

● Pathophysiologic changes
- Weakness due to tissue hypoxia
- Sore tongue due to atrophy of the papillae
- Numbness and tingling in the extremities as a result of interference with impulse transmission from demyelination
- Pale appearance of lips and gums caused by tissue hypoxia
- Faintly jaundiced sclera and pale to bright yellow skin due to hemolysis-induced hyperbilirubinemia
- Nausea, vomiting, anorexia, weight loss, flatulence, diarrhea, and constipation from disturbed digestion due to gastric mucosal atrophy and decreased hydrochloric acid production
- Neurologic symptoms due to interference of nerve impulse transmission from demyelination
    - Lack of coordination, ataxia, impaired fine finger movement, positive Babinski's and Romberg's signs, and light-headedness
    - Altered vision (diplopia, blurred vision), taste, and hearing (tinnitus) and optic muscle atrophy
    - Loss of bowel and bladder control and, in males, impotence (initially affects peripheral nerves but gradually extends to the spinal cord)
    - Irritability, poor memory, headache, depression, and delirium (some symptoms are temporary, but irreversible CNS changes may have occurred before treatment)
- Low hemoglobin level due to widespread destruction of RBCs resulting from increasingly fragile cell membranes
- Palpitations, wide pulse pressure, dyspnea, orthopnea, tachycardia, premature beats and, eventually, heart failure due to compensatory increased cardiac output

● Complications
- Gastric polyps
- Hypokalemia (first week of treatment)
- Permanent CNS symptoms (if the patient isn't treated within 6 months of appearance of symptoms)
- Stomach cancer

● Diagnostic test findings
- Hemoglobin level is decreased (4 to 5 g/µl)
- RBC count is decreased
- Mean corpuscular volume is greater than 120 µl due to increased amounts of hemoglobin in larger-than-normal RBCs
- Serum vitamin B_{12} is less than 0.1 µg/ml
- Bone marrow aspiration shows erythroid hyperplasia (crowded red bone marrow), with increased numbers of megaloblasts but few normally developing RBCs

- Gastric analysis shows absence of free hydrochloric acid after histamine or pentagastrin injection
- Schilling test for excretion of radiolabeled vitamin B_{12} is the definitive test for pernicious anemia
- Serologic findings include intrinsic factor antibodies and antiparietal cell antibodies

● **Treatment**
  - Early parenteral vitamin B_{12} replacement (can reverse pernicious anemia, minimize complications, and possibly prevent permanent neurologic damage)
  - Concomitant iron and folic acid replacement to prevent iron deficiency anemia (rapid cell regeneration, increasing the patient's iron and folate requirements)
  - After initial response, decreasing vitamin B_{12} dosage to monthly self-administered maintenance dose (must be given for life)
  - Bed rest for extreme fatigue until hemoglobin level rises
  - Blood transfusions for dangerously low hemoglobin level
  - Digoxin (Lanoxin), diuretic, and low-sodium diet (if patient is in heart failure)
  - Antibiotics to combat infections

● **Nursing considerations**
  - Patient and family teaching can promote compliance with lifelong vitamin B_{12} replacement
  - If the patient has severe anemia
    - Plan activities, rest periods, and necessary diagnostic tests to conserve the patient's energy
    - Monitor pulse rate often; tachycardia means the patient's activities are too strenuous
  - To ensure accurate Shilling test results, make sure that all urine over a 24-hour period is collected and that specimens are uncontaminated
  - Warn the patient to guard against infections
    - Tell him to report signs of infection promptly, especially pulmonary and urinary tract infections
    - The patient's weakened condition may increase susceptibility
  - Provide a well-balanced diet, including foods high in vitamin B_{12} (meat, liver, fish, eggs, and dried fruits)
  - Offer between-meal snacks, and encourage the family to bring favorite foods from home
  - Because a sore mouth and tongue make eating painful, avoid giving the patient irritating foods
  - Provide diluted mouthwash or, with severe conditions, swab the patient's mouth with water or warm saline solution
  - Warn the patient with a sensory deficit not to use a heating pad because it may cause burns
  - If the patient is incontinent
    - Establish a regular bowel and bladder routine
    - After the patient is discharged, a home health care nurse should follow up on this schedule and make adjustments as needed
  - If neurologic damage causes behavioral problems
    - Assess mental and neurologic status often
    - If necessary, give sedatives, as ordered, and apply a jacket restraint at night

- Stress that vitamin B_{12} replacement isn't a permanent cure and that these injections must be continued for life, even after symptoms subside
- To prevent pernicious anemia, emphasize the importance of vitamin B_{12} supplements for patients who have had extensive gastric resections or who follow strict vegetarian diets

SIDEROBLASTIC ANEMIAS

● **Definition**
- Group of heterogeneous disorders with a common defect that causes failure to use iron in hemoglobin synthesis, despite the availability of adequate iron stores
- May be hereditary or acquired
- If hereditary, commonly responds to treatment with pyridoxine (vitamin B_6)
- If acquired, can be primary or secondary
  - Primary acquired (idiopathic) form
    · Known as *refractory anemia with ringed sideroblasts*
    · Resists treatment
    · Is usually fatal within 10 years of the onset because of complications or a concomitant disease
    · Common in elderly patients
    · Usually associated with thrombocytopenia or leukopenia as part of a myelodysplastic syndrome
  - Secondary acquired form
    · Correction depends on the cause

● **Underlying pathophysiology**
- Normoblasts fail to use iron to synthesize hemoglobin
- Iron is deposited in the mitochondria of normoblasts, which are then termed *ringed sideroblasts*
- Iron toxicity can cause organ damage, which if left untreated, can damage the nuclei of RBC precursors

● **Causes**
- Hereditary form
  - X-linked inheritance
  - Occurs mostly in young males (female carriers usually show no signs of this disorder)
- Primary acquired form
  - Cause unknown
- Secondary acquired form
  - Ingestion of or exposure to toxins (such as alcohol and lead) or drugs (such as isoniazid [Laniazid] and chloramphenicol [Chloromycetin])
  - Other diseases, such as rheumatoid arthritis, lupus erythematosus, multiple myeloma, tuberculosis, and severe infections

● **Pathophysiologic changes**
- Anorexia, fatigue, weakness, dizziness, pale skin and mucous membranes and, occasionally, enlarged lymph nodes due to iron toxicity
- Dyspnea, exertional angina, slight jaundice, and hepatosplenomegaly due to heart and liver failure caused by excessive iron accumulation in these organs
- Other symptoms depending on the underlying cause (secondary sideroblastic anemia)

Key facts about sideroblastic anemias

- Refer to a group of disorders
- Involve a defect that causes normoblasts to fail to use iron to synthesize hemoglobin
- Result in iron being deposited in the mitochondria of normoblasts
- Can lead to iron toxicity and organ damage
- May be hereditary or acquired

Key pathophysiologic changes in sideroblastic anemias

- Fatigue
- Pale skin and mucous membranes
- Dyspnea
- Exertional angina
- Hepatosplenomegaly

Complications
- Acute myelogenous leukemia
- Heart, liver, and pancreatic disease

Diagnostic test findings
- Microscopic examination of bone marrow aspirate stained with Prussian blue or alizarin red dye reveals ringed sideroblasts
- RBC indices are revealed by microscopic examination of blood
  - RBCs are hypochromic or normochromic and slightly macrocytic
  - RBC precursors may be megaloblastic with anisocytosis and poikilocytosis (abnormal variation in shape)
- Hemoglobin level is decreased with high serum iron, transferrin, urobilinogen, and bilirubin levels due to RBC lysis
- Platelet and leukocyte counts are normal with occasional thrombocytopenia or leukopenia
- Serum reticulocyte count is low because young cells die in the marrow

Treatment
- Several weeks of treatment with high doses of pyridoxine for hereditary form
- Removal of the causative drug or toxin, or treatment of the underlying condition (symptoms usually subside in acquired secondary form)
- Folic acid supplements (may be beneficial when concomitant megaloblastic nuclear changes in RBC precursors are present)
- Deferoxamine (Desferal) to treat chronic iron overload as needed
- Palliative measures for patients with primary acquired form
  - Blood transfusions (providing hemoglobin)
  - High doses of androgens
- Phlebotomy to prevent hemochromatosis (the accumulation of iron in body tissues)
  - Increases the rate of erythropoiesis
  - Uses up excess iron stores, reducing serum and total-body iron levels

Nursing considerations
- Administer medications as ordered
- Teach the patient the importance of continuing prescribed therapy, even after he begins to feel better
- Provide frequent rest periods if the patient becomes easily fatigued
- If phlebotomy is scheduled
  - Explain the procedure thoroughly to help reduce anxiety
  - If this procedure must be repeated frequently, provide a high-protein diet to help replace the protein lost during phlebotomy
  - Encourage the patient to follow a similar diet at home
- Always inquire about the possibility of exposure to lead in the home (especially for children) or on the job
- Identify patients who abuse alcohol and refer them for appropriate therapy

DISSEMINATED INTRAVASCULAR COAGULATION

Definition
- Occurs as a complication of diseases and conditions that accelerate clotting

---

Key diagnostic test results for sideroblastic anemias
- Microscopic examination of bone marrow aspirate: Ringed sideroblasts
- Microscopic examination of blood: RBC indices, hypochromic or normochromic and slightly macrocytic RBCs, and possible megaloblastic RBC precursors with abnormal shape

Key treatments for sideroblastic anemias
- High doses of pyridoxine (hereditary form)
- Removal of causative drug or toxin, or treatment of underlying condition
- Deferoxamine
- Phlebotomy

Key nursing considerations for sideroblastic anemias
- Teach patient the importance of continuing prescribed therapy.
- Inquire about exposure to lead.
- Identify patients who abuse alcohol and refer them for therapy.

Key facts about DIC

- Occurs as a complication of diseases and conditions that accelerate clotting
- Results in activation of prothrombin, an excess of thrombin, large usage of coagulation factors, activation of the fibrinolytic system, and hemorrhage

Key pathophysiologic changes in DIC

- Bleeding from surgical or I.V. sites
- GI bleeding
- Cyanotic, cold, mottled fingers and toes
- Confusion
- Severe back, abdominal, and chest pain
- Oliguria

- Causes small blood vessel occlusion, organ necrosis, depletion of circulating clotting factors and platelets, activation of the fibrinolytic system, and consequent severe hemorrhage
- Causes clotting in the microcirculation
  - Usually affects the kidneys and extremities
  - May occur in the brain, lungs, pituitary and adrenal glands, and GI mucosa
- Also called DIC, *consumption coagulopathy,* or *defibrination syndrome*
- Prognosis depends on early detection and treatment, the severity of the hemorrhage, and treatment of the underlying disease

Underlying pathophysiology
- Typical accelerated clotting results in generalized activation of prothrombin and a consequent excess of thrombin
- The thrombin converts fibrinogen to fibrin, producing fibrin clots in the microcirculation
- This process uses large amounts of coagulation factors (especially fibrinogen, prothrombin, platelets, and factors V and VIII), causing hypofibrinogenemia, hypoprothrombinemia, thrombocytopenia, and factor V and VIII deficiencies
- Circulating thrombin also activates the fibrinolytic system, which dissolves fibrin clots into fibrin degradation products
- Hemorrhage may be mostly the result of the anticoagulant activity of fibrin degradation products and the depletion of plasma coagulation factors

Causes
- Disorders that produce necrosis, including extensive burns and trauma, brain tissue destruction, transplant rejection, and hepatic necrosis
- Infection, including gram-negative or gram-positive septicemia and viral, fungal, rickettsial, or protozoal infection
- Neoplastic disease, including acute leukemia, metastatic carcinoma, and aplastic anemia
- Obstetric complications, including abruptio placentae, amniotic fluid embolism, retained dead fetus, septic abortion, and eclampsia
- Other conditions, including heatstroke, shock, poisonous snakebite, cirrhosis, fat embolism, incompatible blood transfusion, cardiac arrest, surgery requiring cardiopulmonary bypass, giant hemangioma, severe venous thrombosis, and purpura fulminans

Pathophysiologic changes
- Abnormal bleeding, cutaneous oozing of serum, petechiae or blood blisters, bleeding from surgical or I.V. sites, bleeding from the GI tract, epistaxis, and hemoptysis caused by the anticoagulant activity of fibrin degradation products and depletion of plasma coagulation factors
- Cyanotic, cold, mottled fingers and toes due to fibrin clots in the microcirculation, resulting in tissue ischemia
- Severe muscle, back, abdominal, and chest pain from tissue hypoxia
- Nausea and vomiting, which may be associated with GI bleeding
- Shock due to hemorrhage
- Confusion, possibly due to cerebral thrombus and decreased cerebral perfusion
- Dyspnea due to poor tissue perfusion and oxygenation
- Oliguria due to decreased renal perfusion

Complications
- Acute tubular necrosis
- Multiple organ failure
- Shock

Diagnostic test findings
- Platelet count is decreased (usually less than 100,000/µl)
- Fibrinogen level is less than 150 mg/dl (levels may be normal if elevated by hepatitis or pregnancy)
- Prothrombin time is greater than 15 seconds
- Partial thromboplastin time is greater than 60 seconds
- Fibrin degradation products are increased (typically greater than 45 mcg/ml)
- D-dimer test (presence of an asymmetrical carbon compound fragment formed in the presence of fibrin split products) is positive at less than 1:8 dilution
- Fibrin monomers reveal diminished levels of factors V and VIII, RBC fragmentation, and hemoglobin level less than 10 g/dl
- Blood urea nitrogen is elevated (greater than 25 mg/dl)
- Serum creatinine is elevated (greater than 1.3 mg/dl)

Treatment
- Prompt recognition and treatment of underlying disorder
- Blood, fresh frozen plasma, platelet, or packed RBC transfusions to support hemostasis in active bleeding
- Heparin
  - Used in early stages to prevent microclotting
  - Used as a last resort in hemorrhage
  - Controversial in acute DIC after sepsis (see *Understanding DIC and its treatment,* page 236)

Nursing considerations
- Avoid dislodging clots, which may cause fresh bleeding
  - Don't scrub bleeding areas
  - Use pressure, cold compresses, and topical hemostatic agents to control bleeding
- Prevent injury
  - Enforce complete bed rest during bleeding episodes
  - If the patient is agitated, pad the side rails
- Check all I.V. and venipuncture sites frequently for bleeding
  - **Apply pressure to injection sites for at least 20 minutes**
  - Post bleeding precaution signs
- Monitor intake and output hourly in acute DIC, especially when administering blood products
- Watch for transfusion reactions and signs of fluid overload
  - To measure the amount of blood lost, weigh dressings and linen and record drainage
  - Weigh the patient daily
- Watch for bleeding from the GI and genitourinary tracts
  - If you suspect intra-abdominal bleeding, measure the patient's abdominal girth at least every 4 hours
  - Monitor closely for signs of shock
- Monitor the results of serial blood studies (particularly hematocrit, hemoglobin level, and coagulation times)

GO WITH THE FLOW

Understanding DIC and its treatment

The prognosis for patients with disseminated intravascular coagulation (DIC) depends on early detection, the severity of the hemorrhage, and treatment of the underlying disease. This flowchart illustrates how DIC progresses and when key treatments should be implemented.

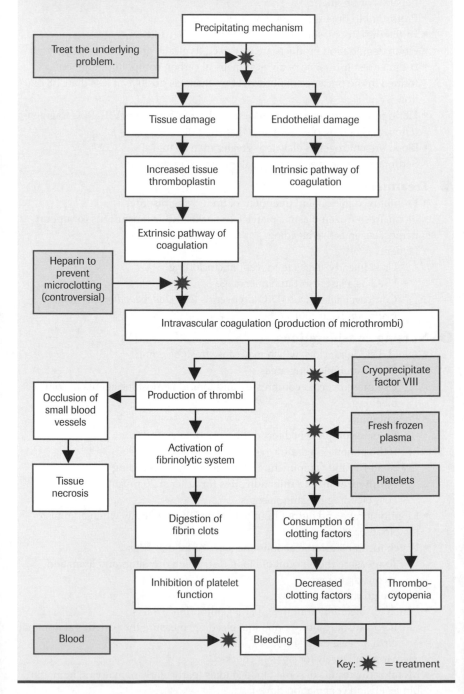

Precipitating mechanism

Treat the underlying problem.

Tissue damage → Increased tissue thromboplastin → Extrinsic pathway of coagulation

Endothelial damage → Intrinsic pathway of coagulation

Heparin to prevent microclotting (controversial)

Intravascular coagulation (production of microthrombi)

Production of thrombi → Occlusion of small blood vessels → Tissue necrosis

Cryoprecipitate factor VIII

Activation of fibrinolytic system

Fresh frozen plasma

Platelets

Digestion of fibrin clots

Consumption of clotting factors

Inhibition of platelet function

Decreased clotting factors

Thrombo-cytopenia

Blood → Bleeding

Key: ✳ = treatment

- Explain all diagnostic tests and procedures to the patient, and allow time for questions
- Provide emotional support for the patient and his family
  – Inform the family of the patient's progress
  – As needed, enlist the help of other members of the health care team in providing support

IDIOPATHIC THROMBOCYTOPENIC PURPURA

Definition
- Deficiency of platelets
- Occurs when the immune system destroys the body's own platelets
- May be acute, as in postviral thrombocytopenia, or chronic, as in essential thrombocytopenia or autoimmune thrombocytopenia
- Prognosis
  – Excellent for acute idiopathic thrombocytopenic purpura (ITP); about four out of five patients recover without treatment
  – Good for chronic ITP; remissions lasting weeks or years are common, especially among women

Underlying pathophysiology
- Circulating immunoglobulin G (IgG) molecules react with host platelets, which are then destroyed by phagocytosis in the spleen and, to a lesser degree, in the liver
- Normally, the life span of platelets in circulation is 7 to 10 days
- In ITP, platelets survive 1 to 3 days or less

Causes
- Drug reactions
- Immunization with a live virus vaccine
- Immunologic disorders
- Viral infection

Pathophysiologic changes
- Nose bleeds; oral bleeding; hemorrhages into the skin, mucous membranes, and other tissues causing red discoloration of skin (purpura); petechiae; and excessive menstrual bleeding caused by decreased platelet levels

Complications
- Cerebral hemorrhage
- Hemorrhage
- Purpuric lesions of vital organs (such as the brain and kidney)

Diagnostic test findings
- Platelet count is less than 20,000/µl
- Bleeding time is prolonged
- Platelets are abnormal in size and appearance
- Hemoglobin level is decreased (if bleeding occurred)
- Bone marrow studies show abundant megakaryocytes (platelet precursor cells) and a circulating platelet survival time of only several hours to a few days
- Humoral tests that measure platelet-associated IgG may help establish the diagnosis; half of patients with ITP have elevated IgG

Key facts about ITP
- Involves a platelet deficiency
- Develops when IgG molecules react with host platelets
- Results in platelets being destroyed by phagocytosis in the spleen and liver

Key pathophysiologic changes in ITP
- Nose bleeds
- Oral bleeding
- Purpura
- Excessive menstrual bleeding

Key diagnostic test results for ITP
- Platelet count: Less than 20,000/µl
- Bone marrow studies: Abundant megakaryocytes, circulating platelet survival time of only several hours to a few days

Key treatments for ITP

- Glucocorticoids and Ig (acute form)
- Blood and blood component transfusions (chronic form)

Key nursing considerations for ITP

- Teach patient to observe for signs of recurrence.
- Tell patient to avoid aspirin and ibuprofen.
- Protect areas of petechiae and ecchymoses from further injury.

Key facts about polycythemia vera

- Involves proliferation or hyperplasia of all bone marrow cells
- Results in abnormally viscous blood and inhibited blood flow
- Can lead to intravascular thrombosis

Treatment

- Acute ITP
  - Glucocorticoids to prevent further platelet destruction
  - Immunoglobulin to prevent platelet destruction
  - Plasmapheresis
  - Platelet pheresis
- Chronic ITP
  - Corticosteroids to suppress phagocytic activity and enhance platelet production
  - Splenectomy (when splenomegaly accompanies the initial thrombocytopenia)
  - Blood and blood component transfusions and vitamin K to correct anemia and coagulation defects
- Alternative treatments
  - Immunosuppressants to help stop platelet destruction
  - High-dose I.V. Ig
  - Immunoabsorption apheresis using staphylococcal protein A columns to remove IgG, thus allowing platelets to grow and function normally

Nursing considerations

- Teach the patient to observe for petechiae, ecchymoses, and other signs of recurrence
- Monitor patients receiving immunosuppressants for signs of bone marrow depression, infection, mucositis, GI ulcers, and severe diarrhea or vomiting
- Tell the patient to avoid aspirin and ibuprofen
- Protect all areas of petechiae and ecchymoses from further injury

POLYCYTHEMIA VERA

Definition

- Chronic disorder characterized by increased RBC mass, erythrocytosis, leukocytosis, thrombocytosis, and increased hemoglobin level, with normal or increased plasma volume
- Also known as *primary polycythemia, erythremia, polycythemia rubra vera, splenomegalic polycythemia,* and *Vaquez-Osler disease*

Underlying pathophysiology

- Uncontrolled and rapid cellular reproduction and maturation cause proliferation or hyperplasia of all bone marrow cells (panmyelosis)
- Increased RBC mass makes the blood abnormally viscous and inhibits blood flow to microcirculation
- Diminished blood flow and thrombocytosis set the stage for intravascular thrombosis

Causes

- Unknown
- Probably related to defects in blood stem cells

Pathophysiologic changes

- Feeling of fullness in the head or headache, tinnitus, weakness, fatigue, syncope due to altered blood volume, as in hypovolemia and hyperviscosity
- Ecchymosis due to hemorrhage

- Ruddy cyanosis (plethora) of the nose and clubbing of the digits due to thrombosis in smaller vessels
- Painful pruritus due to abnormally high concentrations of mast cells in the skin and their release of heparin and histamine
- Vision disturbances resulting from hypervolemia and hyperviscosity (blurring, diplopia, engorged veins of fundus and retina, and congestion of conjunctiva, retina, retinal veins, and oral mucous membranes)

● Complications
- Hemorrhage
- Uric acid stones
- Vascular thromboses

● Diagnostic test findings
- RBC mass reveals increased arterial oxygen saturation in association with splenomegaly or two of the following conditions
  - Platelet count above 400,000/µl
  - WBC count above 10,000/µl in adults
  - Elevated leukocyte alkaline phosphatase level
  - Elevated serum vitamin B_{12} levels of unbound vitamin B_{12}-binding capacity
- Uric acid level is increased
- Blood histamine level is increased
- Serum iron concentration is decreased
- Urinary erythropoietin is decreased or absent
- Bone marrow biopsy shows excess production of myeloid stem cells

● Treatment
- Phlebotomy to reduce RBC mass
- Myelosuppressive therapy with radioactive phosphorus (^{32}P) to suppress erythropoiesis (may increase the risk of leukemia) or hydroxyurea

● Nursing considerations
- If the patient requires phlebotomy
  - Explain the procedure
  - Check blood pressure, pulse rate, and respiratory rate
- During phlebotomy
  - Make sure that the patient is lying down comfortably to prevent vertigo and syncope
  - Stay alert for tachycardia, clamminess, or complaints of vertigo; if these effects occur, the procedure should be stopped
- Immediately after phlebotomy
  - Check blood pressure and pulse rate
  - Have the patient sit up for about 5 minutes before allowing him to walk to prevent vasovagal attack or orthostatic hypotension
  - Have the patient drink 24 oz (710 ml) of juice or water
- Tell the patient to watch for and report signs or symptoms of iron deficiency (pallor, weight loss, weakness, glossitis)
- Take measures to prevent thrombosis
  - Keep the patient active and ambulatory
  - If bed rest is absolutely necessary, prescribe a daily program of active and passive range-of-motion exercises

Key pathophysiologic changes in polycythemia vera
- Ecchymosis
- Ruddy cyanosis of nose
- Painful pruritus
- Vision disturbances

Key diagnostic test results for polycythemia vera
- RBC mass: Increased arterial oxygen saturation in association with splenomegaly or two of the following conditions:
  - Platelet count: Above 400,000/µl
  - WBC count: Above 10,000/µl in adults
  - Leukocyte alkaline phosphatase level: Elevated
  - Serum vitamin B_{12} levels: Elevated unbound vitamin B_{12}-binding capacity

Key treatments for polycythemia vera
- Phlebotomy
- Myelosuppressive therapy

Key nursing considerations for polycythemia vera

Phlebotomy

- Explain phlebotomy procedure to patient.
- Stay alert for tachycardia, clamminess, or complaints of vertigo.
- Afterwards, check blood pressure and pulse rate, have the patient sit up before ambulating, and have him drink 24 oz of juice or water.

Myelosuppressive treatment

- Advise patient to avoid crowds.
- Instruct patient to watch for infection and to report signs of bleeding.
- Tell patient about possible reactions.

Treatment with ^{32}P

- Explain procedure to patient.
- Take blood sample for CBC and platelet count before beginning treatment.
- Maintain radiation precautions.
- Have patient lie down during and after the procedure.

Key facts about secondary polycythemia

- Excessive production of circulating RBCs
- May result from increased production of erythropoietin as a response to such conditions as hypoxia, tumor, or disease

- Watch for complications, such as hypervolemia, thrombocytosis, and signs or symptoms of an impending stroke (decreased sensation, numbness, transitory paralysis, fleeting blindness, headache, and epistaxis)
- Regularly examine the patient closely for bleeding
  - Tell the patient which areas are the most common bleeding sites (such as the nose, gingiva, and skin) so he can check for bleeding
  - Advise him to report abnormal bleeding promptly
- Compensate for increased uric acid production
  - Give additional fluids
  - Administer allopurinol
  - Alkalinize the urine to prevent uric acid calculi
- If the patient has symptomatic splenomegaly, suggest or provide small, frequent meals, followed by a rest period, to prevent nausea and vomiting
- Report acute abdominal pain immediately, which may signal splenic infarction, renal calculi, or abdominal organ thrombosis
- During myelosuppressive treatment
  - Monitor complete blood count (CBC) and platelet count before and during therapy
  - Warn the patient who develops leukopenia that his resistance to infection is low
    - Advise him to avoid crowds
    - Instruct him to watch for signs and symptoms of infection
  - If thrombocytopenia develops, tell the patient to watch for signs of bleeding (blood in urine, nosebleeds, and black stools)
  - Tell the patient about possible reactions (nausea, vomiting, and risk of infection) to alkylating agents
    - Alopecia may follow the use of busulfan, cyclophosphamide, and uracil mustard
    - Sterile hemorrhagic cystitis may follow the use of cyclophosphamide (encouraging fluid intake can prevent it)
  - Watch for and report all reactions
  - If nausea and vomiting occur, begin antiemetic therapy and adjust the patient's diet
- During treatment with ^{32}P
  - Explain the procedure to the patient to relieve anxiety
  - Tell the patient he may require repeated phlebotomies until ^{32}P takes effect
  - Take a blood sample for CBC and platelet count before beginning treatment
  - Remember that the use of ^{32}P requires radiation precautions to prevent contamination
  - Have the patient lie down during I.V. administration (to facilitate the procedure and prevent extravasation) and for 15 to 20 minutes afterward

SECONDARY POLYCYTHEMIA

- ### Definition
  - Excessive production of circulating RBCs due to hypoxia, tumor, or disease
  - Also called *reactive polycythemia*

Underlying pathophysiology

- May result from increased production of the hormone erythropoietin
- Increased erythropoietin stimulates bone marrow to produce RBCs in a compensatory response to several conditions
  - Hypoxemia
  - Hemoglobin abnormalities (such as carboxyhemoglobinemia or carbon monoxide poisoning)
  - Heart failure due to decreased ventilation-perfusion ratio
  - Right-to-left shunting of blood in the heart
  - Central or peripheral alveolar hypoventilation (such as with barbiturate intoxication)
  - Low oxygen content at high altitudes
- Increased production of erythropoietin may also be a response to other conditions
  - Renal, CNS, or endocrine disorders
  - Certain neoplasms, such as renal tumors, uterine myomas, or cerebellar hemangiomas

Causes

- Conditions that cause prolonged tissue hypoxia, such as shock or compression of major blood vessels
- Increased production of erythropoietin
- Recessive genetic trait (rare)

Pathophysiologic changes

- Ruddy cyanotic skin, emphysema, and hypoxemia without hepatomegaly or hypertension due to hypoxia
- Clubbing of the fingers when the underlying cause is cardiovascular

Complications

- Hemorrhage
- Thromboemboli secondary to hemoconcentration

Diagnostic test findings

- Hematocrit and hemoglobin level are elevated
- Mean corpuscular volume and mean corpuscular hemoglobin are elevated
- Urinary erythropoietin is elevated
- Blood histamine is elevated
- Arterial oxygen saturation is normal or low
- Bone marrow biopsy shows hyperplasia or erythroid precursors

Treatment

- Correction of the underlying disease or environmental condition
- Phlebotomy or pheresis to reduce blood volume (used to correct hazardous hyperviscosity or if the patient doesn't respond to treatment of the primary disease)
- Continuous low-flow oxygen therapy to correct severe hypoxia

Nursing considerations

- Keep the patient as active as possible to decrease the risk of thrombosis due to increased blood viscosity
- Reduce calorie and sodium intake to counteract the tendency toward hypertension
- Before phlebotomy, check blood pressure with the patient lying down

Key pathophysiologic changes in secondary polycythemia

- Ruddy, cyanotic skin
- Clubbing of fingers
- Hypoxemia

Key diagnostic test results for secondary polycythemia

- Hematocrit and hemoglobin level: Elevated
- Mean corpuscular volume and mean corpuscular hemoglobin: Elevated
- Arterial oxygen saturation: Normal or low

Key treatments for secondary polycythemia

- Correction of underlying cause
- Low-flow oxygen therapy

Key nursing considerations for secondary polycythemia

- Teach patient about underlying disorder and its relationship to polycythemia.
- Teach patient to recognize symptoms of recurrence.

- After phlebotomy
  - Have the patient drink approximately 24 oz (710 ml) of water or juice
  - To prevent syncope, have the patient sit up for about 5 minutes before walking
- Emphasize the importance of regular blood studies (every 2 to 3 months), even after the disease is controlled
- Teach the patient and his family about the underlying disorder
  - Explain its relationship to polycythemia
  - Explain the measures needed to control both conditions
- Teach the patient to recognize symptoms of recurring polycythemia and the importance of reporting them promptly

SPURIOUS POLYCYTHEMIA

● Definition
- Characterized by an increased hematocrit and a normal or low RBC total mass
- Results from diminished plasma volume and subsequent hemoconcentration
- Also known as *relative polycythemia, stress erythrocytosis, stress polycythemia, benign polycythemia, Gaisböck's disease,* and *pseudopolycythemia*

● Underlying pathophysiology
- There are three possible courses through which this disorder can occur
  - Conditions, such as persistent vomiting or diarrhea, burns, adrenocortical insufficiency, aggressive diuretic therapy, decreased fluid intake, diabetic acidosis, and renal disease, promote severe fluid loss, decrease plasma volume, and lead to hemoconcentration
  - Nervous stress causes hemoconcentration by some unknown mechanism, possibly by temporarily decreasing circulating plasma volume or vascular redistribution of erythrocytes
    - This occurrence is particularly common in middle-aged men who are chronic smokers and have a type A personality (tense, hard driving, and anxious)
  - In many patients, an increased hematocrit merely reflects a normally high RBC mass and low plasma volume
    - This condition is particularly common in normal-weight nonsmokers who have no history of hypertension

● Causes
- Dehydration
- Elevated serum cholesterol and uric acid
- Familial tendency
- Hemoconcentration due to stress
- Hypertension
- Thromboembolic disease

● Pathophysiologic changes
- Headaches, dizziness, and fatigue due to altered circulation secondary to hypovolemia and hyperviscosity
- Ruddy appearance caused by excess RBCs in vasculature
- Slight hypertension, diaphoresis, dyspnea, and tendency to hyperventilate when recumbent due to decreased blood volume
- Cardiac or pulmonary disease related to hypovolemia

● **Complications**
  • Thromboemboli

● **Diagnostic test findings**
  • Hemoglobin level and hematocrit are elevated
  • RBC count is increased
  • RBC mass is normal or decreased
  • Arterial oxygen saturation is normal
  • Bone marrow studies are normal
  • Plasma volume is normal or decreased
  • Serum cholesterol and lipid levels may indicate hyperlipidemia
  • Urine uric acid level may be increased

● **Treatment**
  • Appropriate fluids and electrolytes to correct dehydration
  • Measures to prevent further fluid loss
    – Antidiarrheals if prescribed
    – Avoiding dietary diuretics (such as caffeine) and prescription diuretics as directed
    – Preventing excessive perspiration
    – Staying hydrated

● **Nursing considerations**
  • During rehydration, carefully monitor intake and output to maintain fluid and electrolyte balance
  • Prevent thromboemboli in predisposed patients
    – Suggest regular exercise and a low-cholesterol diet
    – Antilipemics may be necessary
    – Reduced calorie intake may be required for the obese patient
  • Whenever appropriate, suggest counseling about the patient's work habits and lack of relaxation
  • If the patient is a smoker, make sure he understands the importance of smoking cessation
    – Refer him to an antismoking program, if necessary
  • Emphasize the need for follow-up examinations every 3 to 4 months after leaving the hospital
  • Thoroughly explain the disorder, all diagnostic measures, and therapy
    – Answer questions honestly
    – Take care to reassure the patient that he can effectively control symptoms by complying with the prescribed treatment

THROMBOCYTOPENIA

● **Definition**
  • Deficiency of circulating platelets
  • May be congenital or acquired (most common)
  • Poses a serious threat to hemostasis because platelets are needed for coagulation
  • If drug-induced, excellent prognosis if the offending drug — usually carbamazepine (Tegretol) or heparin — is withdrawn

---

Key diagnostic test results for spurious polycythemia

● Hemoglobin level and hematocrit: Elevated
● RBC count: Increased
● RBC mass: Normal or decreased

Key treatment for spurious polycythemia

● Correcting and preventing dehydration

Key nursing considerations for spurious polycythemia

● Monitor intake and output to maintain fluid and electrolyte balance.
● Prevent thromboemboli.

Key facts about thrombocytopenia

● Deficiency of circulating platelets
● Can cause inadequate hemostasis
● Involves four mechanisms: decreased platelet production, decreased platelet survival, pooling of blood in the spleen, and intravascular dilution of circulating platelets

Key pathophysiologic changes in thrombocytopenia

- Petechiae
- Blood-filled blisters in mouth
- Malaise
- Fatigue

Key diagnostic test results for thrombocytopenia

- Platelet count: Usually less than 100,000/µl in adults
- Platelet antibody studies: Reason for low platelet count (helps select treatment)
- Platelet survival studies: Differentiation between ineffective platelet production and platelet destruction

Key treatments for thrombocytopenia

- Treatment of underlying cause
- Corticosteroids
- I.V. gamma globulin
- Splenectomy

● **Underlying pathophysiology**
- Lack of platelets can cause inadequate hemostasis
- Four mechanisms are responsible
  - Decreased platelet production
  - Decreased platelet survival
  - Pooling of blood in the spleen
  - Intravascular dilution of circulating platelets
- Megakaryocytes — giant cells in the bone marrow — produce platelets
- Platelet production decreases when the number of megakaryocytes is reduced or when platelet production becomes dysfunctional (see *What happens in thrombocytopenia*)

● **Causes**
- Blood loss
- Decreased or defective platelet production in the bone marrow (as in leukemia, aplastic anemia, or drug toxicity)
- Increased platelet destruction outside the marrow due to an underlying disorder (such as cirrhosis of the liver, DIC, or severe infection)
- Sequestration (increased amount of blood in a limited vascular area such as the spleen)
- Radiation therapy
- Blood transfusions
- Idiopathic causes

● **Pathophysiologic changes**
- Petechiae or blood blisters, bleeding into the mucous membrane, and large blood-filled blisters in the mouth (in adults) caused by inadequate hemostasis
- Malaise, fatigue, and general weakness resulting from decreased oxygenation

● **Complications**
- Hemorrhage
- Death

● **Diagnostic test findings**
- Platelet count is usually less than 100,000/µl in adults
- Bleeding time is prolonged
- Platelet antibody studies help determine why the platelet count is low and help select treatment
- Platelet survival studies help differentiate between ineffective platelet production and platelet destruction as causes of thrombocytopenia
- Bone marrow studies determine the number, size, and maturity of megakaryocytes in severe diseases, helping identify ineffective platelet production as the cause and ruling out malignant disease

● **Treatment**
- Withdrawing the offending drug or treating the underlying cause
- Corticosteroids to increase platelet production
- Lithium carbonate (Eskalith) or folate to stimulate bone marrow production
- I.V. gamma globulin to increase platelet production
- Platelet transfusion to treat complications of severe hemorrhage
- Splenectomy to correct disease caused by platelet destruction (because the spleen is the primary site of platelet removal and antibody production)

GO WITH THE FLOW

What happens in thrombocytopenia

Thrombocytopenia, a deficiency of circulating platelets, poses a serious threat to hemostasis because platelets are needed for coagulation. Here's what happens.

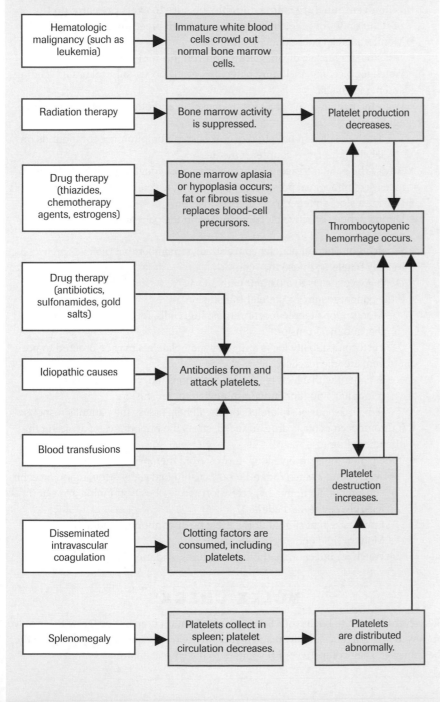

Key nursing considerations for thrombocytopenia

- Take precautions against bleeding.
- Warn patient to avoid aspirin and other drugs that impair coagulation.
- Advise patient to avoid straining during defication and coughing.
- Teach patient receiving long-term steroid therapy cushingoid signs to report.
- When venipuncture is unavoidable, be sure to exert pressure on the puncture site for at least 20 minutes or until bleeding stops.

TOP 5

Items to study for your next test on the hematologic system

1. Facts about RBCs and WBCs
2. Types of anemia and their treatments
3. Pathophysiology of DIC
4. Nursing considerations for transfusions and bleeding precautions
5. Common hematologic diagnostic tests, such as hemoglobin, hematocrit, platelets, and Schilling test

● **Nursing considerations**
- Take every possible precaution against bleeding
  - Protect the patient from trauma
  - Keep the side rails up and pad them, if possible
  - Promote the use of an electric razor and a soft toothbrush
- Avoid invasive procedures, such as venipuncture or urinary catheterization, if possible
- **When venipuncture is unavoidable, be sure to exert pressure on the puncture site for at least 20 minutes or until bleeding stops**
- Monitor platelet count daily
- Test stool for guaiac; dipstick urine and vomitus for blood
- Watch for bleeding, including petechiae, ecchymoses, surgical or GI bleeding, and menorrhagia
- Warn the patient to avoid all forms of aspirin and other drugs that impair coagulation
  - Teach the patient how to recognize aspirin or ibuprofen compounds on labels of over-the-counter remedies
- Advise the patient to avoid straining at stool or coughing, which can lead to increased intracranial pressure, possibly causing cerebral hemorrhage
- Provide a stool softener to avoid constipation
- During periods of active bleeding, maintain the patient on strict bed rest, if necessary
- When administering platelet concentrate, remember that platelets are extremely fragile, so infuse them quickly
- Don't give platelets to a patient with a fever
- If the patient requires a platelet transfusion
  - Monitor for a febrile reaction (flushing, chills, fever, headache, tachycardia, and hypertension)
  - Histocompatibility locus antigen-typed platelets may be ordered to prevent afebrile reaction
  - A patient with a history of minor reactions may benefit from acetaminophen and diphenhydramine before transfusion
  - A 1- to 2-hour postplatelet count will help assess the patient's response
- If thrombocytopenia is drug-induced, stress the importance of avoiding the offending drug
- If the patient must receive long-term steroid therapy
  - Teach him to watch for and report cushingoid signs (acne, moon face, hirsutism, buffalo hump, hypertension, girdle obesity, thinning arms and legs, glycosuria, and edema)
  - Emphasize that steroid doses must be discontinued gradually
  - Monitor fluid and electrolyte balance
  - Watch for infection, pathologic fractures, and mood changes

NCLEX CHECKS

It's never too soon to begin your licensure examination preparation. Now that you've reviewed this chapter, carefully read each of the following questions and choose the best answer. Then compare your responses to the correct answers.

1. Which type of WBCs devours invading organisms by phagocytosis?
☐ 1. Lymphocytes
☐ 2. Eosinophils
☐ 3. Basophils
☐ 4. Monocytes

2. The nurse is preparing to administer supplemental iron I.V. Which statement about iron deficiency anemia is correct?
☐ 1. Thick, tough, flat nails are common in patients who lack adequate iron.
☐ 2. Transferrin is the protein that binds iron for transport to the cells.
☐ 3. Iron-deficient RBCs are characteristically larger and darker than normal RBCs.
☐ 4. Adults receiving less than 10 to 20 mg of iron per day can develop iron deficiency anemia.

3. The nurse is teaching a patient who was prescribed iron supplementation. Which of the following enhances the absorption of iron?
☐ 1. Vitamin C
☐ 2. Vitamin D
☐ 3. Folate
☐ 4. Phosphate

4. The cause of primary acquired sideroblastic anemia is:
☐ 1. unknown.
☐ 2. a genetic defect on the X chromosome.
☐ 3. ingestion of toxins.
☐ 4. rheumatoid arthritis.

5. Your patient has been admitted with a diagnosis of aplastic anemia. Bleeding precautions should be initiated when the platelet count is:
☐ 1. less than 200,000/μl.
☐ 2. less than 100,000/μl.
☐ 3. less than 50,000/μl.
☐ 4. less than 20,000/μl.

6. A patient complains of gradually progressing fatigue, shortness of breath, palpitations, headache, anorexia, and weakness. Which diagnostic test would the nurse expect to be ordered to determine if the patient has folic acid deficiency anemia?
☐ 1. CBC
☐ 2. Schilling test
☐ 3. Chemistry panel with electrolytes and serum calcium
☐ 4. Serum iron, total iron-binding capacity, and ferritin level

7. The organ that's most likely to be affected by DIC is the:
☐ 1. heart.
☐ 2. lung.
☐ 3. kidney.
☐ 4. brain.

8. Which teaching point is appropriate for the patient receiving myelosuppressive treatment for polycythemia vera?

- ☐ 1. Avoid crowds
- ☐ 2. Exercise regularly
- ☐ 3. Reduce fluid intake
- ☐ 4. Eat a high-protein diet

9. When transfusing platelets to a patient with thrombocytopenia, the nurse should:

- ☐ 1. transfuse the platelets slowly.
- ☐ 2. transfuse the platelets quickly.
- ☐ 3. use a blood warmer.
- ☐ 4. infuse the platelets with a solution of dextrose 5% and water.

10. The nurse is teaching a patient about aplastic anemia. Identify where red bone marrow is located.

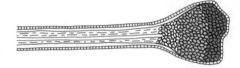

ANSWERS AND RATIONALES

1. CORRECT ANSWER: 4

Monocytes, along with neutrophils, help devour invading organisms by phagocytosis. Lymphocytes are involved in producing antibodies. Eosinophils produce antihistamines and indicate allergic conditions. Basophils become mast cells during an allergic response.

2. CORRECT ANSWER: 2

With iron deficiency anemia, transferrin binds to iron to transport iron to the cells. The RBCs in iron deficiency anemia are paler and smaller, not darker and larger, than normal RBCs. Coarsely ridged, spoon-shaped, thin, brittle nails — not thick, tough, flat nails — are typical in chronic forms of iron deficiency anemia. Adults must receive 1 to 2 mg of iron per day to prevent iron deficiency anemia.

3. CORRECT ANSWER: 1

Vitamin C (ascorbic acid) increases the absorption of iron in the GI tract. Patients with iron deficiency anemia should be encouraged to take their iron supplements with vitamin C. The patient should avoid milk products and antacids because they decrease absorption. Folate and phosphate don't affect iron absorption.

4. CORRECT ANSWER: 1

The cause of primary acquired sideroblastic anemia is unknown. This condition resists treatment and is usually fatal within 10 years of the onset of complications or a concomitant disease. The hereditary form of sideroblastic anemia is caused by a genetic defect on the X chromosome. Secondary acquired sideroblastic anemia is caused by certain chronic diseases, such as rheumatoid arthritis, or ingestion of toxins.

5. CORRECT ANSWER: 4

A normal platelet count is 130,000 to 400,000/µl. If the patient's platelet count is less than 20,000/µl, he's prone to bleeding.

6. CORRECT ANSWER: 2

The Schilling test, which measures the amount of vitamin B_{12} excreted in the urine, distinguishes between folic acid deficiency anemia and pernicious anemia. Significant findings include macrocytosis, decreased reticulocyte count, abnormal platelets, and serum folate level less than 4 mg/ml. CBC alone isn't diagnostic for folic acid deficiency anemia. Chemistry panels and tests for iron storage and production aren't indicated for this type of anemia.

7. CORRECT ANSWER: 3

Kidneys are usually affected by DIC because of the clotting in the microcirculation, which can lead to acute tubular necrosis and renal failure. Complications can also occur in the brain, lungs, pituitary and adrenal glands, and GI mucosa, but the kidneys are the most likely organs to be affected.

8. CORRECT ANSWER: 1

Patients undergoing myelosuppressive therapy have a low WBC count and low resistance to infections. The nurse should instruct such patients to avoid crowds and watch for symptoms of infection. Exercise and a high-protein diet, although part of a healthy lifestyle, aren't required. The patient doesn't need to restrict fluids.

9. CORRECT ANSWER: 2

Platelets are extremely fragile. The nurse should infuse them quickly. Platelets should not be warmed or mixed with another solution for transfusion.

10. CORRECT ANSWER:

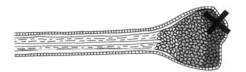

Red bone marrow is located at the ends of the long bones. This marrow is the site of the formation of red blood cells as well as other blood and immune system cells.

7

Immune system

LEARNING OBJECTIVES

After reading this chapter, you should be able to:

- Identify conditions that affect the immune response.
- Describe the relationship between presenting symptoms and pathophysiologic changes for various immune system disorders.
- List possible causes of various immune system disorders.
- Discuss the medications used to treat immune system disorders.
- List nursing considerations for the patient with an immune system disorder.
- Write teaching goals for the patient with an immune system disorder.

CHAPTER OVERVIEW

The body protects itself from infectious organisms and other harmful invaders with three lines of defense: physical barriers to infection (such as skin), the inflammatory response, and the immune response. This chapter reviews key pathophysiologic concepts related to the immune system, and then outlines the underlying pathophysiology, causes, changes, complications, diagnostic test findings, treatment approaches, and nursing considerations associated with common immune system disorders.

PATHOPHYSIOLOGIC CONCEPTS

● **Autoimmune reactions**
- Result when normal defenses become self-destructive
- Lead the body to recognize its own antigens as foreign
- Cause unclear; may result from a combination of factors
  - Genetic (increases the incidence and severity of autoimmune reactions)
  - Hormonal, including estrogen
  - Environmental
- Commonly characterized by B-cell hyperactivity, which may be related to T-cell abnormalities, and hypergammaglobulinemia
- Categorized into three types
  - Autoimmune diseases
  - Immune complex diseases
  - Allergy or hypersensitivity reactions
- May affect almost any tissue or cell in the body

● **Hypersensitivity**
- Exaggerated or inappropriate response that occurs on the second or later exposure to an antigen
- Results in inflammation and destruction of healthy tissue
- May involve an immediate reaction (occurring within minutes to hours of reexposure), or a delayed reaction (occurring several hours after reexposure, being most severe days after the reexposure)
- Classified as one of four types
  - Type I hypersensitivity (immediate type)
    · Examples include allergies to food, pollens, spores, and seasonal exposures
    · Repeated exposure to relatively large doses of an allergen activates T cells, which induce B-cell production of immunoglobulin (Ig) E
    · IgE binds to the fragment c (Fc) receptors on the surface of mast cells
    · When enough IgE has been produced, the person is sensitized to the allergen
    · At the next exposure, the antigen binds with the surface IgE, cross-links the Fc receptors, and causes mast cells to degranulate and release various mediators
      - Rhinorrhea, urticaria, and edema occur
      - Condition may progress to wheezing, bronchial edema, and hypotension
  - Type II hypersensitivity (tissue specific)
    · An antibody directed against cell-surface antigens destroys a target cell
    · Direct tissue damage occurs through several mechanisms
      - Binding of the antigen and antibody activates complement, which ultimately disrupts cellular membranes (complement-mediated lysis)
      - Phagocytic cells with receptors for immunoglobulin (Fc region) and complement fragments envelop and destroy opsonized targets (targets that have been previously bound to opsonin, a

Key facts about autoimmune reactions
● Result when normal defenses become self-destructive
● Cause the body to recognize its own antigens as foreign

Types of autoimmune reactions
● Autoimmune diseases
● Immune complex diseases
● Allergy or hypersensitivity reactions

Key facts about hypersensitivity
● Exaggerated or inappropriate response to an antigen
● Results in inflammation and destruction of healthy tissue

Types of hypersensitivity

Type I
- Immediate
- Includes allergies to food or pollen

Type II
- Tissue specific
- Occurs with mismatched blood transfusions

Type III
- Immune complex–mediated
- Includes vasculitis and renal damage

Type IV
- Delayed
- Cell mediated
- Includes contact dermatitis and latex allergy

substance that enhances phagocytosis), such as red blood cells (RBCs), leukocytes, and platelets
- Cytotoxic T cells and natural killer cells, although not antigen specific, damage tissue by releasing toxic substances that destroy the cells
- Binding causes the target cell to malfunction rather than cause its destruction
- Examples include mismatched blood transfusions, hemolytic disease of the neonate due to ABO or Rh incompatibility, and certain drug reactions
 – Type III hypersensitivity (immune complex–mediated)
- Circulating antigen-antibody complexes (immune complexes) accumulate and are deposited in the tissues, most commonly the renal glomerulus, skin venules, the lungs, joint synovium, and blood vessels
- Immune complexes deposited in the tissues cause indirect damage by activating the complement cascade and causing local inflammation, and then trigger platelet release of vasoactive amines that increase vascular permeability so that more immune complexes accumulate in the vessel walls
- Complement fragments attract neutrophils
- Neutrophils attempt to ingest the immune complexes
  - Generally unsuccessful
  - In the attempt, neutrophils release lysosomal enzymes, which exacerbate the tissue damage
- Examples include vasculitis (seen in systemic lupus erythematosus [SLE]), renal damage (seen in glomerular nephritis), and serum sickness
 – Type IV hypersensitivity (delayed type; cell mediated)
- Involves the processing of the antigen by the macrophages
- Antigen is presented to the T cells
- Cytotoxic T cells, if activated, attack and destroy the target cells directly
- When T cells are activated, they release lymphokines, which recruit and activate other lymphocytes, monocytes, macrophages, and polymorphonuclear leukocytes
- The coagulation, kinin, and complement cascades also contribute to tissue damage
- This response usually occurs 24 to 72 hours after exposure to the antigen
- Examples include Mantoux test reactions, contact dermatitis, and latex allergy

ACQUIRED IMMUNODEFICIENCY SYNDROME

● **Definition**
- Also known as AIDS
- Characterized by gradual destruction of cell-mediated (T-cell) immunity and autoimmunity
- Makes the patient susceptible to opportunistic infections, cancers, and other abnormalities

- Marked by progressive failure of the immune system
- Caused by the human immunodeficiency virus (HIV)
- Transmitted by contact with infected blood or body fluids, including from an infected mother to the fetus, or through infected blood and blood component transfusions (before controls were established in 1985)
- Associated with identifiable high-risk behaviors

Underlying pathophysiology

- HIV enters the body through the transmission of infected blood or body fluids
- Through the action of reverse transcriptase, HIV produces a copy of the viral ribonucleic acid (RNA) and a reverse copy (a mirror image) resulting in the double-stranded viral deoxyribonucleic acid (DNA)
- Viral DNA enters the nucleus of the cell and is incorporated into the host cell's DNA, where it's transcribed into more viral RNA
- If the host cell reproduces, it duplicates the HIV DNA along with its own and passes it on to the daughter cells
- The host cell carries the HIV DNA and, if activated, replicates the virus
- In replication, viral enzymes (proteases) arrange the structural components and RNA into viral particles that move out to the periphery of the host cell, where the virus buds and emerges from the host cell to travel and infect other cells
- HIV replication may lead to cell death, or replication may become latent
- Abnormalities may occur directly through destruction of CD4+ helper T cells, other immune cells, and neuroglial cells, or indirectly through the secondary effects of CD4+ T-cell dysfunction and resulting immunosuppression
- HIV infection involves three types of effects
  - Immunodeficiency (such as opportunistic bacterial and viral infections and unusual cancers)
  - Autoimmunity (such as lymphoid interstitial pneumonitis, arthritis, hypergammaglobulinemia, and production of autoimmune antibodies)
  - Neurologic dysfunction (such as acquired immunodeficiency syndrome [AIDS] dementia complex, HIV encephalopathy, and peripheral neuropathies)
- The infectious process has three phases during which the three types of affects can occur
  - Primary infection
    - Syndrome of fever, fatigue, myalgia, sore throat, lymphadenopathy, GI problems, maculopapular rash, and headache develops
    - Increased viral replication occurs 2 to 4 weeks after exposure to HIV
    - Phase lasts for a few days to 2 weeks
  - Latent phase
    - This is a chronic asymptomatic phase
    - It's characterized by lack of symptoms of disease but gradually falling CD4+ counts
    - Median duration is 10 years
  - Overt AIDS
    - This phase starts when CD4+ count is 200 cells/µl or when patient develops an AIDS-defining illness
    - Death occurs in 2 to 3 years if left untreated

Key facts about AIDS

- Characterized by gradual destruction of T-cell immunity and autoimmunity
- Caused by HIV
- Has three phases: primary infection, latent phase, overt AIDS

Key facts about HIV

- Transmits through infected blood or body fluids
- Creates viral DNA, which enters cell nuclei and incorporates into the host cell's DNA
- Replicates if host cell carrying the HIV DNA is activated
- May lead to cell death or become latent

Causes
- HIV-1 or HIV-2 retrovirus

Pathophysiologic changes
- Persistent generalized lymphadenopathy secondary to impaired function of CD4+ cells
- Nonspecific symptoms, including weight loss, fatigue, night sweats, and fevers related to altered function of CD4+ cells, immunodeficiency, and infection of other CD4+ antigen–bearing cells
- Neurologic symptoms including forgetfulness, imbalance, weakness, and impaired language resulting from HIV encephalopathy and infection of neuroglial cells
- Opportunistic infection, such as cytomegalovirus (CMV), or cancer, such as Kaposi's sarcoma, related to immunodeficiency

Complications
- Repeated opportunistic infections, such as *Pneumocystis carinii* pneumonia, toxoplasmosis, candidiasis, herpes simplex 1 and 2, CMV retinitis, tuberculosis, or Kaposi's sarcoma

Diagnostic test findings
- Diagnosis of AIDS includes one or more of the following test results
  - Enzyme-linked immunosorbent assay and Western blot test detect the presence of HIV antibodies, which indicates HIV infection
  - CD4+ T-cell count is less than 200 cells/μl
  - One or more conditions specified by the Centers for Disease Control and Prevention (CDC) as categories A, B, or C are present (see *Conditions associated with AIDS*)

Treatment
- Primary therapy
  - Use of various combinations of three different types of antiretroviral agents to try to gain the maximum benefit of inhibiting HIV viral replication with the fewest adverse reactions
  - Use of two nucleosides plus one protease inhibitor, or two nucleosides and one nonnucleoside is currently recommended to help inhibit the production of resistant, mutant strains (check CDC Guidelines for the most current treatment recommendations)
- Additional treatment
  - Immunomodulatory agents to boost the immune system weakened by AIDS and retroviral therapy
  - Human granulocyte colony-stimulating growth factor to stimulate neutrophil production (retroviral therapy causes anemia, so patients may receive epoetin alfa)
  - Anti-infective and antineoplastic agents to combat opportunistic infections and associated cancers (some prophylactically to help resist opportunistic infections)
  - Supportive therapy
    - Nutritional support
    - Fluid and electrolyte replacement therapy
    - Pain relief
    - Psychological support

Conditions associated with AIDS

The Centers for Disease Control and Prevention lists acquired immunodeficiency syndrome (AIDS)–associated diseases under three categories.

CATEGORY A
- Persistent generalized lymph node enlargement
- Acute primary human immunodeficiency virus (HIV) infection with accompanying illness
- History of acute HIV infection

CATEGORY B
- Bacillary angiomatosis
- Oropharyngeal or persistent vulvovaginal candidiasis, fever, or diarrhea lasting longer than 1 month
- Idiopathic thrombocytopenic purpura
- Pelvic inflammatory disease, especially with a tubo-ovarian abscess
- Peripheral neuropathy

CATEGORY C
- Candidiasis of the bronchi, trachea, lungs, or esophagus
- Invasive cervical cancer
- Disseminated or extrapulmonary coccoidiomycosis
- Extrapulmonary cryptococcosis
- Chronic interstitial cryptosporidiosis
- Cytomegalovirus (CMV) disease affecting organs other than the liver, spleen, or lymph nodes
- CMV retinitis with vision loss
- Encephalopathy related to HIV
- Herpes simplex infection with chronic ulcers or herpetic bronchitis, pneumonitis, or esophagitis
- Disseminated or extrapulmonary histoplasmosis
- Chronic intestinal isopsoriasis
- Kaposi's sarcoma
- Burkitt's lymphoma or its equivalent
- Immunoblastic lymphoma or its equivalent
- Primary brain lymphoma
- Disseminated or extrapulmonary *Mycobacterium avium* complex or *M. kansasii*
- Pulmonary or extrapulmonary *M. tuberculosis*
- Disseminated or extrapulmonary infection with another species of *Mycobacterium*
- *Pneumocystis carinii* pneumonia
- Recurrent pneumonia
- Progressive multifocal leukoencephalopathy
- Recurrent *Salmonella* septicemia
- Toxoplasmosis of the brain
- Wasting disease caused by HIV

Nursing considerations
- Advise the patient, health care workers, and the public to use precautions in all situations that risk exposure to blood, body fluids, and secretions
- Recognize that a diagnosis of AIDS is profoundly distressing because of the disease's social impact and discouraging prognosis
- Assist the patient to cope with an altered body image, the emotional burden of serious illness, and the threat of death or other issues identified by the patient
- Encourage and assist the patient in learning about AIDS support programs and reputable information sources
- Encourage the patient to obtain CD4+ count and viral load testing every 3 to 4 months

Key nursing considerations for AIDS
- Use precautions in situations that risk exposure to blood, body fluids, and secretions.
- Help patient cope with issues related to illness.
- Refer patient to AIDS support programs.

ALLERGIC RHINITIS

● **Definition**
- Reaction to airborne (inhaled) allergens
- May occur seasonally (hay fever) or year-round (perennial allergic rhinitis) depending on the allergen
- Most common atopic allergic reaction

● **Underlying pathophysiology**
- During primary exposure to an allergen, T cells recognize the foreign allergens and release chemicals that instruct B cells to produce IgE antibodies
- IgE antibodies attach themselves to mast cells
- Mast cells with attached IgE can remain in the body for years, ready to react when they next encounter the same allergen
- The second time the allergen enters the body, it comes into direct contact with the IgE antibodies attached to the mast cells
- This contact stimulates the mast cells to release chemicals, such as histamine, which initiate a response that causes tightening of the smooth muscles in the airways, dilation of small blood vessels, increased mucus secretion in the nasal cavity and airways, and itching

● **Causes**
- IgE-mediated type I hypersensitivity response to an environmental antigen (allergen) in a genetically susceptible person
- Common triggers
  - Perennial allergens and irritants
    - Dust mite excreta, fungal spores, and molds
    - Feather pillows
    - Cigarette smoke
    - Animal dander
  - Windborne pollens
    - Oak, elm, maple, alder, birch, and cottonwood during spring
    - Grasses, sheep sorrel, and English plantain during summer
    - Ragweed and other weeds during autumn

● **Pathophysiologic changes**
- Paroxysmal sneezing, profuse watery rhinorrhea, nasal obstruction or congestion, and pruritus of the nose and eyes caused by histamine release
- Pale, cyanotic, edematous nasal mucosa; red and edematous eyelids and conjunctivae; excessive lacrimation; and headache or sinus pain resulting from histamine response
- Possible dark circles under the patient's eyes ("allergic shiners") because of venous congestion in the maxillary sinuses

● **Complications**
- Nasal polyps, which may result from edema and infection and increase nasal obstruction
- Sinus and middle ear infections due to swelling of the turbinates and mucous membranes

Diagnostic test findings

- Microscopic examination of sputum and nasal secretions reveals large numbers of eosinophils
- IgE levels are normal or elevated

Treatment

- Elimination of environmental antigens, if possible
- Antihistamines to block histamine effects
  - Commonly produce anticholinergic adverse effects (sedation, dry mouth, nausea, dizziness, blurred vision, and nervousness)
  - Fewer adverse effects with the use of newer antihistamines such as fexofenadine (Allegra)
- Injectable steroids, such as triamcinolone acetonide (Kenalog), to provide symptom relief for 6 to 8 weeks
- Inhaled intranasal steroids, such as beclomethasone (Beconase, Vancenase), flunisolide (Nasalide), and fluticasone (Flonase)
  - Provide local anti-inflammatory effects with minimal systemic adverse effects
  - Require consistent use and usually take 2 weeks to relieve symptoms
- Long-term management
  - Immunotherapy
  - Desensitization with injections of extracted allergens, administered before or during allergy season or perennially
    - Seasonal allergies require particularly close dosage regulation

Nursing considerations

- Before desensitization injections, assess the patient's symptom status
- After desensitization injections, watch for adverse reactions, including anaphylaxis and severe localized erythema
  - Keep epinephrine and emergency resuscitation equipment available
  - Observe the patient for 30 minutes after the injection
  - Instruct the patient to call the physician if a delayed reaction should occur
- Monitor the patient's compliance with prescribed drug treatment regimens
  - Note changes in the control of his symptoms
  - Stay alert for signs of drug misuse
- Advise the patient to use intranasal steroids regularly, as prescribed, for optimal effectiveness
- Cromolyn (Nasalcrom) may help prevent allergic rhinitis, but this drug may take up to 4 weeks to produce a satisfactory effect and must be taken regularly during allergy season
- Offer suggestions for reducing environmental exposure to airborne allergens
  - Sleep with the windows closed
  - Avoid the countryside during pollination seasons
  - Use air conditioning to filter allergens and minimize moisture and dust
  - Eliminate items that collect dust easily, such as wool blankets, deep-pile carpets, and heavy drapes, from the home
- In severe and resistant cases, suggest that the patient consider drastic changes in lifestyle, such as relocation to a pollen-free area seasonally or year-round

Key facts about anaphylaxis

- Life-threatening hypersensitivity reaction
- Marked by sudden onset of rapidly progressive urticaria and respiratory distress
- Occurs within minutes or up to 1 hour after reexposure to antigen
- Results when reexposure to antigen activates cellular reactions that trigger mast cell degranulation, which causes release of chemical mediators
- Activates the complement cascade
- Leads to contraction of smooth muscles, increased vascular permeability, and reduction of blood volume

ANAPHYLAXIS

● Definition
- Acute, potentially life-threatening type I (immediate) hypersensitivity reaction
- Marked by the sudden onset of rapidly progressive urticaria (vascular swelling in skin accompanied by itching) and respiratory distress
- If severe, may precipitate vasodilation, peripheral pooling, and relative hypovolemia leading to decreased tissue perfusion and impaired cellular metabolism, systemic shock and, sometimes, death
- Good prognosis with prompt recognition and treatment
- Typically occurs within minutes but can occur up to 1 hour after reexposure to the antigen

● Underlying pathophysiology
- Previous sensitization or exposure to the specific antigen results in IgE production by plasma cells in the lymph nodes and enhancement by helper T cells
- IgE antibodies then bind to membrane receptors on mast cells in connective tissue and to basophils
- On reexposure, the antigen binds to adjacent IgE antibodies or cross-linked IgE receptors, activating a series of cellular reactions that trigger mast cell degranulation
- With degranulation, powerful chemical mediators, such as histamine, eosinophil chemotactic factor of anaphylaxis, and platelet-activating factor, are released from the mast cells
- IgG or IgM enters into the reaction and activates the complement cascade, leading to the release of the complement fractions
- At the same time, two other chemical mediators, bradykinin and leukotrienes, induce vascular collapse by stimulating contraction of smooth muscles and increasing vascular permeability
- Vasodilation, smooth muscle contraction, enhanced vascular permeability, and increased mucus production occurs
- Continued release, along with the spread of these mediators through the body by way of the basophils in the intravascular circulation, triggers the systemic responses
- Increased vascular permeability leads to decreased peripheral resistance and plasma leakage from the intravascular circulation to the extravascular tissues
- Consequent reduction of blood volume causes hypotension, hypovolemic shock, and cardiac dysfunction (see *Understanding anaphylaxis*, pages 260 and 261)

● Causes
- Ingestion of or systemic exposure to sensitizing drugs or other substances
  - Allergen extracts
  - Diagnostic chemicals, such as sulfobromophthalein sodium, sodium dehydrocholate, and radiographic contrast media
  - Enzymes such as L-asparaginase
  - Food additives containing sulfite
  - Food proteins, such as those in legumes, nuts, berries, seafood, and egg albumin
  - Hormones

- Insect venom
- Local anesthetics
- Penicillin or other antibiotics
  - Induce anaphylaxis in 1 to 4 of every 10,000 patients treated
  - Most likely occurs after parenteral administration or prolonged therapy or in patients with an inherited tendency to food or drug allergy
- Polysaccharides
- Salicylates
- Serums (usually horse serum)
- Snakebite venom
- Sulfonamides
- Vaccines
- Idiopathic (cause unknown)

Pathophysiologic changes
- Feeling of impending doom or fright due to activation of IgE and subsequent release of chemical mediators
- Sweating, sneezing, shortness of breath, nasal pruritus, urticaria, and angioedema (swelling of nerves and blood vessels) due to histamine release
- Hypotension, shock, and sometimes cardiac arrhythmias due to increased vascular permeability and subsequent decrease in peripheral resistance and leakage of plasma fluids
- Nasal mucosal edema, profuse watery rhinorrhea, itching, nasal congestion, and sudden sneezing attacks due to histamine release, vasodilation, and increased capillary permeability
- Edema of the upper respiratory tract, resulting in hypopharyngeal and laryngeal obstruction, due to increased capillary permeability and mast cell degranulation
- Hoarseness, stridor, wheezing, and accessory muscle use secondary to bronchiole smooth muscle contraction and increased mucus production
- Severe stomach cramps, nausea, diarrhea, and urinary urgency and incontinence resulting from smooth muscle contraction of the intestines and bladder

Complications
- Respiratory obstruction
- Systemic vascular collapse
- Death

Diagnostic test findings
- None identifies anaphylaxis
- Diagnosis is determined by the rapid onset of severe respiratory or cardiovascular symptoms after exposure to a trigger
- Diagnostic tests may provide some clues to the patient's risk of anaphylaxis
  - Skin tests may show hypersensitivity to a specific allergen
  - Serum IgE levels may be elevated

Treatment
- Immediate administration of epinephrine 1:1,000 aqueous solution to reverse bronchoconstriction and cause vasoconstriction
  - Given I.M. or subcutaneously (subQ) if the patient hasn't lost consciousness and is normotensive

(Text continues on page 262.)

Key pathophysiologic changes in anaphylaxis
- Urticaria
- Angioedema
- Rhinorrhea
- Itching
- Sneezing
- Wheezing

Key treatments for anaphylaxis
- Epinephrine
- CPR (if cardiac arrest occurs)
- Tracheostomy or ET intubation
- Oxygen therapy

TOP 3

Chemical mediators released in anaphylaxis

1. Histamine
2. Serotonin
3. Leukotrienes

Understanding anaphylaxis

An anaphylactic reaction requires previous sensitization or exposure to the specific antigen. Here's what happens next.

1. RESPONSE TO THE ANTIGEN

Immunoglobulin (Ig) M and IgG recognize the antigen as a foreign substance and attach to it.

Destruction of the antigen by the complement cascade begins but remains unfinished, either because of insufficient amounts of the protein catalyst or because the antigen inhibits certain complement enzymes. The patient has no signs and symptoms at this stage.

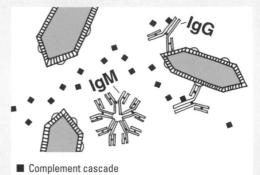

■ Complement cascade

2. RELEASED CHEMICAL MEDIATORS

The antigen's continued presence activates IgE on basophils. The activated IgE promotes the release of mediators, including histamine, serotonin, and leukotrienes. The sudden release of histamine causes vasodilation and increases capillary permeability. The patient begins to have signs and symptoms, including sudden nasal congestion, itchy and watery eyes, flushing, sweating, weakness, and anxiety.

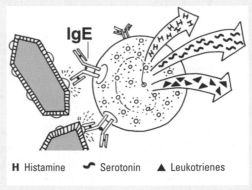

H Histamine   Serotonin   ▲ Leukotrienes

3. INTENSIFIED RESPONSE

The activated IgE also stimulates mast cells in connective tissue along the venule walls to release more histamine and eosinophil chemotactic factor of anaphylaxis (ECF-A). These substances produce disruptive lesions that weaken the venules. Now, red and itchy skin, wheals, and swelling appear, and signs and symptoms worsen.

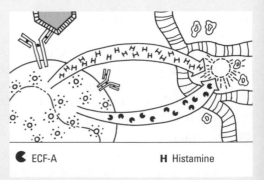

ECF-A   **H** Histamine

4. DISTRESS

In the lungs, histamine causes endothelial cells to burst and endothelial tissue to tear away from surrounding tissue. Fluids leak into the alveoli, and leukotrienes prevent the alveoli from expanding, thus reducing pulmonary compliance. Tachypnea, crowing, accessory muscle use, and cyanosis signal respiratory distress. Resulting neurologic signs and symptoms include changes in level of consciousness, severe anxiety and, possibly, seizures.

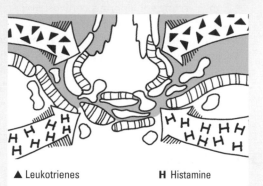

▲ Leukotrienes   H Histamine

5. DETERIORATION

Meanwhile, basophils and mast cells begin to release prostaglandins and bradykinin along with histamine and serotonin. These substances increase vascular permeability, causing fluids to leak from the vessels. Shock, confusion, cool and pale skin, generalized edema, tachycardia, and hypotension signal rapid vascular collapse.

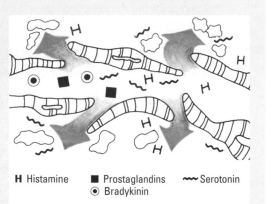

H Histamine   ■ Prostaglandins   ∿ Serotonin
                ◉ Bradykinin

6. FAILED COMPENSATORY MECHANISMS

Damage to the endothelial cells causes basophils and mast cells to release heparin. Additional substances are also released to neutralize the other mediators. Eosinophils release arylsulfatase B to neutralize the leukotrienes, phospholipase D to neutralize heparin, and cyclic adenosine monophosphate and the prostaglandins E_1 and E_2 to increase the metabolic rate. However, these events can't reverse anaphylaxis. Hemorrhage, disseminated intravascular coagulation, and cardiopulmonary arrest result.

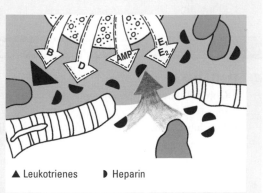

▲ Leukotrienes   ▶ Heparin

Key nursing considerations for anaphylaxis

- Teach patient to avoid exposure to known allergens.
- Instruct patient to wear a medical identification bracelet.

– Given I.V. if the reaction is severe (repeating dosage every 5 to 20 minutes as needed)
- Tracheostomy or endotracheal (ET) intubation and mechanical ventilation to maintain a patent airway
- Oxygen therapy to increase tissue perfusion
- Longer-acting epinephrine, corticosteroids, and diphenhydramine (Benadryl) to reduce the allergic response
- Albuterol (Proventil) mini-nebulizer treatment
- Cimetidine (Tagamet) or other histamine-2 (H_2) receptor antagonists
- Aminophylline to reverse bronchospasm
- Volume expanders to maintain and restore circulating plasma volume
- I.V. vasopressors such as norepinephrine (Levophed) and dopamine (Intropin) to stabilize blood pressure
- Cardiopulmonary resuscitation (CPR) to treat cardiac arrest

● **Nursing considerations**
- Perform measures to prevent anaphylaxis
  - Teach the patient to avoid exposure to known allergens
    - A person allergic to certain foods or drugs must learn to avoid the offending food or drug in all its forms
    - A person allergic to insect stings should avoid open fields and wooded areas during the insect season and carry an Epi-Pen (epinephrine), a spring-activated needle delivering a single dose of 0.3 mg of epinephrine
  - Instruct every patient prone to anaphylaxis to wear a medical identification bracelet identifying his allergies
- If a patient must receive a drug to which he's allergic, prevent a severe reaction by making sure that he receives careful desensitization with gradually increasing doses of the antigen or advance administration of steroids
- A patient with a known allergic history should receive a drug with a high anaphylactic potential only after cautious pretesting for sensitivity
  - Closely monitor the patient during testing
  - Make sure that you have resuscitative equipment and epinephrine ready
- Closely monitor a patient undergoing diagnostic tests that use radiographic contrast media, such as excretory urography, cardiac catheterization, and angiography

ATOPIC DERMATITIS

Key facts about atopic dermatitis

- Characterized by superficial skin inflammation and intense itching
- Typically begins during infancy or early childhood
- Develops when allergic reaction releases inflammatory mediators
- Leads to lesions because of dry skin and decreased threshold for itching

● **Definition**
- Chronic skin disorder characterized by superficial skin inflammation and intense itching
- Typically begins during infancy or early childhood, but may occur at any age
- Most common cause of eczema in children
- May subside spontaneously, followed by exacerbations in late childhood, adolescence, or early adulthood
- Presentation varies
  - In children, appears as a rash primarily on the head, trunk, and extensor surfaces of arms and legs in children
  - In older children and adults, appears as a rash generally found on neck, antecubital and popliteal fossae, hands, and feet

- Involves a personal or family history of asthma or allergic rhinitis in 75% to 80% of affected individuals

Underlying pathophysiology
- The allergic mechanism of hypersensitivity results in a release of inflammatory mediators through sensitized IgE antibodies
- Histamine and other cytokines induce acute inflammation
- Abnormally dry skin and a decreased threshold for itching setup the "itch, scratch, itch" cycle, eventually causing lesions (excoriations, lichenification)

Causes
- Unknown; a genetic predisposition is likely
- Possible contributing factors
    - Chemical irritants
    - Extremes of temperature and humidity
    - Food allergy
    - Infection
    - Psychological stress or strong emotions

Pathophysiologic changes
- Erythematous, weeping lesions caused by vasoconstriction
- Scaly and lichenified lesions located in areas of flexion and extension, such as the neck, antecubital fossa, popliteal folds, and behind the ears, resulting from intense pruritus
- Pink pigmentation and swelling of the upper eyelid and a double fold under the lower lid (Morgan's line or Dennie's sign) in children with atopic dermatitis due to severe pruritus

Complications
- Allergic contact dermatitis
- Bacterial and fungal skin infections
- Ocular disorders
- Scarring
- Severe viral infections

Diagnostic test findings
- History of atopy (hereditary allergy), such as asthma, hay fever, or urticaria
- Complete blood count (CBC) shows increased number of eosinophils
- Serum IgE levels are elevated

Treatment
- Frequent application of nonirritating topical lubricants, especially after bathing or showering, to prevent dry skin, which aggravates itching
- Avoidance of hot tubs to prevent excessive drying of the skin
- Minimizing exposure to allergens and irritants, such as wools and harsh detergents
- Drug therapy depending on disorder's severity and location
    - Topical corticosteroids, such as fluocinolone acetonide (Synalar) and flurandrenolide (Cordran), applied immediately after bathing (for optimal penetration) to treat active dermatitis
    - Topical immunomodulators, such as pimecrolimus (Elidel) and tacrolimus (Protopic) for nonsteroidal treatment of itching and rash

---

Key pathophysiologic changes in atopic dermatitis
- Erythematous, weeping lesions
- Scaly and lichenified lesions
- Morgan's line or Dennie's sign

Key diagnostic test results for atopic dermatitis
- History of hereditary allergy
- Serum IgE level: Elevated

Key treatments for atopic dermatitis
- Topical lubricants
- Topical corticosteroids
- Antihistamines

Key nursing considerations for atopic dermatitis

- Teach patient when and how to apply topical corticosteroids.
- Be alert for signs and symptoms of secondary infection.
- Discourage use of laundry additives.
- Dissuade patient from scratching.

    – Oral antihistamines, especially hydroxyzine (Atarax) and the phenothiazine derivatives, such as methdilazine (Tacaryl) and trimeprazine (Temaril), to help control itching
      • Bedtime dose may reduce involuntary scratching during sleep
    – Antibiotics if secondary infection develops
    – Possible use of phototherapy (ultraviolet light), systemic oral steroids, or coal tar preparations for severe or refractory eczema
- Counseling to help the patient and his caregiver cope with the frustrations of the disorder

Nursing considerations

- Monitor the patient's compliance with drug therapy
- Teach the patient when and how to apply topical corticosteroids
- Emphasize the importance of regular personal hygiene using only lukewarm water with a small amount of a mild, bar soap
- For prevention, use moisturizing creams or ointments with little water content instead of standard lotions
- Be alert for signs and symptoms of secondary infection, and teach the patient how to recognize them as well
- If the patient's diet is modified to exclude food allergens, monitor his nutritional status
- Offer support to help the patient and his family cope with this chronic disorder
- Discourage use of laundry additives, such as fragrances and dyes
- Dissuade the patient from scratching urticaria to help prevent secondary infection

LATEX ALLERGY

Definition

- Type I, IgE-mediated hypersensitivity reaction or type IV cell-mediated response to products that contain natural rubber latex (see *Commonly used sources of latex*)
- Can range from local dermatitis to life-threatening anaphylactic reaction

Underlying pathophysiology

- Type I reaction
    – Mast cells release histamine and other secretory products
    – Vascular permeability increases and vasodilation and bronchoconstriction occur
- Type IV reaction
    – Latex allergy resulting in a type IV delayed hypersensitivity reaction involves chemical sensitivity dermatitis, in which the immune system reacts to the chemicals used in processing rather than the latex itself
    – In a cell-mediated allergic reaction, sensitized T lymphocytes are triggered, stimulating the proliferation of other lymphocytes and mononuclear cells
    – Proliferation of lymphocytes and mononuclear cells results in tissue inflammation and contact dermatitis

Key facts about latex allergy

- Involves type I or type IV hypersensitivity reaction to natural rubber latex
- Causes vasodilation and bronchoconstriction (type I reaction) or tissue inflammation and contact dermatitis (type IV reaction)

Commonly used sources of latex

Many household items and medical supplies contain latex. Use this list to identify common sources of latex to which a patient with a latex allergy may be exposed.

HOUSEHOLD SOURCES
- Buttons on electronic equipment
- Carpet backing
- Clothing, including elastic on underwear
- Computer mouse pads
- Condoms and diaphragms
- Diapers and sanitary and incontinence pads
- Erasers
- Food handled with powdered latex gloves
- Handles on racquets or tools
- Infant feeding nipples and pacifiers
- Non-mylar balloons
- Rubber bands
- Shoe soles
- Sports equipment
- Toys

MEDICAL SOURCES
- Adhesive tape
- Manual resuscitation valve masks
- Bandages
- Bulb syringes
- Dental devices
- Electrode pads
- Facemasks
- Injection ports
- Mattresses on stretchers
- Nonvinyl gloves
- Patient-controlled anesthesia syringes
- Rubber syringe stoppers and medication vial stoppers
- Stethoscope and blood pressure cuff tubing
- Tourniquets
- Urinary catheters
- Wound drains

Causes
- Direct exposure to latex proteins found in natural rubber products
- Exposure to latex particles that are protein bound to other particles (such as the cornstarch from latex, which disperses as gloves are removed)

Pathophysiologic changes
- Hypotension due to vasodilation and increased vascular permeability
- Tachycardia secondary to hypotension
- Urticaria and pruritus due to histamine release
- Difficulty breathing, bronchospasm, wheezing, and stridor secondary to bronchoconstriction
- Angioedema from increased vascular permeability and loss of water to tissues

Complications
- Respiratory obstruction
- Systemic vascular collapse
- Death

Diagnostic test findings
- Diagnosis of latex allergy is based mainly on history and physical assessment
- Radioallergosorbent test shows IgE antibodies specific to latex (safest for use in patients with history of type I hypersensitivity)
- Patch test causes hives along with itching or redness

Key pathophysiologic changes in latex allergy
- Urticaria
- Pruritus
- Wheezing
- Angioedema

Key diagnostic test results for latex allergy
- Radioallergosorbent test: Presence of IgE antibodies specific to latex
- Patch test: Hives accompanied by itching or redness

Key treatments for latex allergy

- Corticosteroids
- Antihistamines
- H_2-receptor antagonists
- Prevention of exposure
- In emergency, epinephrine and airway maintenance

Key nursing considerations for latex allergy

- Make sure items that aren't available latex-free are wrapped in cloth before contact with patient's skin.
- Use powder-free and vinyl gloves.
- Place patient in private room.
- When adding medication to an I.V. bag, inject the drug through the spike port.

In acute emergency

- Immediately administer epinephrine 1:1,000 aqueous solution
- Assist with tracheostomy or ET intubation and mechanical ventilation

● **Treatment**
- Prevention of exposure
  - Use of latex-free products
  - Avoidance of airborne particles to decrease possible exacerbation of hypersensitivity
- Drug therapy, such as corticosteroids, antihistamines, and H_2-receptor antagonists before and after possible exposure to latex, to depress immune response and block histamine release
- If the patient is experiencing an acute emergency
  - Immediately administer epinephrine 1:1,000 aqueous solution
    - Given I.M. or subQ if the patient hasn't lost consciousness and is normotensive
    - Given I.V. if the reaction is severe (repeating dosage every 5 to 20 minutes as needed)
  - Assist with tracheostomy or ET intubation and mechanical ventilation
  - Oxygen therapy to increase tissue perfusion
  - Volume expanders to maintain and restore circulating plasma volume
  - I.V. vasopressors, such as norepinephrine and dopamine, to stabilize blood pressure
  - CPR to treat cardiac arrest
  - Longer-acting epinephrine, corticosteroids, and diphenhydramine to reduce the allergic response (long-term management)
  - Drugs to reverse bronchospasm, including aminophylline and albuterol

● **Nursing considerations**
- Make sure items that aren't available latex-free, such as stethoscopes and blood pressure cuffs, are wrapped in cloth before they come in contact with a hypersensitive patient's skin
- Use powder-free and vinyl gloves
- Place the patient in a private room or with another patient who requires a latex-free environment
- When adding medication to an I.V. bag, inject the drug through the spike port, not the rubber latex port
- Urge the patient to wear an identification tag mentioning his latex allergy
- Teach the patient and his family how to use an epinephrine autoinjector
- Instruct the patient to consider avoiding tomatoes, bananas, avocados, chestnuts, and kiwifruits because they contain some proteins similar to those in rubber
- Teach the patient to be aware of all latex-containing products and to use vinyl or silicone products instead

LUPUS ERYTHEMATOSUS

● **Definition**
- Chronic inflammatory disorder of the connective tissues
- Appears in two forms
  - Discoid, or cutaneous, lupus erythematosus
    - Usually affects only the skin
    - May become systemic

Signs of systemic lupus erythematosus

Diagnosing systemic lupus erythematosus (SLE) is difficult because it commonly mimics other diseases; symptoms may be vague and vary greatly among patients.

For these reasons, the American Rheumatism Association issued a list of criteria for classifying SLE to be used primarily for consistency in epidemiologic surveys. Usually, four or more of these signs are present at some time during the course of the disease:

- malar or discoid rash
- photosensitivity
- oral or nasopharyngeal ulcerations
- nonerosive arthritis (of two or more peripheral joints)
- pleuritis or pericarditis
- profuse proteinuria (more than 0.5 g/day) or excessive cellular casts in the urine
- seizures or psychoses
- hemolytic anemia, leukopenia, lymphopenia, or thrombocytopenia
- anti–double-stranded deoxyribonucleic acid or positive findings of antiphospholipid antibodies (elevated immunoglobulin [Ig] G or IgM anti-cardiolipin antibodies, positive test result for lupus anticoagulant, or false-positive serologic test results for syphilis)
- abnormal antinuclear antibody titer.

- SLE
  - Affects multiple organ systems as well as the skin
  - Can be fatal
- Characterized by recurring exacerbations and remissions; exacerbations especially common during the spring and summer
- The onset of SLE may be acute or insidious and produces no characteristic clinical pattern (see *Signs of systemic lupus erythematosus*)
- Most common in women of childbearing age

Underlying pathophysiology
- Immune dysregulation occurs in the form of autoimmunity
- B-cell hyperactivity causes the body to produce antibodies against components of its own cells, such as the antinuclear antibody (ANA), and the immune complex disease follows
- Antigen-antibody complexes are produced against many different tissue components, such as RBCs, neutrophils, platelets, and lymphocytes, or almost any organ or body tissue, leading to widespread degeneration of connective tissue
- Possible cardiovascular, renal, or neurologic complications can result as well as severe bacterial infections

Causes
- Exact cause unknown
- Contributing factors
  - Abnormal estrogen metabolism
  - Exposure to sunlight or ultraviolet light
  - Genetic predisposition
  - Immunization
  - Physical or mental stress
  - Pregnancy

Key facts about lupus erythematosus
- Inflammatory disorder of connective tissues
- Discoid form: Affects skin only
- SLE: Affects multiple organ systems and skin
- Develops when B-cell hyperactivity causes the body to produce antibodies against its own cells

Factors contributing to lupus erythematosus
- Genetic predisposition
- Physical or mental stress
- Treatment with certain drugs
- Streptococcal or viral infections

- Streptococcal or viral infections
- Treatment with certain drugs, such as procainamide (Pronestyl), hydralazine (Apresoline), anticonvulsants and, less frequently, penicillins, sulfa drugs, and hormonal contraceptives

● Pathophysiologic changes

- Effects throughout all systems resulting from tissue injury, inflammation, and necrosis due to invasion of immune complexes
  - Cardiovascular changes, such as pericarditis, myocarditis, endocarditis, early coronary atherosclerosis, valvular complications, vasculitis (especially in digits) possibly leading to infarctive lesions, necrotic leg ulcers, or digital gangrene, and Raynaud's phenomenon
  - Constitutional changes, including fever, weight loss, malaise, and fatigue
  - Dermatologic changes, such as alopecia, photosensitivity, and malar (classic butterfly pattern, which occurs in less than 50% of patients) and discoid (scaly, papular; mimics psoriasis) rashes
  - Hematologic changes, such as hemolytic anemia, leukopenia, lymphopenia, and thrombocytopenia
  - Musculoskeletal changes, such as polyarthralgia, arthritis, avascular necrosis, and muscle weakness and atrophy
  - Neuropsychiatric changes, such as cognitive dysfunction, depression, psychosis, stroke, and seizures
  - Pulmonary changes, such as pleuritis, pneumonitis, and pulmonary hypertension
  - Renal changes, such as nephritis, glomerulonephritis, microscopic hematuria, pyuria, and urine sediment with cellular casts

● Complications

- Concomitant infections
- Osteonecrosis of the hip from long-term steroid use
- Renal failure
- Urinary tract infections

● Diagnostic test findings

- CBC with differential possibly showing anemia and a decreased white blood cell (WBC) count
- Platelet count may be decreased
- Erythrocyte sedimentation rate (ESR) is elevated
- Serum electrophoresis may show hypergammaglobulinemia
- ANA and lupus erythematosus cell tests are positive in active SLE
- Anti–double-stranded DNA antibody (anti-ds-DNA) is the most specific test for SLE
  - It correlates with disease activity, especially renal involvement
  - It helps monitor response to therapy
  - May be low or absent in remission
- Urine studies show RBCs and WBCs, urine casts and sediment, and significant protein loss (more than 0.5 g/24 hours)
- Serum complement blood studies show decreased serum complement (C3 and C4), indicating active disease
- Chest X-ray shows pleurisy or lupus pneumonitis
- Electrocardiogram (ECG) shows a conduction defect with cardiac involvement or pericarditis

- Kidney biopsy determines the disease stage and extent of renal involvement
- Lupus anticoagulant and anticardiolipin tests are positive in some patients (usually in patients prone to antiphospholipid syndrome of thrombosis, abortion, and thrombocytopenia)

● **Treatment**
  - Palliative care (no cure available)
  - Nonsteroidal anti-inflammatory drugs (NSAIDs), including aspirin, to control arthritis symptoms
  - Topical corticosteroid creams, such as hydrocortisone buteprate (Acticort) or triamcinolone (Aristocort), for acute skin lesions
  - Intralesional corticosteroids or antimalarials, such as hydroxychloroquine sulfate (Plaquenil), to treat refractory skin lesions
  - Systemic corticosteroids to reduce systemic symptoms of SLE, for acute generalized exacerbations, or for serious disease related to vital organ systems, such as pleuritis, pericarditis, lupus nephritis, vasculitis, and central nervous system involvement
  - High-dose steroids and cytotoxic therapy, such as cyclophosphamide (Cytoxan), to treat diffuse proliferative glomerulonephritis
  - Dialysis or kidney transplant for renal failure
  - Antihypertensive drugs and dietary changes to minimize the effects of renal involvement

● **Nursing considerations**
  - Watch for constitutional symptoms (joint pain or stiffness, weakness, fever, fatigue, and chills)
  - Observe for dyspnea, chest pain, and edema of the extremities
  - Note the size, type, and location of skin lesions
  - Check urine for hematuria, scalp for hair loss, and skin and mucous membranes for petechiae, bleeding, ulceration, pallor, and bruising
  - Provide a balanced diet
    – Renal involvement may mandate a low-sodium, low-protein diet
  - Urge the patient to get plenty of rest and schedule diagnostic tests and procedures to allow adequate rest
  - Explain all tests and procedures
  - Apply heat packs to relieve joint pain and stiffness
  - Encourage regular exercise to maintain full range of motion (ROM) and prevent contractures
    – Teach ROM exercises as well as body alignment and postural techniques
    – Arrange for physical therapy and occupational counseling as appropriate
  - Administer prescribed medications
    – Explain their expected benefits
    – Watch for adverse effects, especially when the patient is taking high doses of corticosteroids
    – Advise the patient receiving cyclophosphamide to maintain adequate hydration
    – Give mesna (Mesnex) to prevent hemorrhagic cystitis and ondansetron (Zofran) to prevent nausea and vomiting, as prescribed
  - Monitor the patient's vital signs, intake and output, weight, and laboratory reports
    – Check pulse rate and observe for orthopnea

Key treatments for lupus erythematosus

- NSAIDs
- Corticosteroids, topical and systemic
- Symptom-specific medications, such as antihypertensives and cytotoxins

Key nursing considerations for lupus erythematosus

- Assess patient for renal involvement.
- Monitor for neurologic damage.
- Monitor vital signs and fluid status.
- Watch for adverse effects of drugs, especially corticosteroids.
- Provide adequate rest periods.

– Check stools and GI secretions for blood
- Monitor the patient for hypertension, weight gain, and other signs of renal involvement
- Assess for signs of neurologic damage, such as personality change, paranoid or psychotic behavior, ptosis, or diplopia
  – Take seizure precautions
  – If Raynaud's phenomenon is present, warm and protect the patient's hands and feet
- Refer the patient to the Lupus Foundation of America and the Arthritis Foundation as necessary

RHEUMATOID ARTHRITIS

Definition
- Chronic, systemic inflammatory disease that primarily attacks peripheral joints and the surrounding muscles, tendons, ligaments, and blood vessels
- Characterized by partial remissions and unpredictable exacerbations
- Prevalence increases with age

Underlying pathophysiology
- If rheumatoid arthritis (RA) isn't arrested, the inflammatory process in the joints occurs in four stages
  – First stage
    · Synovitis develops from congestion and edema of the synovial membrane and joint capsule
    · Infiltration by lymphocytes, macrophages, and neutrophils continues the local inflammatory response
    · These cells, as well as fibroblast-like synovial cells, produce enzymes that help to degrade bone and cartilage
  – Second stage
    · Pannus (thickened layers of granulation tissue) covers and invades cartilage
    · Eventually pannus destroys the joint capsule and bone
  – Third stage
    · Fibrous ankylosis (fibrous invasion of the pannus and scar formation) occludes the joint space
    · Bone atrophy and misalignment causing visible deformities and disrupting the articulation of opposing bones results in muscle atrophy and imbalance and, possibly, partial dislocations (subluxations)
  – Fourth stage
    · Fibrous tissue calcifies
    · Bony ankylosis and total immobility results

Causes
- Unknown
- Theories
  – Abnormal immune activation in a genetically susceptible individual leading to inflammation, complement activation, and cell proliferation within joints and tendon sheaths
  – Infection (viral, such as Epstein-Barr, or bacterial), hormone action, or lifestyle factors influencing onset

Key facts about rheumatoid arthritis
- Systemic inflammatory disease
- Affects peripheral joints and surrounding muscles, tendons, ligaments, and blood vessels

Stages of rheumatoid arthritis
- First stage – synovitis develops
- Second stage – pannus invades cartilage
- Third stage – fibrous ankylosis occludes joint
- Fourth stage – fibrous tissue calcifies

– Development of an IgM antibody against the body's own IgG (also called *rheumatoid factor [RF]*), which aggregates into complexes and generates inflammation, causing eventual cartilage damage and triggering other immune responses

● **Pathophysiologic changes**

- Fatigue, malaise, anorexia and weight loss, persistent low-grade fever, lymphadenopathy, and vague articular symptoms resulting from initial inflammatory reactions before the inflammation of the synovium
- Specific localized, bilateral, and symmetric articular symptoms, commonly in the fingers at the proximal interphalangeal, metacarpophalangeal, and metatarsophalangeal joints, possibly extending to the wrists, knees, elbows, and ankles and stiffening of affected joints after inactivity from inflammation and destruction of the synovium
- Spindle-shaped fingers from marked edema and congestion in the joints
- Joint pain and tenderness, at first only with movement but eventually even at rest, due to prostaglandin release, edema, and synovial inflammation and destruction
- Feeling of warmth at joint from inflammation
- Diminished joint function and deformities as synovial destruction continues
- Flexion deformities or hyperextension of metacarpophalangeal joints, subluxation of the wrist, and stretching of tendons pulling the fingers to the ulnar side (ulnar drift), or characteristic swan-neck or boutonnière deformity caused by joint swelling and loss of joint space
- Carpal tunnel syndrome resulting from synovial pressure on the median nerve causing paresthesia in the fingers
- Gradual appearance of rheumatoid nodules (subcutaneous, round or oval, nontender masses), usually on the elbows, hands, or Achilles tendon resulting from destruction of the synovium
- Vasculitis, possibly leading to skin lesions, leg ulcers, and multiple systemic complications due to infiltration of immune complexes and subsequent tissue damage and necrosis in the vasculature
- Pericarditis, pulmonary nodules or fibrosis, pleuritis, or inflammation of the sclera and overlying tissues of the eye resulting from immune complex invasion and subsequent tissue damage and necrosis
- Peripheral neuropathy with numbness or tingling in the feet, or weakness and loss of sensation in the fingers resulting from infiltration of the nerve fibers
- Stiff, weak, or painful muscles secondary to limited mobility and decreased use

● **Complications**

- Fibrosis and ankylosis
- Soft tissue contractures
- Pain
- Joint deformities
- Sjögren's syndrome
- Destruction of second cervical vertebra
- Spinal cord compression
- Temporomandibular joint disease
- Infection
- Osteoporosis

Key pathophysiologic changes in rheumatoid arthritis

- Persistent low-grade fever
- Joint pain and tenderness
- Feeling of warmth at joints
- Gradual appearance of rheumatoid nodules
- Diminished joint function and deformities
- Bilateral and symmetrical symptoms

Common complications of rheumatoid arthritis

- Pain
- Joint deformities
- Fibrosis and ankylosis

Key diagnostic test results for rheumatoid arthritis

- X-ray: Bone demineralization and soft-tissue swelling (early stages); cartilage loss, narrowed joint spaces, cartilage and bone destruction and erosion, subluxations, and deformities (later stages)
- RF titer: Positive (1:160 or higher) in 75% to 80% of patients
- ESR and C-reactive protein: Elevated in 85% to 90% of patients

Key treatments for rheumatoid arthritis

- Salicylates
- NSAIDs
- Corticosteroids
- Antimalarials
- Surgery

- Myositis (inflammation of voluntary muscles)
- Cardiopulmonary lesions
- Lymphadenopathy
- Peripheral neuritis
- Hip joint necrosis

Diagnostic test findings
- X-ray findings depend on disease stage
  - Bone demineralization and soft-tissue swelling appear in early stages
  - Cartilage loss, narrowed joint spaces, and cartilage and bone destruction and erosion, subluxations, and deformities appear in later stages
- RF titer is positive (1:160 or higher) in 75% to 80% of patients
- Synovial fluid analysis reveals increased volume and turbidity but decreased viscosity and elevated WBC count (usually greater than 10,000/µl)
- Serum protein electrophoresis detects elevated serum globulin level
- ESR and C-reactive protein levels show elevations in 85% to 90% of patients
  - It may be useful to monitor response to therapy because elevation frequently parallels disease activity
- CBC usually shows moderate anemia, slight leukocytosis, and slight thrombocytosis

Treatment
- Lifelong treatment and, sometimes, surgery
- Salicylates, particularly aspirin (mainstay of therapy) to decrease inflammation and relieve joint pain
- NSAIDs, such as fenoprofen (Nalfon), ibuprofen (Motrin), and indomethacin (Indocin), and the cyclooxygenase-2 (COX-2) inhibitors celecoxib (Celebrex) and valdecoxib (Bextra) to relieve inflammation and pain
- Antimalarials, such as hydroxychloroquine sulfate (Plaquenil), sulfasalazine (Azulfidine), gold salts, and penicillamine (Cuprimine), to reduce acute and chronic inflammation
- Corticosteroids such as prednisone
  - Used in low doses for anti-inflammatory effects
  - Used in higher doses for immunosuppressive effect on T cells
- Azathioprine (Imuran), cyclosporine (Neoral), and methotrexate (Folex) in early disease for immunosuppression by suppressing T- and B-lymphocyte proliferation, causing destruction of the synovium
- Synovectomy (removal of destructive, proliferating synovium, usually in the wrists, knees, and fingers) to possibly halt or delay the course of the disease
- Osteotomy (cutting of bone or excision of a wedge of bone) to realign joint surfaces and redistribute stress
- Tendon transfers to prevent deformities or relieve contractures
- Joint reconstruction or total joint arthroplasty
  - Metatarsal head and distal ulnar resectional arthroplasty
  - Insertion of a Silastic prosthesis between metacarpophalangeal and proximal interphalangeal joints (severe disease) (see *Preparing for joint replacement*)
- Arthrodesis (joint fusion) for stability and relief from pain (sacrifices joint mobility)

Nursing considerations
- Assess all joints carefully

Preparing for joint replacement

Your patient with rheumatoid arthritis may receive total or partial replacement of a joint with a synthetic prosthesis to restore stability and relieve pain. Joint replacement may also provide an increased sense of independence and self-worth.

PREPARING THE PATIENT FOR RECOVERY

Get the patient ready for the lengthy postoperative recovery and rehabilitation period. He'll probably remain in bed for up to 6 days after surgery. Explain that even while he's confined to bed, he'll begin an exercise program to maintain joint mobility. As appropriate, show him range-of-motion exercises or demonstrate the continuous passive motion device that he'll use during recovery.

Point out that he may not experience pain relief after surgery and that, in fact, pain may actually worsen for several weeks. Reassure him that pain will diminish dramatically when edema subsides. Emphasize that an analgesic will be available if he needs it.

PREPARING THE PATIENT FOR HOME CARE

Reinforce the exercise regimen prescribed by the health care provider and physical therapists. Remind the patient to adhere closely to his schedule and not to rush rehabilitation, no matter how good he feels.

Review prescribed limitations on activity. Depending on the location and extent of surgery, the health care provider may order the patient to avoid bending or lifting, extensive stair climbing, and sitting for prolonged periods (including long car trips or plane flights). He'll also caution against overusing the joint, especially if it's a weight-bearing one.

Caution the patient to promptly report signs and symptoms of possible infection, such as persistent fever and increased pain, tenderness, and stiffness in the joint and surrounding area. Remind him that infection may develop several months after joint replacement.

Tell the patient to report a sudden increase in pain, which may indicate dislodgment of the prosthesis.

Key home care tips after joint replacement
- Instruct patient to maintain exercise regimen prescribed by physical therapist.
- Review prescribed limitations on activity.
- Teach signs and symptoms of joint or incision infection.

- Look for deformities, contractures, immobility, and an inability to perform everyday activities
- Monitor the patient's vital signs, and note weight changes, sensory disturbances, and level of pain
- Administer analgesics, as ordered, and watch for adverse effects
- Provide meticulous skin care
  - Check for rheumatoid nodules as well as pressure ulcers and skin breakdown due to immobility, vascular impairment, corticosteroid treatment, or improper splinting
  - Use lotion or cleaning oil — not soap — for dry skin
- Explain all diagnostic tests and procedures
- Monitor the duration, not the intensity, of morning stiffness because duration more accurately reflects disease severity
- Encourage the patient to take hot showers or baths at bedtime or in the morning to reduce the need for pain medication
- Apply splints as ordered

Key nursing considerations for rheumatoid arthritis
- Assess all joints carefully.
- Administer analgesics.
- Urge patient to perform ADLs.
- Instruct patient to pace daily activities and schedule rest periods.

TOP 3

Ways to avoid joint stress

1. Use the largest joint available for a given task.
2. Slide (don't lift) objects whenever possible.
3. Always use hands toward the center of the body.

- Observe for pressure ulcers if the patient is in traction or wearing splints
- Explain the nature of the disease; RA is a chronic disease that requires major changes in lifestyle
- Encourage a balanced diet
  - Make sure that the patient understands that special diets won't cure RA
  - Stress the need for weight control because obesity adds more stress to joints
- Urge the patient to perform activities of daily living (ADLs), such as dressing and feeding himself
  - Give the patient easy-to-open cartons, lightweight cups, and unpackaged silverware
  - Allow the patient enough time to calmly perform tasks
- Provide emotional support
  - Encourage the patient to discuss his fears concerning dependency, sexuality, body image, and self-esteem
  - Refer the patient to an appropriate social service agency as needed
- Make sure that the patient knows how and when to take prescribed medication and how to recognize possible adverse effects
- Teach the patient how to stand, walk, and sit correctly
  - Tell the patient to sit in chairs with high seats and armrests; he'll find it easier to get up from a chair if his knees are lower than his hips
  - Suggest an elevated toilet seat
- Instruct the patient to pace daily activities
  - Tell him to rest for 5 to 10 minutes out of each hour
  - Advise him to alternate sitting and standing tasks
- Stress the importance of getting adequate sleep and using correct sleeping posture
  - The patient should sleep on his back on a firm mattress
  - He should avoid placing a pillow under his knees, which encourages flexion deformity
- Teach the patient ways to avoid putting undue stress on joints
  - Using the largest joint available for a given task
  - Avoiding positions of flexion and promoting positions of extension
  - Holding objects parallel to the knuckles as briefly as possible
  - Always using his hands toward the center of his body
  - Sliding (not lifting) objects whenever possible
  - Supporting weak or painful joints as much as possible
- Suggest using assistive devices to help with ADLs
  - Dressing aids, such as long-handled shoehorns, reachers, elastic shoelaces, zipper-pulls, and buttonhooks
  - Household items, such as easy-to-open drawers, a handheld shower nozzle, handrails, and grab bars
- Advise the patient who has trouble maneuvering fingers into gloves to wear mittens
- Tell the patient to dress while in a sitting position as often as possible
- Refer the patient to the Arthritis Foundation for more information on coping with the disease

URTICARIA AND ANGIOEDEMA

- **Definition**
  - Urticaria
    - Commonly known as *hives*
    - Is an episodic, usually self-limited skin reaction characterized by local dermal wheals (smooth elevated areas) surrounded by an erythematous flare
  - Angioedema
    - Subcutaneous and dermal eruption
    - Produces deeper, larger wheals (usually on the hands, feet, lips, genitals, and eyelids) and a more diffuse swelling of loose subcutaneous tissue
  - Can occur simultaneously, but angioedema may last longer
  - Are common allergic reactions that may occur in 20% of the general population

- **Underlying pathophysiology**
  - Several mechanisms and underlying disorders may provoke urticaria and angioedema; for example
    - IgE induces release of mediators from cutaneous mast cells
    - IgG or IgM bind to an antigen, resulting in complement activation
  - When urticaria and angioedema are part of an anaphylactic reaction, they almost always persist long after the systemic response has subsided
    - Circulation to the skin is the last to be restored after an allergic reaction
    - Histamine reabsorption at the reaction site is slow
  - Nonallergic urticaria and angioedema may also be related to histamine release by some still-unknown mechanism

- **Causes**
  - Allergy to drugs, foods, insect stings and, occasionally, inhalant allergens (such as animal dander and cosmetics) that provoke an IgE–mediated response to protein allergens (although certain drugs may cause urticaria without an IgE response)
  - External physical stimuli, such as cold (usually in young adults), heat, water, or sunlight

- **Pathophysiologic changes**
  - In urticaria, distinct, raised, evanescent dermal wheals surrounded by an erythematous flare that vary in size resulting from complement activation
  - In angioedema, nonpitted swelling of deep subcutaneous tissue resulting from complement activation
    - Usually develops on the eyelids, lips, genitalia, and mucous membranes
    - Don't itch but may burn and tingle

- **Complications**
  - Skin abrasion and secondary infection due to scratching
  - Life-threatening laryngeal edema, if angioedema involves the upper respiratory tract
  - Severe abdominal colic, with possible GI involvement that can lead to surgery

Key facts about urticaria and angioedema

- Can be part of an anaphylactic reaction

Urticaria
- Commonly known as *hives*
- Characterized by local dermal wheals surrounded by an erythematous flare

Angioedema
- Produces deeper, larger wheals

Key pathophysiologic changes in urticaria and angioedema

- Raised dermal wheals (urticaria)
- Nonpitted swelling of deep subcutaneous tissue (angioedema)

● **Diagnostic test findings**
- Skin testing, an elimination diet, and a food diary (recording time and amount of food eaten and circumstances) can pinpoint provoking allergens
- Decreased serum levels of complement 4 and complement 1 esterase inhibitors confirm the diagnosis

● **Treatment**
- Preventing or limiting contact with triggering factors
- If contact with triggers is unavoidable, desensitization, in which progressively larger doses of specific antigens (determined by skin testing) are injected intradermally, to relieve symptoms
- Hydroxyzine or another antihistamine to ease itching and swelling of urticaria
- Corticosteroid therapy in some patients

● **Nursing considerations**
- When the triggering stimulus has been removed, urticaria usually subsides in a few days
- Drug reactions may persist as long as the drug is in the bloodstream
- Inform patients receiving antihistamines of the possibility of drowsiness
- Inspect the skin for signs of secondary infection caused by scratching
- Instruct the patient to keep his fingernails short to avoid abrading the skin when scratching

VASCULITIS

● **Definition**
- Broad spectrum of disorders characterized by inflammation and necrosis of blood vessels
- Clinical effects depend on the vessels involved and reflect tissue ischemia caused by blood flow obstruction
- Can occur at any age, except for mucocutaneous lymph node syndrome, which occurs only during childhood
- May be a primary disorder or occur secondary to other disorders, such as RA or SLE

● **Underlying pathophysiology**
- Current theory holds that vasculitis is initiated by excessive circulating antigen, which triggers a type III hypersensitivity reaction, causing the formation of soluble antigen–antibody complexes
- These complexes can't be cleared effectively by the reticuloendothelial system, so they're deposited in blood vessel walls
- Increased vascular permeability associated with release of vasoactive amines by platelets and basophils exacerbates this process
- The deposited complexes activate the complement cascade, resulting in chemotaxis of neutrophils, which release lysosomal enzymes
- Lysosomal enzymes cause vessel damage and necrosis, which may precipitate thrombosis, occlusion, hemorrhage, and ischemia
- Another mechanism that may contribute to vascular damage is the cell-mediated (T-cell) immune response
  - Circulating antigen triggers lymphocytes to release soluble mediators, which attract macrophages

– The macrophages release intracellular enzymes, which cause vascular damage
– Macrophages can also transform into the epithelioid and multinucleated giant cells that typify granulomatous vasculitides
– Phagocytosis of immune complexes by macrophages enhances granuloma formation

Causes
• Associated with a history of serious infectious disease, such as hepatitis B or bacterial endocarditis, and high-dose antibiotic therapy

Pathophysiologic changes
• Changes depend on the blood vessels involved (see *Types of vasculitis*, pages 278 and 279)

Complications
• Renal, cardiac, and hepatic involvement that may be fatal if vasculitis is left untreated
• Renal failure, renal hypertension, and glomerulitis
• Fibrous scarring of the lung tissue
• Stroke
• GI bleeding

Diagnostic test findings
• Findings depend on the type of vasculitis (see *Types of vasculitis*, pages 278 and 279)

Treatment
• Primary vasculitis
  – Removal of offending antigen or discontinuation of anti-inflammatory or immunosuppressant drugs, if possible
  – Drug therapy with low-dose cyclophosphamide and daily corticosteroids
  – In rapidly fulminant vasculitis
    · Cyclophosphamide dosage may be increased daily for the first 2 to 3 days, followed by the regular dose
    · Prednisone given in divided doses for 7 to 10 days, with consolidation to a single morning dose by 2 to 3 weeks
    · When the vasculitis appears to be in remission or when prescribed cytotoxic drugs take full effect, tapering of corticosteroids down to a single daily dose
    · Alternate-day schedule of steroids may continue for 3 to 6 months before slow discontinuation of steroids
• Secondary vasculitis
  – Treatment of the underlying disorder

Nursing considerations
• Assess patients with Wegener's granulomatosis for dry nasal mucosa
  – Instill nose drops to lubricate the mucosa and help diminish crusting
  – Irrigate the nasal passages with warm normal saline solution
• Monitor the patient's vital signs
  – Use a Doppler ultrasonic flowmeter, if available, to auscultate blood pressure in patients with Takayasu's arteritis, whose peripheral pulses are generally difficult to palpate

(Text continues on page 280.)

Common complications of vasculitis
• Renal failure
• Stroke
• Lung fibrosis

Key treatments for vasculitis

Primary
• Removal of offending antigen
• Low-dose cyclophosphamide
• Corticosteroids

Secondary vasculitis
• Treatment of underlying disorder

Types of vasculitis

TYPE	VESSELS INVOLVED
Polyarteritis nodosa	Small to medium arteries throughout the body, with lesions that tend to be segmental, occur at bifurcations and branchings of arteries, spread distally to arterioles and, in severe cases, circumferentially involve adjacent veins
Allergic granulomatosus angiitis (Churg-Strauss syndrome)	Small to medium arteries (including arterioles, capillaries, and venules), mainly of the lungs but also other organs
Polyangiitis overlap syndrome	Small to medium arteries (including arterioles, capillaries, and venules) of the lungs and other organs
Wegener's granulomatosis	Small to medium vessels of the respiratory tract and kidney
Temporal arteritis	Medium to large arteries, most commonly branches of the carotid artery
Takayasu's arteritis (aortic arch syndrome)	Medium to large arteries, particularly the aortic arch, its branches and, possibly, the pulmonary artery
Hypersensitivity vasculitis	Small vessels, especially of the skin
Mucocutaneous lymph node syndrome (Kawasaki disease)	Small to medium vessels, primarily of the lymph nodes; may progress to involve coronary arteries
Behçet's syndrome	Small vessels, primarily of the mouth and genitalia but also of the eyes, skin, joints, GI tract, and central nervous system

SIGNS AND SYMPTOMS	DIAGNOSIS
Hypertension, abdominal pain, myalgia, headache, joint pain, and weakness	History of symptoms; elevated erythrocyte sedimentation rate (ESR); leukocytosis; anemia; thrombocytosis; depressed C3 complement; rheumatoid factor more than 1:60; circulating immune complexes; tissue biopsy showing necrotizing vasculitis
Resemblance to polyarteritis nodosa with hallmark of severe pulmonary involvement	History of asthma; eosinophilia; tissue biopsy showing granulomatous inflammation with eosinophilic infiltration
Combined symptoms of polyarteritis nodosa, allergic angiitis, and granulomatosis	Possible history of allergy; eosinophilia; tissue biopsy showing granulomatous inflammation with eosinophilic infiltration
Fever, pulmonary congestion, cough, malaise, anorexia, weight loss, and mild to severe hematuria	Tissue biopsy showing necrotizing vasculitis with granulomatous inflammation; leukocytosis; elevated ESR and immunoglobulin A (IgA) and IgG levels; low titer rheumatoid factor; circulating immune complexes; antineutrophil cytoplasmic antibody in more than 90% of patients
Fever, myalgia, jaw claudication, vision changes, and headache (associated with polymyalgia rheumatica syndrome)	Decreased hemoglobin level; elevated ESR; tissue biopsy showing panarteritis with infiltration of mononuclear cells, giant cells within vessel wall, fragmentation of internal elastic lamina, and proliferation of intima
Malaise, pallor, nausea, night sweats, arthralgia, anorexia, weight loss, pain or paresthesia distal to affected area, bruits, loss of distal pulses, syncope and, if a carotid artery is involved, diplopia and transient blindness; may progress to heart failure or stroke	Decreased hemoglobin level; leukocytosis; positive lupus erythematosus cell preparation and elevated ESR; arteriography showing calcification and obstruction of affected vessels; tissue biopsy showing inflammation of adventitia and intima of vessels, and thickening of vessel walls
Palpable purpura, papules, nodules, vesicles, bullae, ulcers, or chronic or recurrent urticaria	History of exposure to antigen, such as a microorganism or drug; tissue biopsy showing leukocytoclastic angiitis, usually in postcapillary venules, with infiltration of polymorphonuclear leukocytes, fibrinoid necrosis, and extravasation of erythrocytes
Fever; nonsuppurative cervical adenitis; edema; congested conjunctivae; erythema of oral cavity, lips, and palms; and desquamation of fingertips; may progress to arthritis, myocarditis, pericarditis, myocardial infarction, and cardiomegaly	History of symptoms; elevated ESR; tissue biopsy showing intimal proliferation and infiltration of vessel walls with mononuclear cells; echocardiography necessary
Recurrent oral ulcers, eye lesions, genital lesions, and cutaneous lesions	History of symptoms

Key diagnostic test findings for vasculitis

- Tissue biopsy: Confirmation of type of vasculitis
- ESR: Increased in 50% of types
- Blood studies: Elevated WBC count, decreased hemoglobin level, positive rheumatoid factor

Key nursing considerations for vasculitis

- Monitor vital signs and intake and output.
- Monitor patient's WBC count during cyclophosphamide therapy.

TOP 5

Items to study for your next test on the immune system

1. Types of hypersensitivity
2. Common immune system disorders, such as rheumatoid arthritis, allergic rhinitis, and latex allergy
3. Drug therapy for anaphylaxis
4. Diagnostic tests for immune system disorders, such as skin testing, serum IgE, ANA, and RF titer
5. Pathophysiology of AIDS and HIV

- Monitor intake and output
  - Check daily for edema
  - Keep the patient well hydrated (3 qt [3 L] daily) to reduce the risk of hemorrhagic cystitis associated with cyclophosphamide therapy
- Provide emotional support to help the patient and his family cope with an altered body image
- Teach the patient how to recognize drug adverse effects
- Monitor the patient's WBC count during cyclophosphamide therapy to prevent severe leukopenia

NCLEX CHECKS

It's never too soon to begin your licensure examination preparation. Now that you've reviewed this chapter, carefully read each of the following questions and choose the best answer. Then compare your responses to the correct answers.

1. Which type of hypersensitivity involves the release of lymphokine by sensitized T cells?
- ☐ **1.** Type I
- ☐ **2.** Type II
- ☐ **3.** Type III
- ☐ **4.** Type IV

2. A patient is hospitalized to undergo surgery for a herniated disk. The nursing documentation reads as follows:

1/15/05	0915	Received Dilaudid 2 mg I.M. Ⓛ ventrogluteus for
		abdominal incision pain. Tolerated well. ———
		————————————— Pat Sloan, RN
	0940	c/o intense itching "everywhere." Diaphoretic, SOB,
		skin blotchy, and upper anterior torso and face
		covered with hives. Injection site has 4 cm red,
		raised area. BP 90/50, P 140, RR 44 in semi-
		Fowler's position. I.V. of D_5 1/2 NSS infusing at
		125 ml/hour in Ⓛ hand. O_2 sat. 94% via pulse
		oximetry on room air. ——— Pat Sloan, RN

What would the nurse's first action be?
- ☐ **1.** Obtain a stat ECG.
- ☐ **2.** Administer nasal oxygen at 2 L/minute.
- ☐ **3.** Increase the I.V. rate to 500 ml/hour.
- ☐ **4.** Place the patient in Trendelenburg's position.

3. The diagnostic test that's most specific for SLE is:
- ☐ **1.** C-reactive protein.
- ☐ **2.** anti-ds-DNA.
- ☐ **3.** serum electrophoresis.
- ☐ **4.** ANA.

4. Allergic rhinitis is a reaction to what kind of allergens?
- ☐ **1.** Food
- ☐ **2.** Drug
- ☐ **3.** Airborne
- ☐ **4.** Chemical

Heart failure

Heart failure occurs when the heart can't pump enough blood to meet the metabolic needs of the body. It may be classified according to the side of the heart affected.

RIGHT-SIDED HEART FAILURE

Ineffective right ventricular contractility
↓
Failure of right ventricular pumping ability
↓
Decreased cardiac output to lungs
↓
Blood backup into right atrium and peripheral circulation
↓
Weight gain, peripheral edema, and engorgement of kidneys and other organs

LEFT-SIDED HEART FAILURE

Ineffective left ventricular contractility
↓
Failure of left ventricular pumping ability
↓
Decreased cardiac output to body
↓
Blood backup into left atrium and lungs
↓
Pulmonary congestion, dyspnea, and activity intolerance
↓
Pulmonary edema and right-sided heart failure

NORMAL CARDIAC CIRCULATION

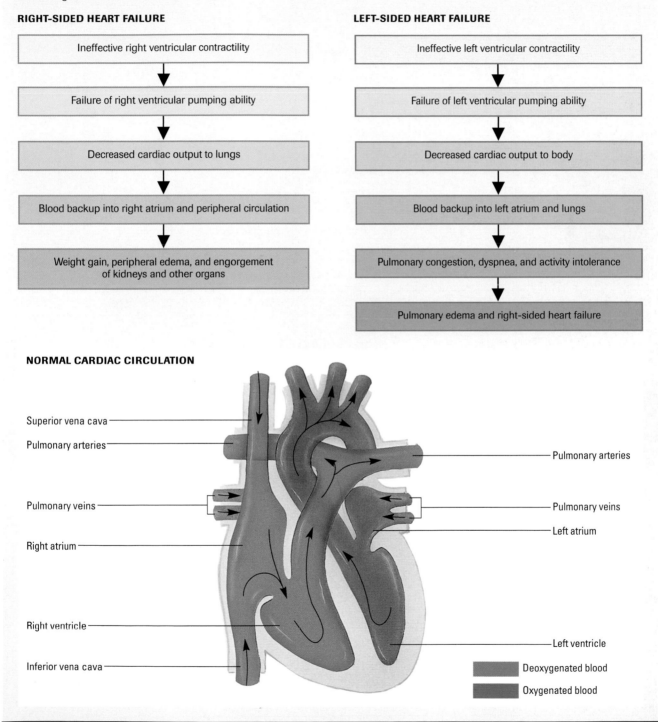

Superior vena cava
Pulmonary arteries
Pulmonary veins
Right atrium
Right ventricle
Inferior vena cava

Pulmonary arteries
Pulmonary veins
Left atrium
Left ventricle

Deoxygenated blood
Oxygenated blood

Complications and symptoms of hypertension

STROKE

Hypertension is the major cause of stroke. The harmful effects of hypertension in the brain may be caused by blood clots that obstruct blood flow to parts of the brain. Aneurysms may burst under increasing pressure, causing hemorrhage and damage to brain tissue.

VASCULAR RETINOPATHY

Interruption in blood supply to the eye from prolonged hypertension can produce vascular retinopathy, which causes retinal vasospasm and consequent damage to and narrowing of the arteriolar lumina. If left untreated, vascular retinopathy can lead to blindness.

RENOVASCULAR HYPERTENSION

The kidneys are vulnerable to variations in blood flow caused by hypertension. They can't function properly if blood flow decreases significantly. If systemic blood pressure rises because of stenosis of the major renal arteries or because of atherosclerosis of their branches, renovascular hypertension occurs. A decrease in blood flow causes the kidneys to release renin, an enzyme that causes blood vessels throughout the body to constrict more, resulting in a further increase in blood pressure. This cycle can be destructive and can lead to heart failure, myocardial infarction (MI), stroke and, sometimes, renal failure.

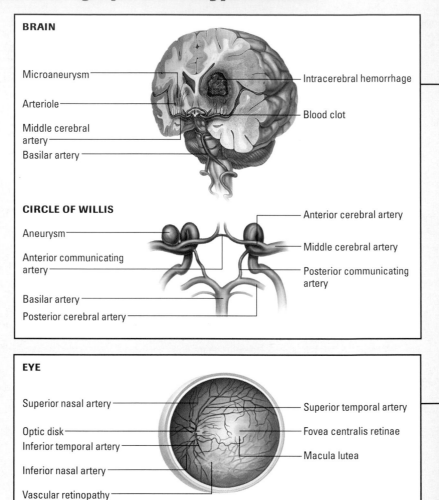

BRAIN

- Microaneurysm
- Arteriole
- Middle cerebral artery
- Basilar artery
- Intracerebral hemorrhage
- Blood clot

CIRCLE OF WILLIS

- Aneurysm
- Anterior communicating artery
- Basilar artery
- Posterior cerebral artery
- Anterior cerebral artery
- Middle cerebral artery
- Posterior communicating artery

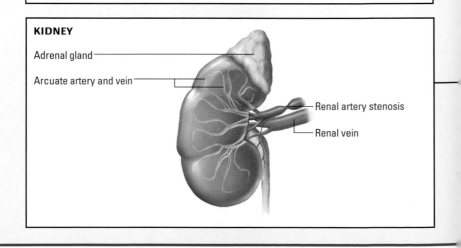

EYE

- Superior nasal artery
- Optic disk
- Inferior temporal artery
- Inferior nasal artery
- Vascular retinopathy
- Superior temporal artery
- Fovea centralis retinae
- Macula lutea

KIDNEY

- Adrenal gland
- Arcuate artery and vein
- Renal artery stenosis
- Renal vein

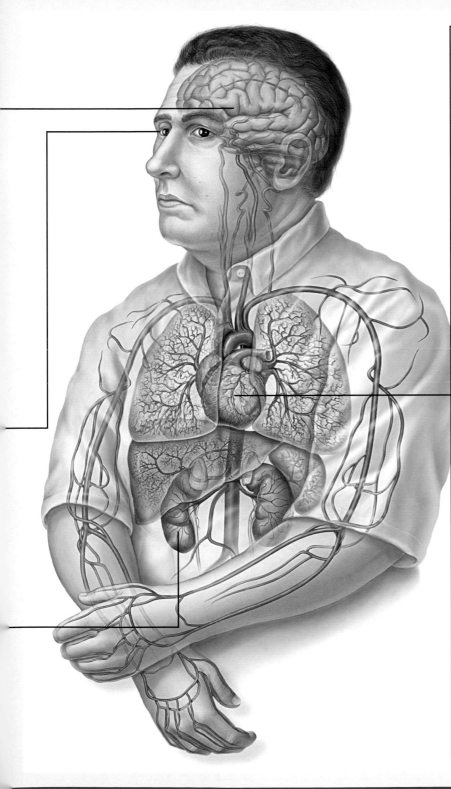

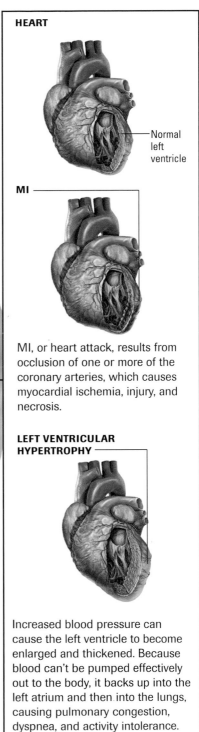

HEART

Normal left ventricle

MI

MI, or heart attack, results from occlusion of one or more of the coronary arteries, which causes myocardial ischemia, injury, and necrosis.

LEFT VENTRICULAR HYPERTROPHY

Increased blood pressure can cause the left ventricle to become enlarged and thickened. Because blood can't be pumped effectively out to the body, it backs up into the left atrium and then into the lungs, causing pulmonary congestion, dyspnea, and activity intolerance.

Hypercholesterolemia

Cholesterol is a lipid whose nucleus is synthesized from fatty acids. It's insoluble in plasma. Therefore, it must be carried in the blood by specialized fat-carrying proteins called *lipoproteins.* Lipoproteins are classified by their density into five types: chylomicrons, very-low-density lipoproteins (VLDLs), intermediate-density lipoproteins (IDLs), low-density lipoproteins (LDLs), and high-density lipoproteins (HDLs). Lipoproteins act as shuttles for fat in the bloodstream.

CHOLESTEROL PATHWAY

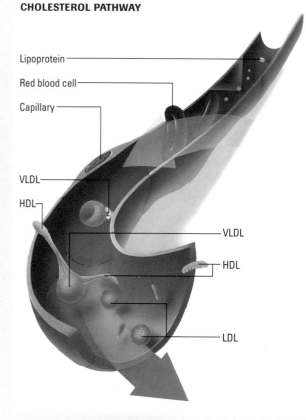

Lipoprotein
Red blood cell
Capillary
VLDL
HDL
VLDL
HDL
LDL

LIPOPROTEIN

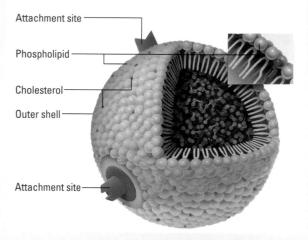

Attachment site
Phospholipid
Cholesterol
Outer shell
Attachment site

CONSEQUENCES OF HYPERCHOLESTEROLEMIA

Hypercholesterolemia is associated with development of atherosclerosis and heart disease. When the levels of cholesterol in the bloodstream are normal, the arterial walls remain smooth and slippery. However, when cholesterol levels are high, excess cholesterol concentrates in the walls of the arteries. Microphages attempt to remove this build-up by forming foam cells with the lipid. These foam cells become trapped in the new plaque matrix, leading to a reduction, and ultimately a blockage, of blood flow.

NORMAL ARTERY

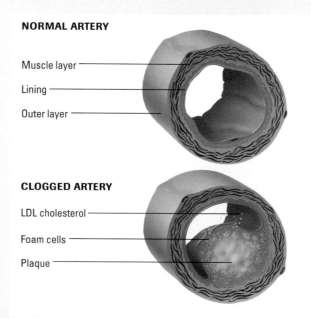

Muscle layer
Lining
Outer layer

CLOGGED ARTERY

LDL cholesterol
Foam cells
Plaque

Cholesterol is transported in the bloodstream primarily by LDLs. VLDLs travel through the bloodstream and attach to the lining of the capillaries. Here, the fatty core, cholesterol, is drawn out. IDLs, smaller lipoproteins, remain in the bloodstream and shed tiny disklike particles of HDL. LDLs remain in the blood and travel back to the liver to be removed by specific receptors on the liver cell. However, if the level of cholesterol in the bloodstream is high, fewer receptors are available on the surface of the liver cell for lipoprotein attachment, thereby interfering with the removal of LDLs.

Asthma

In asthma, bronchial linings overreact to various stimuli, causing episodic smooth muscle spasms that severely constrict the airways. Immunoglobulin (Ig) E antibodies, attached to histamine-containing mast cells and receptors on cell membranes, initiate intrinsic asthma attacks. When exposed to an antigen such as pollen, the IgE antibody combines with the antigen.

On subsequent exposure to the antigen, mast cells degranulate and release mediators. Mast cells in the lung interstitium are stimulated to release histamine and leukotrienes.

Histamine attaches to receptor sites in the larger bronchi, where it causes swelling in smooth muscles. Mucous membranes become inflamed, irritated, and swollen.

Leukotrienes attach to receptor sites in the smaller bronchi and cause local swelling of the smooth muscle. Leukotrienes also cause prostaglandins to travel through the bloodstream to the lungs, where they enhance histamine's effect. Histamine stimulates the mucous membranes to secrete excessive mucus, further narrowing the bronchial lumen. Goblet cells secrete

viscous mucus that's difficult to cough up. Mucosal edema and thickened secretions further block the airways.

On inhalation, the narrowed bronchial lumen can still expand slightly, allowing air to reach the alveoli. On exhalation, increased intrathoracic pressure closes the bronchial lumen completely. Air enters but can't escape. Thus, air is trapped in the alveoli.

Mucus fills the lung bases, inhibiting alveolar ventilation. Blood is shunted to alveoli in other lung parts but still can't compensate for diminished ventilation.

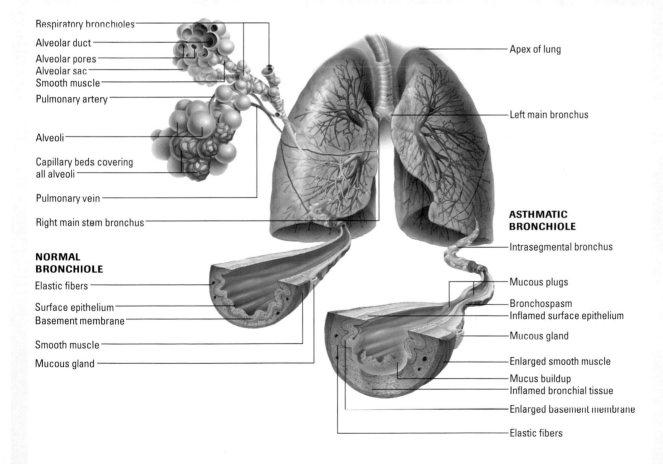

Chronic bronchitis

A form of chronic obstructive pulmonary disease (COPD), bronchitis is inflammation of the bronchi caused by irritants or infection. It may be classified as acute or chronic. In chronic bronchitis, hypersecretion of mucus and chronic productive cough last for 3 months of the year and occur for at least 2 consecutive years. The distinguishing characteristic of bronchitis is airflow obstruction.

Chronic bronchitis occurs when irritants are inhaled for a prolonged time. The irritants inflame the tracheobronchial tree, leading to increased mucus production and a narrowed or blocked airway. As inflammation continues, changes in the cells lining the respiratory tract result in resistance of the small airways and severe ventilation-perfusion ($\dot{V}/\dot{Q}$) imbalance, which decreases arterial oxygenation.

Chronic bronchitis results in hypertrophy and hyperplasia of the mucous glands, increased numbers of goblet cells, ciliary damage, squamous metaplasia of the columnar epithelium, and chronic leukocytic and lymphocytic infiltration of bronchial walls. Hypersecretion of the goblet cells blocks the free movement of cilia, which normally sweep dust, irritants, and mucus away from the airways. With mucus and debris accumulating in the airway, the defenses are altered and the individual is prone to respiratory tract infections.

Additional effects include widespread inflammation, airway narrowing, and mucus within the airways. Bronchial walls become inflamed and thickened from edema and accumulation of inflammatory cells, and the effects of smooth muscle bronchospasm further narrow the lumen. At first, only large bronchi are involved, but eventually all airways are affected. Airways become obstructed and closure occurs, especially on expiration. The gas is then trapped in the distal portion of the lung. Hypoventilation occurs, leading to a $\dot{V}/\dot{Q}$ mismatch and resultant hypoxemia.

CHRONIC BRONCHITIS

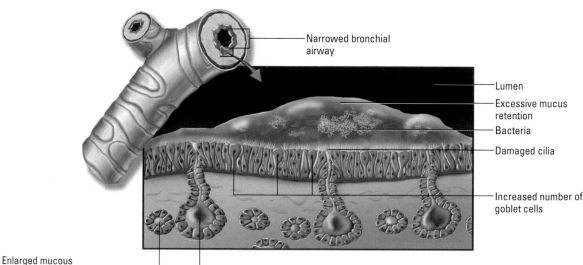

Narrowed bronchial airway

Lumen

Excessive mucus retention

Bacteria

Damaged cilia

Increased number of goblet cells

Enlarged mucous glands

Types of GI ulcers

Ulcers may occur anywhere in the esophagus, stomach, pylorus, duodenum, or jejunum, with the crater of the ulcer penetrating through one or more layers of tissue. If this damage recurs or if healing doesn't take place, the crater may penetrate the wall and extend to adjacent tissues and organs such as the pancreas.

EROSION
Penetration of only the superficial layer

Mucosa

Muscularis mucosa

Submucosa

Oblique muscle

Circular muscle

Longitudinal muscle

Serosa

ACUTE ULCER
Penetration into the
muscular layer

PERFORATING ULCER
Penetration of the wall, creating a passage for gastric
acids, other fluids, and air to enter adjacent spaces

Exudate

Granulation tissue

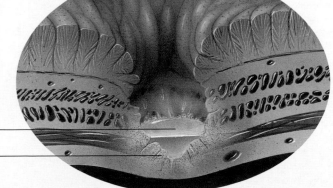

Osteoporosis

Normally, the blood absorbs calcium from the digestive system and deposits it in the bones. In osteoporosis, blood levels of calcium are reduced because of dietary calcium deficiency, inability of the intestines to absorb calcium, or postmenopausal estrogen deficiency. To maintain the blood calcium level as close to normal as possible, resorption from the bones increases, causing osteoporosis.

In addition to enhancing bone resorption, low calcium levels enhance the effects of two other factors: parathyroid hormone (PTH) and vitamin D. PTH is produced by the parathyroid glands, which are buried in the thyroid gland. Vitamin D is supplied by the diet, produced in the skin as a reaction to sunlight, and processed into a very potent form in the liver and kidneys. Both substances stimulate calcium absorption from the intestine and increase resorption from the bone. This results in an increased sacrifice of bone calcium to maintain normal levels of calcium in the blood.

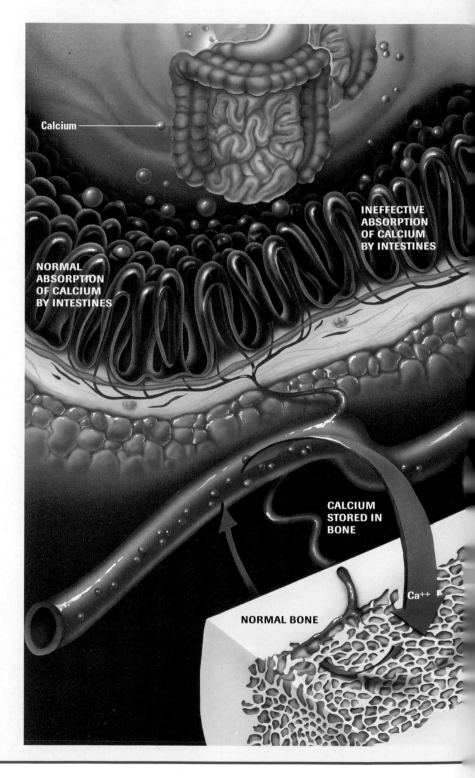

Calcium

INEFFECTIVE ABSORPTION OF CALCIUM BY INTESTINES

NORMAL ABSORPTION OF CALCIUM BY INTESTINES

CALCIUM STORED IN BONE

NORMAL BONE

Ca++

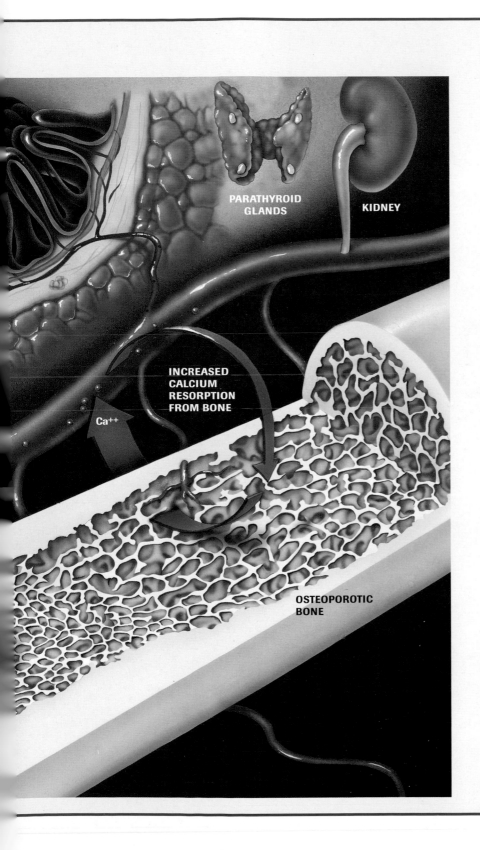

PARATHYROID
GLANDS

KIDNEY

INCREASED
CALCIUM
RESORPTION
FROM BONE

Ca++

OSTEOPOROTIC
BONE

Diabetes mellitus

WHAT IS DIABETES?

Diabetes is the name for a group of chronic or lifelong diseases that affect the way the body uses food to make the energy necessary for life. Primarily, diabetes is a disruption of carbohydrate (sugar and starch) metabolism that also affects fats and proteins. There are two main forms of diabetes (type 1 and type 2) as well as conditions of glucose intolerance, gestational diabetes, and diabetes caused by pancreatic disorders. Regardless of the form, metabolic control under the care of a physician is essential for good health.

WHAT IS INSULIN?

Insulin is an essential hormone produced in the pancreas and released into the bloodstream. Insulin attaches itself to cells at places called *insulin receptors*. When attached, insulin allows sugar or glucose from the food we eat to enter the liver, fat, and muscle cells, where it's used for energy.

TYPE 1 DIABETES MELLITUS

In type 1 diabetes, the pancreas makes little or no insulin. Without insulin, sugar can't enter cells to be used for energy. The body's tissues are starved and blood glucose levels become dangerously high. The disorder usually begins in youth, but it may also occur in older adults. Type 1 diabetes occurs in 5% to 10% of patients with diabetes, who require insulin therapy for treatment.

TYPE 2 DIABETES MELLITUS

In type 2 diabetes, the pancreas produces some insulin, but it's either too little or isn't effective. In addition, insulin receptors that control the transport of glucose into cells may not work properly or are reduced in number. Type 2 diabetes typically develops in people older than age 40. Most newly diagnosed patients with type 2 diabetes are overweight but are able to control their diabetes through diet and weight loss. Some patients may require oral medications or insulin injections to achieve glucose control.

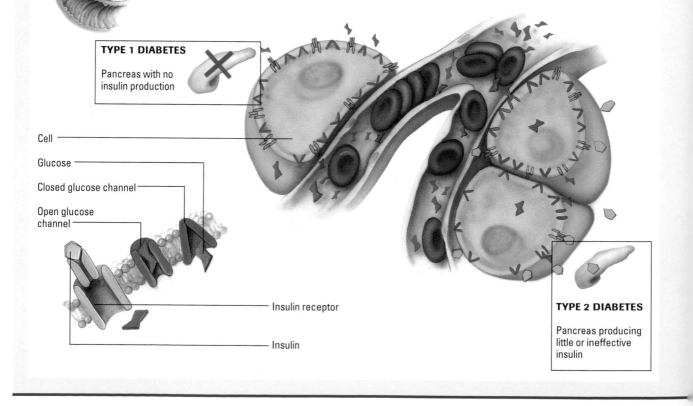

Pancreas

TYPE 1 DIABETES

Pancreas with no insulin production

Cell

Glucose

Closed glucose channel

Open glucose channel

Insulin receptor

Insulin

TYPE 2 DIABETES

Pancreas producing little or ineffective insulin

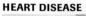

LONG-TERM HEALTH PROBLEMS ASSOCIATED WITH DIABETES

High plasma glucose levels caused by diabetes may damage small and large blood vessels and nerves. Diabetes may also lower the body's ability to fight infection. As a result, people with diabetes are more likely to have serious eye problems, kidney disease, heart attacks, strokes, high blood pressure, poor circulation, tingling in hands and feet, sexual problems, amputations, and infections. Good diabetes control may help prevent these problems or make them less serious.

HEART DISEASE

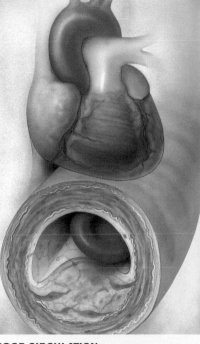

KIDNEY FAILURE

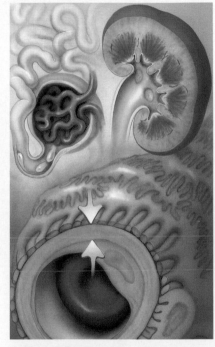

LOSS OF VISION

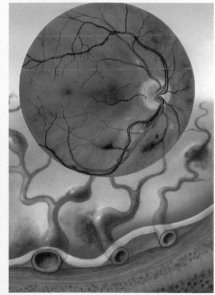

POOR CIRCULATION

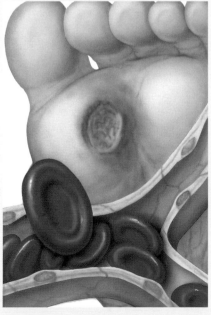

NERVE DAMAGE

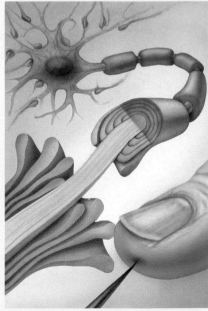

Anaphylaxis

An anaphylactic reaction requires previous sensitization to the specific antigen. The pathophysiology of anaphylaxis is described here.

1. RESPONSE TO ANTIGEN

Immunoglobulins (Ig) M and G recognize and bind to the antigen.

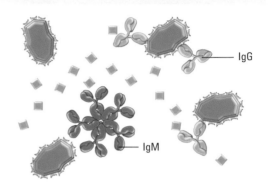

Complement cascade = ▣

2. RELEASE OF CHEMICAL MEDIATORS

Activated IgE on basophils promotes the release of mediators: histamine, serotonin, and leuko-trienes.

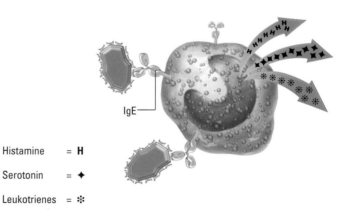

Histamine   = **H**

Serotonin   = ✦

Leukotrienes = ✣

3. INTENSIFIED RESPONSE

Mast cells release more histamine and eosinophil chemotactic factor of anaphylaxis (ECF-A), which create venule-weakening lesions.

ECF-A   = ◗
Histamine   = **H**

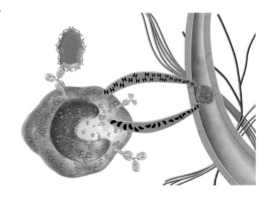

4. RESPIRATORY DISTRESS

In the lungs, histamine causes endothelial cell destruction and fluid leak into alveoli.

Leukotrienes = ❊

Histamine = **H**

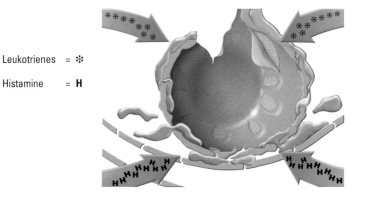

5. DETERIORATION

Meanwhile, mediators increase vascular permeability, causing fluid leak from the vessels.

Bradykinin = ●

Histamine = **H**

Prostaglandins = ✛

Serotonin = ✦

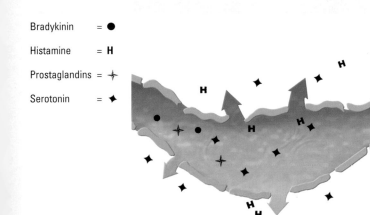

6. FAILURE OF COMPENSATORY MECHANISMS

Endothelial cell damage causes basophils and mast cells to release heparin and mediator-neutralizing substances.

Heparin = ▲

Leukotrienes = ❊

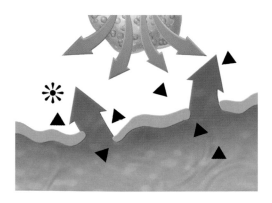

Cancer

CANCER STAGING

The diagnosis of cancer is determined by a biopsy, a microscopic evaluation of sampled tissue. Determining the extent of spread of the malignant cells is called *staging*. Although many different staging systems exist, a four-stage system is typically used.

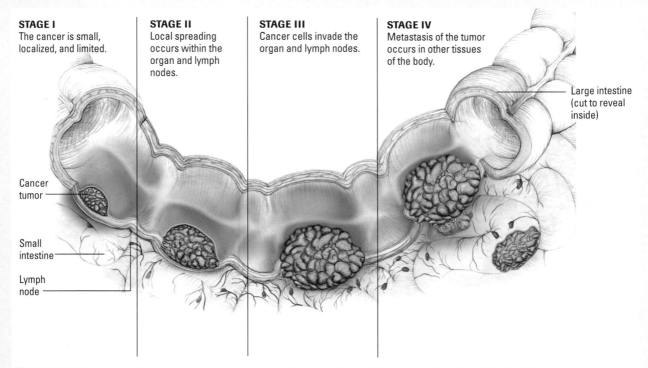

STAGE I
The cancer is small, localized, and limited.

STAGE II
Local spreading occurs within the organ and lymph nodes.

STAGE III
Cancer cells invade the organ and lymph nodes.

STAGE IV
Metastasis of the tumor occurs in other tissues of the body.

Large intestine (cut to reveal inside)

Cancer tumor

Small intestine

Lymph node

CANCER SPREAD

Cancer cells may invade nearby tissues or metastasize to other organs in three ways:

- through the blood—cancer cells may travel through the blood vessels, often to the liver and the lungs
- through the lymphatic system—the lymphatic system plays a key role in the immune system by helping to fight conditions as minor as colds or as serious as cancer; cancer cells may move through the network of channels, from the tissues to the lymph nodes, to the circulatory system, and eventually to other organs
- through seeding—cancer may penetrate an organ, moving into a nearby body cavity such as the chest or abdominal area and spread throughout the area.

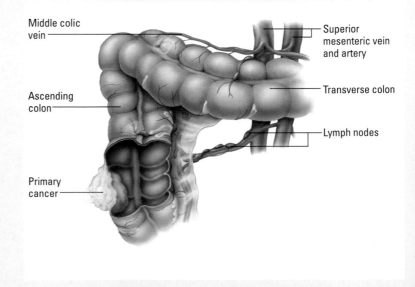

Middle colic vein

Ascending colon

Primary cancer

Superior mesenteric vein and artery

Transverse colon

Lymph nodes

5. A patient receives a desensitization injection. The nurse should monitor the patient for which adverse reaction?
- ☐ **1.** Bruising at the injection site
- ☐ **2.** Localized itching
- ☐ **3.** Anaphylaxis
- ☐ **4.** Nausea and vomiting

6. A patient experiences a skin reaction characterized by dermal wheals surrounded by an erythematous flare. Which term does the nurse use to document this finding?
- ☐ **1.** Urticaria
- ☐ **2.** Angioedema
- ☐ **3.** Atopic dermatitis
- ☐ **4.** Scleroderma

7. A patient experiences anaphylaxis. Which drug should be administered first?
- ☐ **1.** Dopamine
- ☐ **2.** Epinephrine
- ☐ **3.** Aminophylline
- ☐ **4.** Sodium bicarbonate

8. Which type of vasculitis produces hypertension, abdominal pain, myalgia, joint pain, and weakness?
- ☐ **1.** Wegener's granulomatosis
- ☐ **2.** Polyangiitis overlap syndrome
- ☐ **3.** Hypersensitivity vasculitis
- ☐ **4.** Polyarteritis nodosa

9. Which test may be used to monitor therapy in a patient with RA?
- ☐ **1.** CBC
- ☐ **2.** Serum protein electrophoresis
- ☐ **3.** ESR
- ☐ **4.** RF titer

10. Dennie's sign is a symptom seen in which disorder?
- ☐ **1.** Scleroderma
- ☐ **2.** Atopic dermatitis
- ☐ **3.** Urticaria
- ☐ **4.** Vasculitis

ANSWERS AND RATIONALES

1. CORRECT ANSWER: 4
In type IV hypersensitivity, antigen is presented to T cells. These sensitized T cells release lymphokines, which recruit and activate other lymphocytes, monocytes, macrophages, and polymorphonuclear leukocytes.

2. CORRECT ANSWER: 2
The nurse should initiate oxygen therapy in light of the decreasing oxygen saturation level, then immediately notify the physician of the patient's status. Obtaining an ECG would be of no value at this time as the patient may have a severe hypersensitivity reaction and is without signs of cardiac distress. The nurse would be outside

her scope of practice to increase the I.V. rate without a physician's order. Placing the patient in Trendelenburg's position would likely cause increased pulmonary distress and harm the patient.

3. CORRECT ANSWER: 2

The anti-ds-DNA test is the most specific test for SLE. It correlates with disease activity, especially renal involvement, and helps monitor the patient's response to therapy. C-reactive protein, serum electrophoresis, and ANA tests can be abnormal in SLE as well as other autoimmune disorders, so they aren't diagnostic for SLE.

4. CORRECT ANSWER: 3

Airborne or inhaled allergens, such as pollens, can cause a reaction that leads to allergic rhinitis.

5. CORRECT ANSWER: 3

After administering a desensitization injection, the nurse should watch for signs of anaphylaxis and severe localized erythema and have emergency resuscitation equipment available. Bruising at the injection site, localized itching, and nausea and vomiting aren't adverse reactions that occur with a desensitization injection.

6. CORRECT ANSWER: 1

Urticaria produces local dermal wheals with a surrounding erythematous flare. It's caused by an IgE-mediated response to an allergen. Angioedema is a large, circumscribed area of subQ swelling that commonly results from reactions to foods or drugs. Atopic dermatitis involves reddening and inflammation of the skin and intense itching. Scleroderma is a chronic condition characterized by thickening of the skin due to new collagen formation.

7. CORRECT ANSWER: 2

Patients experiencing anaphylaxis require immediate administration of epinephrine 1:1000 aqueous solution to reverse bronchoconstriction and cause vasoconstriction. The drug may be given I.M. or subQ if the patient hasn't lost consciousness and is normotensive, or I.V. if the reaction is severe. Dopamine, aminophylline, and sodium bicarbonate aren't appropriate drugs to treat anaphylaxis.

8. CORRECT ANSWER: 4

Polyarteritis nodosa affects small to medium arteries throughout the body. Lesions tend to be segmental, occur at bifurcations and branching of arteries, spread distally to arterioles and, in severe cases, circumferentially involve adjacent veins. These effects produce the signs and symptoms of hypertension, abdominal pain, myalgia, joint pain, and weakness. Wegener's granulomatosis mainly affects the respiratory tract and kidneys. Polyangiitis overlap syndrome shares many features with polyarteritis nodosa, but also involves pulmonary symptoms. Hypersensitivity vasculitis is evidenced by palpable purpura, papules, ulcers, or chronic or recurrent hives.

9. CORRECT ANSWER: 3

ESR (along with C-reactive protein) is used to monitor response to therapy in patients with RA because elevated results typically parallel disease activity. The RF titer can indicate the presence of disease, but it doesn't help determine the specific degree of inflammation. CBC and protein electrophoresis aren't used to diagnose RA.

10. CORRECT ANSWER: 2

Dennie's sign, or Morgan's line, characterized by pink pigmentation and swelling of the upper eyelid and a double fold under the lower lid, is seen in atopic dermatitis. This disorder usually occurs in children and is due to severe pruritus. Neither sclero-derma nor urticaria results in this specific pattern of inflammation and edema around the eye. Vasculitis affects the arteries, not local tissues.

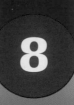

8

Endocrine system

CHAPTER OVERVIEW

The endocrine system consists of glands, specialized cell clusters, hormones, and target tissues. The glands and cell clusters secrete hormones and chemical transmitters in response to stimulation from the nervous system and other sites. Together with the nervous system, the endocrine system regulates and integrates the body's metabolic activities and maintains internal homeostasis on an extracellular and intracellular level. Each target tissue has receptors for specific hormones. Hormones connect with the receptors, and the resulting hormone-receptor complex triggers the target cell's response.

Caring for a patient with an endocrine disorder requires an understanding of the pathophysiologic changes that occur, the signs and symptoms they produce, and the appropriate ways to intervene. The first section of this chapter provides an overview of key pathophysiologic concepts related to the endocrine system. Common endocrine disorders are then defined, and specific pathophysiologic changes, complications, diagnostic test findings, treatments, and nursing considerations are outlined.

PATHOPHYSIOLOGIC CONCEPTS

● **Altered intracellular mechanisms**
  • Involves the inadequate synthesis of the second messenger needed to convert the hormone signal into intracellular effects
  • Two different mechanisms may be involved
    – Faulty response of target cells to water-soluble hormones (peptides) results in a failure to generate the second messenger required to translate the hormone signal into the intracellular effect
    – Abnormal response of the target cell to the second messenger with resultant failure to express the required hormonal effect

● **Altered receptor mechanisms**
  • Associated with water-soluble hormones but involve problems with the receptors, not the cellular mechanism
    – Fewer receptors, resulting in diminished or defective hormone-receptor binding
    – Impaired receptor function, resulting in insensitivity to the hormones
    – Presence of antibodies against specific receptors, either reducing available binding sites or mimicking hormone action and suppressing or exaggerating target cell response
    – Unusual expression of receptor function

ADRENAL HYPOFUNCTION

● **Definition**
  • Chronic condition that results from the partial or complete destruction of the adrenal cortex
  • Classified as primary or secondary
  • Primary adrenal hypofunction or insufficiency (Addison's disease): Originates within the adrenal gland; characterized by decreased secretion of mineralocorticoids, glucocorticoids, and androgens
    – Adrenal crisis (addisonian crisis): Critical deficiency of mineralocorticoids and glucocorticoids; can follow acute stress, sepsis, trauma, surgery, or the omission of steroid therapy in patients with chronic adrenal insufficiency (see *Adrenal crisis: How it happens,* page 286)
  • Secondary adrenal hypofunction: Due to a disorder outside the gland such as impaired pituitary secretion of corticotropin; characterized by decreased glucocorticoid secretion; secretion of aldosterone is commonly unaffected

Key facts about altered intracellular mechanisms
● Involve inadequate synthesis of second messenger
● Impair hormonal signals within the cell

Key facts about altered receptor mechanisms
● Abnormal receptor response to water-soluble hormones

Key facts about adrenal hypofunction
● Results from partial or complete destruction of the adrenal cortex

Primary (Addison's disease)
● Originates within adrenal gland
● Characterized by decreased secretion of mineralocorticoids, glucocorticoids, and androgens
● May lead to addisonian crisis

Secondary
● Develops due to a disorder outside the gland
● Characterized by decreased glucocorticoid secretion

GO WITH THE FLOW

Adrenal crisis: How it happens

Acute adrenal crisis, the most serious complication of Addison's disease, involves a critical deficiency of glucocorticoids and mineralocorticoids. This flowchart highlights the underlying mechanisms responsible for this life-threatening event, which requires prompt assessment and immediate treatment.

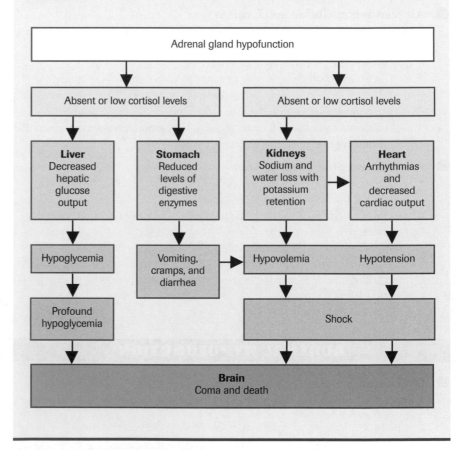

Underlying pathophysiology

- Corticotropin primarily regulates the adrenal release of glucocorticoids (primarily cortisol), mineralocorticoids (including aldosterone), and sex steroids that supplement androgens produced by the gonads
- Corticotropin secretion is controlled by corticotropin-releasing hormone produced by the hypothalamus and by negative feedback control by glucocorticoids
- Autoimmune antibodies can block the corticotropin receptor or bind with corticotropin, preventing it from stimulating adrenal cells
- Addison's disease is a decrease in the biosynthesis, storage, or release of adrenocortical hormones

– In about 80% of patients, an autoimmune process causes partial or complete destruction of both adrenal glands
– All zones of the cortex are involved, causing deficiencies of the adrenocortical secretions, glucocorticoids, androgens, and adrenal cortex
• Manifestations of adrenocortical hormone deficiency become apparent when 90% of the functional cells in both adrenal glands are lost; usually, cellular atrophy is limited to the cortex, although medullary involvement may occur, resulting in catecholamine deficiency
• Cortisol deficiency causes decreased liver gluconeogenesis; the resulting blood glucose levels can become dangerously low in patients who take insulin routinely
• Aldosterone deficiency causes increased renal sodium loss and enhances potassium reabsorption; sodium excretion causes a reduction in water volume that leads to hypotension

Causes
• Primary hypofunction
– Autoimmune process in which circulating antibodies react specifically against the adrenal tissue (most common cause)
• Family history of autoimmune disease (may predispose the patient to Addison's disease and other endocrinopathies)
– Tuberculosis (once the chief cause, now responsible for less than 20% of adult cases)
– Bilateral adrenalectomy
– Hemorrhage into the adrenal gland
– Neoplasms
– Infections (histoplasmosis, cytomegalovirus)
• Secondary hypofunction (glucocorticoid deficiency)
– Hypopituitarism (causing decreased corticotropin secretion)
– Abrupt withdrawal of long-term corticosteroid therapy (long-term, exogenous corticosteroid stimulation suppresses pituitary corticotropin secretion, resulting in adrenal gland atrophy)
– Removal of a corticotropin-secreting tumor
– Exhausted body stores of glucocorticoids in a person with adrenal hypofunction after trauma, surgery, or other physiologic stress

Pathophysiologic changes
• Primary hypofunction
– Weakness; fatigue; weight loss, nausea, vomiting, and anorexia; decreased tolerance for even minor stress resulting from mineralocorticoid or glucocorticoid deficiency
– Conspicuous bronze color of the skin, especially in the creases of the hands and over the metacarpophalangeal joints (hand and finger), elbows, and knees resulting from decreased cortisol levels and simultaneous secretion of excessive corticotropin and melanocyte stimulating hormone
– Darkening of scars, areas of vitiligo (absence of pigmentation), and increased pigmentation of the mucous membranes (especially the buccal mucosa) due to decreased secretion of cortisol, causing simultaneous secretion of excessive corticotropin and melanocyte-stimulating hormone by the pituitary gland

Common causes of adrenal hypofunction
• Autoimmune process (primary)
• Hypopituitarism (secondary)
• Abrupt withdrawal of long-term corticosteroid therapy (secondary)

Key pathophysiologic changes in adrenal hypofunction
• Weakness and fatigue
• Weight loss
• Bronze skin color
• Pigmentation changes
• Orthostatic hypotension
• Decreased cardiac output
• Weak, irregular pulse

– Associated cardiovascular abnormalities, including orthostatic hypotension, decreased cardiac size and output, and weak, irregular pulse due to mineralocorticoid or glucocorticoid deficiency
– Fasting hypoglycemia due to decreased gluconeogenesis
– Craving for salty food due to decreased mineralocorticoid secretion (which normally causes salt retention)
– Normal blood pressure when supine, but marked hypotension and tachycardia after standing for several minutes
– Renin release and resulting increased production of angiotensin II to raise blood pressure is caused by low plasma volume and arteriolar pressure
– Possible decreased hair growth in axillary and pubic areas as well as on the extremities in women due to androgen deficiency (hair loss less noticeable in men because of metabolic effects of testicular androgens)
– In addisonian crisis, profound weakness and fatigue; nausea, vomiting, and dehydration; hypotension; and high fever followed by hypothermia (occasionally) caused by glucocorticoid and mineralocorticoid deficiencies
• Secondary hypofunction
– Similar to signs and symptoms of primary hypofunction, but without hyperpigmentation due to lower corticotropin and melanocyte-stimulating hormone levels
– Possible absence of hypotension and electrolyte abnormalities due to relatively normal aldosterone secretion

Complications
• Hyperpyrexia
• Psychotic reactions
• Inadequate or excessive steroid replacement therapy
• Shock
• Profound hypoglycemia
• Ultimate vascular collapse, renal shutdown, coma, and death (if untreated)

Diagnostic test findings
• Plasma cortisol testing reveals decreased levels (less than 5 mcg/dl in the morning; less than 3 mcg/dl in the evening)
• Comprehensive metabolic panel shows decreased fasting blood glucose level (in some patients) due to increased insulin sensitivity and increased peripheral utilization of glucose; decreased serum sodium and increased serum potassium due to loss of action of aldosterone; increased creatinine and blood urea nitrogen levels due to hypovolemia
• Complete blood count (CBC) reveals elevated hematocrit (due to hypovolemia) and increased lymphocyte and eosinophil counts (due to loss of glucocorticoid function), and decreased hemoglobin level and red blood cells (due to anemia)
• Rapid corticotropin stimulation testing is used to determine corticotropin and aldosterone levels, which are compared to baseline levels obtained before administration of the test dose
– Two criteria required for diagnosis of Addison's disease (equivocal tests may be extended 24 to 48 hours to determine the presence of a secondary adrenocortical insufficiency)

Key diagnostic test results for adrenal hypofunction
• Plasma cortisol level: Decreased
• Rapid corticotropin stimulation test: Failure of cortisol and aldosterone levels to rise
• CT scan: Adrenal calcification and enlargement if cause is infectious; atrophy if cause is primary

- A low aldosterone level (less than 5 ng/100 ml) that fails to increase by at least 4 ng/100 ml 30 or 60 minutes after corticotropin stimulation confirms abnormal mineralocorticoid function of the adrenal cortex
  - Failure of the cortisol level to increase more than 7 mcg/dl above the baseline value indicates abnormal glucocorticoid function
- Metyrapone test confirms or rule outs suspected secondary adrenal hypofunction
  - Used only when the rapid corticotropin stimulation test is normal because the test can be lethal if administered to a patient with Addison's disease
  - Abnormally elevated plasma concentrations of the cortisol precursor 11 deoxycortisol indicate secondary adrenal disease
- Computed tomography (CT) scan shows adrenal calcification if the cause is infectious; enlargement if the cause is infectious, hemorrhagic, or related to infiltrating diseases; and atrophy if the cause is idiopathic autoimmune
- Chest X-ray may show a small heart, common in people with Addison's, or signs of adrenal calcification if cause is infectious

● Treatment

- Lifelong corticosteroid replacement, usually with cortisone or hydrocortisone, both of which have a glucocorticoid effect (primary or secondary adrenal hypofunction)
- Oral fludrocortisone (Florinef), a synthetic mineralocorticoid, to prevent dangerous dehydration, hypotension, hyponatremia, and hyperkalemia (Addison's disease)
- For addisonian crisis: I.V. bolus of hydrocortisone, then follow-up with an I.M. injection or I.V. infusion until the patient's condition stabilizes; 3 to 5 L of I.V. normal saline and glucose solutions may be needed (adrenal crisis; usually subsides quickly)
  - After the crisis, maintenance doses of hydrocortisone to preserve physiologic stability

● Nursing considerations

- During adrenal crisis, monitor the patient's vital signs carefully for signs of shock; watch for hyperkalemia before treatment and hypokalemia after treatment; watch for cardiac arrhythmias due to a serum potassium disturbance
- If the patient also has diabetes, check blood glucose levels periodically because steroid replacement may require an adjustment to the insulin dosage
- Record weight and intake and output because the patient may have volume depletion; until onset of mineralocorticoid effect, force fluids to replace excessive fluid loss
- For the patient receiving maintenance steroid therapy
  - Arrange for a diet that maintains sodium and potassium balances
  - If the patient is anorexic, suggest six small meals per day to increase calorie intake, and keep a late-morning snack available in case the patient becomes hypoglycemic
  - Watch for fluid and electrolyte imbalance, especially if the patient is receiving mineralocorticoids
  - Check for petechiae because the patient may bruise easily

Key treatments for adrenal hypofunction
- Lifelong corticosteroid replacement
- I.V. hydrocortisone (in addisonian crisis)

Key nursing considerations for adrenal hypofunction
- Watch for fluid and electrolyte imbalance in patients receiving steroids.
- Teach patient symptoms of steroid overdose and underdose.
- Warn patient that stress may necessitate additional cortisone to prevent adrenal crisis.
- Check blood glucose levels periodically in patient with diabetes.

During adrenal crisis
- Monitor vital signs.
- Watch for hyperkalemia before treatment; hypokalemia after treatment.
- Watch for cardiac arrhythmias.

– If the patient receives glucocorticoids alone, observe for orthostatic hypotension or electrolyte abnormalities, which may indicate a need for mineralocorticoid therapy

– Teach the patient the symptoms of steroid overdose (swelling, weight gain) and underdose (lethargy, weakness)

– Instruct the patient to always carry a medical identification card

– Explain the importance of taking antacids while on steroids to decrease gastric irritation

– Warn the patient that stress may necessitate additional cortisone to prevent an adrenal crisis

CUSHING'S SYNDROME

● **Definition**
  • Cluster of clinical abnormalities caused by excessive adrenocortical hormones (particularly cortisol) or related corticosteroids and, to a lesser extent, androgens and aldosterone

● **Underlying pathophysiology**
  • Cortisol excess results in anti-inflammatory effects and excessive catabolism of protein and peripheral fat to support hepatic glucose production
  • Mechanism may be corticotropin-dependent (elevated plasma corticotropin levels stimulate the adrenal cortex to produce excess cortisol) or corticotropin-independent (excess cortisol is produced by the adrenal cortex or exogenously administered)
  • Excess cortisol suppresses the hypothalamic-pituitary-adrenal axis (also present in ectopic corticotropin-secreting tumors)

● **Causes**
  • Anterior pituitary hormone (corticotropin) excess
  • Autonomous, ectopic corticotropin secretion by a tumor outside the pituitary gland (usually malignant, frequently oat cell carcinoma of the lung)
  • Excessive glucocorticoid administration, including prolonged use

● **Pathophysiologic changes**
  • Diabetes mellitus with decreased glucose tolerance, fasting hyperglycemia, and glucosuria due to cortisol-induced insulin resistance and increased gluconeogenesis in the liver
  • Muscle weakness due to hypokalemia
  • Loss of muscle mass from increased catabolism
  • Pathologic fractures due to decreased bone mineral ionization, osteopenia, osteoporosis, and skeletal growth retardation in children
  • Purple striae; facial plethora (edema and blood vessel distention); acne; fat pads above the clavicles, over the upper back (buffalo hump), on the face (moon facies), and throughout the trunk (truncal obesity) with slender arms and legs; little or no scar formation; poor wound healing; spontaneous ecchymosis; hyperpigmentation; and fungal skin infections due to decreased collagen and weakened tissues
  • Peptic ulcer, abdominal pain, increased appetite, and weight gain due to increased gastric secretions and pepsin production and decreased gastric mucus

Key facts about Cushing's syndrome
- Caused by excessive adrenocortical hormones (particularly cortisol) or related corticosteroids
- Suppresses the hypothalamic-pituitary-adrenal axis
- Causes anti-inflammatory effects and excessive protein and peripheral fat catabolism

Key pathophysiologic changes in Cushing's syndrome
- Diabetes mellitus
- Muscle weakness and loss of muscle mass
- Pathologic fractures
- Hypertension
- Redistribution of fat
- Poor wound healing
- Emotional lability
- Insomnia

- Irritability and emotional lability, ranging from euphoric behavior to depression or psychosis; insomnia due to the cortisol's role in neurotransmission
- Hypertension due to sodium and secondary fluid retention
- Heart failure, left ventricular hypertrophy, and capillary weakness from protein loss (which leads to bleeding and ecchymosis)
- Increased susceptibility to infection due to decreased lymphocyte production and suppressed antibody formation, decreased resistance to stress, and suppressed inflammatory response that masks even severe infection
- Fluid retention, increased potassium excretion, and ureteral calculi from increased bone demineralization with hypercalciuria
- Clitoral hypertrophy, mild virilism, hirsutism, and amenorrhea or oligomenorrhea in women
- Sexual dysfunction, decreased libido, and impotence in men due to increased androgen production

● Complications
- Osteoporosis
- Infections
- Ureteral calculi
- Metastasis of malignant tumors

● Diagnostic test findings
- Urinalysis reveals free cortisol levels above 150 µg/24 hr
- Dexamethasone suppression test shows failed suppression of plasma cortisol levels
- Serum cortisol testing shows elevated levels in the morning
- Corticotropin testing shows high levels of corticotropin that may be caused by corticotropin-producing tumors in the pituitary gland or another area; low levels of corticotropin may be caused by an adrenal tumor that is making cortisol (corticotropin testing should be separate from the cortisol testing)
- Blood chemistry analysis may show decreased potassium and calcium levels and elevated blood glucose and sodium levels
- Salivary free cortisol analysis (rarely done) reveals an elevated cortisol level
- Inferior petrosal sinus sampling (blood samples taken near the brain) reveal increased corticotropin levels if the source of the increased cortisol is the pituitary gland
- Ultrasonography, CT scan, and magnetic resonance imaging (MRI) show the location of a pituitary or adrenal tumor

● Treatment
- Surgery for tumors of the adrenal and pituitary glands or other tissue such as the lung
- Radiation therapy (tumor)
- Drug therapy, which may include ketoconazole (Nizoral) and aminoglutethimide (Cytadren) to inhibit cortisol synthesis, mitotane (Lysodren) to destroy the adrenocortical cells that secrete cortisol, and bromocriptine (Parlodel) to inhibit prolactin secretion from the pituitary gland

● Nursing considerations
- Frequently monitor the patient's vital signs; carefully observe the hypertensive patient who also has cardiac disease

Key diagnostic test results for Cushing's syndrome

- Urinalysis: Free cortisol levels above 150 µg/24 hr
- Dexamethasone suppression test: Failure to suppress plasma cortisol levels

Key treatments for Cushing's syndrome

- Surgery
- Drug therapy

Key nursing considerations for Cushing's syndrome

- Monitor vital signs, daily weight, and intake and output.
- Tell patient to report physiologically stressful situations, such as infections or pain.
- Instruct patient to watch for signs of steroid underdosage and overdosage.

After surgery
- Watch for signs of shock; give vasopressors and increase rate of I.V. fluids, as ordered.
- Monitor urine output.
- Check vital signs.
- Report signs of increased intracranial pressure.
- Watch for hypopituitarism.

- Check laboratory reports for hypernatremia, hypokalemia, hyperglycemia, and glycosuria
- Because the cushingoid patient is likely to retain sodium and water, check for edema and carefully monitor daily weight and intake and output
  - Provide a diet that's high in protein and potassium but low in calories, carbohydrates, and sodium
- Watch for signs of infection
- If the patient has osteoporosis, perform passive range-of-motion (ROM) exercises carefully because of the severe risk of pathologic fractures
- Because Cushing's syndrome produces emotional lability, record incidents that upset the patient and try to prevent such situations; teach the patient to get needed physical and mental rest by balancing rest and activity periods, utilizing relaxation techniques, and talking with the physician about a sleep aid if needed
- After bilateral adrenalectomy and pituitary surgery
  - Report wound drainage or temperature elevation immediately
  - Use strict sterile technique when changing dressings
  - Administer analgesics and replacement steroids as ordered
  - Watch for signs of shock; monitor urine output and check the patient's vital signs carefully
  - To counteract shock, give vasopressors and increase the rate of I.V. fluids, as ordered
  - Assess neurologic and behavioral status; mitotane, aminoglutethimide, and metyrapone decrease mental alertness and produce physical weakness
  - Check laboratory reports for hypoglycemia due to removal of the source of cortisol, a hormone that maintains blood glucose levels
  - Check for abdominal distention and return of bowel sounds after adrenalectomy
  - After pituitary surgery, immediately report signs of increased intracranial pressure (confusion, agitation, changes in the patient's level of consciousness [LOC], nausea, and vomiting) and watch for hypopituitarism
- For patients treated with steroid replacement therapy
  - Check regularly for signs of adrenal hypofunction (orthostatic hypotension, apathy, weakness, fatigue), which indicate inadequate steroid replacement
  - Advise the patient to take replacement steroids with antacids or meals to minimize gastric irritation; taking two-thirds of the dosage in the morning and the remaining third in the early afternoon is usually helpful (mimics diurnal adrenal secretion)
  - Tell the patient to report physiologically stressful situations, such as infections or pain, which may necessitate increased steroid dosage
  - Instruct the patient to watch closely for signs of inadequate steroid dosage (fatigue, weakness, dizziness) and overdosage (severe edema, weight gain)
  - Warn against abrupt discontinuation of steroids, which may produce a fatal adrenal crisis

DIABETES MELLITUS

● Definition
- Metabolic disorder characterized by hyperglycemia (elevated serum glucose) resulting from lack of insulin, lack of insulin effect, or both
- Four general classifications are recognized:
  - Pre-diabetes (fasting blood glucose > 100 mg/dl and < 126 mg/dl or postprandial blood glucose > 140 mg/dl and < 200 mg/dl)
  - Type 1 (absolute insulin insufficiency)
  - Type 2 (insulin resistance with varying degrees of insulin secretory defects)
  - Gestational (develops during pregnancy)

● Underlying pathophysiology
- Type 1
  - A triggering event, possibly a viral infection, causes production of autoantibodies against beta cells of the pancreas
  - Resultant destruction of beta cells leads to a decline in and an ultimate lack of insulin secretion
  - Insulin deficiency leads to hyperglycemia, enhanced lipolysis (decomposition of fat), and protein catabolism
  - These characteristics occur when more than 90% of beta cells have been destroyed
- Type 2
  - Impaired insulin secretion, inappropriate hepatic glucose production, or peripheral insulin receptor insensitivity leads to hyperglycemia
- Gestational
  - Occurs when a woman not previously diagnosed with diabetes shows glucose intolerance during pregnancy
  - This intolerance may occur if placental hormones counteract insulin, causing insulin resistance

● Causes
- Type 1
  - Autoimmune process triggered by viral or environmental factors
  - Idiopathic (no evidence of autoimmune process)
- Type 2
  - Beta cell exhaustion due to lifestyle choices or hereditary factors
  - Risk factors
    · Obesity
    · Family history
    · Ethnicity (Black, Hispanic, Native American)
    · Pregnancy (infant weighing more than 9 lb [4 kg] at birth)
    · HDL ≤ 35 mg/dl or a triglyceride level ≥ 250 mg/dl
    · Hypertension
    · Age ≥ 45

● Pathophysiologic changes
- Polyuria and polydipsia due to high serum osmolality caused by high serum glucose levels
- Polyphagia (occasional) due to depleted cellular storage of carbohydrates, fats, and proteins

Key facts about diabetes mellitus
- Characterized by hyperglycemia resulting from lack of insulin, lack of insulin effect, or both

Pre-diabetes
- Fasting blood glucose > 100 mg/dl and < 126 mg/dl
- Postprandial blood glucose > 140 mg/dl and < 200 mg/dl

Type 1
- Involves lack of insulin production in pancreas
- Causes hyperglycemia, lipolysis, and protein catabolism

Type 2
- Involves impaired glucose secretion or resistance of peripheral insulin receptors

Gestational
- Occurs during pregnancy
- Involves insulin resistance

TOP 5
Risk factors for type 2 diabetes
1. Obesity
2. Family history
3. Ethnicity (Black, Hispanic, Native American)
4. Pregnancy ending in birth of a neonate weighing more than 9 lb
5. Hypertension

Key pathophysiologic changes in diabetes mellitus
- Polyuria and polydipsia
- Fatigue and lethargy
- Vision changes
- Numbness and tingling
- Slow-healing skin infections or wounds

- Weight loss (usually 10% to 30%; persons with type 1 diabetes typically have almost no body fat at the time of diagnosis) due to prevention of normal metabolism of carbohydrates, fats, and proteins caused by impaired or absent insulin function
- Headaches, fatigue, lethargy, reduced energy levels, and impaired school and work performance due to low intracellular glucose levels
- Muscle cramps, irritability, and emotional lability due to electrolyte imbalance
- Vision changes, such as blurring, due to glucose-induced swelling around the optic nerve
- Numbness and tingling due to neural tissue damage
- Abdominal discomfort and pain due to autonomic neuropathy, causing gastroparesis and constipation
- Nausea, diarrhea, or constipation due to dehydration and electrolyte imbalances or autonomic neuropathy
- Slow-healing skin infections or wounds, itching of skin, and recurrent monilial infections of the vagina or anus due to hyperglycemia

● Complications
- Microvascular disease, including retinopathy, nephropathy, and neuropathy
- Dyslipidemia
- Macrovascular disease, including coronary, peripheral, and cerebral artery disease
- Diabetic ketoacidosis (DKA)
- Hyperosmolar hyperglycemic nonketotic syndrome
- Excessive weight gain
- Skin ulcerations
- Amputation
- Chronic renal failure

● Diagnostic test findings
- Blood testing reveals fasting plasma glucose level of 126 mg/dl or more on at least two occasions; random blood glucose level of 200 mg/dl or more; 2-hour blood glucose test results of 200 mg/dl or more (2 hours after ingesting 75 g of oral dextrose); and increased glycosylated hemoglobin (HbA_{1c}), reflecting glycemic control during the previous 2 to 3 months
- Ophthalmologic examination may show diabetic retinopathy
- Urinalysis reveals elevated acetone and glucose

● Treatment
- Careful monitoring of blood glucose and HbA_{1c} levels
- Individualized meal planning (per American Diabetes Association guidelines) to meet nutritional needs, control blood glucose and lipid levels, and reach and maintain appropriate body weight
  - Weight management: Reduction (obese patient with type 2) or high calorie allotment (type 1), depending on growth stage and activity level
- Regular exercise
- Type 1
  - Insulin replacement (current forms include mixed dose, split mixed-dose, and multiple daily injection regimens and continuous subcutaneous [subQ] insulin infusions)
  - Pancreas transplantation (currently requires chronic immunosuppression) (see *Treatment of type 1 diabetes mellitus,* pages 296 and 297)

Common complications of diabetes mellitus

- Microvascular disease (such as retinopathy, nephropathy, neuropathy)
- Macrovascular disease (such as coronary, peripheral, and cerebral artery disease)

Key diagnostic test results for diabetes mellitus

- Fasting plasma glucose level: 126 mg/dl or more on at least two occasions
- HbA_{1c} level: Increased, reflecting glycemic control during the previous 2 to 3 months

- Type 2
  - Oral antidiabetic drugs to stimulate endogenous insulin production, increase insulin sensitivity at the cellular level, suppress hepatic gluconeogenesis, and delay GI absorption of carbohydrates (drug combinations may be used)
- Gestational
  - Medical nutrition therapy
  - Injectable insulin if glucose level isn't achieved with diet alone (oral antidiabetic agents are teratogenic and are therefore contraindicated during pregnancy)
  - Postpartum counseling to address the high risk of gestational diabetes in subsequent pregnancies and type 2 diabetes later in life

⬤ **Nursing considerations**

- Stress the importance of complying with the prescribed treatment program (diet, exercise, blood glucose monitoring, recognition and treatment of hypoglycemia and hyperglycemia)
- Teach the patient and his family about possible adverse effects of medications
- Watch for complications, especially hypoglycemia (vagueness, slow cerebration, dizziness, weakness, pallor, tachycardia, diaphoresis, seizures, and coma); immediately give carbohydrates, such as fruit juice, hard candy, honey or, if the patient is unconscious, glucagon or dextrose I.V.
- Stay alert for signs of ketoacidosis (acetone breath, dehydration, weak and rapid pulse, Kussmaul's respirations) and hyperosmolar coma (polyuria, thirst, neurologic abnormalities, stupor); these hyperglycemic crises require I.V. fluids and regular insulin
- Teach the patient and his family how to recognize hypoglycemia and ketoacidosis, how to respond, and when to seek medical attention
- Monitor diabetes control by obtaining blood glucose, HbA$_{1c}$, lipid level, and blood pressure measurements regularly
- Watch for diabetic effects on the cardiovascular system and the peripheral and autonomic nervous systems
  - Meticulously treat all injuries, cuts, and blisters
  - Monitor for signs and symptoms of cellulitis (skin reddening and edema, possible blistering or ulceration)
  - Stay alert for signs of urinary tract infection (UTI) and renal disease
- Urge the patient to get regular ophthalmologic examinations to detect diabetic retinopathy
- Assess the patient for signs of diabetic neuropathy (changes in sensation or in motor strength or agility in an extremity)
  - Stress the need for personal safety precautions
  - Minimize complications by maintaining strict blood glucose control
- Teach the patient to care for his feet and inspect for corns, calluses, redness, swelling, bruises, and breaks in the skin, and to report changes to the physician
  - Advise the patient to wear nonconstricting shoes and socks and to avoid walking barefoot
  - Encourage periodic visits to a podiatrist
- Recommend genetic counseling for young adults with diabetes who are planning families

(Text continues on page 298.)

Key treatments for diabetes mellitus

- Insulin replacement (type 1)
- Oral antidiabetics (type 2)
- Meal planning per American Diabetes Association guidelines
- Regular exercise

Key nursing considerations for diabetes mellitus

- Stress the importance of complying with prescribed treatment program.
- Teach patient and family about possible adverse effects of medications.
- Watch for hypoglycemia and ketoacidosis and teach patient and family how to recognize and respond to these complications.
- Monitor blood glucose, HbA$_{1c}$, lipid level, and blood pressure measurements regularly.

GO WITH THE FLOW

Treatment of type 1 diabetes mellitus

This algorithm shows the pathophysiologic process of type 1 diabetes and points for intervention.

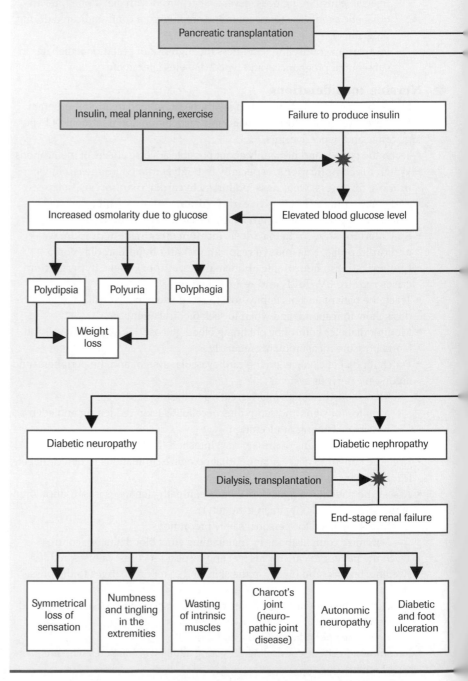

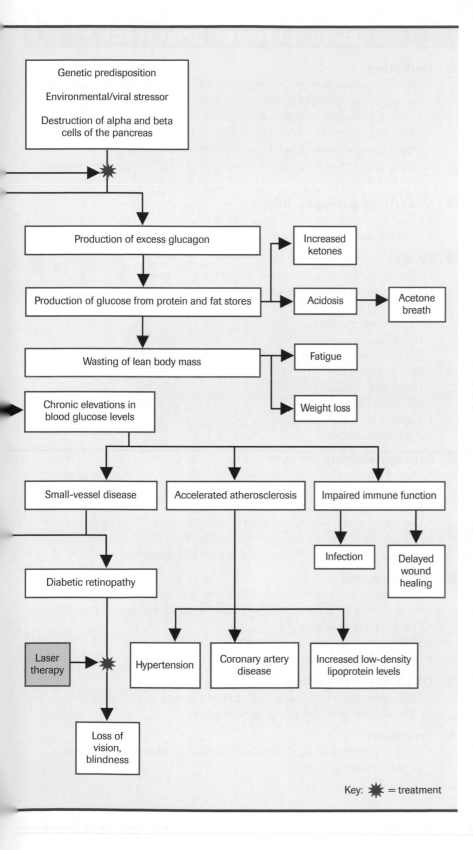

Key: ✸ = treatment

GROWTH HORMONE DEFICIENCY

Key facts about growth hormone deficiency

- Results from hypofunction of anterior pituitary gland
- In children, characterized by subnormal growth rate and delayed bone age
- In adults, characterized by weakness and increased cardio-vascular mortality

Key pathophysiologic changes in growth hormone deficiency

- Short stature
- Reduced muscle mass and increased subcutaneous fat
- Delayed or lack of sexual development

Key diagnostic test result for growth hormone deficiency

- Blood tests: Decreased serum GH and somatomedin C levels

Key treatment for growth hormone deficiency

- Exogenous GH given subQ during puberty

- **Definition**
  - Decreased secretion of growth hormone (GH) resulting from hypofunction of the anterior pituitary gland
  - In children, characterized by subnormal growth rate, delayed bone age, and a subnormal response to at least two stimuli (special test doses of other factors should cause an increase in GH production) to release the hormone
  - Characterized in adults by general weakness and increased cardiovascular mortality

- **Underlying pathophysiology**
  - Absence or deficiency of GH synthesis causes growth failure in children
  - In adults, metabolic derangements decrease GH response to stimulation

- **Causes**
  - Autosomal-recessive, autosomal-dominant, or X-linked trait
  - Pituitary or central nervous system (CNS) tumor
  - Pituitary hypoxic necrosis
  - Pituitary inflammation
  - Hypothalamic failure
  - GH receptor insensitivity
  - Biologically inactive GH
  - Hematologic disorders
  - Idiopathic causes
  - Trauma
  - Pituitary irradiation

- **Pathophysiologic changes**
  - Short stature (two standard deviations less than the predicted mean for age and gender) resulting from GH deficiency
  - Reduced muscle mass and increased subcutaneous fat due to decreased protein synthesis and insufficient muscle anabolism caused by GH deficiency
  - Hypoglycemia (usually in neonates) resulting from GH deficiency
  - Delayed or lack of sexual development from GH deficiency

- **Complications**
  - Short stature and possible related psychosocial difficulties (if untreated)
  - Fatal seizures, especially during periods of stress, due to fasting hypoglycemia
  - Gonadotropin deficiency
  - Multiple pituitary hormone deficiencies
  - Increased cardiovascular mortality (adults)

- **Diagnostic test findings**
  - Blood testing reveals decreased serum GH and somatomedin C levels
  - Xrays show delayed closures of bony epiphyses

- **Treatment**
  - Exogenous GH given subQ up to several times weekly (see *Indications for growth hormone replacement*)

Indications for growth hormone replacement

Recombinant human growth hormone therapy is indicated for the following conditions:
- growth failure in children with inadequate secretion of endogenous growth hormone
- growth failure in children caused by chronic renal insufficiency (until kidney transplantation)
- short stature related to Turner's syndrome
- growth failure in children with Prader-Willi syndrome
- idiopathic short stature in children who are less than 2.25 standard deviations below the mean in height and who are unlikely to catch up
- intrauterine growth restriction (small for gestational age) in children who haven't reached a normal height range by age 2
- lack of endogenous growth hormone deficiency in adults
- acquired immunodeficiency syndrome wasting in adults.

Key nursing considerations for growth hormone deficiency
- Stress the need to take replacement GH as directed and to obtain ongoing follow-up care.

Nursing considerations
- Stress the need to take replacement GH as directed and to obtain ongoing follow-up care

GROWTH HORMONE EXCESS

Definition
- Slow but progressive disease that decreases longevity if untreated (morbidity and mortality tend to be related to coronary artery disease and hypertension)
- Two forms: acromegaly (GH excess that begins in adulthood after epiphyseal closure), or pituitary gigantism (GH excess that's present before closure of the epiphyseal growth plates of the long bones)
- Acromegaly and pituitary gigantism result in increased growth of bone, cartilage, and other tissues as well as increased catabolism of carbohydrates and protein synthesis
- Earliest clinical sign of acromegaly is soft-tissue swelling of the extremities, causing coarsening and hypertrophy of the facial features
- In gigantism, proportional overgrowth of all body tissues starts before epiphyseal closure, causing remarkable height increases — as much as 6" (15.2 cm) per year
  - Affects infants and children, causing them to reach as much as three times the normal height for their age
  - May reach a height of more than 7.5' (228.6 cm) as adults

Underlying pathophysiology
- GH-secreting tumor creates an unpredictable GH secretion pattern, which replaces the usual peaks that occur 1 to 4 hours after the onset of sleep
- Elevated GH and somatomedin levels stimulate tissue growth

Key facts about growth hormone excess
- Results from a GH-secreting tumor

Acromegaly
- Begins in adulthood
- Increases bone density and width
- Increases proliferation of connective and soft tissues

Gigantism
- Starts before epiphyseal closure
- Stimulates linear growth
- Increases bulk of bones and joints
- Causes enlargement of internal organs and metabolic abnormalities

- In pituitary gigantism, because the epiphyseal plates aren't closed, the excess GH stimulates linear growth; it also increases the bulk of bones and joints and causes enlargement of internal organs and metabolic abnormalities
- In acromegaly, the excess GH increases bone density and width and the proliferation of connective and soft tissues

Causes
- Eosinophilic or mixed-cell adenomas of the anterior pituitary gland

Pathophysiologic changes
- Acromegaly
  - Diaphoresis, oily skin, hypermetabolism, hypertrichosis (excessive hair growth), weakness, arthralgia, malocclusion of the teeth, and new skin tags (typical) resulting from GH excess
  - Severe headache, CNS impairment, bitemporal hemianopsia (defective vision), loss of visual acuity, and blindness due to the intrasellar tumor compressing the optic chiasm or nerves
  - Characteristic hulking appearance, with an enlarged supraorbital ridge and thickened ears and nose due to cartilaginous and connective tissue overgrowth
  - Marked prognathism (projection of the jaw) that may interfere with chewing related to cartilage and tissue overgrowth
  - Laryngeal hypertrophy, paranasal sinus enlargement, and thickening of the tongue causing the voice to sound deep and hollow related to GH excess
  - Arrowhead appearance of distal phalanges (on X-rays), and thickened fingers caused by GH excess
  - Irritability, hostility, and various psychological disturbances related to GH excess
  - Bowlegs, barrel chest, arthritis, osteoporosis, kyphosis, hypertension, and arteriosclerosis caused by prolonged effects of excessive GH secretion
  - Glucose intolerance and clinical diabetes mellitus due to action of GH as an insulin antagonist
- Gigantism
  - Backache, arthralgia, and arthritis due to rapid bone growth
  - Excessive height due to rapid growth before epiphyseal plate closure
  - Headache, vomiting, seizure activity, vision disturbances, and papilledema (edema where the optic nerve enters the eye chamber) due to a tumor compressing nerves and tissue in surrounding structures
  - Deficiencies of other hormone systems due to destruction of other hormone-secreting cells by the GH-producing tumor
  - Glucose intolerance and diabetes mellitus due to insulin-antagonistic actions of GH

Complications
- Cardiomegaly
- Hypertension (may increase risk of myocardial infarction or stroke)
- Diabetes mellitus

Key pathophysiologic changes in growth hormone excess

Acromegaly
- Hulking appearance
- Deep-sounding voice
- Headache
- Vision changes
- Irritability and psychological disturbances
- Hypertension
- Arthritis
- Arteriosclerosis
- Diabetes mellitus

Gigantism
- Excessive height
- Arthralgia
- Deficiencies of other hormones

Diagnostic test findings

- Radioimmunoassay reveals elevated plasma GH level (results of random sampling may be misleading because of pulsatile GH secretion)
    - Elevated somatomedin C, a metabolite of GH, is a better diagnostic alternative
- Glucose suppression test is used to confirm the diagnosis (because glucose normally suppresses GH secretion, if glucose infusion doesn't suppress GH to less than 2 ng/ml and the patient has characteristic clinical features, hyperpituitarism is likely)
- Skull X-rays, CT scan, or MRI show the presence and extent of the pituitary lesion
- Bone X-rays show a thickening of the cranium (especially frontal, occipital, and parietal bones) and long bones and osteoarthritis in the spine (supporting the diagnosis)
- Blood testing reveals elevated blood glucose levels

Treatment

- Tumor removal by cranial or transsphenoidal hypophysectomy or by pituitary radiation
- Mandatory surgery for a tumor causing blindness or other severe neurologic disturbances (acromegaly)
- Thyroid, cortisone, and gonadal hormone replacement therapy (postoperative) (see *Teaching your patient about corticosteroids*, page 302)
- Bromocriptine and octreotide (Sandostatin) to inhibit GH synthesis (adjunctive treatment)

Nursing considerations

- Provide emotional support to help the patient cope with an altered body image
- Perform or assist with ROM exercises to promote maximal joint mobility and prevent injury; evaluate muscle weakness, especially in a patient with late-stage acromegaly
- Keep the skin dry; avoid using an oily lotion because the skin is already oily
- If the patient has a hemianopia (loss of half of the visual field in one or both eyes), stand where he can see you
- Reassure the patient's family that mood changes result from the disease and can be modified with treatment
- For the pediatric patient undergoing surgery
    - Provide the child with an age-appropriate explanation
    - Explain to the parents that surgery prevents permanent soft-tissue deformities but won't correct bone changes that have already occurred
    - If needed, arrange for counseling to help the child and his parents cope with these permanent alterations
    - Diligently monitor the child's vital signs and neurologic status after surgery
    - Before discharge, emphasize the importance of continuing hormone replacement therapy

Key diagnostic test results for growth hormone excess

- Glucose suppression test: Doesn't suppress GH to less than 2 ng/ml
- Skull X-rays, CT scan, or MRI: Presence and extent of pituitary lesion

Key treatments for growth hormone excess

- Tumor removal by surgery or radiation
- Postoperative thyroid, cortisone, and gonadal hormone replacement therapy
- Bromocriptine and octreotide

Key nursing considerations for growth hormone excess

- Provide emotional support.
- Perform or assist with ROM.
- Evaluate muscle weakness.
- Instruct patient to get follow-up examinations at least once per year.

TOP 3

Teaching tips about corticosteroids

1. Take the medication exactly as prescribed.
2. Don't stop the drug abruptly.
3. Call the prescriber immediately if vomiting; black, tarry stools; irregular heartbeat; lower extremity swelling; bone pain; markedly increased thirst and urination; severe headache; weight loss, or mood changes occur.

Key facts about hyperparathyroidism

- Results from excessive PTH secretion

Primary
- Develops when parathyroid glands increase PTH secretion
- Causes increased levels of circulating calcium

Secondary
- Develops due to an abnormality outside of the parathyroid gland that causes a low calcium level
- Stimulates compensatory PTH secretion

TIME-OUT FOR TEACHING

Teaching your patient about corticosteroids

Cover these teaching points with a patient who's beginning corticosteroid therapy for the first time:
- Teach your patient to take the drug exactly as prescribed and not to adjust the dose or stop the drug abruptly.
  – Stopping without weaning can precipitate a crisis.
  – Missed doses should be taken as soon as possible but never doubled.
- Instruct your patient to report these major adverse reactions to steroid therapy:
  – nausea, vomiting (especially if emesis looks like coffee grounds), diarrhea, or black tarry stools
  – palpitations or a feeling of irregular heart beat
  – swelling of the feet or lower legs
  – weakness, dizziness, giddiness or depression, or excessive fatigue
  – increased urination, increased thirst, decreased weight, or bad headache
  – bone pain.

- Inform the patient that acne and increased fat on the face and trunk are normal but not serious side effects, as are increased appetite and improved mood.
- Tell the patient that the drug should be taken with food to prevent GI distress, but to avoid caffeine, alcohol, tobacco, and aspirin to avoid further stress on the stomach.
- Suggest that your patient eat foods high in calcium, and encourage him to talk to his physician about whether a calcium supplement would be helpful in maintaining bone strength while on steroid therapy.
- Stress the importance of avoiding sources of infection and keeping wounds clean because of immunosuppression; instruct your patient to see his physician for evaluation of poorly healing wounds.
- Inform the patient to check with his physician before taking over-the-counter or herbal products; make sure that all his healthcare providers are aware that he's taking a corticosteroid.

- Instruct the patient to get follow-up examinations at least once per year because of the slight chance that the tumor that caused the hyperpituitarism may recur

HYPERPARATHYROIDISM

● **Definition**
- Metabolic imbalance that results from excessive parathyroid hormone (PTH) secretion from one or more of the four parathyroid glands
- Classified as primary or secondary

Underlying pathophysiology

- In primary hyperparathyroidism, one or more parathyroid glands enlarge and increase PTH secretion and serum calcium level, or an adenoma secretes PTH; unresponsive to negative feedback of serum calcium
- In secondary hyperparathyroidism, a hypocalcemia-producing abnormality outside the parathyroid glands, such as decreased intestinal absorption of calcium or vitamin D, causes excessive compensatory production of PTH and isn't responsive to PTH
- Increased PTH levels act directly on the bone and the kidney tubules, resulting in an increase in extracellular calcium
- Renal excretion and uptake into the soft tissues or skeleton can't compensate for the excess calcium

Causes

- Adenoma
- Genetic disorders
- Multiple endocrine neoplasia
- Dietary vitamin D or calcium deficiency
- Decreased intestinal absorption of vitamin D or calcium
- Chronic renal failure
- Osteomalacia
- Ingestion of drugs such as phenytoin
- Laxative ingestion
- Idiopathic

Pathophysiologic changes

- Polyuria, nephrocalcinosis, nocturia, polydipsia, dehydration, uremia symptoms, renal colic pain, nephrolithiasis, and renal insufficiency related to hypercalcemia
- Vague aches and pains, arthralgia, and localized swelling due to hypercalcemia
- Chronic lower back pain and increased susceptibility to fractures due to bone degeneration; bone tenderness; chondrocalcinosis (decreased bone mass); osteopenia and osteoporosis, especially of the vertebrae; erosions of the juxtaarticular (adjoining joint) surface; subchondral fractures; traumatic synovitis; and pseudogout caused by hypercalcemia
- Pancreatitis, causing constant, severe epigastric pain that radiates to the back; peptic ulcers, causing abdominal pain, anorexia, nausea, and vomiting resulting from hypercalcemia
- Muscle weakness and atrophy, particularly in the legs, caused by hypercalcemia
- Psychomotor and personality disturbances, emotional lability, depression, slow mentation, poor memory, drowsiness, ataxia, overt psychosis, stupor and, possibly, coma due to excess calcium
- Pruritus caused by ectopic calcifications in the skin
- Skin necrosis, cataracts, calcium microthrombi to the lungs and pancreas, anemia, and subcutaneous calcification due to hypercalcemia
- In secondary hyperparathyroidism: fewer clinical features (may be lack of sufficient calcium instead of excess), possible skeletal deformities of the long

Key pathophysiologic changes in hyperparathyroidism

- Renal insufficiency
- Dehydration
- Osteopenia and osteoporosis
- Pseudogout
- Muscle weakness
- Psychomotor and personality disturbances

bones (such as rickets from vitamin D deficiency), and symptoms of the underlying disease
  – Enlarged glands may not revert to normal size and function even after calcium level has been controlled in the patient with chronic secondary hyperparathyroidism

● **Complications**
  • Pathologic fractures
  • Renal damage
  • UTIs
  • Hypertension
  • Cardiac arrhythmias
  • Insulin hypersecretion, decreased insulin sensitivity
  • Pseudogout

● **Diagnostic test findings**
  • Primary
    – Blood testing reveals increased alkaline phosphatase and serum amylase levels (may indicate acute pancreatitis); elevated total and ionized serum calcium, serum chloride, alkaline phosphatase, and uric acid and creatinine levels (may also increase basal gastric acid secretion and serum immunoreactive gastrin); and decreased serum phosphorus level
    – Radioimmunoassay shows increased serum PTH (confirms the diagnosis)
    – X-rays show diffuse demineralization of bones, bone cysts, outer cortical bone absorption, and subperiosteal erosion of the phalanges and distal clavicles
    – Microscopic bone examination by X-ray spectrophotometry shows increased bone turnover
    – Urine testing reveals an elevated calcium level
  • Secondary
    – Blood testing reveals increased serum PTH and serum calcium levels, variable serum phosphorus level (normal or slightly decreased, especially when the cause is rickets), and osteomalacia or kidney disease (also seen in X-rays and scans showing bony abnormalities or kidney stones)

● **Treatment**
  • Primary
    – Surgery to remove the adenoma or, depending on the extent of hyperplasia, all but half of one gland to produce normal PTH levels (may relieve bone pain within 3 days, but renal damage may be irreversible)
      • I.V. magnesium and phosphate, or sodium phosphate solution by mouth or retention enema (for potential postoperative magnesium and phosphate deficiencies) and, possibly, supplemental calcium, vitamin D, or calcitriol (Calcijex) (serum calcium decreases to low-normal range during the first 4 to 5 days after surgery)
    – Force fluids, limit dietary intake of calcium, and promote sodium and calcium excretion through forced diuresis (using as much as 6 qt [6 L] of urine output in life-threatening circumstances), and use of furosemide (Lasix) or ethacrynic acid (Edecrin) (preoperatively or if surgery isn't feasible or necessary) to lower calcium level

Key diagnostic test results for hyperparathyroidism

- Radioimmunoassay: Increased serum PTH
- Blood testing: Increased total and ionized serum calcium level, decreased serum phosphorus level

Key treatments for hyperparathyroidism

- Increased fluid intake
- Diuretics
- Oral sodium or potassium phosphate, subQ or I.M. calcitonin, and I.V. plicamycin
- Surgery to remove parathyroid tumors or glands

- Oral sodium or potassium phosphate, subQ or I.M. calcitonin (Miacalcin), and I.V. plicamycin (Mithracin) to promote excess calcium excretion
- Secondary
  - Vitamin D to correct the underlying cause of parathyroid hyperplasia; aluminum hydroxide preparation to correct hyperphosphatemia in the patient with kidney disease
  - Dialysis (may be lifelong) in the patient with renal failure to decrease phosphorus level
  - For severe hypercalcemia (serum calcium greater than 14 mg/dl) or for the patient with severe symptoms, calcitonin along with hydration; possible initiation of pamidronate (Aredia) to provide a longer-lasting effect

Nursing considerations
- Obtain pretreatment baseline serum potassium, calcium, phosphate, and magnesium levels
- During hydration to reduce serum calcium level, record intake and output accurately
  - Strain urine to check for calculi
  - Provide at least 3 qt (3 L) of fluid per day, including cranberry or prune juice to increase urine acidity and help prevent calculus formation
- Auscultate breath sounds often, listening for signs of pulmonary edema
- Carefully monitor the patient on cardiac glycosides because an elevated calcium level can rapidly produce toxic effects
- Because the patient is predisposed to pathologic fractures, take safety precautions to minimize the risk of injury
- Watch for signs of peptic ulcer and administer antacids as appropriate
- After parathyroidectomy
  - Check frequently for respiratory distress and keep a tracheotomy tray at the bedside; watch for postoperative complications, such as laryngeal nerve damage or, rarely, hemorrhage
  - Monitor intake and output carefully
  - Check for swelling at the operative site; place the patient in semi-Fowler's position, and support his head and neck with sandbags to decrease edema, which may cause pressure on the trachea
  - Watch for signs of mild tetany such as complaints of tingling in the hands and around the mouth; these symptoms should subside quickly but may be prodromal signs of tetany, so keep calcium gluconate or calcium chloride I.V. available for emergency administration
  - Watch for increased neuromuscular irritability and other signs of severe tetany, and report them immediately
  - Have the patient walk as soon as possible because pressure on the bones speeds up bone recalcification
  - Check laboratory results for low serum calcium and magnesium levels
  - Monitor the patient's mental status and watch for listlessness
- Before discharge, advise the patient of possible adverse effects of drug therapy and the need for periodic follow-up laboratory blood tests
- If hyperparathyroidism isn't corrected surgically, caution the patient to avoid calcium-containing antacids and thiazide diuretics

Key nursing considerations for hyperparathyroidism
- Strain urine to check for calculi.
- Auscultate for signs of pulmonary edema.

After parathyroidectomy
- Check frequently for respiratory distress.
- Check for swelling at the operative site.
- Watch for postoperative complications.
- Watch for signs of tetany.

Key facts about hyperthyroidism

- Overproduction of thyroid hormone
- Also known as *thyrotoxicosis*
- Results when thyroid-stimulating antibodies bind to and stimulate TSH receptors
- Appears most commonly as Graves' disease

Key pathophysiologic changes in hyperthyroidism

- Enlarged thyroid
- Nervousness
- Heat intolerance
- Tremor and palpitations
- Hypertension

Thyroid storm
- Tachycardia
- Vomiting
- High fever
- Vomiting
- Shock
- Coma

HYPERTHYROIDISM

● Definition
- Metabolic imbalance that results from the overproduction of thyroid hormone
- Most common form is Graves' disease, which increases thyroxine (T_4) production, enlarges the thyroid gland (goiter), and causes multiple system changes (see *Other forms of hyperthyroidism*)
- Also known as *thyrotoxicosis*
- Thyroid storm — (an acute, severe exacerbation of thyrotoxicosis) is a medical emergency that may have life-threatening cardiac, hepatic, or renal consequences

● Underlying pathophysiology
- Although the exact mechanism isn't understood, hyperthyroidism has a hereditary component and is occasionally associated with other autoimmune endocrinopathies
- T-cell lymphocytes become sensitized to thyroid antigens and stimulate B-cell lymphocytes to secrete autoantibodies
- Thyroid-stimulating antibodies bind to and stimulate thyroid-stimulating hormone (TSH) receptors of the thyroid gland
- This stimulation increases production of thyroid hormones and cell growth

● Causes
- Genetic factors
- Occasional coexistence with other endocrine abnormalities, such as type 1 diabetes mellitus, thyroiditis, and hyperparathyroidism
- Clinical thyrotoxicosis precipitated by excessive dietary intake of iodine or possibly stress (patients with latent disease)
- Medications, such as lithium and amiodarone
- Toxic nodules or tumors
- Precipitating factors (surgery, infection, toxemia of pregnancy, or DKA)

● Pathophysiologic changes
- Hyperthyroidism
  - Enlarged thyroid (goiter), nervousness, heat intolerance and sweating, weight loss despite increased appetite, frequent bowel movements, tremor and palpitations, and hypertension due to increased amounts of thyroid hormone
  - Exophthalmos (characteristic, but absent in many patients with thyrotoxicosis) caused by cytokine-mediated activation of orbital tissue fibroblasts
  - Difficulty concentrating related to accelerated cerebral function
  - Fine tremor, shaky handwriting, and clumsiness due to increased activity in spinal cord area that controls muscle tone
  - Pretibial myxedema, localized dry, waxy type of swelling with papules or plaques of hyaluronic acid in the dermus due to uncertain cause, probable autoantibodies directed against thyroid antigens
  - Ackopachy, clubbing of the fingers and toes, due to excess thyroid hormone

Other forms of hyperthyroidism

Hyperthyroidism is a metabolic imbalance that results from the overproduction of thyroid hormone (TH). The disorder can take several forms, which are described here:

- *Toxic adenoma,* a small, benign nodule in the thyroid gland that secretes TH, is the second most common cause of hyperthyroidism. The cause of toxic adenoma is unknown; incidence is highest in elderly patients. Clinical effects are essentially similar to those of Graves' disease, except that toxic adenoma doesn't cause ophthalmopathy, pretibial myxedema, or acropachy. The adenoma is confirmed by radioactive iodine (^{131}I) uptake and thyroid scanning, which show a single hyperfunctioning nodule suppressing the rest of the gland. Treatment includes ^{131}I therapy or surgery to remove the adenoma after a euthyroid state is achieved with antithyroid drugs.
- *Thyrotoxicosis factitia* results from chronic ingestion of TH for thyrotropin suppression in patients with thyroid carcinoma or from TH abuse by people who are trying to lose weight.
- *Functioning metastatic thyroid carcinoma* is a rare disease that causes excess TH production.
- *Thyroid-stimulating hormone-secreting pituitary tumor* causes overproduction of TH.
- *Subacute thyroiditis* is a virus-induced, granulomatous inflammation of the thyroid that produces transient hyperthyroidism associated with fever, pain, pharyngitis, and tenderness in the thyroid gland.
- *Silent thyroiditis* is a self-limiting, transient form of hyperthyroidism, with histologic thyroiditis but no inflammatory symptoms.

- Thyroid storm
  - Hypertension, tachycardia, vomiting, high fever, pulmonary edema, shock, tremors, emotional lability, extreme irritability, confusion, delirium, psychosis, apathy, stupor, coma, diarrhea, abdominal pain, nausea and vomiting, jaundice, and hyperglycemia due to increased catecholamine response and hyperthyroid state

Complications
- Muscle wasting, atrophy, and paralysis
- Vision loss or diplopia
- Heart failure, arrhythmias
- Hypoparathyroidism after thyroidectomy
- Hypothyroidism after radioactive iodine (^{131}I) treatment

Diagnostic test findings
- Radioimmunoassay shows increased serum T_4 and triiodothyronine (T_3) levels
- Blood testing reveals decreased TSH level
- Thyroid scan shows an increased uptake of ^{131}I in Graves' disease and, usually, in toxic multinodular goiter and toxic adenoma; low radioactive uptake in thyroiditis and thyrotoxic factitia (test contraindicated in pregnancy)
- Ultrasonography confirms subclinical ophthalmopathy

Key treatments for hyperthyroidism

- Antithyroid drugs
- Surgery
- ^{131}I treatment
- Supportive care (thyroid storm)

Key nursing considerations for hyperthyroidism

- Monitor vital signs, serum electrolyte level, ECG, and LOC.
- Watch for signs of thyroid storm.
- Avoid excessive palpation of thyroid.

After thyroidectomy

- Monitor for respiratory distress.
- Keep tracheotomy tray at bedside.
- Watch for evidence of hemorrhage into the neck.
- Keep patient in semi-Fowler's position, and support his head and neck with sandbags.
- Check for dysphagia or hoarseness.
- Watch for signs of hypocalcemia.

After ^{131}I treatment

- Mix iodide with milk, juice, or water to prevent GI distress.
- Tell patient not to expectorate or cough freely.
- Be aware that traces of iodine may remain in the body for up to 1 week.
- Have patient avoid contact with infants and children for 1 week after treatment.

● **Treatment**
- Antithyroid drugs for new-onset Graves' disease (preferred because of spontaneous remission in many patients; also used to correct the thyrotoxic state in preparation for ^{131}I treatment or surgery)
- Thyroid hormone antagonists, including propylthiouracil and methimazole (Tapazole), to block thyroid hormone synthesis
- Propranolol (Inderal) until antithyroid drugs reach their full effect, to manage tachycardia and other peripheral effects of excessive hypersympathetic activity resulting from blocking the conversion of T_4 to active T_3
- Single oral dose of ^{131}I (treatment of choice for patients not planning to have children; patients of reproductive age must give informed consent for this treatment because ^{131}I concentrates in the gonads)
    - In most patients, hypermetabolic symptoms diminish 6 to 8 weeks after treatment (some require a second dose)
    - Almost all patients treated with ^{131}I eventually become hypothyroid
- Subtotal thyroidectomy to decrease the thyroid gland's capacity for hormone production (patients who refuse or aren't candidates for ^{131}I treatment)
- Iodides (Lugol's solution or saturated solution of potassium iodide), antithyroid drugs, and propranolol to relieve hyperthyroidism preoperatively (if patient doesn't become euthyroid, surgery should be delayed and antithyroid drugs and propranolol given to decrease the systemic effects of thyrotoxicosis)
- Emergency treatment of thyroid storm
    - An antithyroid drug
    - Corticosteroids
    - Supportive measures, including nutrients, vitamins, fluids, oxygen, hypothermia blankets, and sedatives

● **Nursing considerations**
- Monitor serum electrolyte level
- Monitor the electrocardiogram (ECG) for arrhythmias and ST-segment changes
- Check the patient's LOC
- Encourage bed rest, and keep the patient's room cool, quiet, and dark
- Optimize comfort by placing the dyspneic patient in high Fowler's position or help him to sit upright
- Reassure the patient and his family that bizarre behavior will probably subside with treatment, and provide ordered sedatives as necessary
- Provide a balanced diet with six meals per day; if the patient has edema, suggest a low-sodium diet
- If iodide is part of the treatment, mix it with milk, juice, or water to prevent GI distress, and administer it through a straw to prevent tooth discoloration
- Watch for signs of thyroid storm (tachycardia, hyperkinesis, fever, vomiting, hypertension)
- Monitor intake and output to ensure adequate hydration and fluid balance
- Closely monitor the patient's vital signs
- Maintain an I.V. line and give drugs as ordered
- Suggest sunglasses to protect exophthalmic eyes from light; frequently moisten the conjunctivae with isotonic eye drops
- Avoid excessive palpation of the thyroid to avoid precipitating thyroid storm

- After thyroidectomy
  - Monitor for respiratory distress; keep a tracheotomy tray at the bedside
  - Watch for evidence of hemorrhage into the neck such as a tight dressing with no blood on it
  - Change dressings as ordered; check the back of the dressing for drainage
  - Keep the patient in semi-Fowler's position, and support his head and neck with sandbags to ease tension on the incision
  - Check for dysphagia or hoarseness from possible laryngeal nerve injury
  - Watch for signs of hypocalcemia (tetany, numbness), a complication that results from accidental removal of the parathyroid glands during surgery
  - Stress the importance of follow-up after discharge because hypothyroidism may develop 2 to 4 weeks postoperatively
- After drug and ^{131}I therapy
  - Tell the patient not to expectorate or cough freely because his saliva will be radioactive for 24 hours after treatment
  - Stress the need for repeated measurement of serum T_4 levels (the patient shouldn't resume antithyroid therapy)
  - If the patient is taking propylthiouracil or methimazole, monitor CBC periodically, and tell him to take these medications with meals and to avoid over-the-counter cough preparations (many contain iodine)
  - Instruct the patient to report fever, enlarged cervical lymph nodes, sore throat, mouth sores, and other signs of blood dyscrasias and any rash or skin eruptions (signs of hypersensitivity)
  - Watch the patient taking propranolol for signs of hypotension (dizziness, decreased urine output); tell him to change positions slowly)
  - Instruct the patient receiving antithyroid drugs or ^{131}I therapy to report symptoms of hypothyroidism
  - Caution the patient receiving ^{131}I therapy
    - Traces of iodine may remain in the body for up to 1 week; patients may trigger radioactivity sensors, such as in airports, for 3 to 4 days after treatment
    - During the first week after treatment, women shouldn't breast-feed and all patients should avoid close contact with infants and children

HYPOTHYROIDISM IN ADULTS

Definition
- Metabolic imbalance that results from hypothalamic, pituitary, or thyroid insufficiency or resistance to thyroid hormone
- Can progress to life-threatening myxedema coma

Underlying pathophysiology
- Malfunction of the hypothalamus, pituitary, or thyroid gland (all of which are part of the same negative-feedback mechanism) leads to altered levels of T_3, T_4, TSH, or thyrotropin-releasing hormone (TRH)

Key facts about hypothyroidism

- Results from hypothalamic, pituitary, or thyroid insufficiency or resistance to thyroid hormone
- Leads to altered levels of T_3, T_4, TSH, or TRH

- Thyroid malfunction results in inadequate thyroid hormone production despite adequate pituitary stimulation with TSH and adequate hypothalamic stimulation of the pituitary gland with TRH; this leads to low T_3 and T_4 levels and high TSH and TRH levels
- Hypothalamic malfunction manifests as inadequate TRH production; neither the pituitary nor the thyroid glands receive normal stimulation, and their hormone output is decreased as well
- Pituitary malfunction manifests as normal TRH production by the hypothalamus, but abnormal pituitary response
  - The pituitary gland then underproduces TSH and the thyroid gland responds with decreased thyroid hormone production
  - Because of this decreased production, no signal is sent back to the hypothalamus to alter its production of TRH; this leads to low thyroid hormone levels

Causes

- Thyroidectomy
- Radiation therapy (particularly with ^{131}I)
- Chronic autoimmune thyroiditis (Hashimoto's disease)
- Amyloidosis
- Sarcoidosis (rare)
- Pituitary failure to produce TSH (rarely a cause)
- Hypothalamic failure to produce TRH (rarely a cause)
- Inborn errors of thyroid hormone synthesis
- Iodine deficiency (usually dietary)
- Use of antithyroid medications such as propylthiouracil

Pathophysiologic changes

- Weakness, fatigue, forgetfulness, sensitivity to cold, unexplained weight gain, and constipation (typical, vague, early clinical features) due to hypometabolic state
- Characteristic myxedematous signs and symptoms of decreasing mental stability; coarse, dry, flaky, inelastic skin; puffy face, hands, and feet; hoarseness; periorbital edema; upper eyelid droop; dry, sparse hair; and thick, brittle nails (as disorder progresses) due to fluid accumulation
- Decreased cardiac output, slow pulse rate, signs of poor peripheral circulation and, occasionally, an enlarged heart due to cardiovascular involvement related to mucopolysaccharide deposits
- Progressive stupor, hypoventilation, hypoglycemia, hyponatremia, hypotension, and hypothermia due to progression to myxedema coma (usually gradual but may occur abruptly; related to stress aggravating severe or prolonged hypothyroidism)

Complications

- Heart failure
- Myxedema coma
- Infection
- Megacolon
- Organic psychosis
- Infertility
- Hyperlipidemia

Common causes of hypothyroidism

- Thyroidectomy
- Use of antithyroid medications
- Hashimoto's disease
- Iodine deficiency

Key pathophysiologic changes in hypothyroidism

- Weakness and fatigue
- Forgetfulness
- Unexplained weight gain
- Constipation
- Periorbital edema
- Decreased cardiac output
- Progressive stupor (myxedema coma)

Thyroid test results in hypothyroidism

DYSFUNCTION INVOLVEMENT	THYROTROPIN RELEASING HORMONE	THYROID-STIMULATING HORMONE	TH (TRIIODOTHYRONINE [T_3] AND THYROXINE [T_4])
Hypothalamus	Low	Low	Low
Pituitary gland	High	Low	Low
Thyroid gland	High	High	Low
Peripheral conversion of thyroid hormone (TH)	High	Low or normal	T_3 and T_4 low, but reverse-T_3 elevated

Diagnostic test findings

- Radioimmunoassay shows low T_3 and T_4 levels
- Blood testing reveals increased TSH level when hypothyroidism is caused by thyroid disorder and decreased TSH when the cause is a hypothalamic or pituitary disorder (rare)
- Thyroid panel differentiates between primary hypothyroidism (thyroid gland hypofunction), secondary hypothyroidism (pituitary hyposecretion of TSH), tertiary hypothyroidism (hypothalamic hyposecretion of TRH), and euthyroid sick syndrome (impaired peripheral conversion of thyroid hormone due to a suprathyroidal illness such as severe infection) (see *Thyroid test results in hypothyroidism*)
- Blood testing reveals elevated serum cholesterol, alkaline phosphatase, and triglyceride levels and low serum sodium level
- Arterial blood gas (ABG) analysis shows decreased pH and increased partial pressure of carbon dioxide (indicating respiratory acidosis [myxedema coma])

Treatment

- Gradual thyroid hormone replacement with synthetic T_4 and, occasionally, T_3
- Surgical excision, chemotherapy, or radiation for tumors

Nursing considerations

- Provide a high-bulk, low-calorie diet and encourage activity to combat constipation and promote weight loss; administer cathartics and stool softeners as needed
- After thyroid replacement begins, watch for signs and symptoms of hyperthyroidism, such as restlessness, sweating, and excessive weight loss
- Tell the patient to report signs of aggravated cardiovascular disease, such as chest pain and tachycardia
- To prevent myxedema coma, tell the patient to continue his course of thyroid medication even if his symptoms subside
- Caution the patient to report infection immediately and to inform all prescribing physicians about the underlying hypothyroidism
- Provide supportive care for patients with myxedema coma

Key diagnostic test results for hypothyroidism

- Radioimmunoassay: Low T_3 and T_4 levels
- Thyroid panel: Source of deficient thyroid hormone

Key treatments for hypothyroidism

- Hormone replacement therapy

Key nursing considerations for hypothyroidism

- Watch for signs and symptoms of hyperthyroidism during hormone replacement therapy.
- Tell patient to continue course of thyroid medication even if symptoms subside.
- Monitor ABG values to determine if ventilatory assistance is needed.
- Monitor vital signs for adverse cardiac effects of levothyroxine.

Key facts about SIADH

- Characterized by impaired water excretion with normal sodium excretion
- Causes dilutional hyponatremia
- Results when excessive ADH secretion is triggered by nonphysiologic causes, such as neoplasms or certain drugs

– Check frequently for signs of decreasing cardiac output
– Monitor temperature until stable (provide extra blankets and clothing and a warm room to compensate for hypothermia; rapid rewarming may cause vasodilation and vascular collapse)
– Record intake and output and daily weight; as treatment begins, urine output should increase and body weight should decrease (if not, report this immediately)
– Turn the edematous, bedridden patient every 2 hours, and provide skin care
– Avoid sedation when possible or reduce the dosage because hypothyroidism delays metabolism of many drugs
– Maintain a patent I.V. line, and monitor serum electrolyte level carefully when administering I.V. fluids
– **Monitor the patient's vital signs carefully when administering levothyroxine (Levoxyl, Synthroid) because rapid correction of hypothyroidism can cause adverse cardiac effects (report chest pain or tachycardia immediately, and watch for hypertension and heart failure in the elderly patient)**
– Check ABG values for hypercapnia, metabolic acidosis, and hypoxia to determine whether the severely myxedematous patient requires ventilatory assistance
– Administer corticosteroids as ordered
– Because myxedema coma may have been precipitated by an infection, check possible sources, such as blood and urine, and obtain sputum cultures

SYNDROME OF INAPPROPRIATE ANTIDIURETIC HORMONE

● Definition
- Usually results when excessive antidiuretic hormone (ADH) secretion is triggered by stimuli other than increased extracellular fluid osmolality and decreased extracellular fluid volume
  – Characterized by impaired water excretion with normal sodium excretion, resulting in dilutional hyponatremia
- Relatively common complication of surgery or critical illness
- Also known as SIADH

● Underlying pathophysiology
- In the presence of excessive ADH, excessive water reabsorption from the distal convoluted tubule and collecting ducts causes hyponatremia and normal to slightly increased extracellular fluid volume

● Causes
- Oat cell carcinoma of the lung
- Neoplastic diseases
- CNS disorders, including brain tumor or abscess, stroke, head injury, and Guillain-Barré syndrome
- Pulmonary disorders, including pneumonia, tuberculosis, lung abscess, aspergillosis, bronchiectasis, and positive-pressure ventilation

- Drugs that either increase ADH production or potentiate ADH action, such as antidepressants, nonsteroidal anti-inflammatory drugs, chlorpropamide (Diabinese), vincristine (Oncovin), cyclophosphamide (Cytoxan), carbamazepine (Tegretol), clofibrate (Atromid-S), metoclopramide (Reglan), and morphine (MSIR, Oramorph, Roxanol)
- Miscellaneous conditions, including psychosis, myxedema, acquired immunodeficiency syndrome, physiologic stress (as from surgery or severe infection), and pain

Pathophysiologic changes

- Thirst, anorexia, fatigue, and lethargy (first signs), followed by vomiting and intestinal cramping due to hyponatremia and electrolyte imbalance manifestations
- Weight gain, edema, water retention, and decreased urine output due to hyponatremia
- Restlessness, confusion, anorexia, headache, irritability, decreasing reflexes, seizures, and coma due to electrolyte imbalances, worsening with the degree of water intoxication
- Decreased deep tendon reflexes resulting from hyponatremia and electrolyte imbalances

Complications

- Cerebral edema
- Brain herniation
- Central pontine myelinosis

Diagnostic test findings

- Blood testing reveals elevated serum ADH, serum osmolality less than 280 mOsm/kg of water, and serum sodium less than 135 mEq/L (lower values indicate worse condition)
- Urinalysis reveals an elevated sodium level (more than 20 mEq/L) and increased osmolality (greater than 150 mOsm/kg)

Treatment

- Restricted water intake (500 to 1,000 ml/day) as symptomatic treatment
- **Administration of 200 to 300 ml of 3% saline solution to slowly and steadily increase the serum sodium level (severe water intoxication); too rapid a rise may result in cerebral edema**
- Correction of the underlying cause, when possible
- Surgical resection, irradiation, or chemotherapy to alleviate water retention for syndrome of inappropriate antidiuretic hormone resulting from cancer
- Demeclocycline (Declomycin) to block the renal response to ADH (if fluid restriction is ineffective)
- Furosemide (Lasix) with normal or hypertonic saline to maintain urine output and block ADH secretion

Nursing considerations

- Closely monitor and record intake and output, vital signs, and daily weight; watch for hyponatremia
- Observe for restlessness, irritability, seizures, heart failure, and unresponsiveness due to hyponatremia and water intoxication

Key pathophysiologic changes in SIADH

- Thirst, anorexia, fatigue, and lethargy (first signs)
- Decreasing reflexes
- Seizures

Key diagnostic test results for SIADH

- Blood testing: Elevated serum ADH, serum osmolality less than 280 mOsm/kg of water, serum sodium less than 135 mEq/L

Key treatments for SIADH

- Correction of underlying cause
- Furosemide with normal or hypertonic saline solution

Key nursing considerations for SIADH

- Monitor and record intake and output, vital signs, and daily weight.
- Watch for hyponatremia.
- Monitor for symptoms of water intoxication.

TOP 6

Items to study for your next test on the endocrine system

1. Source, target organs or structures, and functions of hormones, such as cortisol, aldosterone, GH, and TSH
2. Pathophysiologic changes associated with diabetes mellitus
3. Differences between Addison's disease and Cushing's syndrome
4. Common treatments for endocrine disorders
5. Nursing considerations for patients with endocrine disorders
6. Major teaching points for patients receiving corticosteroids

• To prevent water intoxication, explain to the patient and his family why he must restrict his intake

NCLEX CHECKS

It's never too soon to begin your licensure examination preparation. Now that you've reviewed this chapter, carefully read each of the following questions and choose the best answer. Then compare your responses with the correct answers.

1. A client is being evaluated for weakness, fatigue, anorexia, and nausea, with a 15 lb [6.8 kg] weight loss in 1 month, blood pressure of 90/56 mm Hg standing and 120/70 mm Hg sitting, and severe anxiety. The diagnosis after testing is addisonian crisis. The nurse explains that the source of the pathophysiologic changes causing adrenal crisis is:

☐ 1. an autoimmune process.
☐ 2. an infection.
☐ 3. exhausted stores of glucocorticoids.
☐ 4. lack of thyroid hormones.

2. When caring for a patient with Cushing's syndrome, it's important to monitor the laboratory reports for hypokalemia, hypocalcemia, and:

☐ 1. hypoglycemia.
☐ 2. hypernatremia.
☐ 3. hyponatremia.
☐ 4. hypochloridemia.

3. A client with type 1 diabetes mellitus has been treated for weakness, increased edema, muscle twitching, and an irregular pulse. Place these pathophysiologic changes in chronological order to demonstrate the sequence leading to these diabetic complications.

1. Diabetic nephropathy	
2. Chronic elevation in blood glucose levels	
3. Small-vessel disease	
4. Destruction of alpha and beta cells of the pancreas	
5. Glomerular filtration rate of 15% of normal (end-stage renal disease)	
6. Failure to produce insulin	

4. A client with diabetes complains of fatigue, lethargy, and headaches. The nurse teaches the client that these symptoms are the result of which pathophysiologic change?

- [ ] **1.** Low intracellular glucose levels
- [ ] **2.** Electrolyte imbalances
- [ ] **3.** Neural tissue damage
- [ ] **4.** Depleted cellular storage of protein

5. A client comes to the physician for a check-up because of bone aches. The physician suspects acromegaly. The nurse is aware that the earliest clinical sign of acromegaly is:

- [ ] **1.** irritability.
- [ ] **2.** barrel chest.
- [ ] **3.** bowlegs.
- [ ] **4.** coarse facial features.

6. A client is being treated for pseudogout. The nurse plans interventions based on the knowledge that pseudo gout is a complication of:

- [ ] **1.** hypoparathyroidism.
- [ ] **2.** hyperparathyroidism.
- [ ] **3.** hypopituitarism.
- [ ] **4.** GH deficiency.

7. In teaching a client about hypothyroidism, the nurse explains that the disorder is a result of a malfunction of the pituitary gland, thyroid gland, or:

- [ ] **1.** pancreas.
- [ ] **2.** parathyroid glands.
- [ ] **3.** adrenal glands.
- [ ] **4.** hypothalamus.

8. The nurse instructs a client with hyperthyroidism that a single dose of ^{131}I will usually cause hypermetabolic symptoms to diminish in:

- [ ] **1.** 4 to 6 weeks.
- [ ] **2.** 6 to 8 weeks.
- [ ] **3.** 4 to 6 months.
- [ ] **4.** 6 to 8 months.

9. The nurse caring for a client with thyroid storm would expect to see hyperkinesis, fever, vomiting, and:

- [ ] **1.** hypertension.
- [ ] **2.** hypotension.
- [ ] **3.** bradycardia.
- [ ] **4.** tachypnea.

10. A 10-year-old client is being evaluated for GH deficiency. The nurse will review the results of which test or finding to best confirm the diagnosis?

- [ ] **1.** Plasma GH level
- [ ] **2.** CT scan of the skull
- [ ] **3.** Radioimmunoassay of plasma GH level
- [ ] **4.** Insulin suppression test

ANSWERS AND RATIONALES

1. CORRECT ANSWER: 3

The pathophysiologic abnormality behind adrenal crisis is a critical deficiency of glucocorticoids as well as mineralocorticoids, generally following acute stress, severe infections, such as sepsis, trauma, or surgery, or the omission of steroid therapy in patients who have chronic adrenal insufficiency. About 80% of clients with the disorder have an underlying autoimmune cause. Lack of thyroid hormones is indicative of hypothyroidism.

2. CORRECT ANSWER: 2

Hypernatremia can occur in Cushing's syndrome due to bone demineralization and fluid retention. Hyperglycemia—not hypoglycemia—occurs in Cushing's syndrome. The chloride level may remain normal or be slightly increased due to the increase—not decrease—in the sodium level.

3. CORRECT ANSWER:

| 4. Destruction of alpha and beta cells of the pancreas |
| 6. Failure to produce insulin |
| 2. Chronic elevation in blood glucose levels |
| 3. Small-vessel disease |
| 1. Diabetic nephropathy |
| 5. Glomerular filtration rate of 15% of normal (end-stage renal disease) |

The pathophysiologic pathway leading to chronic kidney failure begins with pancreatic failure of alpha and beta cells. Blood glucose control with insulin, proper diet, and exercise can prevent the small-vessel disease that damages the kidney and other organs. Kidney dialysis or transplant can prevent end-stage renal failure.

4. CORRECT ANSWER: 1

Headaches, fatigue, lethargy, and reduced energy levels are all due to low intracellular glucose levels. Insulin deficiency compromises the cells' access to essential nutrients for fuel and storage. Electrolyte and protein storage depletion aren't typical of diabetes. Neural tissue damage is generally peripheral, as in peripheral neuropathy, not central to the brain itself.

5. CORRECT ANSWER: 4

The earliest clinical sign of acromegaly is coarsened and hypertrophied (enlarged supraorbital ridge, thickened ears and nose) facial features. This enlargement is related to soft tissue swelling and overgrowth of cartilage. Irritability, barrel chest, and bowlegs are all late signs of the disorder.

6. CORRECT ANSWER: 2

Pseudogout is a complication of hyperparathyroidism and is caused by an increased calcium level. Hypoparathyroidism, hypopituitarism, and decreased GH wouldn't involve increased calcium, which could precipitate a goutlike episode.

7. CORRECT ANSWER: 4

Hypothyroidism is a result of hypothalamus, pituitary, or thyroid insufficiency, or resistance to thyroid hormone, all of which are part of the same negative feedback mechanism. The pancreas is involved in insulin production and secretion. The parathyroid glands are implicated in calcium excess, and the adrenal glands secrete corticosteroids.

8. CORRECT ANSWER: 2

A single oral dose of ^{131}I is the treatment of choice for hyperthyroidism for clients not planning to have children. In most clients, hypermetabolic symptoms diminish 6 to 8 weeks after such treatment; however, some clients may require a second dose.

9. CORRECT ANSWER: 1

Hypertension, not hypotension, can occur in thyroid storm due to increased catecholamine response and a hyperthyroid state. Tachycardia is another common finding.

10. CORRECT ANSWER: 3

Radioimmunoassay of plasma GH level is more accurate than routine plasma GH level due to the frequent fluctuations of GH. A glucose suppression test can help confirm this diagnosis because glucose normally suppresses GH. X-ray and CT scan of the skull may demonstrate pituitary tumors or coarsening of the skull bone.

9

Renal and urinary systems

LEARNING OBJECTIVES

After studying this chapter, you should be able to:

- Describe the relationship between presenting signs and symptoms and the pathophysiologic changes for any renal or urinary system disorder.

- Identify conditions that alter renal function.

- List three probable causes for any renal or urinary disorder.

- Discuss medications that may be used in a patient with a renal or urinary disorder.

- List treatments for a patient with a renal or urinary disorder.

- Write three teaching goals for a patient with a renal or urinary disorder.

CHAPTER OVERVIEW

The kidneys, urethra, ureters, and urinary bladder are essential parts of the body's waste management system as well as its fluid and electrolyte maintenance system. Caring for a patient with a renal or urinary system disorder requires an understanding of the pathophysiologic changes that occur, the signs and symptoms they produce, and the appropriate ways to intervene. The first section of this chapter provides an overview of how osmotic pressure changes and obstruction can affect the renal and urinary systems. Common renal and urinary disorders are then defined, and underlying pathophysiology, causes, pathophysiologic changes, complications, diagnostic test findings, treatments, and nursing considerations are outlined.

PATHOPHYSIOLOGIC CONCEPTS

● **Altered capillary pressure**
- Capillary pressure and glomerular filtration rate (GFR) in the kidneys vary directly with mean arterial pressure (MAP)
  - Normal MAP ranges from 80 to 180 mm Hg; normal GFR is about 120 ml/min
  - GFR decreases steeply if MAP decreases to less than 80 mm Hg
  - Autoregulation of afferent and efferent arterioles affects capillary pressure in the nephron (see *Structure of the nephron,* page 320)
- Increased sympathetic activity and angiotensin II constrict afferent and efferent arterioles, decreasing capillary pressure
- Prostaglandin-mediated relaxation of afferent arterioles and angiotensin II–mediated constriction of efferent arterioles maintain GFR
- Decreased cardiac output diminishes renal perfusion (inadequate renal perfusion accounts for 40% to 80% of acute renal failure)
  - Hypovolemia may reduce circulating blood volume and decrease MAP, decreasing capillary pressure as well
  - Prolonged renal hypoperfusion causes acute tubular necrosis (ATN)
- Drugs that block prostaglandin production (nonsteroidal anti-inflammatory drugs) can cause vasoconstriction and acute renal failure during hypotension
- Emboli or thrombi, aortic dissection, or vasculitis can occlude renal arteries

● **Altered interstitial fluid colloid osmotic pressure**
- Injury to glomeruli or peritubular capillaries can increase interstitial fluid colloid osmotic pressure, drawing fluid out of glomerulus and peritubular capillaries
  - Swelling and edema occur in Bowman's space and in the interstitial space surrounding the collecting tubules
  - Increased interstitial fluid pressure opposes glomerular filtration, causes collapse of surrounding nephron tubules and peritubular capillaries, and leads to hypoxia and renal cell injury or death
  - When cells die, intracellular enzymes are released, stimulating immune and inflammatory reactions
  - Increased interstitial fluid pressure interferes with (duplicative) tubular resorption, rendering the kidney incapable of regulating fluid volume and electrolyte composition
- Glomerular disease disrupts the basement membrane, allowing leakage of large proteins
  - Plasma osmotic pressure decreases and edema results as fluid moves from capillaries into the interstitium
  - Consequent activation of the renin-angiotensin and sympathetic nervous systems increases renal salt and water resorption, which further contributes to edema

● **Obstruction**
- Causes urine to accumulate behind blockage in the urinary tract, leading to infection or damage
- May be congenital or acquired, acute or chronic
  - Acute: complete obstruction increases pressure transmitted to the proximal tubule, inhibiting glomerular filtration

Key facts about altered capillary pressure

- Has direct relationship with MAP
- Affected by autoregulation of afferent and efferent arterioles
- Results when increased sympathetic activity and angiotensin II constrict afferent and efferent arterioles
- Prostaglandin-mediated relaxation of afferent arterioles and angiotensin II-mediated constriction of efferent arterioles maintain GFR

Key facts about altered interstitial fluid colloid osmotic pressure

- If increased, caused by injury to glomeruli or peritubular capillaries
- If decreased, caused by glomerular disease, which causes fluid to move from capillaries into interstitium

Key facts about urinary obstruction

- Causes urine to accumulate behind a blockage in the urinary tract, leading to infection or damage
- May be congenital or acquired, acute or chronic

Key facts about
the nephron

- Kidneys' basic functional unit
- Site of urine formation
- Consists of glomerulus and collecting ducts

Structure of the nephron

The nephron, the kidneys' basic functional unit and the site of urine formation, consists of the glomerulus and a series of collecting ducts. The glomerulus, a cluster of capillaries fed by the afferent arteriole, and the proximal and distal convoluted tubules are located in the cortex of the kidney. The long loops of Henle, together with their accompanying blood vessels and collecting tubules, form the renal pyramids in the medulla of the kidney. The renal artery and its offshoots within the kidneys carry fluid, electrolytes, waste products of metabolism, acids, and bases into the nephron where osmotic pressures selectively cause these items to be retained for excretion through the collecting tubules or returned to the circulation via the venous system.

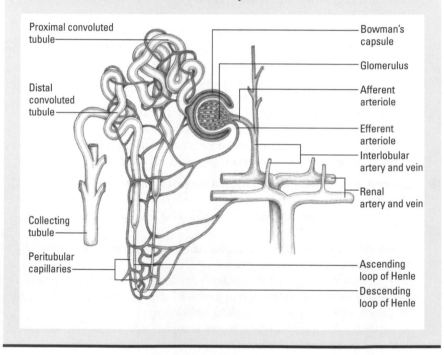

- Chronic: partial obstruction compresses structures as urine accumulates, and results in papillary and medullary infarct; underlying tubular damage decreases the kidney's ability to function
- Tubular obstruction increases interstitial fluid pressure; if unrelieved, the nephron and capillaries collapse and irreversible renal damage results
  - Relief is usually followed by copious diuresis of sodium and water and a return to a normal GFR

ACUTE PYELONEPHRITIS

Key facts about acute pyelonephritis

- Sudden inflammation of kidney caused by bacteria
- May lead to colonies of bacterial infection within 24 to 48 hours
- May occur due to vesicoureteral reflux

Definition
- Sudden inflammation of the kidney caused by bacteria
- One of the most common renal diseases
- May affect one or both kidneys

- Primarily affects the interstitial area and the renal pelvis or, less commonly, the renal tubules

Underlying pathophysiology

- Infection spreads from the bladder to the ureters and then to the kidneys; may occur due to vesicoureteral reflux
- Vesicoureteral reflux may result from congenital weakness at the junction of the ureter and the bladder
- Bacteria refluxed to intrarenal tissues may create colonies of infection within 24 to 48 hours

Causes

- Bacterial infection of the kidneys caused by
  - *Escherichia coli* (most common causative organism)
  - Klebsiella
  - Proteus
  - Pseudomonas
  - *Staphylococcus aureus*
  - *Enterococcus faecalis*

Pathophysiologic changes

- Urinary urgency and frequency, dysuria (burning during urination), nocturia, and hematuria (usually microscopic but may be gross) due to bacterial invasion
- Cloudy urine that has an ammonia-like or fishy odor due to bacterial by-products
- Temperature of 102° F (38.9° C) or higher, shaking chills, nausea and vomiting, flank pain, anorexia, and general fatigue related to inflammation and infection

Complications

- Septic shock
- Chronic pyelonephritis
- Chronic renal insufficiency

Diagnostic test findings

- Urinalysis and urine culture and sensitivity tests reveal pyuria, significant bacteriuria, low specific gravity and osmolality, slightly alkaline urine pH, or proteinuria, glycosuria, and ketonuria (less frequent)
- Blood testing shows elevated white blood cell (WBC) and neutrophil counts and erythrocyte sedimentation rate
- Computed tomography (CT) scan may reveal calculi, tumors, or cysts in the kidneys and urinary tract
- Excretory urography may show asymmetrical kidneys

Treatment

- Antibiotic therapy appropriate for the specific infecting organism after identification by urine culture and sensitivity studies
- Broad-spectrum antibiotics (usually) when the infecting organism can't be identified
  - Antibiotic therapy used with caution in pregnant and elderly patients
- Urinary analgesics such as phenazopyridine (Prodium, Pyridium)
- Surgery to relieve an obstruction or correct an anomaly (may be necessary if infection is caused by an obstruction or vesicoureteral reflux)

Key pathophysiologic changes in acute pyelonephritis

- Urinary urgency and frequency
- Dysuria
- Hematuria
- Temperature of 102° F (38.9° C) or higher
- Flank pain

Key diagnostic test results for acute pyelonephritis

- Urinalysis and urine culture and sensitivity tests: Pyuria and bacteriuria

Key treatments for acute pyelonephritis

- Antibiotic therapy
- Urine reculturing 1 week after treatment and periodically thereafter for those with higher risk of recurrence

Chronic pyelonephritis

Chronic pyelonephritis is a persistent kidney inflammation that can scar the kidneys and may lead to chronic renal failure. Its etiology may be bacterial, metastatic, or urogenous. This disease is most common in patients who are predisposed to recurrent acute pyelonephritis, such as those with urinary obstructions or vesicoureteral reflux.

Patients with chronic pyelonephritis may have a childhood history of unexplained fevers or bed-wetting. Clinical effects may include flank pain, anemia, low urine specific gravity, proteinuria, leukocytes in urine and, especially in late stages, hypertension. Uremia rarely develops from chronic pyelonephritis unless structural abnormalities exist in the excretory system. Bacteriuria may be intermittent. When no bacteria are found in the urine, diagnosis depends on excretory urography (the renal pelvis may appear small and flattened) and renal biopsy.

Effective treatment requires control of hypertension, elimination of the existing obstruction (when possible), and long-term antimicrobial therapy.

- Short term follow-up treatment including urine reculturing 1 week after drug therapy stops
- Long-term follow-up (periodic urine cultures) for patients at high risk for recurring urinary tract and kidney infections, such as those with a long-term indwelling catheter or those on maintenance antibiotic therapy (recurrent episodes of acute pyelonephritis can eventually result in chronic pyelonephritis) (see *Chronic pyelonephritis*)

Nursing considerations
- Administer antipyretics for fever
- Force fluids to achieve urine output of more than 2,000 ml per day to help empty the bladder of contaminated urine and prevent calculi formation (discourage intake of more than 2 to 3 qt [2 to 2.8 L] because this may decrease the effectiveness of the antibiotics)
- Provide an acid-ash diet to prevent calculus formation (see *Your renal patient's diet*)
- Teach the proper technique for collecting a clean-catch urine specimen
- Stress the need to complete prescribed antibiotic therapy even after symptoms subside
- Take steps to prevent recurrent-acute or chronic pyelonephritis
  - Observe strict sterile technique during catheter insertion and care
  - Teach female patients to prevent bacterial contamination by wiping the perineum from front to back after defecation
  - Advise routine checkups for patients with a history of urinary tract infections (UTIs), and teach them to recognize signs of infection (cloudy urine, burning on urination, urgency, and frequency, especially when accompanied by flank pain and a low-grade fever)

TIME-OUT FOR TEACHING

Your renal patient's diet

Your patient may be given one of several different diets depending on the cause and extent of renal insufficiency. Here are a few of the special diets you may need to explain to your patient.

TYPE OF DIET	PURPOSE AND INSTRUCTIONS
Acid-ash	• Used to acidify the urine to prevent calcific kidney stones • Eat meat, fish, eggs, and cereals • Minimize fruits and vegetables • Eliminate cheese and milk (dairy)
Low-oxalate	• Used to prevent oxalate kidney stones • Eliminate potatoes, beans, fiber vegetables, sweet fruits and teas, chocolate, and sweets in general
High-calorie, low-protein	• Used to decrease protein load and maintain weight in renal insufficiency and failure (degree of protein limitation varies with extent of disease) • Eat beef, pork, poultry, fish, egg whites, and milk (for protein) • Consume fruit drinks and lemonade, chewy fruit snacks, sorbet, honey, corn syrup, and butter or margarine (for protein-free calories) • Minimize or eliminate legumes, nuts, and nut-butters
Low-potassium	• Used to decrease potassium, which is generally retained in renal failure • Eat (in moderation) green beans, wax beans, fresh peas, mashed potatoes, apples, and pears • Avoid avocados, bananas, cantaloupe and melon, orange and grapefruit (fruits and juices), peaches, dried fruit, beans (except green and wax), split peas, broccoli, greens, spinach, tomatoes in any form, potatoes of any kind and in any form (except mashed), molasses, nuts, chocolate, and salt substitutes
Low-phosphorus	• Used to decrease phosphorus, which is generally retained in renal failure (found in almost all foods so medication may also be used) • Eliminate beans (red, black, white), black-eyed peas, lima beans, cheese, milk, desserts made with milk, chocolate, yogurt, sardines, liver, and nuts

ACUTE RENAL FAILURE

● **Definition**
  • Sudden interruption of renal function
  • Can be caused by obstruction, poor circulation, or underlying kidney disease
  • Classified as prerenal, intrarenal, or postrenal
  • Usually reversible with treatment but, if not treated, may progress to end-stage renal disease, prerenal azotemia (build up of urea and other nitrogenous waste in the blood), and death
  • Normally occurs in three distinct phases: oliguric, diuretic, and recovery

Key facts about acute renal failure
● Sudden interruption of renal function

Prerenal failure
● Occurs when diminished blood flow to kidneys leads to hypoperfusion

Intrarenal failure
● Results from damage to filtering structures of the kidneys
● Causes hypotension, ischemia, and necrosis

Postrenal failure
● Results from bilateral obstruction of urine

Phases of acute renal failure

Oliguric phase
- Phase lasts for a few days or several weeks
- Urine output drops below 400 ml/day
- Cellular injury and necrosis occur

Diuretic phase
- Phase lasts for days or weeks
- Urine output increases to more than 400 ml/day
- GFR may be normal or increased
- High BUN levels produce osmotic diuresis

Recovery phase
- Phase lasts for 3 to 12 months or longer
- Renal function returns to normal or near-normal

- Oliguric phase
  - May last for a few days or several weeks
  - Urine output drops below 400 ml/day
  - Fluid volume excess, azotemia, and electrolyte imbalance occur
  - Local mediators are released, causing intrarenal vasoconstriction
  - Medullary hypoxia causes cellular swelling and adherence of neutrophils to capillaries and venules
  - Hypoperfusion occurs
  - Cellular injury and necrosis occur
- Diuretic phase
  - May last for days or weeks
  - Kidneys become unable to conserve sodium and water
  - Urine output gradually increases to more than 400 ml/day
  - GFR may be normal or increased, although tubular transport systems remain abnormal
  - High blood urea nitrogen (BUN) levels produce osmotic diuresis and consequent deficits of potassium, sodium, and water
- Recovery phase
  - May last for 3 to 12 months or longer
  - Renal function gradually returns to normal or near-normal

● Underlying pathophysiology
- Prerenal failure
  - Ensues when a condition that diminishes blood flow to the kidneys leads to hypoperfusion
  - When renal blood flow is interrupted, so is oxygen delivery
  - The ensuing hypoxemia and ischemia can rapidly and irreversibly damage the kidney; the tubules are most susceptible to hypoxemia's effects
  - Azotemia is a consequence of renal hypoperfusion, and the impaired blood flow results in a decreased GFR and increased tubular reabsorption of sodium and water
  - A decrease in the GFR causes electrolyte imbalance and metabolic acidosis
  - Usually, restoring renal blood flow and glomerular filtration reverses azotemia
- Intrarenal failure
  - Results from damage to the filtering structures of the kidneys
  - Causes are classified as nephrotoxic, inflammatory, or ischemic
  - When the damage is caused by nephrotoxicity or inflammation, the basement membrane (delicate layer under the epithelium) becomes irreparably damaged, typically leading to chronic renal failure
  - Severe or prolonged lack of blood flow caused by ischemia may lead to renal damage (ischemic parenchymal injury) and excess nitrogen in the blood (intrinsic renal azotemia)
  - ATN, the precursor to intrarenal failure, can result from ischemic damage to renal parenchyma during unrecognized or poorly treated prerenal failure or from obstetric complications
  - Fluid loss causes hypotension, which leads to ischemia; the ischemic tissue generates toxic oxygen-free radicals, which cause swelling, injury, and necrosis

- Postrenal failure
  - Bilateral obstruction of urine outflow leads to postrenal failure
  - The cause may be in the bladder, ureters, or urethra

Causes
- Prerenal failure
  - Cardiovascular: Antihypertensive drugs, arrhythmias that cause reduced cardiac output, arterial embolism, arterial or venous thrombosis, cardiogenic shock, cardiac tamponade, eclampsia, heart failure, malignant hypertension, myocardial infarction, vasculitis
  - Fluid imbalance: Burns, dehydration, diuretic overuse, hemorrhage, hypovolemic shock
  - Other: Disseminated intravascular coagulation, sepsis, trauma, tumor
- Intrarenal failure
  - Renal: Acute glomerulonephritis, acute interstitial nephritis, acute pyelonephritis, bilateral renal vein thrombosis, malignant nephrosclerosis, nephrotoxins, poorly treated prerenal failure, renal myeloma
  - Other: Crush injuries, myopathy, obstetric complications, polyarteritis nodosa, sickle cell disease, systemic lupus erythematosus (SLE), transfusion reaction, vasculitis
- Postrenal failure
  - Bladder, ureteral, and urethral obstruction

Pathophysiologic changes
- Oliguria, azotemia and, rarely, anuria due to decreased blood flow within the kidneys (early signs)
- Electrolyte imbalance and metabolic acidosis related to impaired fluid balance
- Anorexia, nausea, vomiting, diarrhea or constipation, stomatitis, hematemesis, dry mucous membranes, uremic breath related to fluid and electrolyte imbalance and urea buildup
- Headache, drowsiness, irritability, confusion, peripheral neuropathy, seizures, and coma due to altered cerebral perfusion and azotemia
- Dry skin, pruritus, pallor, purpura and, rarely, uremic frost due to buildup of urea and decreased hemoglobin and clotting factors
- Pulmonary edema and Kussmaul's respirations caused by altered volume state
- Hypotension (early in the disease)
- Hypertension, arrhythmias, fluid overload, heart failure, systemic edema, anemia, and altered clotting mechanisms related to altered volume status (later in the disease)

Complications
- Infection
- Metabolic acidosis
- Heart failure
- Hypertensive crisis
- Electrolyte imbalance
- Renal shutdown

Diagnostic test findings
- Blood testing shows elevated BUN, serum creatinine, and potassium levels; decreased hematocrit, bicarbonate, and hemoglobin levels; and low blood pH

- Urinalysis shows casts, cellular debris, and decreased specific gravity; in glomerular diseases, proteinuria and urine osmolality close to serum osmolality; urine sodium level less than 20 mEq/L if oliguria results from decreased perfusion, and more than 40 mEq/L if the cause is intrarenal
- Creatinine clearance testing measures GFR and reflects the number of remaining functioning nephrons
- Electrocardiography (ECG) shows tall, peaked T waves, a widening QRS complex, and disappearing P waves if hyperkalemia is present
- Ultrasonography, X-rays of the abdomen, kidney-ureter-bladder (KUB) radiography, excretory urography, renal scanning, retrograde pyelography, CT scan, and nephrotomography may reveal the cause of renal failure

Treatment
- High-calorie diet low in protein, sodium, and potassium to meet metabolic needs
- Electrolyte and I.V. therapy monitoring to maintain and correct fluid and electrolyte balance
- Fluid restriction to minimize edema
- Diuretic therapy to treat oliguric phase
- Sodium polystyrene sulfonate (Kayexalate) by mouth or rectally (enema) to reverse mild hyperkalemia
- Hypertonic glucose, insulin, and sodium bicarbonate I.V. for more severe hyperkalemic symptoms
- Hemodialysis or peritoneal dialysis to correct electrolyte and fluid imbalances

Nursing considerations
- Measure and record intake and output
- Weigh the patient daily
- Assess hemoglobin level and hematocrit and replace blood components as ordered
  - Use packed red blood cells (RBCs) instead of whole blood if the patient is prone to heart failure and can't tolerate the additional fluid volume
- Monitor the patient's vital signs; report signs of pericarditis (pleuritic chest pain, tachycardia, pericardial friction rub), inadequate renal perfusion (hypotension), and acidosis
- Maintain proper electrolyte balance; watch for symptoms of hyperkalemia (malaise, anorexia, paresthesia, or muscle weakness) and ECG changes (tall, peaked T waves; widening QRS segment; and disappearing P waves), and report them immediately
- Monitor potassium and glucose levels in a patient receiving hypertonic glucose and insulin infusions
- When giving sodium polystyrene sulfonate rectally, make sure that the patient doesn't retain it and become constipated (to prevent bowel perforation)
- Maintain nutritional status
  - Provide a high-calorie, low-protein, low-sodium, and low-potassium diet with vitamin supplements
  - Give the anorexic patient small, frequent meals
- Use sterile technique because the patient with acute renal failure is highly susceptible to infection
- Perform passive range-of-motion (ROM) exercises and help the patient walk as soon as possible

Key treatments for acute renal failure
- High-calorie diet that's low in protein, sodium, and potassium
- Electrolyte and I.V. therapy
- Fluid restriction
- Diuretic therapy (oliguric phase)
- Hemodialysis or peritoneal dialysis (if severe)

Key nursing considerations for acute renal failure
- Measure and record intake and output.
- Weigh patient daily.
- Monitor vital signs.
- Maintain proper electrolyte balance.

Peritoneal dialysis
- Watch for complications, such as peritonitis.
- Watch for signs of infection.

Hemodialysis
- Weigh patient before and after hemodialysis.
- Watch for complications such as septicemia.
- Check blood access site every 2 hours for patency and signs of clotting.
- Don't use the arm with the shunt or fistula for taking blood pressures or drawing blood.

- Provide good skin care; add lubricating lotion to the bath water to combat skin dryness
- Provide frequent oral hygiene; if stomatitis occurs and an antibiotic solution is ordered, have the patient swish the solution around in his mouth before swallowing
- Monitor for GI bleeding by guaiac-testing stools for blood
  - Give aluminum hydroxide-based antacids, as needed; magnesium-based antacids can cause serum magnesium levels to rise to critical levels
- Use appropriate safety measures; a patient with central nervous system (CNS) involvement may be dizzy or confused
- Provide emotional support to the patient and his family, and clearly explain all procedures
- During peritoneal dialysis
  - Elevate the head of the bed to reduce pressure on the diaphragm and aid respiration
  - Watch for signs of infection (cloudy drainage, elevated temperature) and bleeding
  - If pain occurs, reduce the amount of dialysate
  - Monitor the diabetic patient's blood glucose and administer insulin as ordered
  - Watch for complications, such as peritonitis, atelectasis, hypokalemia, pneumonia, and shock
- If the patient requires hemodialysis
  - Weigh the patient before beginning dialysis
  - Check the blood access site (arteriovenous fistula, subclavian or femoral catheter) every 2 hours for patency and signs of clotting
  - Don't use the arm with the shunt or fistula for taking blood pressures or drawing blood
  - During dialysis, monitor the patient's vital signs, clotting times, blood flow, function of the vascular access site, and arterial and venous pressures
    - Watch for complications, such as septicemia, embolism, hepatitis, and rapid fluid and electrolyte loss
    - After dialysis, monitor the patient's vital signs and the vascular access site; weigh the patient; and watch for signs of fluid and electrolyte imbalances
- Use standard precautions when handling blood and other body fluids

ACUTE TUBULAR NECROSIS

- **Definition**
  - Most common cause of acute renal failure in critically ill patients
  - Injures the nephron's tubular segment, causing renal failure and uremic syndrome
  - Also known as *acute tubulointerstitial nephritis*, or ATN

- **Underlying pathophysiology**
  - Results from ischemic or nephrotoxic injury, most commonly in debilitated patients, such as the critically ill or those who have undergone extensive surgery

Key facts about ATN

- Results from ischemic or nephrotoxic injury
- Leads to renal failure and uremic syndrome

Ischemic injury
- Involves patches of necrosis in straight portions of proximal tubules
- Creates lesions that destroy the tubular epithelium and basement membrane

Nephrotoxic injury
- Involves necrosis in tubular epithelium only
- May be reversible

- In ischemic injury, necrosis typically develops as patches in straight portions of the proximal tubules, creating deep lesions that destroy the tubular epithelium and basement membrane (in areas without lesions, tubules usually are dilated)
- With nephrotoxic injury, necrosis occurs only in the epithelium of the tubules, leaving the basement membrane of the nephrons intact; consequently, the damage may be reversible (the tubules maintain a more uniform appearance)

Causes
- Ischemic injury
    - Circulatory collapse, severe hypotension
    - Trauma, hemorrhage, severe dehydration
    - Cardiogenic or septic shock
    - Reaction to surgery, anesthetics, or transfusion
- Nephrotoxic injury
    - Toxic chemical ingestion or inhalation
    - Hypersensitivity reaction of kidneys to antibiotics, radiographic contrast agents

Pathophysiologic changes
- Decreased urine output (generally the first recognizable effect); hyperkalemia (with characteristic ECG changes); elevated serum creatinine and BUN levels; edema; dry mucous membranes and skin; possible CNS changes, including lethargy or twitching, due to a marked decrease in glomerular filtration (oliguric or decreased urine output phase may not be present in some patients because of higher levels of glomerular filtration)
- Uremic syndrome resulting from inability of the nephrons to process urea from protein metabolism for excretion, with nausea, vomiting, headache, vertigo, dimmed vision, and confusion, which may progress to uremic seizures or coma
- Diuresis due to return of BUN and creatinine levels to normal (recovery phase)

Complications
- Heart failure; uremic pericarditis
- Pulmonary edema; uremic lung
- Anemia
- Anorexia, intractable vomiting
- Poor wound healing due to debilitation

Diagnostic test findings
- Urinalysis reveals sediment containing RBCs and casts, and dilute urine of a low specific gravity (1.010), low osmolality (less than 400 mOsm/kg), and a high sodium level (40 to 60 mEq/L)
- Blood testing reveals elevated BUN and serum creatinine levels, anemia, defects in platelet adherence, metabolic acidosis, and hyperkalemia
- ECG may show arrhythmias (due to electrolyte imbalances) and, with hyperkalemia, widening QRS segment, disappearing P waves, and tall, peaked T waves

Treatment
- Acute phase

Key pathophysiologic changes in ATN

- Decreased urine output
- Dry mucous membranes and skin
- Possible CNS changes
- Nausea and vomiting
- Headache
- Vertigo
- Dimmed vision
- Confusion
- Possible uremic seizures or coma

Key diagnostic test results for ATN

- Urinalysis: Sediment containing RBCs and casts, low specific gravity, osmolality less than 400 mOsm/kg, high sodium level (40 to 60 mEq/L)
- Blood testing: Elevated BUN and serum creatinine levels, anemia, defects in platelet adherence, metabolic acidosis, hyperkalemia

- Vigorous supportive measures until normal kidney function resumes
- Initially, possible administration of diuretics and infusion of a large volume of fluids to flush tubules of cellular casts and debris and to replace fluid loss (risk of fluid overload with this treatment)
- Long-term fluid management
  - Daily replacement of projected and calculated losses (including insensible loss)
- Other appropriate measures to control complications
  - Transfusion of packed RBCs for anemia; epoetin alfa to stimulate RBC production as an alternative to blood transfusion
  - Administration of antibiotics for infection
  - Emergency I.V. administration of 50% glucose, regular insulin, and sodium bicarbonate for hyperkalemia
  - Sodium polystyrene sulfonate with sorbitol by mouth or rectally (by enema) to reduce extracellular potassium levels
  - Peritoneal dialysis or hemodialysis if the patient is catabolic or if hyperkalemia and fluid volume overload aren't controlled by other measures

Nursing considerations
- Maintain fluid balance
  - **Watch for fluid overload, a common complication of therapy**
  - Record intake and output, including wound drainage, nasogastric output, and hemodialysis and peritoneal dialysis balances
  - Weigh the patient daily
- Monitor hemoglobin level and hematocrit, and administer blood products as needed
  - Use fresh packed cells instead of whole blood to prevent fluid overload and heart failure
- Maintain electrolyte balance
  - Monitor laboratory results and report imbalances
  - Enforce dietary restriction of foods containing sodium and potassium, such as bananas, orange juice, and baked potatoes, and check for potassium content in prescribed medications (for example, penicillin G potassium)
  - Provide adequate calories and essential amino acids while restricting protein intake to maintain an anabolic state; total parenteral nutrition may be indicated in a severely debilitated or catabolic patient
- Use sterile technique because the debilitated patient is vulnerable to infection; immediately report fever, chills, delayed wound healing, or flank pain if the patient has an indwelling catheter
- Watch for complications, such as worsening of anemia or acidosis
  - Watch for signs of diminishing renal perfusion (hypotension and decreased urine output)
  - Encourage coughing and deep breathing to prevent pulmonary complications
- Perform passive ROM exercises
- Provide good skin care
- Provide reassurance and emotional support, and fully explain each procedure
- To prevent ATN, make sure that the patient is well hydrated before surgery or after X-rays that involve use of a contrast medium; administer mannitol (Os-

Key treatments for ATN
- Supportive measures (early phase)
- Possible administration of diuretics and I.V. fluids (early phase)
- Transfusion of packed RBCs (if severe anemia occurs)
- Sodium polystyrene sulfonate with sorbitol
- I.V. administration of 50% glucose, regular insulin, and sodium bicarbonate (for hyperkalemia)

Key nursing considerations for ATN
- Maintain fluid balance.
- Watch for complications, such as worsening of anemia or acidosis.

mitrol), as ordered, to the high-risk patient before and during these procedures
- Carefully monitor patients receiving blood transfusions to detect early signs of transfusion reaction (fever, rash, chills), and discontinue such transfusions immediately

CHRONIC RENAL FAILURE

● Definition
- Usually the end result of gradual tissue destruction and loss of renal function
- Can also result from a rapidly progressing disease of sudden onset that destroys the nephrons and causes irreversible kidney damage
- Fatal without treatment (maintenance on dialysis or a kidney transplant can sustain life)

● Underlying pathophysiology
- Typically progresses through four stages
  - Reduced renal reserve: GFR of 60% to 89% of normal
  - Renal insufficiency: GFR of 30% to 59% of normal
  - Renal failure: GFR of 15% to 29% of normal
  - End-stage renal disease: GFR less than 15% of normal
- Nephron damage is progressive; the damaged nephrons can't function and don't recover
- The kidneys can maintain relatively normal function until about 75% of the nephrons are nonfunctional (few symptoms develop until less than 25% of glomerular filtration remains)
- Surviving nephrons hypertrophy and increase their rate of filtration, reabsorption, and secretion; compensatory excretion continues as GFR diminishes
- The normal parenchyma then deteriorates rapidly, and symptoms worsen as renal function decreases
- As GFR decreases, plasma creatinine levels increase proportionately without regulatory adjustment
- As sodium delivery to the nephron increases, less is reabsorbed, and sodium deficits and volume depletion follow; the kidney becomes incapable of concentrating and diluting urine
  - If *tubulointerstitial disease* is the cause, primary damage to the tubules — the medullary portion of the nephron — precedes failure, as do such problems as renal tubular acidosis, salt wasting, and difficulty diluting and concentrating urine
    - Tubulointerstitial injury occurs from toxic or ischemic tubular damage, and debris and calcium deposits obstruct the tubules; the resulting defective tubular transport is associated with interstitial edema, leukocyte infiltration, and tubular necrosis
  - If *vascular or glomerular damage* is the primary cause, proteinuria, hematuria, and nephrotic syndrome are more prominent
    - Vascular injury causes diffuse or focal ischemia of the renal parenchyma, associated with thickening, fibrosis, or focal lesions of renal blood vessels; decreased blood flow then leads to tubular atrophy, interstitial fibrosis, and functional disruption of glomerular filtration, medullary gradients, and concentration

- Structural changes trigger an inflammatory response; fibrin deposits begin to form around the interstitium, and microaneurysms result from vascular wall damage and increased pressure secondary to obstruction or hypertension
- Eventual loss of the nephron triggers compensatory hyperfunction of uninjured nephrons, which initiates a positive-feedback loop of increasing vulnerability
- Eventually, the healthy glomeruli become sclerotic, stiff, and necrotic; toxins accumulate and potentially fatal changes ensue in all major organ systems

Causes
- Chronic glomerular disease (glomerulonephritis)
- Chronic infection, such as chronic pyelonephritis and tuberculosis
- Congenital anomalies (polycystic kidney disease)
- Vascular disease (hypertension, nephrosclerosis)
- Obstruction (renal calculi)
- Collagen disease such as SLE
- Nephrotoxic agents (long-term aminoglycoside therapy)
- Endocrine disease (diabetic nephropathy)

Pathophysiologic changes
- Hypervolemia due to increased proteins
- Hypocalcemia and hyperkalemia due to electrolyte imbalance
- Azotemia due to retention of nitrogenous wastes from protein metabolism
- Metabolic acidosis due to loss of bicarbonate
- Bone and muscle pain and fractures caused by calcium-phosphorus imbalance and consequent parathyroid hormone imbalances
- Peripheral neuropathy due to accumulation of toxins
- Dry mouth, fatigue, and nausea due to hyponatremia
- Hypotension due to sodium loss, early finding
- Altered mental state due to hyponatremia and toxin accumulation
- Lethargy and dizziness due to uremic toxins shortening RBC survival time
- Irregular heart rate due to hyperkalemia
- Kussmaul's respirations due to metabolic acidosis
- Hypertension due to fluid overload
- GI bleeding, hemorrhage, and bruising; gum soreness and bleeding due to thrombocytopenia and platelet defects
- In end-stage renal failure, stomatitis, uremic fetor, peptic ulcer, and pancreatitis due to retention of metabolic acids and other metabolic waste products
- Yellow-bronze skin due to altered metabolic processes
- Dry, scaly skin and severe itching due to uremic frost
- Muscle cramps and twitching, including cardiac irritability, due to hyperkalemia
- Growth retardation in children from endocrine abnormalities induced by renal failure
- Impaired bone growth and bowlegs in children due to vitamin D deficiency contributing to hypocalcemia
- Infertility, decreased libido, amenorrhea, and impotence due to endocrine disturbances
- Pain, burning, and itching in legs and feet associated with peripheral neuropathy
- Infection related to decreased macrophage activity

Key pathophysiologic changes in chronic renal failure
- Hypervolemia
- Hypocalcemia and hyperkalemia
- Azotemia
- Hypertension
- GI and gum bleeding
- Growth retardation in children

● **Complications**
- Anemia
- Peripheral neuropathy
- Cardiopulmonary complications
- GI complications
- Sexual dysfunction
- Skeletal defects
- Paresthesia
- Motor nerve dysfunction, such as footdrop and flaccid paralysis
- Pathologic fractures

● **Diagnostic test findings**
- Arterial blood gas analysis reveals decreased pH and bicarbonate level
- Blood testing reveals elevated BUN, creatinine, low sodium level, and potassium levels; increased aldosterone secretion; low hemoglobin level and hematocrit; decreased RBC survival time; mild thrombocytopenia; platelet defects; and hyperglycemia
- Urinalysis aids in diagnosis (specific gravity fixed at 1.010, proteinuria, glycosuria, RBCs, leukocytes, casts, or crystals, depending on the cause)
- KUB radiography, excretory urography, nephrotomography, renal scanning, or renal arteriography shows reduced kidney size
- Renal biopsy may be performed to identify the underlying disease
- EEG may be performed to identify metabolic encephalopathy

● **Treatment**
- Diet
  - Low-protein diet to limit accumulation of end-products of protein metabolism that the kidneys can't excrete
  - High-protein diet for patients on continuous peritoneal dialysis
  - High-calorie diet to prevent ketoacidosis and tissue atrophy
  - Sodium, potassium, and phosphorus restrictions to prevent elevated levels
  - Fluid restrictions to maintain fluid balance
- Medications
  - Loop diuretics, such as furosemide (Lasix), to maintain fluid balance
  - Cardiac glycosides, such as digoxin (Digitek, Lanoxin), to mobilize fluids causing edema
  - Calcium carbonate (Caltrate) or calcium acetate (PhosLo) to treat renal osteodystrophy by binding phosphate and supplementing calcium
  - Antihypertensives to control blood pressure and edema
  - Antiemetics to relieve nausea and vomiting
  - Famotidine (Pepcid) or ranitidine (Zantac) to decrease gastric irritation
  - Methylcellulose or docusate to prevent constipation
  - Iron and folate supplements or RBC transfusion to treat anemia
  - Synthetic erythropoietin to stimulate the bone marrow to produce RBCs; conjugated estrogens, and desmopressin (DDAVP, Stimate) to combat hematologic effects
  - Antipruritics, such as trimeprazine (Temaril) or diphenhydramine (Benadryl), to relieve itching
  - Phosphate-removing drugs to decrease serum phosphate levels

- Supplementary vitamins, particularly vitamin B and D, and essential amino acids to ensure adequate intake
- Oral or rectal cation exchange resins, such as sodium polystyrene sulfonate, and I.V. calcium gluconate, sodium bicarbonate, 50% dextrose, and regular insulin to reverse hyperkalemia
- Dialysis for hyperkalemia and fluid imbalances
- Emergency pericardiocentesis or surgery for cardiac tamponade
- Intensive dialysis and thoracentesis to relieve pulmonary edema and pleural effusion
- Peritoneal or hemodialysis to help control end-stage renal disease
- Kidney transplantation (usually the treatment of choice if a donor is available)

● Nursing considerations

- Bathe the patient daily using superfatted soaps, oatmeal baths, and skin lotion without alcohol to ease pruritus; provide good perineal care using mild soap and water; and turn the patient often and use a convoluted foam mattress to prevent skin breakdown
- Provide good oral hygiene by encouraging or performing frequent brushing with a soft brush or sponge tip to reduce breath odor and providing sugarless hard candy and mouthwash to minimize the metallic taste in the mouth and alleviate thirst
- Offer small, nutritious, and palatable meals
  - Encourage intake of high-calorie foods and instruct the outpatient to avoid high-sodium and high-potassium foods
  - Encourage adherence to fluid and protein restrictions
  - To prevent constipation, stress the need for exercise and sufficient dietary bulk
- Monitor for signs of hyperkalemia (cramping of the legs and abdomen and diarrhea); as potassium levels rise, watch for muscle irritability and a weak pulse rate
  - Monitor the ECG for tall, peaked T waves; widening QRS segment; prolonged PR interval; and disappearance of P waves
- Carefully assess the patient's hydration status; check for jugular vein distention, auscultate the lungs for crackles, carefully measure daily intake and output, record daily weight, and document peripheral edema
- Monitor for bone or joint complications
  - Prevent pathologic fractures by turning the patient carefully and ensuring his safety
  - Provide passive ROM exercises for a bedridden patient
- Encourage deep breathing and coughing to prevent pulmonary congestion, auscultate the lungs often, stay alert for clinical effects of pulmonary edema (dyspnea, restlessness, crackles), and administer diuretics and other medications as ordered
- Maintain strict sterile technique; use a micropore filter during I.V. therapy
  - Watch for signs of infection (listlessness, high fever, leukocytosis) during hospitalization and urge the outpatient to avoid contact with infected people during the cold and flu season
- **Carefully observe and document seizure activity; infuse sodium bicarbonate for acidosis and sedatives or anticonvulsants for seizures as ordered**

Key nursing considerations for chronic renal failure
- Carefully observe and document seizure activity.
- Provide good skin care and oral hygiene.
- Monitor for signs of hyperkalemia.
- Assess hydration status.
- Observe for signs of bleeding.

Key nursing considerations for the dialysis patient
- Explain procedure and care for vascular access site.
- Regularly check vascular access site and extremity.
- Don't use extremity for other procedures.
- Use standard precautions when handling body fluids and needles.
- Perform patient teaching, including drug therapy and nutrition.

– Pad the side rails and keep an oral airway and suction setup at the bedside
– Assess the patient's neurologic status periodically, and check for Chvostek's and Trousseau's signs (indicators of low serum calcium levels)
• Observe for signs of bleeding (prolonged bleeding at puncture sites and at the vascular access site used for hemodialysis), monitor hemoglobin level and hematocrit, and check stool, urine, and vomitus for blood
• Report signs of pericarditis, such as a pericardial friction rub and chest pain
• If the patient requires dialysis
– Explain the procedure, and make sure that he understands how to protect and care for the vascular access site
– Check the vascular access site every 2 hours for patency, and check the extremity for adequate blood supply and intact nervous function (temperature, pulse rate, capillary refill, and sensation)
  • If a fistula is present, feel for a thrill and listen for a bruit; use a gentle touch to avoid occluding the fistula
  • Report signs of possible clotting
– Don't use the arm with the vascular access site to take blood pressure readings, draw blood, or give injections because these procedures may rupture the fistula or occlude blood flow
– Withhold the 6 a.m. (or morning) dose of antihypertensive medication on the morning of dialysis, and instruct the discharged patient to do the same
– Use standard precautions when handling body fluids and needles
– Monitor hemoglobin level and hematocrit
– After dialysis
  • Check for disequilibrium syndrome, a result of sudden correction of blood chemistry abnormalities (symptoms range from headache to seizures)
  • Check for excessive bleeding from the dialysis site; apply a pressure dressing or absorbable gelatin sponge, as indicated
  • Monitor blood pressure carefully
– Refer the patient to appropriate counseling agencies for assistance in coping with chronic renal failure

GLOMERULONEPHRITIS

● **Definition**
• Bilateral inflammation of the glomeruli, typically following a streptococcal infection
• Also called *acute poststreptococcal glomerulonephritis*
• Most common in boys ages 3 to 7 but can occur at any age
• Recovery in up to 95% of children and 70% of adults; others, especially elderly patients, may progress to chronic renal failure within months
• Rapidly progressive glomerulonephritis (RPGN) — also called *subacute, crescentic,* or *extracapillary glomerulonephritis* — most commonly occurs between ages 50 and 60
  – May be idiopathic or associated with a proliferative glomerular disease such as poststreptococcal glomerulonephritis

Key facts about glomerulonephritis

● Bilateral inflammation of glomeruli
● Typically follows streptococcal infection
● Most common in boys ages 3 to 7 but can occur at any age
● May be classified as RPGN, which commonly occurs between ages 50 and 60
● Develops when antigen-antibody complexes lodge in glomerular capillaries, causing injury
● Leads to activation complement, leukocytes, and fibrin and release of lysosomal enzymes that damage glomerular cell walls
● Leads to platelet aggregation, platelet degranulation, and increased cell wall permeability
● Diminishes renal blood flow and GFR

Characteristics of glomerular lesions

The types of glomerular lesions and their characteristics include:
- diffuse — relatively uniform, and involve most or all glomeruli (for example, glomerulonephritis)
- focal — involve only some glomeruli (others are normal)
- segmental-local — involve only one part of the glomerulus
- mesangial — deposits of immunoglobulins in the mesangial matrix
- membranous — thickening of the glomerular capillary wall
- proliferative — increased number of glomerular cells
- sclerotic — glomerular scarring from previous glomerular injury
- crescent — accumulation of proliferating cells in Bowman's space.

- Goodpasture's syndrome, a rare type of RPGN, occurs most commonly in men ages 20 to 30
- Chronic glomerulonephritis, a slowly progressive disease characterized by inflammation, sclerosis, scarring and, eventually, renal failure, generally remains undetected until the progressive phase, which is usually irreversible

Underlying pathophysiology
- In nearly all types of glomerulonephritis, the epithelial or podocyte layer of the glomerular membrane is disturbed, resulting in a loss of negative charge across the membrane (see *Characteristics of glomerular lesions*)
- Acute poststreptococcal glomerulonephritis results from the entrapment and collection of antigen-antibody complexes in the glomerular capillary membranes, after endogenous or exogenous infection with group A-beta streptococci
- Circulating antigen-antibody complexes become lodged in the glomerular capillaries, causing glomerular injury and the release of immunologic substances that lyse cells and increase membrane permeability
- Antibody damage to basement membranes contribute to crescent formation
- Antibody or antigen-antibody complexes in the glomerular capillary wall activate biochemical mediators of inflammation — complement, leukocytes, and fibrin
- Activated complement attracts neutrophils and monocytes, which release lysosomal enzymes that damage the glomerular cell walls and cause proliferation of the extracellular matrix, affecting glomerular blood flow
- Membrane permeability is increased, causing a loss of negative charge across the glomerular membrane as well as enhanced protein filtration
- This process leads to platelet aggregation, platelet degranulation, and release of substances that increase glomerular permeability; protein molecules and RBCs can now pass into the urine, resulting in proteinuria or hematuria
- Activation of the coagulation system leads to fibrin deposits in Bowman's space, contributing to crescent formation and diminished renal blood flow and GFR
- In Goodpasture's syndrome, antibodies are produced against the pulmonary capillaries and glomerular basement membrane, and diffuse intracellular anti-

Key facts about Goodpasture's syndrome
- Rare form of RPGN
- Most common in men ages 20 to 30
- Produces antibodies against pulmonary capillaries and glomerular basement membrane
- Leads to rapid renal failure

body proliferation in Bowman's space leads to crescent formation composed of fibrin and endothelial, mesangial, and phagocytic cells
- These cells compress the glomerular capillaries, diminish blood flow, and cause extensive scarring of the glomeruli; GFR is reduced, and renal failure occurs within weeks or months
- When nephritis results from immunoglobulin (Ig) A nephropathy, or Berger's disease (usually idiopathic), the plasma IgA level is elevated, and IgA and inflammatory cells are deposited into Bowman's space; the result is sclerosis and fibrosis of the glomerulus and a reduced GFR
- Lipid nephrosis causes disruption of the capillary filtration membrane and loss of its negative charge; this increased permeability with resultant loss of protein leads to nephrotic syndrome
- In membranous glomerulopathy, an inflammatory process causes thickening of the glomerular capillary wall; increased permeability and proteinuria lead to nephrotic syndrome

● Causes
- Acute glomerulonephritis and RPGN
  - Streptococcal infection of the respiratory tract
  - Impetigo
  - IgA nephropathy (Berger's disease)
  - Lipid nephrosis
- Chronic glomerulonephritis
  - Membranoproliferative glomerulonephritis
  - Membranous glomerulopathy
  - Focal glomerulosclerosis
  - RPGN
  - Poststreptococcal glomerulonephritis
  - SLE
  - Goodpasture's syndrome
  - Hemolytic uremic syndrome

● Pathophysiologic changes
- Decreased urination or oliguria due to decreased GFR
- Smoky or coffee-colored urine due to hematuria
- Dyspnea and orthopnea due to pulmonary edema secondary to hypervolemia
- Periorbital edema due to hypervolemia
- Mild to severe hypertension due to decreased GFR, sodium or water retention, and inappropriate release of renin
- Bibasilar crackles due to hypervolemia and heart failure

● Complications
- Pulmonary edema
- Heart failure
- Sepsis
- Renal failure
- Severe hypertension
- Cardiac hypertrophy

Key pathophysiologic changes in glomerulonephritis
- Oliguria
- Bibasilar crackles
- Hypertension

Diagnostic test findings

- Blood testing reveals elevated antistreptolysin-O titers (in 80% of patients); elevated electrolyte, BUN, and creatinine levels; and decreased serum protein and hemoglobin levels (in chronic glomerulonephritis)
- Streptozyme analysis (a hemagglutination test that detects antibodies to several streptococcal antigens) shows elevated antibody levels
- Blood studies reveal elevated anti-DNase B titers (indicating previous infection with group A beta-hemolytic streptococcus) and low levels of serum complement (indicating recent streptococcal infection)
- Urinalysis shows RBCs, WBCs, mixed cell casts, and protein (indicating renal failure and fibrin-degradation products and C3 protein)
- Throat culture reveals group A beta-hemolytic streptococcus
- KUB X-rays show bilateral kidney enlargement (acute glomerulonephritis)
- X-rays of the kidney show symmetric contraction with normal pelves and calyces (chronic glomerulonephritis)
- Renal biopsy confirms the diagnosis or assesses renal tissue status

Treatment

- Treatment of the primary disease to alter the immunologic cascade (see *Treating renal failure in glomerulonephritis,* page 338)
- Antibiotics for 7 to 10 days to treat infections contributing to ongoing antigen-antibody response
- Anticoagulants to control fibrin crescent formation in RPGN
- Bed rest to reduce metabolic demands
- Fluid restrictions to decrease edema
- Dietary sodium restriction to prevent fluid retention
- Correction of electrolyte imbalances
- Loop diuretics, such as metolazone (Zaroxolyn) or furosemide, to reduce extracellular fluid overload
- Vasodilators, such as hydralazine (Apresoline) or nifedipine (Procardia), to decrease hypertension
- Dialysis or kidney transplantation for chronic glomerulonephritis
- Corticosteroids to decrease antibody synthesis and suppress the inflammatory response
- Plasmapheresis (possibly combined with corticosteroids and cyclophosphamide [Cytoxan]) in RPGN to suppress rebound antibody production

Nursing considerations

- Check the patient's vital signs and electrolyte values; monitor intake and output and daily weight; and assess renal function daily through serum creatinine, BUN, and urine creatinine clearance levels
  - **Watch for and immediately report signs of acute renal failure (oliguria, azotemia, acidosis); monitor for ascites and edema**
- Consult the dietitian to provide a diet high in calories and low in protein, sodium, potassium, and fluids
- Provide good skin care and oral hygiene
- Instruct the patient to continue taking prescribed antihypertensives as scheduled, even if he's feeling better, and to report adverse effects

GO WITH THE FLOW

Treating renal failure in glomerulonephritis

This flowchart shows the pathophysiologic occurrences in glomerulonephritis and the treatments that can alter the course of the disorder.

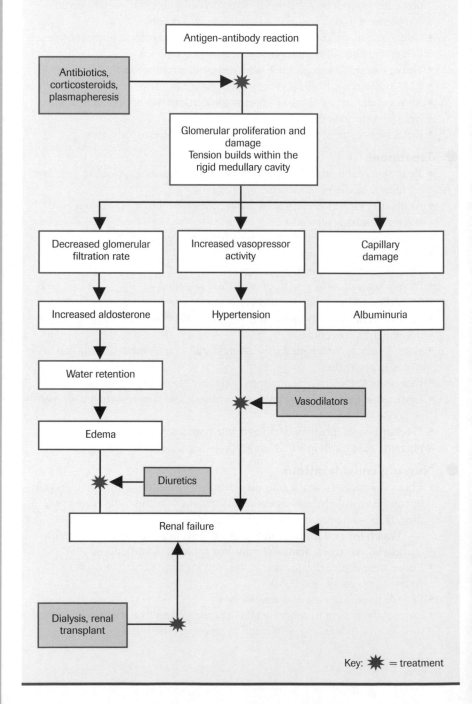

- Advise the patient to take diuretics in the morning, so he won't have to disrupt his sleep to void; teach him how to assess ankle edema
- Protect the debilitated patient against secondary infection by providing good nutrition, using good hygienic technique, and preventing contact with infected people
- Allow the patient to gradually resume normal activities as symptoms subside
- Advise the patient to immediately report signs of infection (fever, sore throat)
- Stress the need for follow-up examinations to detect chronic renal failure
- Encourage pregnant women with a history of glomerulonephritis to have frequent medical evaluations (pregnancy further stresses the kidneys and increases the risk of chronic renal failure)
- Explain all necessary procedures beforehand, and answer the patient's questions about them

NEPHROTIC SYNDROME

Definition
- Characterized by marked proteinuria, hypoalbuminemia, hyperlipidemia, and edema
- Results from a defect in the permeability of glomerular vessels
- Some forms may eventually progress to end-stage renal failure

Underlying pathophysiology
- Regardless of the cause, the injured glomerular filtration membrane allows the loss of plasma proteins, especially albumin and immunoglobulin
- Metabolic, biochemical, or physiochemical disturbances in the glomerular basement membrane result in the loss of negative charge as well as increased permeability to protein
- Hypoalbuminemia results from urinary loss and decreased hepatic synthesis of replacement albumin; increased plasma concentration and low molecular weight accentuate albumin loss, stimulating the liver to synthesize lipoprotein (with consequent hyperlipidemia) and clotting factors
- Decreased dietary intake, as with anorexia, malnutrition, or concomitant disease, further contributes to decreased plasma albumin levels
- Loss of immunoglobulin also increases susceptibility to infections

Causes
- Lipid nephrosis (nil lesions) (main cause in children younger than age 8)
- Membranous glomerulonephritis (most common lesion in adult idiopathic nephrotic syndrome)
- Focal glomerulosclerosis
- Membranoproliferative glomerulonephritis
- Metabolic diseases such as diabetes mellitus
- Collagen-vascular disorders, such as SLE and periarteritis nodosa
- Circulatory diseases, such as heart failure, sickle cell anemia, and renal vein thrombosis
- Nephrotoxins, such as mercury, gold, and bismuth
- Infections, such as tuberculosis and enteritis
- Allergic reactions
- Pregnancy

Key facts about nephrotic syndrome
- Results from a defect of glomerular vessel permeability
- Causes loss of plasma proteins, especially albumin and immunoglobulin

Common causes of nephrotic syndrome
- Lipid nephrosis (in children younger than age 8)
- Membranous glomerulonephritis
- Diabetes mellitus
- Collagen-vascular disorders
- Tuberculosis
- Nephrotoxins

Key pathophysiologic changes in nephrotic syndrome

- Periorbital or dependent edema
- Ascites
- Orthostatic hypotension

Key diagnostic test results for nephrotic syndrome

- Urine testing: High protein levels
- Blood testing: Increased serum cholesterol, phospholipid, and triglyceride levels; decreased serum albumin levels
- Renal biopsy: Histologic identification of lesion

Key treatments for nephrotic syndrome

- Corticosteroids
- Diuretics
- Sodium-restricted diet that includes 0.6 g of protein/kg of body

- Hereditary nephritis
- Neoplastic diseases such as multiple myeloma

● **Pathophysiologic changes**
- Periorbital edema due to fluid overload (generally occurs in the morning)
- Mild to severe dependent edema of the ankles or sacrum due to hypoalbuminemia and water and sodium retention
- Orthostatic hypotension due to fluid imbalance
- Ascites due to fluid imbalance and hypoalbuminemia
- Swollen external genitalia due to edema in dependent areas
- Respiratory difficulty due to pleural effusion
- Anorexia due to edema of intestinal mucosa
- Pallor due to hypochromic anemia from excessive urinary excretion of transferrin
- Shiny skin with prominent veins due to fluid imbalance
- Diarrhea due to edema of intestinal mucosa
- Frothy urine in children due to protein excretion
- Change in hair quality related to protein deficiency
- Pneumonia due to susceptibility to infections

● **Complications**
- Malnutrition
- Infection
- Coagulation disorders
- Thromboembolic vascular occlusion (especially in the lungs and legs)
- Accelerated atherosclerosis
- Acute renal failure

● **Diagnostic test findings**
- Urine testing shows protein (consistent, heavy proteinuria [24-hour protein more than 3.5 mg/dl]), hyaline, granular and waxy fatty casts, and oval fat bodies
- Blood testing reveals increased serum cholesterol, phospholipid (especially low-density and very low-density lipoproteins), and triglyceride levels and decreased serum albumin levels
- Renal biopsy enables histologic identification of the lesion

● **Treatment**
- Correction of underlying cause, if possible
- Diet that includes 0.6 g of protein/kg of body weight and restricted sodium intake
- Diuretics to diminish edema
- Antibiotics to treat infection
- 8-week course of a corticosteroid, such as prednisone (Deltasone), followed by maintenance therapy or a combination of prednisone and azathioprine (Imuran) or cyclophosphamide
- Treatment for hyperlipidemia (usually unsuccessful)
- Paracentesis for ascites
- Thoracentesis for pleural effusion

● **Nursing considerations**
- Frequently check urine protein (urine containing protein appears frothy)

- Measure blood pressure while the patient is supine and while he's standing; immediately report a drop that exceeds 20 mm Hg
- Monitor and document the location and degree of edema
- After kidney biopsy, watch for bleeding and shock
- Monitor intake and output, and check weight at the same time each morning (after the patient voids and before he eats)
- Ask the dietitian to plan a moderate-protein, low-sodium diet
- Provide good skin care (especially because of edema)
- Avoid thrombophlebitis by encouraging activity and exercise, and provide antiembolism stockings as ordered
- Teach the patient and his family how to recognize adverse drug effects, such as bone marrow toxicity and cushingoid symptoms from long-term steroid therapy
- Monitor for and teach the patient about other steroid-related complications, including masked infections, increased susceptibility to infections, ulcers, GI bleeding, steroid-induced diabetes, and steroid crisis (may occur if the drug is discontinued abruptly)
  – To prevent GI complications, administer steroids with an antacid or with cimetidine or ranitidine; explain that adverse effects will subside when steroid therapy is discontinued
- Offer the patient and his family reassurance and support, especially during the acute phase when edema is severe and the patient's body image changes

NEUROGENIC BLADDER

Definition
- Bladder dysfunction caused by an interruption of normal bladder innervation by the nervous system
- Can be hyperreflexic (hypertonic, spastic, or automatic) or flaccid (hypotonic, atonic, or autonomous)

Underlying pathophysiology
- In hyperreflexic dysfunction, an upper motor neuron lesion (at or above T12) causes spastic neurogenic bladder, with spontaneous contractions of detrusor muscles, increased intravesical voiding pressure, bladder wall hypertrophy with trabeculation, and urinary sphincter spasms
- In flaccid dysfunction, a lower motor neuron lesion (at or below S2) affects the spinal reflex that controls micturition; the result is a flaccid neurogenic bladder with decreased intravesical pressure, increased bladder capacity, residual urine retention, and poor detrusor contraction (the bladder may not empty spontaneously)
- Upper motor neuron (cortical) dysfunction may originate in the brain in the pontine micturition center (located in the pons) with interruption of the efferent nerves resulting in loss of voluntary control, or voiding may be incomplete; sensory neuron interruption in lower motor pathways may lead to dribbling and overflow incontinence (see *Types of neurogenic bladder,* page 342)

Causes
- Stroke
- Brain tumor (meningioma and glioma)
- Parkinson's disease

Common causes of neurogenic bladder

- Spinal cord dysfunctions
- Diabetes mellitus
- Multiple sclerosis

Types of neurogenic bladder

NEURAL LESION	TYPE	CAUSE
Upper motor	Uninhibited	• Lack of voluntary control in infancy • Multiple sclerosis
	Reflex or automatic	• Spinal cord transection • Cord tumors • Multiple sclerosis
Lower motor	Autonomous	• Sacral cord trauma • Tumors • Herniated disk • Abdominal surgery with transection of pelvic parasympathetic nerves
	Motor paralysis	• Lesions at levels S2, S3, S4 • Poliomyelitis • Trauma • Tumors
	Sensory paralysis	• Posterior lumbar nerve roots • Diabetes mellitus • Tabes dorsalis

- Multiple sclerosis
- Dementia
- Incontinence associated with aging
- Spinal stenosis causing cord compression
- Arachnoiditis
- Cervical spondylosis
- Spina bifida
- Poliomyelitis
- Myelopathies from hereditary or nutritional deficiencies
- Tabes dorsalis
- Diabetes mellitus
- Metabolic disturbances, such as hypothyroidism or uremia
- Acute infectious diseases such as Guillain-Barré syndrome
- Heavy metal toxicity
- Chronic alcoholism
- Collagen diseases such as SLE
- Vascular diseases such as atherosclerosis
- Distant effects of certain cancers such as primary oat cell carcinoma
- Herpes zoster
- Sacral agenesis (absence of a completely formed sacrum)

Key pathophysiologic changes in neurogenic bladder

- Varying degrees of incontinence
- Frequent UTIs
- Autonomic dysreflexia (when bladder is distended and lesion is at upper thoracic or cervical level)

● **Pathophysiologic changes**
- Some degree of incontinence, changes in initiation or interruption of micturition, and an inability to completely empty the bladder due to interruption of the efferent nerves at the cortical motor neuron
- Frequent UTIs due to urine retention

- Hyperactive autonomic reflexes (autonomic dysreflexia) when the bladder is distended and the lesion is at the upper thoracic or cervical level
- Severe hypertension, bradycardia, and vasodilation (blotchy skin) above the level of the lesion
- Piloerection and profuse sweating above the level of the lesion
- Involuntary or frequent, scant urination without a feeling of bladder fullness; spontaneous spasms (caused by voiding) of the arms and legs; and increased anal sphincter tone due to severe hyperreflexic neurogenic bladder
- Voiding and spontaneous contractions of the arms and legs due to tactile stimulation of the abdomen, thighs, or genitalia
- Overflow incontinence and diminished anal sphincter tone due to flaccid neurogenic bladder
- Greatly distended bladder without a feeling of fullness due to sensory impairment

Complications
- Incontinence
- Residual urine retention
- UTI
- Calculus formation
- Renal failure

Diagnostic test findings
- Voiding cystourethrography evaluates bladder neck function, vesicoureteral reflux, and continence
- Urodynamic studies evaluate how urine is stored in the bladder, how well the bladder empties urine, and the rate of movement of urine out of the bladder during voiding
- Urine flow study (uroflow) shows diminished or impaired urine flow
- Cystometry evaluates bladder nerve supply, detrusor muscle tone, and intravesical pressures during bladder filling and contraction
- Urethral pressure profile determines urethral function with respect to length and outlet pressure resistance
- Sphincter electromyelography correlates neuromuscular function of the external sphincter with bladder muscle function during bladder filling and contraction and is used to evaluate how well the bladder and urinary sphincter muscles work together
- Videourodynamic studies correlate visual documentation of bladder function with pressure studies
- Retrograde urethrography shows strictures and diverticula

Treatment
- Teach the patient intermittent self-catheterization to empty the bladder if medications are ineffective
- Anticholinergics and alpha-adrenergic stimulators for hyperreflexic neurogenic bladder
- Teach the patient Credé's method to assist in emptying the bladder (pressing on the suprapubic area with a downward motion to express urine from the bladder)
- Terazosin (Hytrin) and doxazosin (Cardura) to facilitate bladder emptying

Key diagnostic test results for neurogenic bladder
- Voiding cystourethrography: Evaluation of bladder neck function, vesicoureteral reflux, and continence
- Urodynamic studies: Bladder handling of urine
- Cystometry: Evaluation of bladder nerve supply, detrusor muscle tone, and intravesical pressures
- Sphincter electromyelography: Correlation between neuromuscular function of external sphincter and bladder muscle function

Key treatments for neurogenic bladder
- Anticholinergics
- Terazosin and doxazosin
- Intermittent self-catheterization (if drugs are ineffective)

Key nursing considerations for neurogenic bladder

- Watch for signs of infection.
- Teach patient and family about intermittent self-catheterization as needed.

- Propantheline (Pro-Banthine), flavoxate (Urispas), dicyclomine (Bentyl), imipramine (Tofranil), and pseudoephedrine (Sudafed) to facilitate urine storage
- Surgery to correct structural impairment through transurethral resection of the bladder neck, urethral dilation, external sphincterotomy, or urinary diversion procedures
- Implantation of an artificial urinary sphincter (may be necessary if permanent incontinence follows surgery)

● Nursing considerations

- Explain diagnostic tests clearly so the patient understands the procedures, the time involved, and the possible results
- Use strict sterile technique during insertion of an indwelling catheter; don't interrupt the closed drainage system for any reason, obtain urine specimens with a syringe and small-bore needle inserted through the aspirating port of the catheter itself, and irrigate in the same manner if ordered
- Clean the catheter insertion site with soap and water at least twice per day; don't allow the catheter to become encrusted
    - Use a sterile applicator to apply antibiotic ointment around the meatus after catheter care
    - Keep the drainage bag below the tubing, and don't raise the bag above the level of the bladder

Renal calculi

Renal calculi vary in size and type. Small calculi may remain in the renal pelvis or may pass down the ureter. A staghorn calculus (a cast of the calyceal and pelvic collecting system) may develop from a calculus that stays in the kidney.

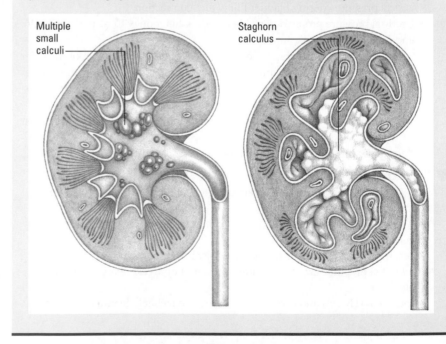

Multiple small calculi

Staghorn calculus

- Clamp the tubing or empty the bag before transferring the patient to a wheelchair or stretcher to prevent accidental urine reflux
    - Empty the bag as needed
- Watch for signs of infection (fever, cloudy or foul-smelling urine), and encourage the patient to drink plenty of fluids to prevent calculus formation and infection from urinary stasis (see *Renal calculi*)
- Encourage mobility; perform passive ROM exercises if necessary
- If a urinary diversion procedure is to be performed, arrange for consultation with an enterostomal therapist
- Teach the patient and his family evacuation techniques, as necessary (Credé's method, intermittent catheterization)
- Counsel the patient regarding sexual activities and provide emotional support

POLYCYSTIC KIDNEY DISEASE

- **Definition**
    - Inherited disorder characterized by multiple, bilateral, grapelike clusters of fluid-filled cysts that enlarge the kidneys, compressing and eventually replacing functioning renal tissue
    - Progression may be slow, even after symptoms of renal insufficiency appear
    - After uremia symptoms develop, polycystic disease usually is fatal within 4 years, unless the patient receives dialysis
    - Three genetic variants of the autosomal dominant form have been identified

- **Underlying pathophysiology**
    - Grossly enlarged kidneys are caused by multiple spherical cysts (distributed evenly throughout the cortex and medulla), a few millimeters to centimeters in diameter, that contain straw-colored or hemorrhagic fluid; hyperplastic polyps and renal adenomas are common
    - Renal parenchyma may have varying degrees of tubular atrophy, interstitial fibrosis, and nephrosclerosis; the cysts cause elongation of the pelvis, flattening of the calyces, and indentations in the kidney
    - Characteristically, an affected infant shows signs of respiratory distress, heart failure and, eventually, uremia and renal failure; accompanying hepatic fibrosis and intrahepatic bile duct abnormalities may cause portal hypertension and bleeding varices
    - About 10 years after symptoms appear, progressive compression of kidney structures by the enlarging mass causes renal failure
    - Cysts also form elsewhere — such as on the liver, spleen, pancreas, and ovaries; intracranial aneurysms, colonic diverticula, and mitral valve prolapse also occur
    - In the autosomal-recessive form, death in the neonatal period is most commonly due to pulmonary hypoplasia

- **Causes**
    - Inherited as an autosomal-dominant (adult type) or autosomal-recessive trait (infantile type)

- **Pathophysiologic changes**
    - In neonates

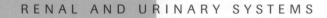

– Pronounced epicanthic folds (vertical fold of skin on either side of the nose); a pointed nose; small chin; and floppy, low-set ears (Potter facies), due to genetic abnormalities
– Huge, bilateral, symmetrical masses on the flanks that are tense and can't be transilluminated due to kidney enlargement
– Respiratory distress due to renal failure
– Uremia due to renal failure
- In adults
  – Hypertension due to activation of the renin-angiotensin system
  – Lumbar pain due to the enlarging kidney mass
  – Widening abdominal girth due to enlarged kidneys
  – Swollen or tender abdomen caused by the enlarging kidney mass, worsened by exertion and relieved by lying down
  – Grossly enlarged kidneys on palpation due to fluid-filled cysts within the kidneys

Complications
- Pyelonephritis
- Recurrent hematuria
- Life-threatening retroperitoneal bleeding from cyst rupture
- Proteinuria
- Colicky abdominal pain from ureteral passage of clots or calculi
- Renal failure

Diagnostic test findings
- Excretory or retrograde urography shows enlarged kidneys with elongation of the pelvis, flattening of the calyces, and indentations in the kidney caused by cysts
- Excretory urography in a neonate shows poor excretion of contrast medium
- Ultrasonography and CT and radioisotope scans show kidney enlargement and cystic damage; CT scan and magnetic resonance imaging show multiple areas of cystic damage
- Urinalysis and creatinine clearance tests show nonspecific results that indicate abnormalities

Treatment
- Antibiotics for infections
- Adequate hydration to maintain fluid balance
- Surgical drainage of cystic abscess or retroperitoneal bleeding
- Surgery for intractable pain (uncommon symptom) or analgesics for abdominal pain
- Dialysis or kidney transplantation for progressive renal failure
- Nephrectomy not recommended (disease occurs bilaterally, and the infection could recur in the remaining kidney)

Nursing considerations
- Refer the young adult patient or the parents of infants for genetic counseling
- Carefully assess the patient's lifestyle and his physical and mental status; determine how rapidly the disease is progressing, and use this information to plan individualized care

- Provide appropriate care and patient and family teaching (dialysis, kidney transplantation) as the disease progresses
- Explain all diagnostic procedures to the patient (or the parents if the patient is an infant)
- Before a procedure involving an iodine-based contrast medium, determine whether the patient has ever had an allergic reaction to iodine or shellfish (even if the patient has no history of allergy, monitor for allergic reactions during and after undergoing the procedures)
- Administer antibiotics as ordered for UTIs; stress to the patient or parents the need to take the medication exactly as prescribed, even if symptoms are minimal or absent

NCLEX CHECKS

It's never too soon to begin your licensure examination preparation. Now that you've reviewed this chapter, carefully read each of the following questions and choose the best answer. Then compare your responses with the correct answers.

1. A client is diagnosed with acute renal failure. During the physical examination, the client complains of left-sided back pain. Identify the area you should percuss to evaluate the left kidney for tenderness.

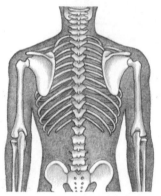

2. A client requests information on glomerulonephritis. The nurse teaches that glomerular lesions formed by accumulation of proliferating cells in Bowman's space are known as:

- ☐ **1.** proliferative.
- ☐ **2.** segmental-local.
- ☐ **3.** crescent.
- ☐ **4.** mesangial.

3. The nurse treating a client with acute renal failure observes the client's MAP. The nurse is aware that GFR will decrease sharply if MAP falls below:

- ☐ **1.** 60 mm Hg.
- ☐ **2.** 80 mm Hg.
- ☐ **3.** 100 mm Hg.
- ☐ **4.** 120 mm Hg.

TOP 6

Items to study for your next test on the renal and urinary systems

1. Pathophysiologic processes involved in acute renal failure, glomerulonephritis, and polycystic kidney disease
2. Common tests used to diagnose urinary dysfunction
3. Signs, symptoms, and care of the patient with neurogenic bladder
4. Nursing considerations for the patient with ATN
5. Treatment options for renal and urinary disorders
6. Effects of upper motor dysfunction versus lower motor dysfunction in neurogenic bladder

4. The nurse teaches a client on antibodies that sudden inflammation that affects the renal pelvis is known as:

☐ **1.** nephrotic syndrome.
☐ **2.** ATN.
☐ **3.** acute pyelonephritis.
☐ **4.** glomerulonephritis.

5. A nurse in the emergency department observes a client for acute renal failure. The nurse will assess for oliguria and what other finding?

☐ **1.** Hypertension
☐ **2.** Confusion
☐ **3.** Nausea
☐ **4.** Azotemia

6. An important nursing consideration to prevent ATN in a client preoperatively is to make sure that the client is:

☐ **1.** well sedated.
☐ **2.** well hydrated.
☐ **3.** hypotensive.
☐ **4.** afebrile.

7. When the GFR is 30% to 59% of normal during chronic renal failure, the client is experiencing:

☐ **1.** reduced renal reserves.
☐ **2.** renal insufficiency.
☐ **3.** renal failure.
☐ **4.** end-stage renal disease.

8. A client is being treated for nephrotic syndrome. The nurse would expect to see proteinuria, hyperlipidemia, edema, and:

☐ **1.** hypoalbuminemia.
☐ **2.** hyperalbuminemia.
☐ **3.** hypokalemia.
☐ **4.** hyperkalemia.

9. After a car accident, a client is diagnosed with a fracture of the fourth thoracic vertebra with severance of the spinal cord. The nurse would expect to see which type of neurogenic bladder?

☐ **1.** Sensory paralysis
☐ **2.** Autonomous
☐ **3.** Uninhibited
☐ **4.** Reflex

10. While caring for a client with acute renal failure, the nurse should expect that hypertonic glucose, insulin infusions, and sodium bicarbonate will be used to treat which complication?

☐ **1.** Hyperkalemia
☐ **2.** Hypocalcemia
☐ **3.** Hyperlipidemia
☐ **4.** Hyponatremia

ANSWERS AND RATIONALES

1. CORRECT ANSWER:

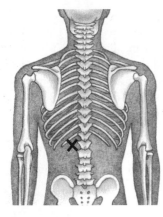

To evaluate renal tenderness, a sign of acute renal failure, percuss the costovertebral angle (the angle over each kidney that's formed by the border of the lowest rib and the vertebral column). Place the palm of one hand over the costovertebral angle and strike it with the fist of the other hand. The patient shouldn't experience discomfort with this procedure.

2. CORRECT ANSWER: 3

In glomerulonephritis, diffuse intracellular antibody proliferation in Bowman's space leads to a crescent-shaped structure that obliterates the space. These crescent lesions compress the glomerular capillaries, diminish blood flow, and cause extensive scarring of the glomeruli. In proliferative lesions, excess glomerular cells form throughout the kidney, whereas the term mesangial is related to deposition of immunoglobulins in the mesangial matrix. Segmental-local lesions involve only one part of the glomerulus.

3. CORRECT ANSWER: 2

Capillary pressure reflects MAP. Therefore, if MAP decreases to less than 80 mm Hg, the GFR will decrease steeply. The normal range for MAP is 80 to 180 mm Hg. At these levels, the body can regulate changes in capillary pressure through the afferent and efferent arterioles.

4. CORRECT ANSWER: 3

Acute pyelonephritis is a sudden inflammation caused by bacteria. It primarily affects the interstitial area and the renal pelvis or, less commonly, the renal tubules. Glomerulonephritis manifests as damage to the epithelial layer of the glomerular membrane and the collection of antigen-antibody complexes in the glomerular capillary membranes. ATN is common in the critically ill and involves injury to the nephron's tubular segment. Nephrotic syndrome results from a defect in the permeability of glomerular vessels.

5. CORRECT ANSWER: 4

Oliguria and azotemia are the early signs of acute renal failure and are caused by decreased blood flow to the kidneys; this, in turn, decreases urine output and GFR. Azotemia results when glomeruli can't properly process proteins — such as urea — for excretion, and these proteins and other nitrogenous wastes build up in the bloodstream.

6. CORRECT ANSWER: 2

To prevent ATN, it's important to make sure that the patient is well hydrated before surgery. ATN can result from ischemic injury due to surgery, particularly if the patient is dehydrated. Hypotension can cause decreased renal perfusion. Fever alone without dehydration would not lead to ATN, and sedation is irrelevant and expected before surgery.

7. CORRECT ANSWER: 2

Chronic renal failure occurs in four stages: Reduced renal reserves, renal insufficiency, renal failure, and end-stage renal disease. In the renal insufficiency phase, the GFR is 30% to 59% of normal. The GFR in the reduced renal reserve stage is 60% to 89% of normal. Renal failure is characterized by a GFR of 15% to 29% of normal, and end-stage renal disease is defined as a GFR of less than 15% of normal.

8. CORRECT ANSWER: 1

Regardless of the cause, the injured glomerular filtration membrane in nephrotic syndrome allows the loss of plasma proteins, especially albumin, causing hypoalbuminemia. Hyperkalemia, not hypokalemia, is a consequence of acute and chronic renal failure.

9. CORRECT ANSWER: 4

Reflex (or automatic) neurogenic bladder is caused by interruption of the efferent nerves at the cortical or upper motor neuron level such as with spinal cord transection resulting in loss of voluntary bladder control. The uninhibited type is also an upper motor neuron disease that can also be found in multiple sclerosis. In infancy, this lack of voluntary control is normal. Sensory paralysis and autonomous neurogenic bladder disease results from lower motor neuron dysfunction.

10. CORRECT ANSWER: 1

Hyperkalemia is a common complication of acute renal failure. Glucose administration and regular insulin infusions (with sodium bicarbonate, if necessary) can temporarily prevent cardiac arrest by moving potassium into the cells and temporarily reducing serum potassium levels. Less critical levels of hyperkalemia may be treated with oral sodium polystyrene sulfonate.

10

Integumentary system

LEARNING OBJECTIVES

After studying this chapter, you should be able to:

● Describe the relationship between presenting signs and symptoms and the pathophysiologic changes that occur with any integumentary disorder.

● Identify conditions that lead to the formation of skin lesions.

● List three probable causes of any integumentary disorder.

● Identify treatments for a patient with an integumentary disorder.

● Write three teaching goals for a patient with an integumentary disorder.

● Identify classes of medication that may improve inflammatory reactions of the skin.

CHAPTER OVERVIEW

The skin is the largest organ of the body and plays an important role in protecting internal structures from heat, light, and infection. The skin also aids in temperature regulation. Caring for a patient with an integumentary disorder requires an under standing of the pathophysiologic changes that occur, the signs and symptoms they produce, and the appropriate ways to intervene. The beginning section of this chapter provides an overview of the pathophysiology of inflammatory skin reactions and lesion formation. Common integumentary disorders are defined, and underlying pathophysiology, causes, pathophysiologic changes, complications, diagnostic test findings, treatments, and nursing considerations are outlined.

PATHOPHYSIOLOGIC CONCEPTS

● **Inflammation of the skin**
- Reaction of vascularized tissue to injury
- Skin changes caused by inflammatory response
- Increased immunoglobulin E (IgE) activity resulting from immune response to an infectious organism, trauma, extreme heat or cold, chemical irritation, or ischemic changes

● **Lesion formation**
- Primary skin lesions appear on previously healthy skin in response to disease or external irritation, such as chemical or radiant exposure
  - Classified as macules, papules, plaques, patches, nodules, tumors, wheals, comedones, cysts, vesicles, pustules, and bullae
- Modified lesions (secondary skin lesions)
  - Result from rupture, mechanical irritation, extension, invasion, or normal or abnormal healing of primary lesions
  - Classified as atrophy, erosions, ulcers, scales, crusts, excoriation, fissures, lichenification, and scars

ACNE

● **Definition**
- Chronic inflammatory disease of the sebaceous glands
- Usually associated with a high rate of sebum secretion; occurs on areas of the body that have sebaceous glands, such as the face, neck, chest, back, and shoulders
- Two types
  - Inflammatory (pustules, papules, and nodules)
    · Hair follicle is blocked by sebum, causing bacteria to grow and eventually rupture the follicle
  - Noninflammatory (closed and open comedones)
    · Follicle remains dilated but doesn't rupture

● **Underlying pathophysiology**
- Androgens stimulate sebaceous gland growth and sebum production, which is secreted into dilated hair follicles that contain bacteria
- The bacteria (usually *Propionibacterium acne* and *Staphylococcus epidermis*) are normal skin flora that secrete lipase
- Lipase interacts with sebum to produce free fatty acids, which provoke inflammation
- Hair follicles also produce more keratin, which joins with the sebum to form a plug in the dilated follicle

● **Causes**
- Possible causes include increased activity of sebaceous glands and blockage of the pilosebaceous ducts (hair follicles)
- Predisposing factors
  - Heredity
  - Androgen stimulation

Key facts about skin inflammation

- Increased IgE activity
- Results from an immune response

Key facts about lesion formation

Primary skin lesions
- Appear on previously healthy skin
- Include macules, nodules, tumors, and cysts

Secondary skin lesions
- Result from rupture, mechanical irritation, extension, invasion, or healing of primary lesions
- Include atrophy, ulcers, and scars

Key facts about acne

- Chronic inflammatory disease of sebaceous glands
- Develops when androgens stimulate sebaceous gland growth and sebum production

Inflammatory
- Blocks hair follicles with sebum, causing bacteria to grow and rupture the follicles

Noninflammatory
- Involves dilated follicles that don't rupture

- Certain drugs, including corticosteroids, corticotropin, androgens, iodides, bromides, trimethadione, phenytoin (Dilantin), isoniazid (Laniazid), lithium (Eskalith), and halothane
- Cobalt irradiation
- Hyperalimentation
- Exposure to heavy oils, greases, or tars
- Trauma or rubbing from tight clothing
- Comedogenic cosmetics
- Emotional stress
- Tropical climate
- Hormonal contraceptives (flare-ups are common during first few menses after starting or discontinuing)

● **Pathophysiologic changes**
- The acne plug appears as a closed or open comedo
  - Closed comedo, or whitehead (not protruding from the follicle and covered by the epidermis), forms due to sebaceous gland inflammation
  - Open comedo, or blackhead (protruding from the follicle and not covered by the epidermis), forms due to sebaceous gland inflammation
    - Melanin or pigment of the follicle causes the black color
- Characteristic acne pustules, papules or, in severe forms, acne cysts or abscesses (chronic, recurring lesions producing acne scars) form due to rupture or leakage of an enlarged plug into the epidermis
- In women, severity increases just before or during menstruation (when estrogen levels are lowest)

● **Complications**
- Acne conglobata (severe cystic form of acne with thickened, nodular scars, usually sparing the face)
- Scarring (when acne is severe)
- Abscesses or secondary bacterial infections
- Lowered self-esteem

● **Diagnostic test findings**
- Clinical appearance of characteristic acne lesions confirms the diagnosis, especially in adolescents
- Culture and sensitivity of pustules or abscesses reveals causative organism of secondary bacterial infection

● **Treatment**
- Topical
  - Antibacterial agents, such as benzoyl peroxide (Benzac 5 or 10), clindamycin (Cleocin), or erythromycin and benzoyl peroxide (Benzamycin), alone or with tretinoin (Retin-A; retinoic acid)
  - Keratolytic agents, such as benzoyl peroxide and tretinoin, dry and peel the skin to help open blocked follicles, moving the sebum up to the skin level
- Systemic
  - Antibiotics, usually tetracycline (Sumycin), to decrease bacterial growth
  - Cultures to identify a possible secondary bacterial infection (looking for exacerbation of pustules or abscesses while on tetracycline or erythromycin therapy)

Key pathophysiologic changes in acne

- Closed or open comedos
- Pustules or papules
- Acne cysts (severe forms)

Key treatments for acne

Topical
- Antibacterials
- Keratolytic agents

Systemic
- Antibiotics
- Isotretinoin

– Oral isotretinoin (Accutane) to inhibit sebaceous gland function and keratinization
– For females, antiandrogens, birth control pills, such as norgestimate and ethinyl estradiol (Ortho Tri-Cyclen), or spironolactone (Aldactone)
• Other (mechanical, surgical, injections)
– Cleaning with an abrasive sponge to dislodge superficial comedones
– Surgery to remove comedones and to open and drain pustules
– Dermabrasion (for severe acne scarring) with a high-speed metal brush to smooth the skin (performed only by a dermatologist or plastic surgeon)
– Bovine collagen injections into the dermis beneath the scarred area to fill in affected areas and even out the skin surface (not recommended by all dermatologists)

● **Nursing considerations**
• Check the patient's drug history because certain medications, such as hormonal contraceptives, may cause flare-ups
• Try to identify predisposing factors that may be eliminated or modified
• Try to identify eruption patterns (seasonal or monthly)
• Teach the patient about the causes of acne, explain the importance of practicing good personal hygiene to prevent secondary infections, and provide written instructions for treatment
• Instruct the patient receiving tretinoin to apply it at least 30 minutes after washing his face and at least 1 hour before bedtime; warn against using it around the eyes or lips
– Tell the patient that the skin should look pink and dry after treatment; skin that appears red or starts to peel may indicate the need to weaken the preparation or apply it less often
– Advise the patient to avoid exposure to sunlight or to use sunscreen
– If the prescribed regimen includes benzoyl peroxide, teach the patient to avoid skin irritation by using one preparation in the morning and the other at night
• Instruct the patient to take tetracycline on an empty stomach and not to take it with antacids or milk (tetracycline interacts with their metallic ions and is then poorly absorbed)
– Instruct the patient to avoid vitamin A supplements, which can worsen adverse effects
– Teach the patient how to deal with the dry skin and mucous membranes that usually occur during treatment; maintain good hydration and use a clinically approved oil-free moisturizer (see *Teaching your patient about skin care*)
• Take appropriate precautions for female patients taking isotretinoin
– Obtain informed consent
– Ensure that Food and Drug Administration-approved manufacturer recommendations regarding the severe risk of teratogenicity are followed
  • Perform pregnancy testing before dispensing and throughout the treatment period
  • Caution the patient to use two highly effective forms of contraception during treatment
• For all patients taking isotretinoin

Key nursing considerations for acne

• Try to identify and eliminate predisposing factors.
• Teach about acne's causes and the importance of good personal hygiene.
• Advise patient using tretinoin to avoid exposure to sunlight or to use sunscreen.
• Instruct patient taking tetracycline to take it on an empty stomach and to avoid vitamin A supplements.
• Advise patient taking isotretinoin to use two forms of contraception during treatment.
• Monitor liver function and lipid levels in patients taking isotretinoin.

Teaching points about wound healing

1. Keep wound moist.
2. Keep wound clean.

TIME-OUT FOR TEACHING

Teaching your patient about skin care

Skin is the body's largest organ and one of the most essential in preventing infection and protecting delicate tissues from heat, light, radiant light, and infective injury. However, most patients don't care for their skin well or recognize which problems should be reported to their health care practitioner. You can promote good skin care and develop teaching moments during many other aspects of care. Here are some basic topics to cover.

MOISTURE
Dry skin is more prone to cuts and irritants than is moist, healthy skin. Dry heat, cold, frequent use of soaps or chemicals, and the effects of aging all contribute to dry skin. Teach your patient to use moisturizers frequently and consistently when dry skin is noted.

WOUND HEALING
Like healthy skin, wounds require moisture to heal. Scabs function as sealants to maintain the body's own moisture in wound beds. Injuries that are too deep or too extensive to scab well should be kept moist with the use of an antibiotic ointment and protective dressing or a special hydrocolloid dressing (now available over the counter). Wounds must also be kept clean, but excessive use of betadine, alcohol-based products, or full-strength hydrogen peroxide can be too harsh or drying to healing tissues. Teach your patient that a physician should evaluate wounds that develop pus, involve punctures, are deep into the dermis or subcutaneous layers, or fail to heal.

WHAT TO REPORT
Teach your patient to report the following to a health care provider for evaluation:
- red, raised, blistered areas that appear suddenly, commonly in a line, and may be painful — possible herpes zoster, which requires immediate care for treatment to be effective
- a rash that hasn't responded to self-care for 2 weeks — possible contact dermatitis, eczema, systemic lupus erythematosus (depending on location), yeast infection, or impetigo
- bull's eye-type, round rash, even if tick exposure isn't identified — possible Lyme disease
- a lesion noted in the genital area — possible sexually transmitted disease
- a mole or wart that has changed in color or shape, or has become infected and won't heal — possible skin cancer
- presence of small, round, purplish lesions or bruises without known injury — possible liver disease or a hematologic disorder.

- Dispense only a 30-day supply; don't exceed a 16- to 20-week course for patients with severe papulopustular or cystic acne not responding to conventional therapy (due to severe adverse reactions)
- Monitor liver function and lipid levels; obtain a serum triglyceride level before and periodically during treatment
• Inform the patient that acne takes a long time to clear — even years for complete resolution; offer emotional support

Key facts about burns

- Denature cellular proteins
- Lead to loss of collagen cross-linking, causing intravascular fluid to move into interstitial spaces
- Cause cellular injury, triggering the release of mediators that increase in capillary permeability

Ways to classify burns

Amount of BSA affected

- Major — more than 10% of adult's BSA; more than 20% of child's BSA
- Moderate — 3% to 10% of adult's BSA; 10% to 20% of child's BSA
- Minor — less than 3% of adult's BSA; less than 10% of child's BSA

Body tissues involved

- First-degree (superficial) — limited to epidermis
- Second-degree (partial thickness) — affects epidermis and part of the dermis
- Third-degree (full thickness) — damage extends through subcutaneous tissue to muscle and bone

BURNS

● **Definition**
- Classified as first-, second-, or third-degree
  - First-degree (superficial) — limited to the epidermis, most common example is sunburn
  - Second-degree (partial thickness) — damage to the epidermis and part of the dermis
  - Third-degree (full thickness) — damage extends through deeply charred subcutaneous tissue to muscle and bone
- Classified by amount of body surface area (BSA) affected (see *Using the Rule of Nines and the Lund-Browder chart,* pages 358 and 359)
  - Major — more than 10% of an adult's BSA; more than 20% of a child's BSA
  - Moderate — 3% to 10% of an adult's BSA; 10% to 20% of a child's BSA
  - Minor — less than 3% of an adult's BSA; less than 10% of a child's BSA

● **Underlying pathophysiology**
- The injuring agent denatures cellular proteins; some cells die because of traumatic or ischemic necrosis
- Loss of collagen cross-linking also occurs with denaturation, creating abnormal osmotic and hydrostatic pressure gradients, which cause the movement of intravascular fluid into interstitial spaces
- Cellular injury triggers the release of mediators of inflammation, contributing to local and, in major burns, systemic increases in capillary permeability
- Specific pathophysiologic events depend on the cause and classification of the burn
  - First-degree burns cause localized injury or destruction to the epidermis only, by direct (such as chemical spill) or indirect (such as sunlight) contact; the barrier function of the skin remains intact, and the burns aren't life-threatening
  - Second-degree burns involve destruction to the epidermis and dermis
    - Thin-walled, fluid-filled blisters develop within a few minutes of the injury
    - As the blisters break, the nerve endings are exposed to the air
    - Some sensory neurons undergo extensive destruction in the area of the burn; the areas around the burn remain very sensitive to pain
    - Hair follicles remain intact (hair will grow again), but the barrier function of the skin is lost
  - Third-degree burns extend through the epidermis and dermis, and into the subcutaneous tissue layer or beyond (involve muscle, bone, and interstitial tissues)
    - Within only hours, fluids and protein shift from capillary to interstitial spaces, causing edema
    - The immediate immunologic response makes sepsis a potential threat
    - All usual functions of the skin are destroyed (the wound will require grafting to replace the skin); nerve death makes the areas less painful
    - Finally, an increased calorie demand for healing increases the metabolic rate

Causes

- Thermal burns (most common type)
  - Residential fires
  - Automobile accidents
  - Playing with matches
  - Improper handling of firecrackers
  - Improper handling of gasoline
  - Scalding and kitchen accidents
  - Abuse (most common in children and elderly patients)
  - Self-inflicted
  - Clothes that catch fire
- Chemical burns
  - Contact, ingestion, inhalation, or injection of acids, alkalis, or vesicants
- Electrical burns
  - Contact with faulty electrical wiring or high-voltage power lines
  - Chewing on electrical cords (young children)
- Friction or abrasion burns
  - Skin rubbing harshly against a coarse surface
- Radiant burns
  - Sunburn from excessive ultraviolet light exposure
  - Radiation from nuclear agents

Pathophysiologic changes

- In first-degree burns, localized pain and erythema (usually without blisters) in the first 24 hours and chills, headache, localized edema, and nausea and vomiting (due to more severe first-degree burn)
- In second-degree burns, thin-walled, fluid-filled blisters appearing within minutes of the injury, with mild to moderate edema and pain and a white, waxy appearance to the damaged area
- In third-degree burns, white, brown, or black leathery tissue and visible thrombosed vessels due to destruction of skin elasticity (dorsum of hand most common site of thrombosed veins), without blisters
- In electrical burns, silver-colored, raised area, usually at the site of electrical contact
- Singed nasal hairs, mucosal burns, voice changes, coughing, wheezing, soot in the mouth or nose, and darkened sputum due to smoke inhalation and pulmonary damage
- Hypotension secondary to shock or hypovolemia

Complications

- Loss of function (burns to face, hands, feet, and genitalia)
- Total occlusion of circulation in affected extremity (due to edema from circumferential burns)
- Airway obstruction (neck burns) or restricted respiratory expansion (chest burns)
- Pulmonary injury
- Acute respiratory distress syndrome
- Greater damage than indicated by the surface burn (electrical and chemical burns) or internal tissue damage along conduction pathway (electrical burns)
- Cardiac arrhythmias

(Text continues on page 360.)

Common causes of thermal burns

- Residential fires
- Automobile accidents
- Scalding and kitchen accidents
- Abuse (most common in children and elderly patients)

Key pathophysiologic changes in burns

First-degree
- Localized pain and erythema
- Localized edema

Second-degree
- Blisters
- White, waxy appearance in damaged area

Third-degree
- White, brown, or black leathery tissue without blisters
- Visible thrombosed vessels

Using the Rule of Nines and the Lund–Browder chart

You can quickly estimate the extent of an adult patient's burn by using the Rule of Nines. This method divides an adult's body surface area (BSA) into percentages. To use this method, mentally transfer your patient's burns to the body chart shown here, and then add up the corresponding percentages for each burned body section. The total, an estimate of the extent of your patient's burn,

RULE OF NINES CHART

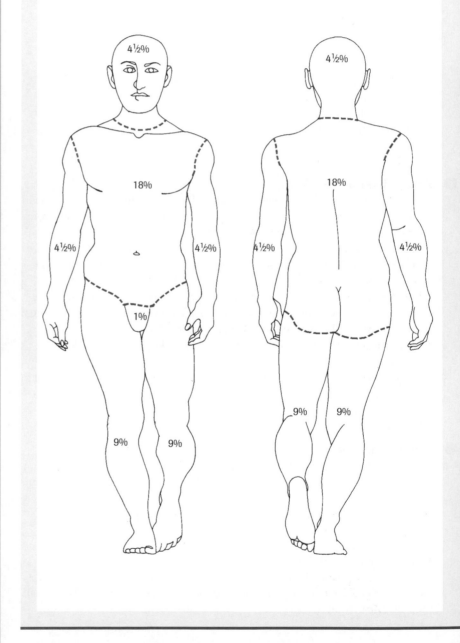

enters into the formula to determine his initial fluid replacement needs.

You can't use the Rule of Nines for infants and children because their body section percentages differ from those of adults. For example, an infant's head accounts for about 17% of his total BSA, compared to only 7% for an adult. Instead, use the Lund-Browder chart shown here.

LUND-BROWDER CHART

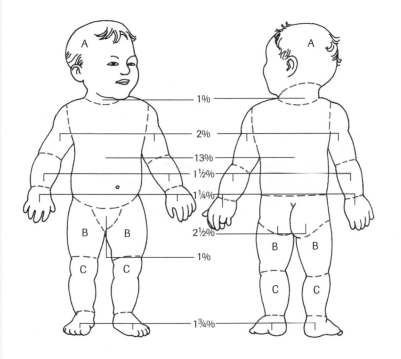

1%	
2%	
13%	
1½%	
1¼%	
2½%	
1%	
1¾%	

RELATIVE PERCENTAGES OF AREAS BY AGE

AT BIRTH	0–1 YR	1–4 YRS	5–9 YRS	10–15 YRS	ADULT
A: Half of head					
9½%	8½%	6½%	5½%	4½%	3½%
B: Half of thigh					
2½%	3½%	4%	4¼%	4½%	4¾%
C: Half of leg					
2½%	2½%	2¾%	3%	3¼%	3½%

- Infected burn wound
- Stroke, heart attack, or pulmonary embolism
- Peptic ulcer disease or ileus
- Burn shock, possibly leading to kidney damage and renal failure
- Disseminated intravascular coagulation (more severe burn states)

● **Diagnostic test findings**
- Wound size and classification are used to diagnose and determine the extent of injury
  - Size
    - Percentage of BSA covered by the burn using the Rule of Nines
    - Percentage of BSA covered by the burn using the Lund-Browder chart (more accurate because it allows BSA changes with age); correlation of the burn's depth and size to estimate its severity
- Arterial blood gas (ABG) levels show evidence of smoke inhalation; may show decreased alveolar function and hypoxia
- Complete blood count (CBC) shows decreased hemoglobin level and hematocrit if blood loss occurs
- Additional blood testing reveals abnormal electrolytes due to fluid losses and shifts, increased blood urea nitrogen (BUN) with fluid losses, decreased blood glucose level in children (due to limited glycogen), and increased carboxyhemoglobin
- Urinalysis shows myoglobinuria and hemoglobinuria
- Electrocardiography may show myocardial ischemia, injury, or arrhythmia, especially in electrical burns
- Fiber-optic bronchoscopy shows airway edema

● **Treatment**
- Initial treatment (based on type of burn)
  - **Maintaining an open airway; assessing airway, breathing, and circulation; checking for smoke inhalation; assisting with endotracheal intubation; and giving 100% oxygen (first immediate treatment for moderate and major burns)**
  - Removing smoldering clothing (first soaking in saline solution if clothing is stuck to the patient's skin), rings, and other constricting items
  - Immersing the burned area in cool water (55° F [12.8° C]) or applying cool compresses (minor burns)
  - Administering pain medication as needed or anti-inflammatory medications
  - Covering the area with an antimicrobial agent and a nonstick, bulky dressing (after debridement); prophylactic tetanus injection as needed
  - Controlling active bleeding
  - Covering partial-thickness burns over 30% of BSA or full-thickness burns over 5% of BSA with a clean, dry, sterile bed sheet (because of drastic reduction in body temperature, large burns should *not* be covered with saline-soaked dressings)
  - **Immediate I.V. therapy to prevent hypovolemic shock and maintain cardiac output (lactated Ringer's solution or a fluid replacement formula; additional I.V. lines may be needed)**
  - Antimicrobial therapy (all patients with major burns)

- CBC, electrolyte, glucose, BUN, and serum creatinine levels; ABG analysis; typing and cross-matching; and urinalysis for myoglobinuria and hemoglobinuria
- Close monitoring of intake and output, frequent checking of the patient's vital signs (every 15 minutes), and possible insertion of an indwelling urinary catheter
- Nasogastric tube insertion to decompress the stomach and avoid aspiration of stomach contents
- Wound irrigation with copious amounts of normal saline solution (chemical burns)
- Surgical intervention, including skin grafts and more thorough surgical cleaning (major burns)

● Nursing considerations
- Don't treat the burn wound in a patient being transferred to a specialty facility within 4 hours; instead, wrap the patient in a sterile sheet and blanket for warmth, elevate the burned extremity, and prepare the patient for transport
- Upon discharge or during prolonged care
  - Explain the need for increased calorie intake due to an increased metabolic rate to promote healing and recovery
  - Give the patient complete discharge instructions for home care
    - Stress the importance of keeping the dressing clean and dry, elevating the burned extremity for the first 24 hours, and having the wound rechecked in 1 to 2 days
    - Stress the importance of taking pain medication as needed, especially before dressing changes

CELLULITIS

● Definition
- Infection of the dermis or subcutaneous layer of the skin
- May follow damage to the skin, such as a bite or wound
- Persons with other contributing health factors, such as diabetes, immunodeficiency, impaired circulation, and neuropathy, have an increased risk of developing or spreading cellulitis to other areas of the body

● Underlying pathophysiology
- As the offending organism invades the compromised area, it overwhelms the defensive cells (neutrophils, eosinophils, basophils, and mast cells), which break down the cellular components that normally contain and localize the inflammation
- As cellulitis progresses, the organism invades tissue around the initial wound site
- As cellulitis spreads, fever, erythema, and lymphangitis may occur

● Causes
- Bacterial and fungal infections, commonly group A streptococcus and *Staphylococcus aureus*

● Pathophysiologic changes
- Erythema and edema due to inflammatory responses to the injury (classic signs)

Key nursing considerations for burns
- Give patient home care instructions. (Keep dressing clean and dry, elevate burned extremity for first 24 hours, have wound rechecked in 1 to 2 days.)
- Stress the importance of taking pain medication as needed.

Key facts about cellulitis
- Infection of dermis or subcutaneous layer of skin
- Commonly caused by group A streptococcus and *Staphylococcus aureus* infections
- Overwhelms defensive cells of compromised area, allowing infection to spread
- Progresses by invading tissue around initial wound site

Key pathophysiologic changes in cellulitis
- Erythema and edema
- Fever and warmth in affected area

Key diagnostic test results for cellulitis

- Culture and Gram stain: Positive for offending organism

Key treatments for cellulitis

- Oral or I.V. penicillin (unless patient has a known penicillin allergy)
- Warm soaks
- Elevation of infected extremity

Key nursing considerations for cellulitis

- Assess patient for enlarged affected area or intensification of pain.
- Teach patient to maintain good skin hygiene.
- Emphasize the importance of complying with treatment.

Key facts about contact dermatitis

- Sharply demarcated skin inflammation
- Results from contact with irritating chemical or atopic allergen

- Pain at the site and possibly surrounding area due to inflammation
- Fever and warmth in affected area due to temperature increase caused by infection

● Complications
- Sepsis (untreated cellulitis)
- Progression of cellulitis to involve more tissue
- Local abscesses
- Thrombophlebitis
- Lymphangitis (recurrent cellulitis)

● Diagnostic test findings
- Culture and Gram stain results from abscess and bulla fluid are positive for the offending organism
- Blood testing reveals a mildly elevated erythrocyte sedimentation rate (ESR), and a white blood cell (WBC) count showing mild leukocytosis with a left shift

● Treatment
- Oral or I.V. penicillin (drug of choice for initial treatment) unless the patient has a known penicillin allergy
- Warm soaks to help relieve pain and decrease edema by increasing vasodilation
- Pain medication as needed to promote comfort
- Elevation of the infected extremity to promote comfort and decrease edema
- Modified bed rest
- Protective footwear for ambulation

● Nursing considerations
- Assess the patient for an enlarged affected area or a worsening of pain
- Administer antibiotics, analgesics, and warm soaks as ordered
- Emphasize the importance of complying with treatment to prevent relapse
- To prevent recurrence, teach the patient to maintain good general hygiene and to carefully clean abrasions and cuts; urge the patient to obtain prompt treatment to prevent the spread of infection
- Explain the importance of range-of-motion (ROM) exercises to prevent deep vein thrombosis
- Encourage patients with diabetes and neuropathy to see a podiatrist on a regular basis

CONTACT DERMATITIS

● Definition
- Sharply demarcated skin inflammation
- Results from contact with irritating chemical or atopic allergen
- Produces varying symptoms, depending on the type and degree of exposure

● Underlying pathophysiology
- Contact with chemical irritants results in sharply demarcated skin inflammation
- Contact with mild irritants, such as detergents or solvents, results in erythema and small vesicles that ooze, scale, and itch

- Contact with strong irritants, such as acids and alkalis, causes blisters and ulceration
- With allergen contact
  - Sensitization is followed by cell-mediated type IV hypersensitivity (with repeated exposure)
  - Clearly defined erythema and lesions (small, oozing vesicles) with straight lines appear after the point of contact (classic mild reaction)
  - Marked erythema, blistering, and edema occur in a severe reaction

Causes
- Mild irritants (chronic exposure to detergents or solvents)
- Strong irritants (damage from or contact with acids or alkalis)
- Allergens (sensitization after repeated exposure)

Pathophysiologic changes
- Erythema and small vesicles that ooze, scale, and itch due to cellular infiltration in the dermis by a mild irritant
- Blisters and ulcerations due to cellular infiltration in the dermis by a strong irritant
- Clearly defined lesions with straight lines following points of contact (classic response); marked erythema, blistering, and edema of affected areas (severe response) due to cellular infiltration in dermis by allergen

Complications
- Secondary bacterial infections requiring antibiotic treatment
- Generalized skin eruptions due to autosensitization

Diagnostic test findings
- A detailed history is obtained to determine the irritant or allergen
- Patch testing identifies allergens

Treatment
- Elimination of known allergens
- Decreased exposure to irritants (wearing protective clothing such as gloves and washing immediately after contact with irritants or allergens)
- Topical anti-inflammatory agents (such as steroids); systemic steroids for edema and bullae; and antihistamines and local applications of Burow's solution (for blisters)
- Antibiotics for secondary infections
- Avoidance of excessive hand washing and drying and of accumulation of soaps and detergents under rings

Nursing considerations
- Warn the patient that drowsiness is possible with the use of antihistamines to relieve daytime itching; if itching interferes with sleep, suggest methods for inducing natural sleep, such as drinking a glass of warm milk, to prevent overuse of sedatives
- Assist the patient in scheduling daily skin care
- Keep the patient's fingernails short to limit excoriation and secondary infections caused by scratching
- Apply cool, moist compresses to relieve itching and burning

Key pathophysiologic changes in contact dermatitis
- Erythema and small vesicles that ooze, scale, and itch (with mild irritants)
- Blisters and ulcerations (with strong irritants)

Key diagnostic test results for contact dermatitis
- Patch testing: Identification of allergens

Key treatments for contact dermatitis
- Elimination of known allergens
- Topical anti-inflammatory drugs
- Systemic steroids (for severe reaction)

Key nursing considerations for contact dermatitis
- Apply cool, moist compresses.
- Keep patient's fingernails short to limit secondary infections caused by scratching.

Key facts about folliculitis, furuncles, and carbuncles

- Inflammatory reactions to infection within the hair follicle
- Most commonly caused by *Staphylococcus aureus*

Key pathophysiologic changes in folliculitis, furuncles, and carbuncles

- Pustules (folliculitis)
- Hard, painful, pus-filled nodules that rupture (furuncles)
- Deep abscesses draining through multiple openings (carbuncles)

FOLLICULITIS, FURUNCLES, AND CARBUNCLES

● **Definition**
- Folliculitis: Bacterial infection of a hair follicle that causes a pustule to form; infection can be superficial (follicular impetigo or Bockhart's impetigo) or deep (sycosis barbae)
- Furuncles: A form of deep folliculitis; also known as *boils*
- Carbuncles: A group of interconnected furuncles (see *Follicular skin infection*)

● **Underlying pathophysiology**
- The affecting organism enters the body, usually at a break in the skin barrier such as a wound site
- The organism then causes an inflammatory reaction within the hair follicle

● **Causes**
- Coagulase-positive *Staphylococcus aureus* (most common cause of folliculitis, furuncles, and carbuncles)
- Other causes
  - *Klebsiella, Enterobacter,* or *Proteus* organisms, which cause gram-negative folliculitis in patients on long-term antibiotic therapy such as for acne
  - *Pseudomonas aeruginosa* (thrives in a warm environment with a high pH and low chlorine content — "hot tub folliculitis")
- Predisposing risk factors
  - Infected wound
  - Poor hygiene
  - Debilitation
  - Tight clothes
  - Friction
  - Immunosuppressive therapy
  - Exposure to certain solvents
  - Diabetes

● **Pathophysiologic changes**
- Folliculitis
  - In children, pustules on the scalp, arms, and legs due to infection
  - In adults, pustules on the trunk, buttocks, scalp, arms, and legs due to infection
- Furuncles
  - Hard, painful nodules (commonly on the neck, face, axillae, and buttocks) that enlarge for several days and then rupture, discharging pus and necrotic material; after the nodules rupture, pain subsides but erythema and edema persist for days or weeks due to bacterial infection
- Carbuncles
  - Extremely painful, deep abscesses draining through multiple openings onto the skin surface, usually around several hair follicles
  - Accompanying fever and malaise due to infection

● **Complications**
- Scarring
- Bacteremia or cellulitis
- Metastatic seeding of a cardiac valve defect or arthritic joint

Follicular skin infection

The degree of hair follicle involvement in bacterial skin infection ranges from superficial erythema and pustules in a single follicle to deep abscesses (carbuncles) involving several follicles.

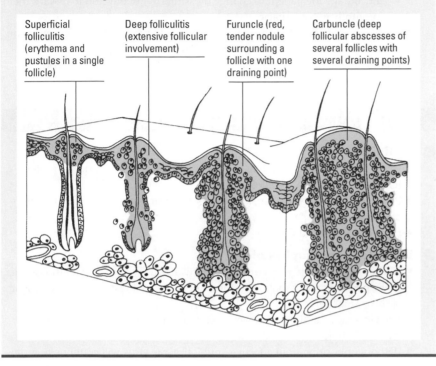

Superficial folliculitis (erythema and pustules in a single follicle)

Deep folliculitis (extensive follicular involvement)

Furuncle (red, tender nodule surrounding a follicle with one draining point)

Carbuncle (deep follicular abscesses of several follicles with several draining points)

● **Diagnostic test findings**
  • Wound cultures of the infected site reveal the infecting organism
  • Blood testing may show elevated WBCs

● **Treatment**
  • Cleaning the infected area thoroughly with antibacterial soap and water
  • Applying warm, wet compresses to promote vasodilation and drainage from the lesions
  • Topical antibiotics, such as mupirocin (Bactroban) ointment or clindamycin (Cleocin T) or erythromycin (Emgel, Staticin) solution
  • Folliculitis (extensive infection)
    – Systemic antibiotics, such as cefazolin (Ancef) or dicloxacillin (Dycill)
  • Furuncles
    – Warm, wet compresses, followed by incision and drainage of ripe lesions, and systemic antibiotics
  • Carbuncles
    – Systemic antibiotic therapy; incision and drainage

● **Nursing considerations**
  • Caution the patient never to squeeze a boil because this may cause it to rupture into the surrounding area and result in scarring

Key nursing considerations for folliculitis, furuncles, and carbuncles

- Teach patient how to prevent spreading bacteria.

- Teach the patient how to prevent spreading bacteria to family members
  - Discourage sharing towels and washcloths; instruct the patient to launder these items in hot water before reusing
  - Instruct the patient to change his clothes and bedding daily, and to wash them in hot water
  - Encourage the patient to change dressings frequently and to discard them promptly in paper bags
- Advise the patient with recurrent furunculosis to have a physical examination because an underlying disease, such as diabetes, may be present
- Caution the patient that trauma resulting from hairstyles, such as "corn-rowing," can cause folliculitis

HERPES ZOSTER

● Definition
- Acute inflammation caused by infection with herpes virus varicella-zoster (chickenpox virus); also called *shingles*
- Produces localized vesicular skin lesions and severe neuralgic pain in peripheral areas
- Usually occurs in adults

● Underlying pathophysiology
- Herpes zoster erupts when the virus reactivates after dormancy in the ganglia of the posterior nerve roots or in the cerebral ganglia (extramedullary ganglia of the cranial nerves)
- The virus may multiply as it reactivates, and antibodies remaining from the initial infection may neutralize it
- Without opposition from effective antibiotics, the virus will continue to multiply in the ganglia, destroying neurons and spreading down the sensory nerves to the skin (see *A look at herpes zoster*)

● Causes
- Reactivation of varicella virus

● Pathophysiologic changes
- Fever and malaise; eruption of small, red, nodular skin lesions on painful areas due to viral reactivation
  - Lesions commonly spread unilaterally around the thorax or vertically over the arms or legs; nodules quickly become vesicles filled with clear fluid or pus
- Severe deep pain, pruritus, and paresthesia or hyperesthesia due to innervation arising in inflamed root ganglia
  - Usually on trunk; occasionally on arms and legs in dermatonal distribution
- Eye pain, corneal and scleral damage (possible), impaired vision due to trigeminal ganglion involvement, conjunctivitis, extraocular weakness, ptosis, and paralytic mydriasis due to oculomotor involvement (rare)
- Complete recovery in most patients, but with possible permanent manifestations (scarring, vision impairment [with corneal damage], or persistent neuralgia)

Key facts about herpes zoster

- Caused by infection with herpes virus varicella-zoster
- Produces vesicular skin lesions and severe neuralgic pain

Key pathophysiologic changes in herpes zoster

- Small, red, nodular skin lesions on painful areas
- Possible eye pain and corneal and scleral damage
- Possible persistent neuralgia

A look at herpes zoster

These characteristic herpes zoster lesions are fluid-filled vesicles that dry and form scabs after about 10 days. Unilateral vesicular lesions in a dermatomal pattern should rapidly lead to a diagnosis of herpes zoster.

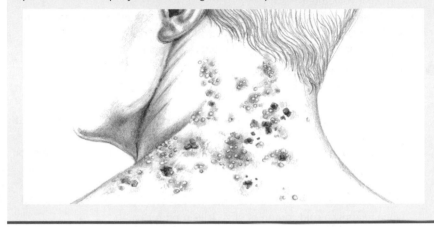

● Complications
- Deafness
- Bell's palsy
- Secondary skin infection
- Postherpetic neuralgia
- Meningoencephalitis
- Cutaneous dissemination
- Ocular involvement with facial zoster
- Hepatitis
- Pneumonitis
- Peripheral motor weakness
- Guillain-Barré syndrome
- Cranial nerve syndrome

● Diagnostic test findings
- Vesicular fluid and infected tissue analyses show eosinophilic inclusions and varicella virus
- Staining antibodies from vesicular fluid and identification under fluorescent light aids in differentiating herpes zoster from herpes simplex virus
- Specific antibody immune globulin measurement of varicella antibodies reveals elevated levels
- Cerebrospinal spinal fluid (CSF) analysis demonstrates increased protein levels and, possibly, pleocytosis
- Lumbar puncture indicates increased CSF pressure

● Treatment
- Antiviral agent (acyclovir [Zovirax], treatment of choice) to help stop rash progression, prevent visceral complications, and shorten duration of pain and symptoms in adults with normal immune function; may be given I.V. to prevent life-threatening disease in immunocompromised patients

Key diagnostic test results for herpes zoster
- Vesicular fluid and infected tissue analyses: Presence of varicella virus
- Antibody immune globulin: Elevated varicella antibody level

Key treatments for herpes zoster
- Antiviral agent
- Cortisone
- Possibly, tricyclic antidepressants, anticonvulsant agents, or a nerve block

Key nursing considerations for herpes zoster

- Maintain meticulous hygiene.
- With open lesions, follow contact isolation precautions.
- Explain local treatment of vesicles to the patient.

Key facts about pressure ulcers

- Localized areas of cellular necrosis
- Occur most commonly on skin and subcutaneous tissue over bony prominences
- Develop when pressure causes ischemia and hypoxemia to tissues
- Result in accumulation of waste products and toxins at the site and cell death

- Calamine lotion (or another antipruritic) and analgesics (aspirin, acetaminophen, codeine) to relieve itching and neuralgic pain
- System antibiotics to treat bacteria-infected, ruptured vesicles
- Immediate follow-up with an ophthalmologist and instillation of idoxuridine (Herplex) ointment (or another antiviral agent) to treat trigeminal zoster with corneal involvement
- Corticosteroids (cortisone) or, possibly, tricyclic antidepressants, anticonvulsant agents, or a nerve block to reduce inflammation and help the patient cope with intractable pain of postherpetic neuralgia

● Nursing considerations

- Maintain meticulous hygiene to prevent spreading the infection to other parts of the body
- With open lesions, follow contact isolation precautions to prevent the spread of infection
- Teach the patient to use a soft toothbrush, eat soft foods, and use a saline- or bicarbonate-based mouthwash and oral anesthetics to decrease discomfort from oral lesions
- Explain local treatment of vesicles, the need to avoid scratching lesions, and when to apply a cold compress (if vesicles rupture)

PRESSURE ULCERS

● Definition

- Commonly called *pressure sores* or *bedsores*
- Localized areas of cellular necrosis that occur most commonly on the skin and subcutaneous tissue over bony prominences
- Most pressure ulcers develop over five body locations: Sacral area, greater trochanter, ischial tuberosity, heel, and lateral malleolus
- May be superficial (caused by local skin irritation with subsequent surface maceration) or deep, originating in underlying tissue
  - Partial-thickness ulcers usually involve the dermis and epidermis (with treatment, heal within a few weeks)
  - Full-thickness ulcers also involve the dermis and epidermis (damage is more severe and complete)

● Underlying pathophysiology

- A pressure ulcer is caused by an injury to the skin and its underlying tissues
- The pressure exerted on the area causes ischemia and hypoxemia to the affected tissues because of decreased blood flow to the site
- As the capillaries collapse, thrombosis occurs, which subsequently leads to tissue edema and progression to tissue necrosis
- Ischemia adds to an accumulation of waste products at the site; this, in turn, leads to the production of toxins
- The toxins further break down the tissue and eventually lead to cell death
- Deep lesions commonly go undetected until they penetrate the skin, when they have usually already caused subcutaneous damage (see *Four stages of pressure ulcers,* pages 370 and 371)

● Causes

- Immobility and decreased level of activity

- Friction or shearing forces causing damage to the epidermal and upper dermal skin layers
- Constant moisture on the skin causing tissue maceration
- Impaired hygiene status, such as with urinary or fecal incontinence, leading to skin breakdown
- Malnutrition (associated with pressure ulcer development)
- Medical conditions, such as diabetes and orthopedic injuries (may be predisposing factors)
- Psychological factors, such as depression and chronic emotional stress

● **Pathophysiologic changes**
- Blanching erythema, varying from pink to bright red depending on the patient's skin color; in dark-skinned people, purple discoloration or a darkening of normal skin color (first clinical sign) due to impaired skin capillary pressure
- Pain at the site and surrounding area due to inflammation
- Localized edema due to the inflammatory response
- Increased body temperature due to initial inflammatory response (in more severe cases, cool skin due to more severe damage or necrosis)
- Nonblanching erythema (more severe cases), ranging from dark red to purple; or cyanotic, caused by deeper dermal involvement
- Blisters, crusts, or scaling as the skin deteriorates and the ulcer progresses due to inflammatory reaction
- Dusky-red appearance (usually), minimal bleeding, warm to the touch, and possibly mottled (deep ulcer originating at the bony prominence below the skin surface) due to inflammatory reaction
- Possible foul-smelling, purulent drainage from the ulcerated lesion due to infection
- Eschar tissue on and around the lesion due to the necrotic tissue that prevents healthy tissue growth

● **Complications**
- Progression to a more severe state (greatest risk)
- Secondary infections such as sepsis
- Loss of limb from bone involvement (osteomyelitis)

● **Diagnostic test findings**
- Wound culture shows exudate or evidence of infection
- Blood testing reveals elevated WBC count (with infection) and ESR
- Total serum protein and serum albumin analysis reveals low levels, indicating severe hypoproteinemia

● **Treatment**
- Repositioning by the caregiver every 2 hours (or more often if indicated) with support of pillows for immobile patients; a pillow and encouragement to change position for those able to move
- Movement and ROM exercises to promote circulation
- Foam, gel, or air mattress on bed to aid in healing (by reducing pressure on the ulcer site) and reduce the risk of additional ulcers
- Foam, gel, or air cushion on chairs and wheelchairs as indicated
- Nutritional assessment and dietary consultation as indicated; nutritional supplements, such as vitamin C and zinc, for the malnourished patient; serum albumin; protein markers; and body weight monitoring

---

Key pathophysiologic changes in pressure ulcers

- Blanching erythema
- Localized edema
- Nonblanching erythema (more severe cases)
- Eschar tissue on and around lesion
- Possible foul-smelling drainage

Key diagnostic test results for pressure ulcers

- Wound culture: Exudate or evidence of infection
- Blood testing: Elevated WBC count (with infection) and ESR

Key treatments for pressure ulcers

- Repositioning every 2 hours
- Foam, gel, or air mattress
- Nutritional assessment and dietary consultation
- Dressings and wound care appropriate for ulcer stage

Pressure ulcer stages

Stage I
- Skin is intact and red
- Ulcer resolves with removal of pressure

Stage II
- Skin breaks appear
- Ulcer penetrates dermis and subcutaneous fat layer

Stage III
- Ulcerated hole with purulent drainage develops
- Eschar develops

Stage IV
- Ulcer penetrates through all tissue layers to bone
- Tissue becomes necrotic
- Tunnels may develop

Four stages of pressure ulcers

To protect your patient from pressure ulcer complications, learn to recognize the four stages of pressure ulcer formation.

STAGE I
The skin is red and intact and doesn't blanche with external pressure. The skin feels warm and firm. Usually, the sore reverses after pressure is removed.

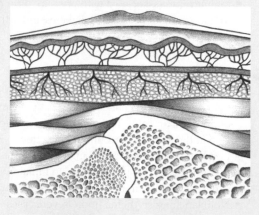

STAGE II
Skin breaks appear and discoloration may occur. Penetrating to the subcutaneous fat layer, the sore is painful and visibly swollen. The ulcer may be characterized as an abrasion, blister, or shallow crater. If pressure is removed, the sore may heal within 1 to 2 weeks.

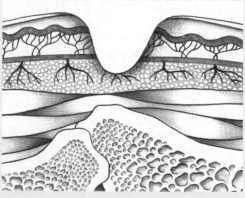

- Adequate fluid intake (I.V. if indicated); increased fluids for a dehydrated patient
- Good skin care and hygiene practices (for example, meticulous hygiene and skin care for the incontinent patient to prevent tissue and skin breakdown)
- For stage II ulcers, covering ulcer with transparent film, polyurethane foam, or hydrocolloid dressing
- For stage II or III ulcers, loosely filling wound with saline- or gel-moistened gauze, managing exudate with absorbent dressing (moist gauze or foam), and covering the site with a secondary dressing
- For deeper wounds (some stage III or stage IV), surgical debridement of necrotic tissue, as indicated, to allow healing
- Clean, bulky dressing (for certain types of ulcers such as decubiti)

● Nursing considerations
- Check the skin of bedridden or other high-risk patients for possible changes in color, turgor, temperature, and sensation; assess for pain and examine an existing ulcer for change in size or degree of damage

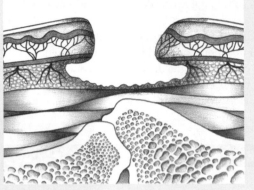

STAGE III

A hole develops that oozes foul-smelling, yellow or green fluid. The ulcer extends into the muscle and may develop a black, leathery crust (eschar) at its edges and, eventually, at the center. Undermining may or may not be present. The ulcer isn't painful, but healing may take months.

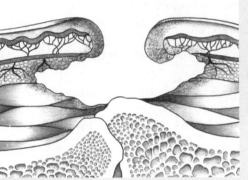

STAGE IV

The ulcer destroys tissue from the skin to the bone and becomes necrotic. Findings include foul drainage and deep tunnels that extend from the ulcer. The ulcer may take months or even a year to heal.

- Prevent pressure ulcers by repositioning the bedridden patient at least every 2 hours around the clock
  - To minimize the effects of a shearing force, use a footboard and raise the head of the bed to an angle not exceeding 60 degrees
  - Use a draw or pull sheet to turn the patient or to pull him up
  - Keep the patient's knees slightly flexed for short periods
  - Perform passive ROM exercises, or encourage the patient to do active exercises, if possible
  - Use pressure relief aids on the patient's bed (immobilized patients)
    - When using pressure relief aids or topical agents, explain their function to the patient
- Provide meticulous skin care, keeping the skin clean and dry without the use of harsh soaps
  - Gently massage the skin around (not on) the affected area to promote healing

Key nursing considerations for pressure ulcers

- Reposition bedridden patient at least every 2 hours.
- Provide meticulous skin care.
- Encourage adequate intake of nutritious food and fluids.

– Thoroughly rub moisturizing lotions into the skin to prevent maceration of the skin surface
– Change bedding frequently for patients who are diaphoretic, incontinent, or who have large amounts of drainage from wounds, suture lines, or drain sites; use a fecal incontinence bag for patients who are incontinent of stool
- Clean open lesions with a 3% solution of hydrogen peroxide or normal saline solution
- When needed, apply porous dressings, taped lightly to healthy skin
- Encourage adequate intake of nutritious food and fluids to maintain body weight and promote healing; consult with the dietitian to provide a diet that promotes granulation of new tissue; encourage the debilitated patient to eat frequent, small meals that provide protein- and calorie-rich supplements; and assist weakened patients with their meals

PSORIASIS

Definition
- Chronic, recurrent disease marked by epidermal proliferation and characterized by recurring partial remissions and exacerbations
- Flare-ups commonly related to specific systemic and environmental factors, but may be unpredictable
- Widespread involvement is called *exfoliative* or *erythrodermic psoriasis*

Underlying pathophysiology
- A skin cell normally takes 14 days to move from the basal layer to the stratum corneum, where it's sloughed off after 14 days of normal wear and tear; thus, the life cycle of a normal skin cell is 28 days, while that of a psoriatic skin cell is only 4 days
- This markedly shortened cycle doesn't allow time for the cell to mature
- Consequently, the stratum corneum becomes thick and flaky, producing the cardinal manifestations of psoriasis

Causes
- Probable immune disorder possibly mediated by the T cells of the dermis
- Probable genetic disorder, as shown in the human leukocyte antigen (HLA)-B13, -B17, and -Cw6 histocompatibility tissue types present in families known to have the disease
- Environmental factors, such as climate (cold weather tends to exacerbate psoriasis); infection; smoking; alcoholism; and ultraviolet light
- Isomorphic effect or Koebner's phenomenon, in which lesions develop at sites of injury due to trauma
- Flare-up of guttate (drop-shaped) lesions due to infections, especially beta-hemolytic streptococci
- Other contributing factors
  – Pregnancy
  – Endocrine changes
  – Emotional stress

Key facts about psoriasis
- Marked by abnormal epidermal proliferation
- Result of shortened skin cell life (4 days), which doesn't allow time for cell to mature
- Causes stratum corneum to become thick and flaky

Key pathophysiologic changes in psoriasis
- Itching and occasional pain
- Erythematous and well-defined lesions
- Plaques with silver scales that flake off easily or thicken

Pathophysiologic changes

- Itching and occasional pain from dry, cracked, encrusted lesions (most common)
- Erythematous and usually well-defined plaques (psoriatic lesions), sometimes covering large areas of the body
  - Lesions most commonly on the scalp, chest, elbows, knees, back, and buttocks; plaques with characteristic silver scales that either flake off easily or thicken, covering the lesion; scale removal can produce fine bleeding; occasional small guttate lesions (usually thin and erythematous, with few scales), either alone or with plaques due to inflammatory reaction by T cells in dermis

Complications

- Spreading to fingernails, producing small indentations or pits and yellow or brown discoloration; occurs in about 60% of patients; (no effective topical treatment)
  - Accumulation of thick, crumbly debris under the nail, causing it to separate from the nail bed (onycholysis)
- Infection, secondary to scratching
- Psoriasis becoming pustular (rare) and taking one of two forms
  - Localized, pustular psoriasis, with pustules on the palms and soles that remain sterile until opened
  - Generalized pustular (Von Zumbusch's) psoriasis, typically occurring with fever, leukocytosis, and malaise, with groups of pustules coalescing to form lakes of pus on red skin (also remain sterile until opened), commonly involving the tongue and oral mucosa
- Erythrodermic psoriasis (least common form), an inflammatory form of the disorder characterized by periodic fiery erythema and exfoliation of the skin with severe itching and pain
- Arthritic symptoms, usually in one or more joints of the fingers or toes, the larger joints, or sometimes the sacroiliac joints, which may progress to spondylitis, and morning stiffness (some patients)

Diagnostic test findings

- Skin biopsy is performed to help rule out other disease
- Serum uric acid analysis reveals a level that's usually elevated in severe cases due to accelerated nucleic acid degradation, but without indications of gout
- Genetic testing may reveal HLA-Cw6, -B13, and -Bw57 in early-onset, familial psoriasis

Treatment

- Ultraviolet B (UVB) or natural sunlight exposure to retard rapid cell production to the point of minimal erythema
  - Tar preparations or crude coal tar applications to the affected areas about 15 minutes before exposure to UVB, or left on overnight and wiped off the next morning
  - Gradually increasing exposure to UVB (outpatient treatment or day treatment prevents the need for long hospitalizations and prolongs remission)
- Steroid creams and ointments applied twice daily, preferably after bathing to facilitate absorption, and overnight use of occlusive dressings to control symptoms
- Intralesional steroid injection for small, recalcitrant plaques

Key diagnostic test results for psoriasis

- Skin biopsy: Rules out other disease
- Genetic testing: Presence of HLA-Cw6, -B13, and -Bw57 (early-onset, familial psoriasis)

Key treatments for psoriasis

- UVB or natural sunlight
- Tar preparations before UVB exposure
- Topical and systemic steroids
- Aspirin and local heat (psoriatic arthritis)

- Anthralin ointment (Anthra-Derm) or paste mixture for well-defined plaques (not applied to unaffected areas due to injury and staining of normal skin); petroleum jelly around affected skin before applying anthralin
- Anthralin at night and systemic steroids during the day
- Calcipotriene ointment (Dovonex), a vitamin D analogue (best when alternated with a topical steroid)
- Goeckerman regimen (combines tar baths and UVB treatments) to help achieve remission and clear the skin in 3 to 5 weeks (severe, chronic psoriasis)
- Ingram technique (variation of the Goeckerman regimen using anthralin instead of tar)
- Administration of psoralens (plant extracts that accelerate exfoliation) with exposure to high-intensity ultraviolet A (UVA) light (psoralen plus UVA [PUVA] therapy)
- A cytotoxin, usually methotrexate (Mexate) as last-resort treatment for refractory psoriasis
- Acitretin (Soriatane), a retinoid compound, for extensive psoriasis
- Cyclosporine (Neoral), an immunosuppressant, in resistant cases
- Low-dose antihistamines, oatmeal baths, emollients, and open, wet dressings to help relieve pruritus
- Aspirin and local heat to help alleviate the pain of psoriatic arthritis; non-steroidal anti-inflammatory drugs in severe cases
- Tar shampoo followed by a steroid lotion to treat psoriasis of the scalp

Nursing considerations
- Make sure that the patient understands his prescribed therapy; provide written instructions to avoid confusion
  - Teach correct application of prescribed ointments, creams, and lotions (for example, a steroid cream should be applied in a thin film and rubbed gently into the skin until the cream disappears)
    - Explain that all topical medications, especially those containing anthralin and tar, should be applied with a downward motion to avoid rubbing them into the follicles; gloves must be worn because anthralin stains and injures the skin
    - Teach the patient to dust himself with powder after application to prevent anthralin from rubbing off on his clothes
    - Caution the patient to never put an occlusive dressing over anthralin; suggest using mineral oil, then soap and water, to remove anthralin
  - Caution the patient to avoid scrubbing his skin vigorously to prevent Koebner phenomenon; if a medication has been applied to the scales to soften them, suggest that the patient use a soft brush to remove them
- Watch for adverse effects, especially allergic reactions to anthralin; atrophy and acne from steroids; and burning, itching, nausea, and squamous cell epitheliomas from PUVA therapy
- Initially, evaluate the patient's red blood cell, WBC, and platelet counts because cytotoxins may cause hepatic or bone marrow toxicity
  - Explain that liver biopsy may be done to assess the effects of methotrexate
  - Strongly caution the patient taking methotrexate not to drink alcohol due to the increased risk of hepatotoxicity
- Caution the patient undergoing PUVA therapy to stay out of the sun on the day of treatment, and to protect his eyes with sunglasses that block out UVA rays for 24 hours after treatment; tell him to wear goggles during exposure to this light

Key nursing considerations for psoriasis
- Teach correct application of prescribed ointments, creams, and lotions.
- Watch for adverse effects of medications.
- Refer patient to National Psoriasis Foundation.

- Be aware that psoriasis can cause psychological problems; assure the patient that psoriasis isn't contagious; and reassure him that, although exacerbations and remissions occur, they're controllable with treatment (make sure that the patient understands that there's no cure)
- Help the patient learn effective stress management techniques and coping mechanisms; explain the relationship between psoriasis and arthritis, but point out that psoriasis causes no other systemic disturbances
- Refer all patients to the National Psoriasis Foundation, which provides information and directs patients to local chapters for information and support

NCLEX CHECKS

It's never too soon to begin your licensure examination preparation. Now that you've reviewed this chapter, carefully read each of the following questions and choose the best answer. Then compare your responses with the correct answers.

1. The organism responsible for hot tub folliculitis is:
- ☐ **1.** *S. aureus.*
- ☐ **2.** *Klebsiella.*
- ☐ **3.** *Proteus.*
- ☐ **4.** *Pseudomonas aeruginosa.*

2. The nurse is caring for a 7-year-old child who has extensive burns to the back of the head and neck, the back, and the right buttock. Using the Lund-Browder chart shown here, what percentage of BSA is affected?

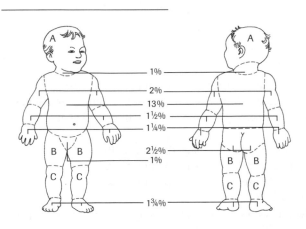

1%
2%
13%
1½%
1¼%
2½%
1%
1¾%

3. Inflammatory reactions of the skin are related to the activity of which immunoglobulin?
- ☐ **1.** A
- ☐ **2.** E
- ☐ **3.** G
- ☐ **4.** M

4. The nurse is teaching a client about oral isotretinoin. Which instruction should the nurse include?
- ☐ **1.** Take medication on an empty stomach.
- ☐ **2.** Test for pregnancy throughout treatment.
- ☐ **3.** Have coagulation studies drawn periodically.
- ☐ **4.** Use vitamin supplements.

TOP 5

Items to study for your next test on the integumentary system

1. Pressure ulcer stages
2. Treatments for acne
3. Teaching points for proper skin care
4. Pathophysiology of psoriasis
5. Common diagnostic tests for integumentary disorders

5. When teaching a client about taking tetracycline for the treatment of acne, the nurse should be sure to tell the client to take the medication:
- [ ] **1.** with milk.
- [ ] **2.** with an antacid.
- [ ] **3.** on a full stomach.
- [ ] **4.** on an empty stomach.

6. A burn that affects the epidermis and dermis is considered:
- [ ] **1.** minor.
- [ ] **2.** second-degree.
- [ ] **3.** thermal.
- [ ] **4.** third-degree.

7. The first treatment for major burns is to:
- [ ] **1.** control active bleeding.
- [ ] **2.** administer pain medication.
- [ ] **3.** maintain an open airway.
- [ ] **4.** immerse the burned area in cool water.

8. The nurse identifies the classic signs of cellulitis as:
- [ ] **1.** fever and warmth.
- [ ] **2.** erythema and edema.
- [ ] **3.** pain at the site.
- [ ] **4.** abscesses.

9. A client is being treated for herpes zoster. The nurse prepares to administer what type of therapy?
- [ ] **1.** Antiviral agents
- [ ] **2.** Antipruritics
- [ ] **3.** Corticosteroids
- [ ] **4.** Antibiotics

10. A client complains of pain and erythema of the right hip. The nurse notes that the area looks abraded, but the skin is firm and without visible drainage. It whitens and the skin stays depressed for 50 seconds after you touch the area. What is the nurse's first nursing intervention?
- [ ] **1.** Apply warm compresses to encourage drainage of the furuncle.
- [ ] **2.** Apply cold compresses to relieve pain and inflammation.
- [ ] **3.** Teach the client ROM exercises and proper use of skin moisturizers to improve circulation.
- [ ] **4.** Illustrate to the client how pressure affects skin over bony prominences and how to relieve this pressure effectively.

ANSWERS AND RATIONALES

1. CORRECT ANSWER: 4
P. aeruginosa thrives in a warm environment with a high pH and low chlorine content such as a hot tub. *S. aureus* is the most common infectious agent for folliculitis; *Klebsiella* and *Proteus* are less common infective agents of the skin.

2. CORRECT ANSWER: 22%
The back of the head in a 7-year-old is 5½%. The neck is 1%. The back is 13% and the right buttock is 2½%.

3.   CORRECT ANSWER: 2

IgE activity is increased from immune response to infectious organisms, trauma, extreme heat or cold, chemical irritation, or ischemic changes.

4.   CORRECT ANSWER: 2

Because isotretinoin, used to treat acne, is known to cause severe birth defects, it's recommended that women have pregnancy testing before the drug is dispensed and that testing be repeated throughout treatment. The female patient must agree to use two primary forms of contraception for 1 month before and 1 month after therapy as well as consistently throughout treatment. The drug is best absorbed following a high-fat meal. Patients must avoid vitamin A and must have frequent tests for elevated lipids and liver enzymes and a decreased WBC count. Alterations in coagulation haven't been documented.

5.   CORRECT ANSWER: 4

Tetracycline should be taken on an empty stomach. It shouldn't be taken with antacids or milk because it interacts with their metallic ions and is then poorly absorbed.

6.   CORRECT ANSWER: 2

Second-degree burns involve destruction of the epidermis and dermis, producing blisters, and mild to moderate edema and pain. Minor or superficial burns are first-degree burns that affect only the epidermis. Third-degree, or major burns, affect the epidermis, dermis, and subcutaneous tissues. The term *thermal* refers to the cause of the burn, not the type.

7.   CORRECT ANSWER: 3

Maintaining an open airway, assisting with endotracheal intubation (if needed), and providing 100% oxygen is the first immediate treatment for major burns.

8.   CORRECT ANSWER: 2

As an organism invades a compromised area of the skin, it causes local inflammation. This inflammatory response produces the classic signs of cellulitis, erythema, and edema. Some patients experience pain with cellulitis, and fever and local warmth due to infection aren't uncommon. Local abscesses may develop in severe cases.

9.   CORRECT ANSWER: 1

Antiviral agents, such as acyclovir, are the treatment of choice for herpes zoster. They help stop rash progression, prevent visceral complications, and shorten the duration of pain and other symptoms in adults.

10.   CORRECT ANSWER: 4

The first goal is to teach the patient about pressure ulcers and methods to relieve the pressure in the affected area. A secondary intervention might be to teach other methods to improve skin care and circulation to the area. Warm and cold compresses are more appropriate for comedones and injuries than for pressure ulcers.

Reproductive system

CHAPTER OVERVIEW

The reproductive system comprises the female and male organs involved in human regeneration, each gender having a unique physiology and specific role in the reproductive process. In addition to the specific organs themselves, various factors — including hormonal triggers, neurologic and vascular function, and psychogenic influences — are essential to maintaining optimal reproductive health.

Caring for a patient with a reproductive disorder requires an understanding of the normal mechanisms involved in reproduction, the pathophysiologic changes that can occur, signs and symptoms of disease or dysfunction, and appropriate ways to intervene. This first section of this chapter provides a brief overview of key pathophysiologic concepts related to reproductive system disorders. Common reproductive system disorders are then defined, and underlying pathophysiology, causes, pathophysiologic changes, complications, diagnostic test findings, treatments, and nursing considerations are outlined.

PATHOPHYSIOLOGIC CONCEPTS

● **Hormonal alterations**
  - In females, hormonal alterations typically involve a defect or malfunction of the hypothalamic-pituitary-ovarian axis; ovarian control is related to a system of negative and positive feedback, mediated by estrogen production
    – May cause infertility due to insufficient gonadotropin secretions (luteinizing hormone [LH] and follicle-stimulating hormone [FSH])
    – May cause sporadic inhibition of ovulation related to hormonal imbalance in gonadotropin production and regulation or abnormalities in the adrenal or thyroid gland that adversely affect hypothalamic-pituitary functioning
    – Possible causes of insufficient gonadotropin levels
      • Infections
      • Tumors
      • Neurologic disease of the hypothalamus or pituitary gland
  - In males, hormonal alterations may result in hypogonadism (abnormal decrease in gonad size and function)
    – Results from decreased androgen production
    – May impair spermatogenesis, causing infertility
    – May inhibit the development of normal secondary sex characteristics

● **Male structural alterations**
  - Structural defects may be congenital or acquired
  - Benign prostatic hyperplasia (BPH) — common with aging — involves prostate enlargement due to androgen-induced growth of prostate cells; it may result in urinary obstructive symptoms
  - Urethral stricture involves narrowing of the urethra from scarring related to trauma

● **Menstrual alterations**
  - Menopause marks cessation of ovarian function
    – Results from a complex continuum of physiologic changes (climacteric) caused by the normal, gradual decline of ovarian function
    – Most dramatic climacteric change: cessation of ovulation and, consequently, cessation of menstruation
    – Considered to have occurred after 1 year without menstruation (amenorrhea); in the United States, average age at time of menopause is 51 years
  - Premature menopause (gradual or abrupt cessation of menses before age 35) occurs without apparent cause; it affects about 5% of women in the United States
  - Induced menopause may follow radiation therapy or surgical procedures such as removing both ovaries (bilateral oophorectomy)

Key facts about hormonal alterations

- In females, typically involve a defect or malfunction of the hypothalamic-pituitary-ovarian axis
- In males, involve decreased androgen production, causing hypogonadism

Key facts about male structural alterations

- May be congenital or acquired
- Include BPH and urethral stricture

Key facts about menstrual alterations

Menopause
- Cessation of ovarian function
- Results from physiologic changes caused by decline of ovarian function

Premature menopause
- Cessation of menses before age 35
- Occurs without apparent cause

Induced menopause
- May follow radiation therapy or surgical procedures

ABNORMAL UTERINE BLEEDING

● **Definition**
- Abnormal endometrial bleeding without recognizable organic lesions
- Accounts for almost 25% of gynecologic surgical procedures
- Good prognosis with correction of hormonal imbalance or structural abnormality

● **Underlying pathophysiology**
- Irregular bleeding is associated with hormonal imbalance and anovulation (failure of ovulation to occur)
- When progesterone secretion is absent but estrogen secretion continues, the endometrium proliferates and becomes hypervascular
- When ovulation doesn't occur, the endometrium is randomly broken down, and exposed vascular channels cause prolonged, excessive bleeding
- In most cases of abnormal uterine bleeding, the endometrium shows no pathologic changes; however, in chronic, unopposed estrogen stimulation (as from a hormone-producing ovarian tumor), the endometrium may show hyperplastic or malignant changes

● **Causes**
- Imbalance in the hormonal-endometrial relationship, with persistent and unopposed stimulation of the endometrium by estrogen (usual cause)
  - Disorders that cause sustained, high estrogen levels
    - Polycystic ovary syndrome
    - Obesity
    - Immaturity of the hypothalamic-pituitary-ovarian mechanism (postpubertal teenagers)
    - Anovulation (women in their late thirties or early forties)
- Other causes
  - Trauma (foreign object insertion or direct trauma)
  - Endometriosis
  - Coagulopathy, such as thrombocytopenia or leukemia (rare)
  - Drug-induced coagulopathy

● **Pathophysiologic changes**
- Metrorrhagia (episodes of vaginal bleeding between menses) related to hormonal imbalances
- Hypermenorrhea (heavy or prolonged menses longer than 8 days, also incorrectly termed menorrhagia) related to hormonal imbalances
- Chronic polymenorrhea (menstrual cycle shorter than 18 days) or oligomenorrhea (infrequent menses) related to hormonal imbalances
- Fatigue due to anemia
- Oligomenorrhea and infertility due to anovulation

● **Complications**
- Iron-deficiency anemia (blood loss of more than 1.6 L over a short time)
- Hemorrhagic shock due to excessive blood loss
- Right-sided heart failure (rare) due to hypovolemia
- Endometrial adenocarcinoma due to chronic estrogen stimulation

● **Diagnostic test findings**
- Blood testing reveals decreased serum progesterone level

- Hemoglobin level and hematocrit determine the need for blood transfusion or iron supplementation
- Dilatation and curettage (D&C) or in-office endometrial biopsy is used to rule out endometrial hyperplasia or endometrial adenocarcinoma in women age 35 and older

Treatment
- High-dose, combination estrogen-progestogen therapy (hormonal contraceptives) to control endometrial growth and reestablish a normal cyclic pattern of menstruation (usually given four times daily for 5 to 7 days even though bleeding usually stops in 12 to 24 hours; drug choice and dosage determined by the patient's age and cause of bleeding); maintenance therapy with lower-dose combination hormonal contraceptives
- Progesterone therapy (alternative for many women who shouldn't take estrogen such as those at risk for thrombophlebitis)
- I.V. estrogen followed by progestogen (if oral drug therapy is ineffective) or combination hormonal contraceptives if the patient is young (more likely to be anovulatory) and severely anemic
- D&C (temporary treatment; not clinically useful for long-term recovery)
- Iron supplementation or transfusions of packed red blood cells (RBCs) or whole blood, as indicated, to treat anemia caused by recurrent or excessive bleeding

Nursing considerations
- Tell the patient to record the dates of bleeding episodes and the number of pads she saturates per day (helps to assess the pattern and amount of bleeding), and instruct her not to use tampons
- Instruct the patient to report abnormal bleeding immediately to help rule out major hemorrhagic disorders such as those that occur in abnormal pregnancy (see *When is uterine bleeding abnormal?*)

TIME-OUT FOR TEACHING
When is uterine bleeding abnormal?

Is your patient uncertain about whether her uterine bleeding episodes signify a temporary upset in her menstrual cycle or an ongoing disorder requiring treatment? If so, teach her that the answers to three basic questions will help her determine if she needs to seek medical help.

QUESTIONS ABOUT BLEEDING CHARACTERISTICS	ANSWERS REQUIRING MEDICAL ATTENTION
• When does it occur?	• Between menstrual periods • After sexual intercourse • More than 1 year after the last menstrual period (menopause)
• How long does it last?	• Prolonged (more than 8 days) or *consistently* heavy period • *Consistently* short menstrual cycle (fewer than 18 days)
• How much bleeding occurs?	• Consistent, bloody discharge • Hemorrhaging

---

Key diagnostic test results for abnormal uterine bleeding
- Blood testing: Decreased serum progesterone level
- D&C or endometrial biopsy: Ruling out of endometrial hyperplasia or endometrial adenocarcinoma

Key treatments for abnormal uterine bleeding
- Combination estrogen-progestogen therapy
- Progesterone therapy
- Iron supplementation or transfusions of packed RBCs or whole blood

TOP 3

Questions to ask patients about uterine bleeding
1. When does it occur?
2. How long does it last?
3. How much bleeding occurs?

Key nursing considerations for abnormal uterine bleeding

- Tell patient to record dates of bleeding episodes and number of pads she saturates per day.
- Instruct patient to report abnormal bleeding immediately.
- Teach patient how to minimize blood flow.
- Explain importance of hormonal therapy.

Key facts about amenorrhea

- Abnormal absence or suppression of menstruation

Primary
- Absence of menarche in females age 16 and older
- Involves hypothalamic-pituitary-ovarian axis dysfunction

Secondary
- Occurs for at least 3 months after onset of menarche
- Results from hypogonadotropic-hypoestrogenic anovulation, uterine factors, cervical stenosis, or premature ovarian failure

- Encourage the patient to have an annual Papanicolaou (Pap) test and pelvic examination to prevent abnormal bleeding due to organic causes and to identify early stages of cancer
- Teach the patient how to minimize blood flow by avoiding strenuous activity and lying down with her feet elevated
- Explain the importance of following the prescribed hormonal therapy, and instruct the patient to take her medication as directed
- Administer antiemetics, if ordered (may be prescribed for more aggressive hormonal dosing)
- Explain the purpose and procedure involved with D&C or endometrial biopsy, if ordered
- Stress the need for regular examinations to assess the effectiveness of treatment

AMENORRHEA

● Definition
- Abnormal absence or suppression of menstruation
- Primary amenorrhea: absence of menarche (beginning of menstruation) in an adolescent (age 16 and older)
- Secondary amenorrhea: cessation of menstruation for at least 3 months after the normal onset of menarche

● Underlying pathophysiology
- Absence of menstruation is normal before puberty, after menopause, and during pregnancy and lactation; at any other time it's abnormal and therefore pathologic
- In primary amenorrhea, the hypothalamic-pituitary-ovarian axis is dysfunctional
  - Caused by anatomic defects of the central nervous system (CNS)
  - Results in the ovary's failure to receive hormonal signals that normally initiate the development of secondary sex characteristics and the beginning of menstruation
- Secondary amenorrhea can result from various factors
  - Hypogonadotropic-hypoestrogenic anovulation
  - Uterine factors (as with Asherman's syndrome, in which the endometrium is sufficiently scarred that no functional endometrium exists)
  - Cervical stenosis
  - Premature ovarian failure

● Causes
- Autoimmune disease
- Hormonal abnormalities
- Infection (mumps, oophoritis)
- Lack of ovarian response to gonadotropins
- Constant presence of progesterone or other endocrine abnormalities
- Absence of a uterus
- Endometrial damage
- Ovarian, adrenal, or pituitary tumors

- Emotional disorders such as anorexia nervosa
- Malnutrition or obesity
- Excessive exercise

● **Pathophysiologic changes**
- Absence of menstruation due to underlying cause
- Vasomotor flushes, vaginal atrophy, hirsutism (abnormal hairiness), and acne (secondary amenorrhea) related to underlying cause

● **Complications**
- Infertility
- Endometrial adenocarcinoma (amenorrhea associated with anovulation that gives rise to unopposed estrogen stimulation of the endometrium)

● **Diagnostic test findings**
- Pregnancy testing rules out (or detects) pregnancy
- Gonadotropin testing reveals elevated pituitary gonadotropin levels; failure of gonadotropin secretion is evidenced by low pituitary gonadotropin levels
- Thyroid testing reveals abnormal (high or low) levels
- X-rays, laparoscopy, and biopsy identifies ovarian, adrenal, and pituitary tumors
- "Ferning" of cervical mucus on microscopic examination shows an estrogen effect
- Vaginal cytologic examination, endometrial biopsy, and serum progesterone and androgen analysis identifies the dominant or missing hormones
- Urine testing reveals elevated urinary 17-ketosteroid levels with excessive androgen secretion
- Plasma FSH analysis suggests primary ovarian failure (level higher than 50 IU/L) or indicates possible hypothalamic or pituitary abnormality (normal or low level)

● **Treatment**
- Appropriate hormone replacement to reestablish menstruation
- Treatment of an underlying cause not related to hormone deficiency (for example, surgery for amenorrhea due to a tumor or obstruction)
- Inducing ovulation using clomiphene citrate (Clomid)
  - For women with an intact pituitary gland
  - May be successful for secondary amenorrhea due to gonadotropin deficiency, polycystic ovarian disease, or excessive weight loss or gain (if weight is normalized)
- FSH and human menopausal gonadotropins (Pergonal) for pituitary disease
- Improving nutritional status and normalizing weight
- Modification of exercise routine, if needed
- Treatment of emotional disorder, if needed

● **Nursing considerations**
- Explain all diagnostic procedures and treatments to the patient
- Provide emotional support; psychiatric counseling may be necessary if amenorrhea results from emotional disturbances or eating disorders
- After treatment, teach the patient how to keep an accurate record of her menstrual cycles to aid in the early detection of recurrent amenorrhea

---

Key pathophysiologic changes in amenorrhea
- Absence of menstruation
- Vasomotor flushes
- Acne

Key diagnostic test results for amenorrhea
- Gonadotropin testing: Elevated or low pituitary gonadotropin levels
- Urine testing: Elevated urinary 17-ketosteroid levels and excessive androgen secretion
- Plasma FSH analysis: Level higher than 50 IU/L in primary ovarian failure; normal or low level in possible hypothalamic or pituitary abnormality

Key treatments for amenorrhea
- Hormone replacement
- Clomiphene citrate
- Treatment of an underlying cause not related to hormone deficiency

Key nursing considerations for amenorrhea
- Teach patient how to keep an accurate record of her menstrual cycles.
- Explain all procedures and treatments to patient.

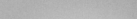

Key facts about BPH

- Enlargement of the prostate
- Compresses the urethra and causes urinary obstruction
- Involves nodular hyperplasia, which compresses the remaining normal gland
- May lead to bladder distention

Key pathophysiologic changes in BPH

- Reduced urinary stream and force
- Frequent urination
- Urinary urgency
- Nocturia

BENIGN PROSTATIC HYPERPLASIA

- **Definition**
  - Enlargement of the prostate gland sufficient to compress the urethra and cause overt urinary obstruction

- **Underlying pathophysiology**
  - Regardless of the cause, BPH begins with nonmalignant changes in peri-urethral glandular tissue
  - Growth of the fibroadenomatous nodules (masses of fibrous glandular tissue) progresses to compress the remaining normal gland (nodular hyperplasia); hyperplastic tissue is mostly glandular, with some fibrous stroma and smooth muscle
  - As the prostate enlarges, it may extend into the bladder and obstruct urinary outflow by compressing or distorting the prostatic urethra
  - Periodic increases in sympathetic stimulation of the smooth muscle of the prostatic urethra and bladder neck occur
  - Progressive bladder distention may cause a pouch to form in the bladder that retains urine when the rest of the bladder empties
  - Retained urine may lead to calculus formation or cystitis

- **Causes**
  - Possible aging-related changes in hormone activity
  - Arteriosclerosis
  - Inflammation
  - Metabolic or nutritional disturbances
  - Positive family history

- **Pathophysiologic changes**
  - Reduced urinary stream caliber and force, urinary hesitancy, and difficulty starting micturition (resulting in straining, feeling of incomplete voiding, and an interrupted stream) due to enlarged prostate gland
  - Frequent urination with nocturia, sense of urgency, dribbling, urine retention, incontinence, and possible hematuria due to increased obstruction and prostate size
  - Visible midline mass above the symphysis pubis due to an incompletely emptied bladder

- **Complications**
  - Complete urinary obstruction
  - Infection
  - Hydronephrosis
  - Renal insufficiency and renal failure
  - Renal calculi
  - Hemorrhage
  - Shock

- **Diagnostic test findings**
  - Digital rectal examination allows estimation of the size, symmetry, and consistency of the prostate gland
  - Prostate-specific antigen (PSA) level is typically slightly elevated and helps to rule out prostatic carcinoma

- Urinalysis and urine cultures usually show hematuria, pyuria and, with bacterial count more than 100,000/µl, urinary tract infection (UTI)
- Blood testing may reveal elevated blood urea nitrogen (BUN) and serum creatinine levels, suggesting renal dysfunction
- Post-void residual urine testing measures residual urine in the bladder
- Excretory urography rules out urinary tract obstruction, hydronephrosis, calculi, or tumors as well as filling and emptying defects in the bladder
- Cystoscopy (if the patient has complications) rules out other causes of urinary tract obstruction, such as neoplasm or calculi
- Cystourethroscopy (if the patient has severe symptoms) provides a definitive diagnosis; shows prostate enlargement, bladder wall changes, and a raised bladder; and helps determine the best surgical procedure
- Transrectal ultrasonography assesses the size and structure of the prostate and bladder

● Treatment

- Symptomatic or surgical treatment depending on the size of the enlarged prostate, the patient's age and health, and the extent of obstruction
- Even spacing of fluid intake throughout the day (to prevent bladder distention); limitation of nighttime fluids (if the patient has nocturia)
- Antimicrobials to treat UTIs
- Alternative treatments for mild symptoms
  - Gentle prostate massages by a urologist to decrease prostatic congestion
  - Cold sitz baths for 3 to 8 minutes to stimulate blood flow to the prostate and bladder
  - Regular ejaculation to help relieve prostatic congestion
  - Herbal supplements, such as saw palmetto (inhibits the conversion of testosterone to dihydrotachysterol, thus preventing enlargement), pygeum, and stinging nettles to relieve symptoms
- Alpha-adrenergic blockers, such as terazosin (Hytrin), doxazosin (Cardura), and tamsulosin (Flomax), to improve urine flow rates and relieve bladder outlet obstruction by relaxing the smooth muscle of the prostate and bladder neck
- Finasteride (Proscar) or dutasteride (Avodart) to reduce prostate size in some patients
- Continuous drainage with an indwelling urinary catheter to alleviate urine retention when other treatments are ineffective
- Surgery (the only effective therapy to relieve acute urine retention, hydronephrosis, severe hematuria, recurrent UTIs, and other severe or intolerable symptoms and complications)
- Minimally invasive surgical techniques
  - Transurethral resection of the prostate (TURP) if the prostate weighs less than 2 oz (56.7 g); tissue is removed with a wire loop and electric current using a resectoscope
  - Transurethral needle ablation (TUNA) to burn away well-defined regions of the prostate, thereby improving urine flow with less risk of incontinence and impotence than with TURP
  - Transurethral microwave treatment to destroy portions of the prostate with heat; similar to TUNA and with fewer adverse effects than TURP
  - Transurethral laser excision to reduce prostate size

Key diagnostic test results for BPH

- Digital rectal examination: Estimation of size, symmetry, and consistency of prostate gland
- PSA level: Typically slightly elevated; helps rule out prostatic carcinoma
- Cystourethroscopy: Visualization of prostate enlargement, bladder wall changes, and a raised bladder

Key treatments for BPH

- Finasteride
- Surgery, including TURP and suprapubic resection

– Prostatic stents to maintain urethral patency in patients with urethral stricture (balloon dilatation of the urethra found ineffective, and discontinued)
- Open surgical techniques (used when gland is very large or if the patient has complicating factors such as bladder damage)
  – Suprapubic (transvesical) resection: most common; useful for prostatic enlargement causing pouching within the bladder
  – Retropubic (extravesical) resection: allows direct visualization; potency and continence are usually maintained

● **Nursing considerations**
- Monitor the patient's vital signs, intake and output, and daily weight, watching closely for signs of postobstructive diuresis (such as increased urine output and hypotension) that may lead to serious dehydration, reduced blood volume, shock, electrolyte loss, and anuria
- Insert an indwelling urinary catheter for urine retention (usually difficult in a patient with BPH); use of coude catheter may make insertion easier
- Assist with suprapubic cystostomy using a local anesthetic (watching for rapid bladder decompression that can cause temporary hypotension) if the catheter can't be passed transurethrally
- Provide appropriate postoperative care
  – **Watch for and prevent postoperative complications, observe for immediate dangers of prostatic bleeding (shock, hemorrhage), check the catheter often (every 15 minutes for the first 2 to 3 hours) for patency and urine color, and check dressings for bleeding**
  – Keep the three-way catheter (if used for continuous bladder irrigation) open at a rate sufficient to maintain clear, light-pink returns, and watch for fluid overload from absorption of the irrigating fluid into the systemic circulation
  – Observe the indwelling catheter closely (if used); if the catheter becomes clogged due to clots, irrigate with 80 to 100 ml of normal saline solution, as ordered, maintaining strict sterile technique
  – Watch for signs of septic shock (most serious complication of prostatic surgery); immediately report severe chills, sudden fever, tachycardia, hypotension, or other signs of shock, and start a rapid infusion of I.V. antibiotics, as ordered
  – Watch for signs and symptoms of a pulmonary embolus, heart failure, or renal failure, and monitor the patient's vital signs, central venous pressure, and arterial pressure continuously
  – Administer belladonna and opium suppositories (B & O Supprettes) or other anticholinergics, as ordered, to relieve painful bladder spasms that commonly occur after TURP
  – Administer analgesic suppositories after open surgical procedures (except perineal prostatectomy) to control incisional pain; be aware that suppositories and rectal temperatures are sometimes contraindicated after open prostatic procedures
  – Continue infusing I.V. fluids until the patient can drink sufficient fluids (2 to 3 L/day) to maintain adequate hydration
  – Administer stool softeners and laxatives, as ordered, to prevent straining; don't check for fecal impaction because a rectal examination may precipitate bleeding

---

Key postoperative nursing considerations for BPH

- Watch for and prevent postoperative complications.
- Check the catheter for patency.
- Irrigate the catheter if it becomes clogged.
- Administer belladonna and opium suppositories or other anticholinergics.
- Infuse I.V. fluids until patient can drink sufficient fluids.
- Administer stool softeners and laxatives.
- Reinforce activity restrictions.
- Instruct patient to avoid bladder irritants.
- Teach patient Kegel exercises.
- Instruct patient about prescribed antibiotic regimen.

- Reassure the patient that temporary frequency, dribbling, and occasional hematuria will probably occur after the catheter is removed
- Reinforce activity restrictions, such as avoiding lifting, strenuous exercise, and long automobile rides (can increase bleeding tendency); caution the patient to restrict sexual activity for several weeks after discharge
- Instruct the patient to avoid bladder irritants, such as alcohol, caffeine, and citrus products
- Instruct the patient about the prescribed oral antibiotic regimen and indications for using gentle laxatives
- Urge the patient to seek immediate medical care if he can't void, passes bloody urine, or develops a fever
- Encourage annual digital rectal exams and screening for PSA levels to identify possible cancer
- Teach the patient to perform Kegel exercises to strengthen sphincter tone and reduce urine leakage

CRYPTORCHIDISM

Definition
- Congenital disorder in which one or both testes fail to descend into the scrotum, remaining in the abdomen or inguinal canal or at the external ring of the inguinal canal
- Most commonly affects the right testis, although it may be bilateral
- True undescended testes — testes remain along the path of normal descent
- Ectopic testes — testes deviate from the path of normal descent

Underlying pathophysiology
- A prevalent but still unsubstantiated theory links undescended testes to development of the gubernaculum, a fibromuscular band that connects the testes to the scrotal floor (this band probably helps pull the testes into the scrotum by shortening as the fetus grows)
- Cryptorchidism may result from inadequate testosterone levels or a defect in the testes or the gubernaculum
- Because the testes are maintained at a higher temperature by being within the body, spermatogenesis is impaired, leading to reduced fertility

Causes
- Hormonal factors (testosterone deficiency)
- Structural factors
- Genetic predisposition
- Prematurity (premature neonates are most commonly affected because testes normally descend into the scrotum around 28 weeks' gestation)
- Prenatal exposure to diethylstilbestrol

Pathophysiologic changes
- Testis on the affected side not palpable in the scrotum; underdeveloped scrotum due to unilateral cryptorchidism
- Scrotum enlarged on the unaffected side due to compensatory hypertrophy (occasionally)
- Infertility after puberty due to absence of spermatogenesis (uncorrected bilateral cryptorchidism) despite normal testosterone levels

Key facts about cryptorchidism
- Congenital disorder marked by failure of one or both testes to descend into scrotum
- May be linked to gubernaculum development

Key pathophysiologic changes in cryptorchidism
- Nonpalpable testis on affected side
- Enlarged scrotum on unaffected side

Complications

- Sterility, significantly increased risk of testicular cancer, and increased vulnerability of the testes to trauma when bilateral cryptorchidism isn't treated by early adolescence

Diagnostic test findings

- Buccal smear (cells from oral mucosa) analysis determines the genetic sex (a male sex chromatin pattern)
- Serum gonadotropin analysis confirms the presence of testes by showing the presence of circulating hormone

Treatment

- Surgical correction (orchiopexy) to secure the testes in the scrotum and to prevent sterility
  - Generally indicated if the testes don't descend spontaneously by age 1
  - Usually performed before age 4; optimum age is 1 to 2 years because about 40% of undescended testes can no longer produce viable sperm by age 2
- Human chorionic gonadotropin (hCG) I.M. to stimulate descent (rarely used); ineffective for testes located in the abdomen

Nursing considerations

- Provide information on causes, available treatments, and the possible effect on reproduction; emphasize that the testes may descend spontaneously (especially in premature infants)
- Prepare the child for surgery (if necessary) using age-appropriate explanations and terms the child understands
  - Tell the child that a rubber band may be taped to his thigh for about 1 week after surgery to keep the testis in place
  - Explain to the child that his scrotum may swell but shouldn't be painful
  - Reassure the child that he won't feel pain during surgery
- Provide appropriate care after orchiopexy
  - Monitor the patient's vital signs and intake and output, check dressings, encourage coughing and deep breathing, and watch for urine retention
  - Keep the operative site clean, and teach the child to wipe from front to back after defecation
  - Maintain tension on the applied rubber band to keep the testis in place and make sure that it isn't too tight
  - Encourage the parents to participate in postoperative care, such as bathing and feeding the child; urge the child to do as much for himself as possible (age-appropriate)

DYSMENORRHEA

Definition

- Painful menstruation associated with ovulation and unrelated to pelvic disease
- The most common gynecologic complaint
- Can occur as a primary disorder or secondary to an underlying disease
  - Primary dysmenorrhea is self-limiting; prognosis is generally good

---

Key diagnostic test results for cryptorchidism

- Serum gonadotropin analysis: Presence of circulating hormone

Key treatments for cryptorchidism

- Surgical correction

Key postoperative nursing considerations for cryptorchidism

- Monitor intake and output and check dressings.
- Watch for urine retention.
- Maintain tension on the applied rubber band.

Key facts about dysmenorrhea

- Painful menstruation associated with ovulation
- Results from increased prostaglandin secretion or sensitivity
- Causes intense muscle contractions and hypoxia, which cause pain
- May be primary (unrelated to an identifiable cause) or secondary (related to other gynecologic disorders)

Causes of pelvic pain

The characteristic pelvic pain of dysmenorrhea must be distinguished from the acute pain caused by normal processes (such as ovulation and uterine contractions during pregnancy) and many disorders, including:

- GI disorders — appendicitis, acute diverticulitis, acute or chronic cholecystitis, chronic cholelithiasis, acute pancreatitis, peptic ulcer perforation, and intestinal obstruction
- urinary tract disorders — cystitis and renal calculi
- reproductive disorders — acute salpingitis, chronic inflammation, degenerative fibroids, and ovarian cyst torsion
- pregnancy disorders: impending abortion (pain and bleeding early in pregnancy), ectopic pregnancy, abruptio placentae, uterine rupture, leiomyoma degeneration, and toxemia.

- – Prognosis for secondary dysmenorrhea depends on the underlying disorder

● Underlying pathophysiology
- Pain results from increased prostaglandin secretion or sensitivity to prostaglandin in menstrual blood, which intensifies normal uterine contractions
- Prostaglandins intensify myometrial smooth muscle contraction and uterine blood vessel constriction, thereby worsening the uterine hypoxia normally associated with menstruation (prostaglandins and their metabolites can also cause GI disturbances, headache, and syncope)
- A combination of intense muscle contractions and hypoxia causes the intense pain of dysmenorrhea
- Because dysmenorrhea almost always follows an ovulatory cycle, primary and secondary forms are rare during the anovulatory cycle of menses

● Causes
- Primary dysmenorrhea — excess prostaglandins without other gynecologic abnormalities; is unrelated to an identifiable cause
  - Possible contributing factors
    - Hormonal imbalance
    - Psychogenic factors such as depression
- Secondary dysmenorrhea — may be related to other gynecologic disorders
  - Endometriosis
  - Cervical stenosis
  - Uterine leiomyomas (benign fibroid tumors)
  - Pelvic inflammatory disease
  - Pelvic tumors (see *Causes of pelvic pain*)

● Pathophysiologic changes
- Sharp, intermittent, cramping, lower abdominal pain (usually radiating to the back, thighs, groin, and vulva), typically starting with or immediately before menstrual flow and peaking within 24 hours (due to excess prostaglandin production)
- Characteristic signs and symptoms suggestive of premenstrual syndrome (urinary frequency, nausea, vomiting, diarrhea, headache, backache, chills, ab-

Key pathophysiologic changes in dysmenorrhea

- Sharp, intermittent, cramping, lower abdominal pain that radiates

dominal bloating, painful breasts, depression, and irritability) due to excess prostaglandin production

● **Complications**
- Dehydration

● **Diagnostic test findings**
- Pelvic examination helps to determine the cause
- Laparoscopy, hysteroscopy, or pelvic ultrasonography may be used to diagnose the underlying disorder in secondary dysmenorrhea

● **Treatment**
- Nonsteroidal anti-inflammatory drugs (NSAIDs) for mild to moderate pain (most effective when taken 24 to 48 hours before onset of menses); inhibit prostaglandin synthesis through suppression of the enzyme cyclooxygenase, thus decreasing the severity of uterine contractions
- Calcium to prevent and ameliorate uterine muscle spasms
- Opioids for severe pain (infrequently used)
- Heat applied locally to the lower abdomen (may relieve discomfort in mature women; should be used cautiously in young adolescents because appendicitis may mimic dysmenorrhea)
- Exercise (may reduce prostaglandin production by reducing endometrial hyperplasia)
- Primary dysmenorrhea
  - Hormonal contraceptives to relieve pain by suppressing ovulation and inhibiting endometrial prostaglandin synthesis (patients attempting pregnancy should rely on antiprostaglandin therapy)
- Secondary dysmenorrhea
  - Identification and correction of underlying cause
  - May include surgical treatment of underlying disorders, such as endometriosis or uterine leiomyomas (after conservative therapy fails)

● **Nursing considerations**
- Obtain a complete history, focusing on the patient's gynecologic complaints; includes detailed information on symptoms of pelvic disease, such as excessive bleeding, changes in bleeding pattern, vaginal discharge, and dyspareunia (painful intercourse)
- Provide thorough patient teaching, including an explanation of normal female anatomy and physiology as well as the nature of dysmenorrhea (depending on the circumstances, may include providing the adolescent patient with information on pregnancy and contraception)
- Encourage the patient to keep a detailed record of her menstrual cycle and symptoms and to seek medical care if symptoms persist
- Encourage the patient to start a regular fitness program; explain that aerobic exercise stimulates endorphin release, helping to relieve her discomfort
- Advise the patient about dietary modifications and vitamin therapy
  - Increase dietary intake of whole grains and green, leafy vegetables
  - Decrease intake of caffeine, chocolate, alcohol, saturated fats, and refined sugar products
  - Increase intake of omega-3 polyunsaturated fatty acids, magnesium, calcium, and B vitamins (help to decrease uterine spasms and cramping)

Key diagnostic test results for dysmenorrhea

- Pelvic examination: Determination of cause

Key treatments for dysmenorrhea

- NSAIDs
- Local heat
- Hormonal contraceptives
- Identification and correction of underlying cause (secondary form)

Key nursing considerations for dysmenorrhea

- Encourage patient to keep a detailed record of her menstrual cycle.
- Encourage patient to start a regular fitness program.
- Advise patient about dietary modifications and vitamin therapy.

ENDOMETRIOSIS

● Definition
- Presence of endometrial tissue outside the lining of the uterine cavity
- Displaced endometrial tissue generally confined to the pelvic area (usually around the ovaries, uterovesical peritoneum, uterosacral ligaments, and cul de sac) but can appear anywhere in the body
- May occur at any age, including adolescence
- May be present in as many as 50% of infertile women

● Underlying pathophysiology
- Displaced endometrial tissue responds to hormonal stimulation the same way the endometrium does, but more unpredictably
- The endometrial cells respond to estrogen and progesterone with proliferation and secretion
- During menstruation, the ectopic tissue bleeds, causing inflammation of the surrounding tissues
- This inflammation causes fibrosis, leading to adhesions that produce pain and infertility

● Causes
- Unknown
- Main theories
  - Retrograde menstruation with implantation at ectopic sites (retrograde menstruation alone may not be sufficient for endometriosis to occur because it occurs in women with no clinical evidence of endometriosis)
  - Genetic predisposition and depressed immune system (may predispose the patient to endometriosis)
  - Coelomic metaplasia (repeated inflammation inducing metaplasia of mesothelial cells to the endometrial epithelium)
  - Lymphatic or hematogenous spread (extraperitoneal disease)
  - Undifferentiated embryonic peritoneal tissue cells that remain dormant until hormones stimulate their response

● Pathophysiologic changes
- Dysmenorrhea, abnormal uterine bleeding, and infertility (classic symptoms); pain that begins 5 to 7 days before menses peaks and lasts for 2 to 3 days (varies among patients) due to implantation of ectopic tissues and adhesions
- Infertility and profuse menses due to ectopic tissue in ovaries and oviducts
- Deep-thrust dyspareunia due to ectopic tissue in ovaries or cul de sac
- Suprapubic pain, dysuria, and hematuria due to ectopic tissue in the bladder
- Abdominal cramps, pain on defecation, and constipation; bloody stools from bleeding of ectopic endometrium in the rectosigmoid musculature due to ectopic tissue in the large bowel and appendix
  - Bleeding from endometrial deposits in these areas during menses; pain on intercourse due to ectopic tissue in cervix, vagina, and perineum

● Complications
- Infertility
- Chronic pelvic pain
- Ovarian carcinoma (rare)

Key facts about endometriosis
- Presence of endometrial tissue outside lining of uterine cavity
- Responds to hormonal stimulation unpredictably
- Causes inflammation of surrounding tissues during menstruation because ectopic tissue bleeds

Key pathophysiologic changes in endometriosis
- Dysmenorrhea
- Abnormal uterine bleeding
- Infertility
- Abdominal cramps
- Pain on defecation

Key diagnostic test results for endometriosis

- Laparoscopy or laparotomy: Presence of endometrial tissue outside the uterus; only definitive way to diagnose endometriosis

Key treatments for endometriosis

- Androgens
- Progestins
- Laparoscopic removal of endometrial implants
- Total abdominal hysterectomy

Key nursing considerations for endometriosis

- Inform patient taking danazol about pseudomenopause and other adverse effects.
- Advise adolescents to use sanitary napkins instead of tampons.

● **Diagnostic test findings**
- Laparoscopy or laparotomy is the only definitive way to diagnose endometriosis
- Biopsy at the time of laparoscopy is helpful in confirming the diagnosis (in some instances, diagnosis is confirmed by visual inspection)
- Empiric trial of gonadotropin-releasing hormone (GnRH) agonist therapy confirms or refutes the impression of endometriosis before resorting to laparoscopy (controversial, but may be cost-effective)

● **Treatment**
- Androgens, such as danazol (Danocrine), to inhibit the anterior pituitary gland
- Progestins and continuous combined hormonal contraceptives (pseudopregnancy regimen) to relieve symptoms by causing a regression of endometrial tissue
- GnRH agonists to induce pseudomenopause (medical oophorectomy), causing remission of the disease (commonly used)
- Laparoscopic removal of endometrial implants with conventional or laser techniques (no benefit shown for laser laparoscopy over electrocautery or suture methods)
- Presacral neurectomy for central pelvic pain (effective in up to 50% of appropriate candidates)
- Laparoscopic uterosacral nerve ablation (as an alternative to presacral neurectomy) for central pelvic pain; definitive studies supporting its efficacy are lacking)
- Total abdominal hysterectomy with or without bilateral salpingo-oophorectomy
- Treatment of last resort for women who don't want to have children or for extensive disease
- Unclear whether ovarian conservation is appropriate (success rates vary)

● **Nursing considerations**
- Tell patients undergoing laparoscopy that they may experience pain in the shoulders from gas pumped into the abdomen (to separate the organs and prevent accidental puncture) as well as some discomfort at the laparoscope insertion site
- Advise the patient to avoid undergoing minor gynecologic procedures immediately before and during menstruation because this may promote spread of endometrial tissue
- Advise adolescents to use sanitary napkins instead of tampons (can help prevent retrograde flow in girls with a narrow vagina or small introitus)
- Advise the patient who wants children not to postpone childbearing (because infertility is a possible complication) (see *Teaching patients with endometriosis*)
- Recommend an annual pelvic examination and Pap test to all patients
- Inform the patient taking danazol that ovulation and menstruation will stop, resulting in pseudomenopause (therapy typically lasts from 6 to 9 months)
  - Advise the patient about expected adverse affects (acne, decreased breast size, edema, flushing, sweating, voice deepening, and weight gain)
  - Inform the patient that virilization effects may be irreversible

TIME-OUT FOR TEACHING

Teaching patients with endometriosis

Include information about these topics when teaching patients with endometriosis about their condition:
- pathophysiology and possible causes
- importance of treatment to prevent or postpone such complications as infertility or endometrioma rupture
- medications to relieve pain
- rationale for using hormonal contraceptives and other hormonal therapies
- surgery, including therapeutic laparoscopy, total hysterectomy and bilateral salpingo-oophorectomy, and presacral neurectomy
- other topics, including the effects of pregnancy on endometriosis, relief of dyspareunia, and dietary prevention of anemia.

ERECTILE DYSFUNCTION

Definition
- Form of impotence characterized by a male's inability to attain or maintain penile erection sufficient to complete intercourse
- Primary impotence — the patient has never achieved a sufficient erection
- Secondary impotence (more common) — the patient has succeeded in completing intercourse in the past
- Transient periods of impotence experienced by about one-half of all adult men (not considered a form of erectile dysfunction)

Underlying pathophysiology
- Neurologic dysfunction results in the absence of the autonomic signal and, in combination with vascular disease, interferes with arteriolar dilation
- Blood is shunted around the sacs of the corpus cavernosum into medium-sized veins, which prevents the sacs from filling completely
- Perfusion of the corpus cavernosum is initially compromised because of partial obstruction of small arteries, leading to the loss of erection before ejaculation
- Psychogenic causes may exacerbate emotional problems in a circular pattern: anxiety causes fear of erectile dysfunction, which causes further emotional problems

Causes
- Psychogenic causes (20% of cases)
- Organic causes (80% of cases)
  - Chronic diseases that cause neurologic and vascular impairment, such as cardiopulmonary disease, diabetes, multiple sclerosis, or renal failure
  - Cirrhosis
  - Spinal cord trauma
  - Complications of surgery, particularly radical prostatectomy
  - Drug- or alcohol-induced dysfunction
  - Genital anomalies or CNS defects (rare)

Key facts about erectile dysfunction
- Inability to attain or maintain penile erection sufficient to complete intercourse
- Psychogenic or organic causes
- Results from absence of autonomic signal and vascular disease, which interferes with arteriolar dilation
- Prevents sacs of corpus cavernosum from filling completely because blood is shunted

TOP 3

Organic causes of erectile dysfunction
1. Cardiopulmonary disease
2. Diabetes
3. Multiple sclerosis

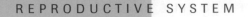

Key pathophysiologic changes in erectile dysfunction

- Feelings of anxiety
- Perspiration
- Palpitations

Key diagnostic test results for erectile dysfunction

- Blood testing: Decreased testosterone, prolactin, and thyroid levels
- Ultrasonography: Evaluation of vascular function

Key treatments for erectile dysfunction

Psychogenic
- Sex therapy

Organic
- Sildenafil
- Testosterone supplementation
- Psychological counseling

Key nursing considerations for erectile dysfunction

- Assess patient's sexual history during initial history.
- Provide discharge instructions about resuming sexual activity.

● **Pathophysiologic changes**
- Feelings of anxiety, perspiration, palpitations, and loss of interest in sexual activity before the sexual encounter (due to psychogenic erectile dysfunction)

● **Complications**
- Depression
- Infertility

● **Diagnostic test findings**
- Blood testing may reveal decreased testosterone, prolactin, and thyroid levels; glycosylated hemoglobin, serum chemistries, lipid profile, and a PSA test may be done to evaluate possible causes
- Ultrasonography is used to evaluate vascular function
- Angiography is used to evaluate vaso-occlusive disease
- Direct injection of Alprostadil (Caverject, Edex) into the corpora is used to evaluate erectile quality
- Nocturnal penile tumescence testing helps distinguish psychogenic impotence from organic impotence

● **Treatment**
- Psychogenic impotence
  – Sex therapy with both partners (course and content of therapy depend on the specific cause of dysfunction and nature of the relationship)
  – Teaching the patient to improve verbal communication skills, eliminate unreasonable guilt, or reevaluate attitudes toward sex and sexual roles
- Organic impotence
  – Reversing the cause, if possible
  – Sildenafil (Viagra) or similar agents to cause vasodilation within the penis (contraindicated in patients taking nitrates)
  – Yohimbine (Aphrodyne, Yocon), an adrenergic antagonist, to enhance parasympathetic neurotransmission
  – Testosterone supplementation for hypogonadal men (not for men with prostate cancer)
  – Alprostadil
  – Surgically inserted inflatable or noninflatable penile implants
  – Psychological counseling to help the couple deal realistically with their situation and explore alternatives for sexual expression

● **Nursing considerations**
- Assess the patient's sexual history during the initial nursing history; help the patient to feel comfortable discussing his sexuality and, when appropriate, refer him for further evaluation or treatment
- Instruct the patient undergoing penile implant surgery to avoid intercourse until the incision heals (usually in 6 weeks)
- Refer the patient (or couple) for psychological counseling, as needed
- Provide information about resuming sexual activity as part of discharge instructions for the postoperative patient and any patient with a condition that requires modification of daily activities (includes cardiac disease, diabetes, hypertension, and chronic obstructive pulmonary disease [COPD])

FIBROCYSTIC BREAST CHANGES

● **Definition**
  - Disorder marked by the development of one or more palpable benign lumps or other changes in breast tissue
  - Breast typically becomes lumpy and tender approximately 1 week before menses begins; may occur in one or both breasts

● **Underlying pathophysiology**
  - Cyclical increases in estrogen underlie most benign breast symptoms
  - Just before menstruation, the breasts may retain water, causing painful swelling
  - One or more cysts may form, and the amount of fibrous breast tissue may increase
  - Cysts tend to enlarge and become tender just before menstruation, and then shrink or disappear afterward

● **Causes**
  - Unknown
    - Factors that may be related
      · Abnormal hormone production
      · Hypersensitive breast tissues that overrespond to normal hormone levels
      · Cyclic increases in estrogen

● **Pathophysiologic changes**
  - Tenderness or pain of the breast due to nerve irritation and inflammation associated with edema
  - Breast lumpiness due to increase in fibrous tissue

● **Complications**
  - Atypical hyperplasia

● **Diagnostic test findings**
  - Mammography aids in the diagnosis and location of cysts
  - Ultrasonography aids in differentiating between fluid-filled and solid cysts
  - Needle aspiration or biopsy determines if a cyst is benign or malignant

● **Treatment**
  - Application of local heat or cold to reduce tenderness
  - Administration of prescribed analgesics and diuretics
  - Drainage of fibrocystic lumps
  - Surgical removal of lumps (only if a cyst can't be aspirated or a solid mass remains after aspiration)
  - Danazol for severe cases that can't be relieved by conservative measures; provides an antiestrogenic effect and reduces hormonal stimulation of the breast, thereby helping to reduce breast pain and nodularity
  - Hormonal contraceptives to help relieve breast tenderness
  - Vitamin A, E, or B complex to relieve fluid engorgement

● **Nursing considerations**
  - Teach the patient to perform monthly breast self-examinations
  - Encourage the patient to wear a supportive bra (reduces tension on the ligaments that support the breasts)

Key facts about fibrocystic breasts

● Marked by palpable benign lumps or other changes in breast tissue
● Involves cyclical increases in estrogen
● May lead to cysts, which enlarge and become tender just before menstruation

Key pathophysiologic changes in fibrocystic breasts

● Breast pain or tenderness
● Breast lumpiness

Key diagnostic test results for fibrocystic breasts

● Mammography: Location of cysts
● Ultrasonography: Differentiation between fluid-filled and solid cysts

Key treatments for fibrocystic breasts

● Analgesics and diuretics
● Drainage of fibrocystic lumps

Key nursing considerations for fibrocystic breasts

- Teach patient to perform monthly breast self-examinations.
- Instruct patient to reduce intake of caffeine and salt.

Key facts about uterine fibroid disease

- Characterized by fibroids, the most common benign tumors in women, in the uterus
- Classified as intramural, submucosal, or subserous
- May lead to a large uterine cavity, increasing the endometrial surface area and causing abnormal uterine bleeding

Key pathophysiologic changes in uterine fibroid disease

- Abnormal bleeding
- Pain
- Pelvic pressure

- Instruct the patient to reduce her intake of caffeine and salt, especially premenstrually (salt reduction can help prevent fluid retention that causes breast discomfort)
- Teach the patient to avoid sleeping in a prone position (puts pressure on the cysts)
- Encourage the patient to join a scheduled exercise and activity program to help reduce breast tenderness and bloating
- Caution the patient taking danazol about the drug's harsh adverse effects such as virilization, and inform her that signs and symptoms may return, requiring another course of therapy

FIBROID DISEASE OF THE UTERUS

● Definition
- Disease characterized by the appearance of fibroids (benign tumors) in the uterus
- Fibroids also known as *uterine leiomyomas, myomas,* and *fibromyomas*
  - Most common benign tumors in women
  - Composed of smooth muscle
  - Usually occur in the uterine corpus, although they may appear on the cervix or on the round or broad ligament
  - Become malignant (leiomyosarcoma) in fewer than 0.1% of patients

● Underlying pathophysiology
- Fibroids are classified according to location
  - Intramural — within the uterine wall
  - Submucosal — protruding into the endometrial cavity
  - Subserous — protruding from the serosal surface of the uterus
- Fibroids vary greatly in size and usually appear firm, surrounded by a pseudocapsule composed of compressed but otherwise normal uterine myometrium
- The uterine cavity may become larger, increasing the endometrial surface area; this can cause increased uterine bleeding

● Causes
- Unknown
  - Possible contributing factors
    - Several growth factors, including epidermal growth factor
    - Steroid hormones, including estrogen and progesterone (fibroids typically arise after menarche and regress after menopause, implicating estrogen as a promoter of fibroid growth)

● Pathophysiologic changes
- Abnormal bleeding, typically menorrhagia due to disrupted submucosal vessels (most common symptom)
- Pain due to torsion of a pedunculated (stemmed) subserous tumor or fibroids undergoing degeneration
- Pelvic pressure (indication for treatment, depending on severity) resulting in mild hydronephrosis due to impingement on adjacent viscera

● Complications
- Recurrent spontaneous abortion
- Preterm labor

- Malposition of the fetus
- Anemia secondary to excessive bleeding
- Bladder compression
- Infection (if tumor protrudes out of the vaginal opening)
- Secondary infertility (rare)
- Bowel obstruction

● Diagnostic test findings

- Blood studies show anemia from abnormal bleeding (may support the diagnosis)
- Bimanual examination reveals an enlarged, firm, nontender, and irregularly contoured uterus (also seen with adenomyosis and other pelvic abnormalities)
- Ultrasonography allows accurate assessment of the dimension, number, and location of tumors
- Magnetic resonance imaging provides especially sensitive fibroid imaging
- Endometrial biopsy rules out endometrial cancer in patients over age 35 with abnormal uterine bleeding
- Laparoscopy corroborates other findings

● Treatment

- GnRH agonists to rapidly suppress pituitary gonadotropin release
  - Leads to profound hypoestrogenemia, a 50% reduction in uterine volume (peak effects occurring in week 12 of therapy), reduced tumor size before surgery and reduced blood loss during surgery, and increased preoperative hematocrit
  - Best used preoperatively or for up to 6 months in perimenopausal women who might soon experience natural menopause (and thus avoid surgery)
- NSAIDs for dysmenorrhea or pelvic discomfort
- Hysterectomy for symptomatic women who have completed childbearing (considered the definitive treatment, but not the only available option)
- Abdominal, laparoscopic, or hysteroscopic myomectomy (removal of tumors in the uterine muscle) for patients of any age who want to preserve their uterus
- Myolysis (outpatient laparoscopic procedure to treat fibroids without hysterectomy or major surgery) to coagulate fibroids and preserve the patient's uterus and childbearing potential
- Uterine artery embolization (radiologic procedure) to block uterine arteries using small pieces of polyvinyl chloride
  - Promising alternative to surgery in many women
  - To date, no long-term studies to confirm appropriateness for women desiring future childbearing or to establish long-term success or adverse effects
  - Recent anecdotal data suggest decreased time to menopause after embolization
- Blood transfusions for patients with severe anemia due to excessive bleeding

● Nursing considerations

- Make sure that the patient understands the purpose and effects of surgery or a medical procedure she's scheduled to have
  - If undergoing hysterectomy or oophorectomy, explain the effects on menstruation, menopause, sexual activity, and hormonal balance

---

Key diagnostic test results for uterine fibroid disease

- Bimanual examination: Enlarged, firm, nontender, and irregularly contoured uterus
- Ultrasonography: Dimension, number, and location of tumors

Key treatments for uterine fibroid disease

- GnRH agonists
- NSAIDs
- Myomectomy
- Hysterectomy

Key nursing considerations for uterine fibroid disease

- Explain surgery's effects on menstruation, menopause, sexual activity, and hormonal balance.
- Tell patient to report abnormal bleeding or pelvic pain immediately.

- – If undergoing multiple myomectomy, explain that pregnancy is still possible, although cesarean delivery may be necessary
- – Reassure the patient that she won't experience premature menopause if her ovaries are left intact
- Tell the patient to immediately report abnormal bleeding or pelvic pain
- Administer iron supplements and blood transfusions, as ordered, in a patient with severe anemia due to excessive bleeding
- Encourage the patient to verbalize her feelings and concerns related to the disease process and its effects on her life

GYNECOMASTIA

● Definition
- Benign enlargement of breast tissue in males
- Commonly a bilateral condition (usually unilateral in men over age 50)
- Usually resolves spontaneously in 6 to 12 months

● Underlying pathophysiology
- Gynecomastia results from a disturbance in the normal ratio of active androgen to estrogen
- This hormonal imbalance causes proliferation of the fibroblastic stroma and duct system of the breast

● Causes
- Testicular tumors
- Obesity
- Pituitary tumors
- Some hypogonadism syndromes
- Liver disease, which causes an inability to break down normal male estrogen secretions
- Chronic renal failure
- COPD
- Various drugs and treatments (see *Drugs and treatments causing gynecomastia*)

● Pathophysiologic changes
- Enlarged breast tissue (at least ¾" [2 cm] in diameter), either unilateral or bilateral, beneath the areola due to hormonal imbalance

● Complications
- Malignant changes in breast tissue
- Impaired self-esteem (in some)

● Diagnostic test findings
- Biopsy rules out cancer
- Blood testing reveals excessively high estrogen levels and normal testosterone levels associated with drug- and tumor-induced hyperestrogenism

● Treatment
- Usually resolves spontaneously without treatment
- Treatments (when indicated)
  - – Treating underlying cause to reduce excess breast tissue
  - – Resection of extra breast tissue for cosmetic reasons
  - – Short course of clomiphene or tamoxifen (Nolvadex)

Drugs and treatments causing gynecomastia

In addition to the common medical causes of gynecomastia, various drugs and treatments may lead to breast enlargement in men.

DRUGS
When gynecomastia is an effect of drugs, it's typically painful and unilateral. Estrogens used to treat prostate cancer, including diethylstilbestrol (DES) and estramustine (Emcyt), directly affect the estrogen-androgen ratio. Drugs that have an estrogen-like effect, such as cardiac glycosides and human chorionic gonadotropin, may do the same.

Regular use of alcohol, marijuana, or heroin reduces plasma testosterone levels, possibly causing gynecomastia. Other drugs — such as flutamide (Eulexin), cyproterone (Androcur), spironolactone (Aldactone), cimetidine (Tagamet), and ketoconazole (Nizoral) — can produce gynecomastia by interfering with androgen production or action. Some common drugs, including phenothiazines, tricyclic antidepressants, and antihypertensives, can produce gynecomastia, but it isn't known how.

TREATMENTS
Gynecomastia may develop within weeks of starting hemodialysis for chronic renal failure. In men on hemodialysis, testosterone levels can decrease while luteinizing hormone and follicle-stimulating hormone levels are normal or elevated. This may lead to hyperprolactinemia, causing gynecomastia.

● Nursing considerations
- Apply cold compresses to the patient's breasts and administer analgesics to make him as comfortable as possible during early stages
- Prepare the patient for diagnostic tests, including chest and skull X-rays and blood hormone levels and treatments
- Provide emotional support and reassurances that time or treatment can reduce gynecomastia (the condition may alter the patient's body image)

HERPES SIMPLEX TYPE 2

● Definition
- Recurrent viral infection, also known as *genital herpes*
- After initial infection with herpes simplex virus (HSV), the patient becomes a carrier susceptible to recurrent attacks
  - Type-1 strain (HSV-1) — usually produces lesions on the skin or mucous membranes of the lips and mouth
  - Type-2 strain (HSV-2) — produces lesions on the genitals
- Recurrent infections may be provoked by fever, menses, stress, heat, cold, lack of sleep, smoking, sun exposure, and contact with reactivated disease (kissing, sharing cosmetics, sexual intercourse, oral sex)

● Underlying pathophysiology
- Virus enters the mucosal surfaces or abraded skin sites and initiates replication in cells of the epidermis and dermis

Key nursing considerations for gynecomastia
- Apply cold compresses.
- Administer analgesics.
- Provide emotional support.

Key facts about herpes simplex type 2
- Recurrent viral infection
- Enters mucosal surfaces or abraded skin and replicates
- Infects sensory or autonomic nerve endings
- Two strains: HSV-1 (lesions on skin or mucous membranes of lips and mouth) and HSV-2 (lesions on genitals)

- Replication continues to permit infection of sensory or autonomic nerve endings
- Virus enters the neuronal cell, is transported intra-axonally to nerve cell bodies in ganglia (where the virus establishes latency), and spreads via the peripheral sensory nerves (see *Understanding the genital herpes cycle*)

● Causes
- Type 1 herpesvirus hominis, which is transmitted primarily by contact with oral secretions
- Type 2 herpesvirus hominis, which is transmitted by contact with genital secretions

● Pathophysiologic changes
- Initially, pain, tingling, and itching in genital area followed by eruption of localized, fluid-filled vesicles due to viral penetration of skin, viral replication, and entry into cutaneous neurons
- Dysuria and dyspareunia due to painful lesions
- Malaise, fever, leukorrhea (in females), and lymphadenopathy due to progression of viral infection
- Sore throat, fever, anorexia, adenopathy, increased salivation, severe mouth pain, halitosis, and small vesicles on an erythematous base (possibly present on pharyngeal and oral mucosa) due to primary perioral HSV
- Photophobia, excessive tearing, follicular conjunctivitis, chemosis, blepharitis, vesicles on eyelids, lethargy and fever, regional adenopathy due to primary ocular infection

● Complications
- Primary HSV infection during pregnancy: abortion, premature labor, microcephaly, and uterine growth retardation
- Congenital herpes transmitted during vaginal birth: subclinical neonatal infection, severe infection with seizures, chorioretinitis, skin vesicles, and hepatosplenomegaly
- HSV-1 causing life-threatening, nonepidemic encephalitis in infants
- Gingivostomatitis in children ages 1 to 3
- Blindness from ocular infection
- Increased risk of cervical cancer
- Urethral stricture from recurrent genital herpes
- Perianal ulcers
- Colitis
- Esophagitis
- Pneumonitis
- Neurologic disorders
- Uremia with multiple organ involvement

● Diagnostic test findings
- Tissue culture shows isolation of virus (gold standard)
- Straining of scrapings from the base of the lesion demonstrates characteristic giant cells or intranuclear inclusions of HSV infection
- Tissue analysis shows HSV antigens or deoxyribonucleic acid in scrapings from lesions

---

Key pathophysiologic changes in herpes simplex type 2

- Pain, tingling, and itching in genital area
- Malaise
- Fever

Key diagnostic test results for herpes simplex type 2

- Tissue culture: Isolation of virus

GO WITH THE FLOW

Understanding the genital herpes cycle

After a patient is infected with genital herpes, a latency period follows. The virus takes up permanent residence in the nerve cells surrounding the lesions, and intermittent viral shedding may take place.

Repeated outbreaks may develop at any time, again followed by a latent stage during which the lesions heal completely. Outbreaks may recur as often as three to eight times per year.

Although the cycle continues indefinitely, some people remain symptom-free for years.

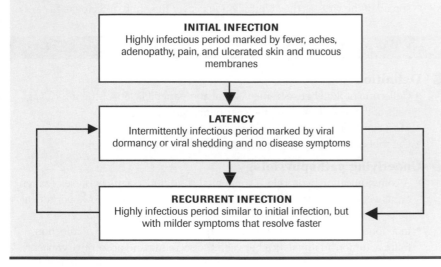

Treatment
- Antiviral drugs (acyclovir, valacyclovir, famciclovir) to decrease disease severity and shorten duration of lesions, decrease viral shedding, and decrease frequency of recurrence by inhibiting viral replication
- Analgesics and antipyretics to relieve pain and reduce fever
- Warm baths, cool compresses, or topical anesthetics to help reduce pain
- Colloidal oatmeal (Aveeno) and Burow's solution to help reduce burning and itching
- Education and counseling about care measures during outbreaks, prevention of secondary or recurrent herpes infections (including eye infections), measures to avoid infecting others (avoiding sexual activity during the active stage), and risk of fetal infection

Nursing considerations
- Encourage the patient to drink 8 to 12 glasses of fluid daily if urination causes pain
- Recommend bed rest for 1 to 2 days if the patient has a severe case with many painful lesions
- Encourage the use of sunscreen to prevent sun-induced recurrences
- Teach the patient to keep lesions dry, except for applying topical drugs

Key treatments for herpes simplex type 2
- Antiviral drugs
- Analgesics
- Antipyretics

Key nursing considerations for herpes simplex type 2
- Advise patient to avoid all sexual contact during outbreaks.
- Teach patient that drugs can't cure herpes, but they can shorten the course of the outbreak.
- Recommend using cool compresses or sitz baths.
- Teach proper hand-washing technique.
- Instruct patient to keep lesions dry.

- Teach the patient that medications can't cure herpes, but they can shorten the course of the outbreak and delay recurrences
- Explain that aspirin, acetaminophen (Tylenol), or ibuprofen (Advil) may be recommended to relieve pain and reduce fever
- Tell the patient that a topical anesthetic, such as lidocaine (Xylocaine), may be ordered for painful skin lesions; lidocaine mouthwash may be ordered for mouth and throat ulcers
- Recommend the use of cool compresses or sitz baths several times per day
- Teach proper hand-washing technique
- Advise the patient to avoid all sexual contact during outbreaks of active infection; stress that the disease can be active and transmissible before lesions are visible
- Teach the patient that the use of condoms may not be sufficient to prevent spread of the virus as they typically don't cover the entire infected area

HYDROCELE

Definition
- Collection of fluid between the visceral and parietal layers of the tunica vaginalis of the testicle or along the spermatic cord
- Most common form of scrotal swelling
- Described as communicating or noncommunicating

Underlying pathophysiology
- A communicating hydrocele, a congenital condition, occurs because of patency between the scrotal sac and the peritoneal cavity, which allows peritoneal fluids to collect in the scrotum
- In a noncommunicating hydrocele, fluid accumulates because of infection, trauma, tumor, an imbalance between the secreting and absorptive capacities of scrotal tissue, or an obstruction of lymphatic or venous drainage in the spermatic cord
  - Leads to displaced fluid in the scrotum, outside the testes
  - Subsequent swelling results, causing reduced blood flow to the testes

Causes
- Congenital malformation (infants)
- Trauma to the testes or epididymis
- Infection of the testes or epididymis
- Testicular tumor

Pathophysiologic changes
- Scrotal swelling and feeling of heaviness due to fluid accumulation
- Inguinal hernia (commonly present in congenital hydroceles)
- Testicular enlargement (from slightly larger than the testes to the size of a grapefruit or larger) due to fluid accumulation
- Fluid collection, with either flaccid or tense mass, due to patency between the scrotal sac and the peritoneal cavity
- Pain due to acute epididymal infection or testicular torsion
- Scrotal tenderness due to severe swelling

Complications
- Epididymitis

Key facts about hydrocele

- Collection of fluid between visceral and parietal layers of tunica vaginalis or along spermatic cord
- Causes scrotal swelling
- May be communicating (involving patency between scrotal sac and peritoneal cavity) or noncommunicating (caused by infection, trauma, tumor, scrotal tissue imbalance, or drainage obstruction in spermatic cord)

Key pathophysiologic changes in hydrocele

- Scrotal swelling
- Feeling of heaviness
- Inguinal hernia

- Testicular atrophy

- ● **Diagnostic test findings**
  - Transillumination is used to distinguish between a fluid-filled and solid mass (tumor doesn't transilluminate)
  - Ultrasonography is used to visualize the testes and determine the presence of a tumor
  - Fluid biopsy determines the cause and differentiates between normal and cancerous cells

- ● **Treatment**
  - Usually no treatment for congenital hydrocele; condition commonly resolves spontaneously by age 1
  - Surgical repair to avoid strangulation of the bowel (inguinal hernia with bowel present in the sac)
  - Aspiration of fluid and injection of sclerosing drug into the scrotal sac for a tense hydrocele that impedes blood circulation or causes pain
  - Excision of the tunica vaginalis for recurrent hydroceles
  - Suprainguinal excision for a testicular tumor detected by ultrasound

- ● **Nursing considerations**
  - Place a rolled towel between the patient's legs, and elevate the scrotum to help reduce severe swelling
  - Advise the patient with mild or moderate swelling to wear a loose-fitting athletic supporter lined with soft cotton dressings
  - Encourage sitz baths, and apply heat or ice packs to decrease inflammation
  - Administer analgesics, such as acetaminophen or ibuprofen, as ordered

OVARIAN CYSTS

- ● **Definition**
  - Nonneoplastic (usually) sacs on an ovary
    - Contain fluid or semisolid material
    - Usually small and produce no symptoms
    - Should be investigated thoroughly to rule out cancer
    - May occur as a single cyst or multiple cysts (polycystic ovarian disease)
  - Types of ovarian cysts
    - Follicular cysts: can develop anytime, including in utero, but most common in women of reproductive age
    - Theca-lutein (luteal) cysts: occur in women of reproductive age
    - Granulosa-lutein cysts: occur within the corpus luteum primarily in women of reproductive age

- ● **Underlying pathophysiology**
  - Follicular cysts are generally very small and arise from follicles that overdistend, either because they haven't ruptured or have ruptured and resealed before their fluid was reabsorbed
  - Luteal cysts develop if a mature corpus luteum persists abnormally and continues to secrete progesterone
    - Consist of blood or fluid that accumulates in the cavity of the corpus luteum
    - Are typically more symptomatic than follicular cysts

Key pathophysiologic changes in ovarian cysts

- Mild pelvic discomfort
- Lower back pain
- Abnormal uterine bleeding

Key diagnostic test results for ovarian cysts

- Pelvic examination: Presence of a mass or an enlarged ovary
- Ultrasound and laparoscopy: Presence of a cyst

Key treatments for ovarian cysts

- In some cases, no treatment
- Analgesics
- Laparoscopy or exploratory laparotomy

- When ovarian cysts persist into menopause, they secrete excessive amounts of estrogen in response to the hypersecretion of FSH and LH that normally occurs during menopause

Causes

- Enlargement of the ovaries caused by excessive accumulation of blood during the hemorrhagic phase of the menstrual cycle can produce granulosa-lutein cysts
  - Considered functional, nonneoplastic cysts
  - Arise during some variation in the ovulatory process in the corpus luteum
- High levels of circulating gonadotropins due to excessive stimulation of the theca intima may produce theca-lutein cysts
  - Commonly bilateral and filled with clear, straw-colored liquid
  - Usually associated with hydatidiform mole, choriocarcinoma, or hormone therapy (with hCG or clomiphene citrate)

Pathophysiologic changes

- Mild pelvic discomfort, lower back pain, dyspareunia, or abnormal uterine bleeding secondary to a disturbed ovulatory pattern related to large or multiple cysts
- Acute abdominal pain similar to that of appendicitis due to torsion of ovarian cysts
- Unilateral pelvic discomfort due to granulosa-lutein cysts appearing early in pregnancy and growing as large as 2″ to 2½″ (5 to 6 cm) in diameter
- Delayed menses followed by prolonged or irregular bleeding due to granulosa-lutein cysts (in nonpregnant women)

Complications

- Torsion or rupture of cyst
- Infertility
- Amenorrhea
- Secondary dysmenorrhea
- Oligomenorrhea

Diagnostic test findings

- Pelvic examination reveals a mass or enlarged ovary
- hCG titer reveals an elevated level (theca-lutein cyst)
- Urinalysis reveals slightly elevated urine 17-ketosteroids (polycystic ovarian disease)
- Ultrasound and laparoscopy reveals the presence of a cyst

Treatment

- No treatment needed in some cases; cysts tend to disappear spontaneously within one to two menstrual cycles (persistent cysts [follicular] should be excised to rule out cancer)
- Hormonal treatment (commonly used, but no proven benefit)
- Analgesics to relieve symptoms (functional cysts that occur during pregnancy); cysts usually diminish during the third trimester, rarely requiring surgery
- Elimination of hydatidiform mole, destruction of choriocarcinoma, or discontinuation of hCG or clomiphene citrate therapy (theca-lutein cysts)
- Laparoscopy or exploratory laparotomy with possible ovarian cystectomy or oophorectomy for persistent or suspicious (possibly malignant) cyst

– May be performed during pregnancy, if necessary
– Optimal timing for surgery during pregnancy is second trimester
- Culdocentesis and draining of intraperitoneal fluid from ruptured ovarian cysts (may be performed in emergency department or office setting)
- Surgery for ongoing hemorrhage from ruptured luteal cyst

Nursing considerations
- Explain to the patient the nature of the cyst, the need for intervention, and how long the condition may last
- Provide appropriate preoperative care
  – Explain the procedure to the patient, and advise her about any expected discomfort
  – Watch for signs of cyst rupture, such as increasing abdominal pain, distention, and rigidity
  – Monitor the patient's vital signs for fever, tachypnea, or hypotension (possibly indicating peritonitis or intraperitoneal hemorrhage)
- Provide appropriate postoperative care
  – Encourage frequent movement in bed and early ambulation, as ordered, to prevent pulmonary embolism
  – Provide emotional support, offering appropriate reassurance if the patient fears cancer or infertility
  – Advise the patient to gradually increase her activities at home over 4 to 6 weeks after surgery

POLYCYSTIC OVARIAN SYNDROME

Definition
- Metabolic disorder characterized by multiple ovarian cysts
- Produces a syndrome of hormonal disturbances that includes insulin resistance, obesity, hirsutism, acne, and ovulation and fertility problems
- Most common in women under age 30
- With appropriate treatment, good prognosis for ovulation and fertility

Underlying pathophysiology
- As with all anovulation syndromes, the pulsatile release of GnRH is lacking
- Although initial ovarian follicle development is normal, many small follicles begin to accumulate because there's no selection of a dominant follicle
- These follicles may respond abnormally to hormonal stimulation, causing an abnormal pattern of estrogen secretion during the menstrual cycle
- These endocrine abnormalities may cause cystic abnormalities or polycystic ovarian syndrome, in which muscle and adipose tissue are resistant to the effects of insulin, and lipid metabolism is abnormal

Causes
- Precise cause unknown
- Theories
  – Abnormal enzyme activity triggering excess androgen secretion from the ovaries and adrenal glands
  – Endocrine abnormalities
  – Genetic links

Key nursing considerations for ovarian cysts
- Watch for signs of cyst rupture.
- Monitor patient's vital signs.

After surgery
- Encourage ambulation.
- Provide emotional support.
- Advise patient to gradually increase activities.

Key facts about polycystic ovarian syndrome
- Results from lack of pulsatile release of GnRH
- Involves accumulation of many small follicles, which cause abnormal estrogen secretion during menstrual cycle
- May cause abnormal lipid metabolism and insulin resistance

Pathophysiologic changes
- Mild pelvic discomfort, lower back pain, and dyspareunia due to multiple ovarian cysts
- Abnormal uterine bleeding secondary to disturbed ovulatory pattern
- Hirsutism and male-pattern hair loss due to abnormal pattern of estrogen secretion
- Obesity due to abnormal hormone regulation
- Acne due to excess sebum production caused by disturbed androgen secretion

Complications
- Increased risk of endometrial carcinoma
- Increased risk of cardiovascular disease and type 2 diabetes mellitus due to hypertension and insulin resistance
- Secondary amenorrhea
- Oligomenorrhea
- Infertility

Diagnostic test findings
- Urine testing reveals slightly elevated urinary 17-ketosteroid level
- Blood testing reveals an elevated LH to FSH ratio (usually 3:1 or greater), and elevated testosterone and androstenedione levels
- Direct visualization by laparoscopy rules out paraovarian cysts of the broad ligament, salpingitis, endometriosis, and neoplastic cysts
- Ultrasonography or surgery allows visualization of the ovary (commonly done for another condition), which may confirm the presence of ovarian cysts

Treatment
- Monitoring of the patient's weight to maintain a normal body mass index (helps reduce risks associated with insulin resistance, which may cause spontaneous ovulation in some women)
- Clomiphene citrate to induce ovulation
- Medroxyprogesterone (Provera) for 10 days each month (for patients wanting to become pregnant)
- Low-dose hormonal contraceptives to treat abnormal bleeding (for patients who require reliable contraception)
- Hysterectomy with bilateral salpingo-oophorectomy for refractory pain and bleeding

Nursing considerations
- Provide appropriate preoperative care
  - Watch for signs of cyst rupture, such as increasing abdominal pain, distention, and rigidity
  - Monitor the patient's vital signs for fever, tachypnea, or hypotension (possibly indicating peritonitis or intraperitoneal hemorrhage)
- Provide appropriate postoperative care
  - Encourage frequent movement in bed and early ambulation, as ordered, to prevent pulmonary embolism
  - Provide emotional support, offering appropriate reassurance if the patient fears cancer or infertility

Key pathophysiologic changes in polycystic ovarian syndrome
- Mild pelvic discomfort
- Lower back pain
- Dyspareunia
- Obesity
- Abnormal uterine bleeding

Key diagnostic test results for polycystic ovarian syndrome
- Blood testing: Elevated ratio of LH to FSH (3:1 or greater), elevated testosterone and androstenedione levels
- Ultrasonography or surgery: Confirmation of presence of ovarian cysts

Key treatments for polycystic ovarian syndrome
- Clomiphene citrate
- Low-dose hormonal contraceptives
- Hysterectomy with bilateral salpingo-oophorectomy

Key nursing considerations for polycystic ovarian syndrome
- Watch for signs of cyst rupture.

After surgery
- Encourage early ambulation.
- Provide emotional support.

PROSTATITIS

● **Definition**
  • Condition marked by inflammation of the prostate gland; may be acute or chronic
    – Acute: easy to recognize and treat
    – Chronic: less recognizable; most common cause of recurrent UTIs in men
  • Common disease classifications
    – Bacterial prostatitis
    – Granulomatous (tuberculous) prostatitis
    – Nonbacterial prostatitis
    – Prostatodynia (painful prostate)

● **Underlying pathophysiology**
  • Spasms in the genitourinary tract or tension in the pelvic floor muscles may cause inflammation and nonbacterial prostatitis
  • Bacterial prostatic infections can result from a previous or concurrent infection; bacteria ascend from the infected urethra, bladder, lymphatics, or blood through the prostatic ducts and into the prostate
  • Infection stimulates an inflammatory response in which the prostate becomes larger, tender, and firm; inflammation is usually limited to a few of the gland's excretory ducts

● **Causes**
  • Bacterial prostatitis: *Escherichia coli* (80% of cases), *Klebsiella, Enterobacter, Proteus, Pseudomonas, Streptococcus, Chlamydia trachomatis, Neisseria gonorrhoeae,* or *Staphylococcus*
    – Probable modes of spread to the prostate
      · Ascending urethral infection or through the bloodstream
      · Invasion of rectal bacteria through lymphatics
      · Reflux of infected urine from bladder into prostate ducts
      · Infrequent or excessive sexual intercourse
      · Procedures, such as cystoscopy or catheterization (less common)
      · Bacterial invasion from the urethra (chronic prostatitis)
  • Granulomatous prostatitis: *Mycobacterium tuberculosis*
  • Nonbacterial prostatitis: exact cause unknown; possible causes include infection by protozoa or virus
  • Prostatodynia: exact cause unknown

● **Pathophysiologic changes**
  • Chills due to inflammation
  • Lower back pain, especially when standing, due to compression of the prostate gland
  • Perineal fullness, suprapubic tenderness, and frequent and urgent urination due to compression of the prostate gland
  • Dysuria, nocturia, and urinary obstruction due to blocked urethra by enlarged prostate
  • Cloudy urine due to infection
  • Fever, myalgia, fatigue, and arthralgia due to systemic infection
  • Recurrent symptomatic cystitis due to chronic prostatitis

Key facts about prostatitis

● Marked by inflammation of prostate gland
● Classified as bacterial, granulomatous, nonbacterial, or prostatodynia
● If bacterial, results from an infection that travels through prostatic ducts into the prostate, stimulating an inflammatory response

Key pathophysiologic changes in prostatitis

● Chills
● Lower back pain
● Perineal fullness

- Evidence of UTI (such as urinary frequency, burning, and cloudy urine) due to infection in chronic prostatitis
- Painful ejaculation, bloody semen, persistent urethral discharge, and sexual dysfunction due to compression of the prostate gland

Complications

- UTI (common)
- Infected and abscessed testis (removed surgically)

Diagnostic test findings

- Rectal examination findings vary with the type of prostatitis
  - Very tender, warm, and enlarged prostate (acute prostatitis)
  - Firm, irregularly shaped, and slightly enlarged prostate due to fibrosis (chronic bacterial prostatitis)
  - Normal prostate gland (nonbacterial prostatitis)
- Pelvic X-ray shows prostatic calculi
- Urine culture analysis identifies the causative organism; the urine culture is negative in prostatodynia
- Meares-Stamey four-glass test (involves comparing urine cultures obtained from four specimens) shows a significant increase in colony count, confirming prostatitis (needed for definitive diagnosis)
- Prostatic smears show inflammatory cells in nonbacterial prostatitis and an absence of inflammatory cells in prostatodynia
- PSA test rules out prostate cancer
- Prostate tissue biopsy reveals *M. tuberculosis* (granulomatous prostatitis)
- Urodynamic evaluation reveals detrusor hyperreflexia and pelvic floor myalgia (from chronic spasms)
- White blood cell count may be elevated, especially with fever

Treatment

- Acute prostatitis
  - Co-trimoxazole (Bactrim, Septra) orally for 30 days (for culture showing sensitivity)
  - I.V. co-trimoxazole or I.V. gentamicin (Garamycin) plus ampicillin and sulbactam (Unasyn) until sensitivity test results are known
  - Parenteral therapy for 48 hours to 1 week, then an oral agent for 30 more days (with favorable test results and clinical response)
  - Doxycycline (Vibramycin) or tetracycline (Sumycin) for patients with multiple sex partners
  - Bed rest
  - Adequate hydration
  - Analgesics, antipyretics, and anti-inflammatory drugs for symptom relief
  - Sitz baths to reduce discomfort
  - Stool softeners as necessary
- Chronic prostatitis
  - Co-trimoxazole for at least 6 weeks (for prostatitis due to *E. coli*)
  - Adequate hydration (instruct the patient to drink at least eight glasses of water daily)
  - Regular, careful massage of the prostate to relieve discomfort (vigorous massage may cause secondary epididymitis or septicemia)
  - Regular ejaculation to help drain prostatic secretions

Key diagnostic test results for prostatitis

- Rectal examination: Tender, warm, and enlarged prostate (acute prostatitis); firm, irregularly shaped, and slightly enlarged prostate (chronic bacterial prostatitis)
- Urine culture: Identification of causative organism; negative in prostatodynia

Key treatments for prostatitis

Acute
- Co-trimoxazole
- Adequate hydration
- Analgesics

Chronic
- Adequate hydration
- Regular, careful massage of the prostate

- Granulomatous prostatitis: antitubercular drug combinations to help relieve symptoms
- Nonbacterial prostatitis: anticholinergics and analgesics to help relieve symptoms
- Prostatodynia: alpha-adrenergic blockers and muscle relaxants to relieve pain
- Continuous, low-dose anabolic steroid therapy (effective in some men)
- Surgery (if drug therapy is unsuccessful)
  - TURP, removing all infected tissue (not usually performed on young adults; may cause retrograde ejaculation and sterility)
  - Total prostatectomy (curative but may cause impotence and incontinence)

Nursing considerations
- Ensure bed rest and adequate hydration
- Provide stool softeners and administer sitz baths as ordered
- Prepare to assist with suprapubic needle aspiration of the bladder or a suprapubic cystostomy, as necessary
- Emphasize the need for strict adherence to the prescribed drug regimen
  - Advise the patient to drink at least eight glasses of water per day
  - Have the patient report adverse drug reactions
- Instruct the patient to avoid lifting, strenuous exercise, and long automobile rides after surgery; tell him to avoid sexual activity for several weeks after discharge

TESTICULAR TORSION

Definition
- Abnormal twisting of the spermatic cord due to rotation of a testis or the mesorchium (fold in the area between the testis and epididymis), which causes strangulation
- Almost always (90%) unilateral
- Causes extreme pain and eventual infarction of the testis if left untreated
- Onset may be spontaneous or may follow physical exertion or trauma
- Greatest risk during the neonatal period, and again between ages 12 and 18 (puberty), but may occur at any age; infants with torsion of one testis have a greater incidence of torsion of the other testis later in life than do males in the general population

Underlying pathophysiology
- Normally, the tunica vaginalis envelops the testis and attaches to the epididymis and spermatic cord; normal contraction of the cremaster muscle causes the left testis to rotate counterclockwise and the right testis to rotate clockwise
- In testicular torsion, the testis rotates on its vascular pedicle and twists the arteries and vein in the spermatic cord, causing an interruption of circulation to the testis
- Vascular engorgement and ischemia develop, causing scrotal swelling unrelieved by rest or elevation of the scrotum
- In intravaginal torsion (most common type of testicular torsion in adolescents), testicular twisting may result from an abnormality of the tunica, in which the testis is abnormally positioned, or from a narrowing of the mesentery support

Extravaginal torsion

In extravaginal torsion, rotation of the spermatic cord above the testis causes strangulation and, eventually, infarction of the testis.

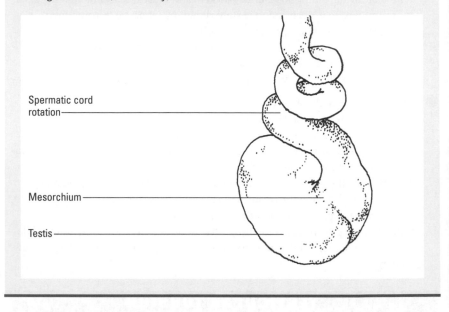

Spermatic cord rotation

Mesorchium

Testis

- In extravaginal torsion (most common in neonates), loose attachment of the tunica vaginalis to the scrotal lining causes spermatic cord rotation above the testis; sudden, forceful contraction of the cremaster muscle may precipitate this condition (see *Extravaginal torsion*)

● **Causes**
  - Congenital anomaly
  - Trauma
  - Sexual activity
  - Undescended testicle
  - Exercise

● **Pathophysiologic changes**
  - Excruciating pain in the affected testis or iliac fossa of the pelvis due to testicular torsion
  - Edematous, elevated, and ecchymotic scrotum with loss of the cremasteric reflex (stimulation of the skin on the inner thigh retracts the testis on the same side) on the affected side due to torsion
  - Abdominal pain due to torsion
  - Nausea and vomiting due to pain

● **Complications**
  - Testicular infarction and necrosis
  - Infertility

Diagnostic test findings
- Doppler ultrasonography helps distinguish testicular torsion from strangulated hernia, undescended testes, or epididymitis (absent blood flow and avascular testis in torsion)

Treatment
- Orchiopexy (fixation of viable testis to the scrotum and prophylactic fixation of the contralateral testis)
- Orchiectomy (excision of a nonviable testis) to decrease the risk of autoimmune response to necrotic testis and its contents, damage to unaffected testis, and subsequent infertility
- Manual, counterclockwise manipulation of the testis to improve blood flow before surgery (not always possible)

Nursing considerations
- Promote the patient's comfort before and after surgery; administer pain medication, as ordered, and provide emotional support
- Provide appropriate postoperative care
  - Administer pain medication as ordered
  - Monitor voiding
  - Apply an ice bag with a cover to reduce edema and to protect the wound from contamination
  - Allow the patient to perform as many normal daily activities as possible

TOXIC SHOCK SYNDROME

Definition
- Acute bacterial infection caused by toxin-producing, penicillin-resistant strains of *Staphylococcus aureus* (toxic shock syndrome [TSS] toxin-1 and staphylococcal enterotoxins B and C)
- Primarily affects menstruating women under age 30; associated with continuous use of tampons during menstrual period
- Incidence peaked in mid-1980s; has since declined (probably because of withdrawal of high-absorbency tampons from the market)

Underlying pathophysiology
- For illness to develop, the patient must be infected with a toxigenic strain of *S. aureus,* and must lack the antibodies to that strain (see *Toxic shock syndrome: How it happens,* page 412)

Causes
- Penicillin-resistant *S. aureus*

Pathophysiologic changes
- Intense myalgia, temperature over 104° F (40° C), vomiting, diarrhea, headache, decreased level of consciousness, and vaginal hyperemia and discharge due to toxin-producing infection
- Deep-red rash (especially on palms and soles) that develops within hours of onset and desquamates later due to hypersensitivity reaction to toxin
- Severe hypotension, hypovolemic shock, and possible renal failure due to disease progression

GO WITH THE FLOW

Toxic shock syndrome: How it happens

In toxic shock syndrome, toxin-producing bacterial pathogens are introduced into the vagina by way of contaminated fingers or a tampon applicator, and the menstrual flow provides a medium for bacterial growth

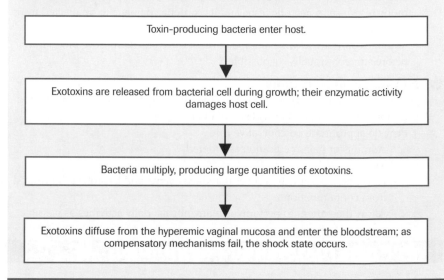

Toxin-producing bacteria enter host.

↓

Exotoxins are released from bacterial cell during growth; their enzymatic activity damages host cell.

↓

Bacteria multiply, producing large quantities of exotoxins.

↓

Exotoxins diffuse from the hyperemic vaginal mucosa and enter the bloodstream; as compensatory mechanisms fail, the shock state occurs.

Complications
- Septic abortions
- Musculoskeletal and respiratory infections
- Staphylococcal bacteremia
- Renal and myocardial dysfunction
- Acute respiratory distress syndrome
- Desquamation of the skin
- Peripheral gangrene
- Muscle weakness
- Neuropsychiatric dysfunction

Diagnostic test findings
- Vaginal smear identifies *S. aureus* from vaginal discharge or infection site, supporting the diagnosis
- Urinalysis shows pyuria
- Blood testing reveals elevated BUN and serum creatinine levels, and low levels of serum albumin, serum calcium, and serum phosphorus
- Complete blood count shows leukocytosis or leukopenia
- Platelet count shows thrombocytopenia

Treatment
- Beta-lactamase-resistant antistaphylococcal antibiotics (oxacillin, nafcillin) I.V. to eliminate infection
- Fluid replacement with I.V. solutions and colloids to reverse shock
- Pressor agents (dopamine [Intropin]) to treat shock unresponsive to fluid replacement
- Dialysis (may be necessary) for kidney dysfunction
- I.V. immunoglobulin (in some cases) to neutralize circulating toxins

Nursing considerations
- Monitor the patient's intake and output, and replenish fluids I.V. as needed
- Use standard precautions for any vaginal discharge and lesion drainage
- Monitor the patient's vital signs and electrolyte, cardiovascular, pulmonary, and neurologic status
- Advise the patient to avoid using tampons (especially superabsorbent) because of the risk of recurrent TSS

VARICOCELE

Definition
- A mass of dilated and tortuous varicose veins in the spermatic cord
- Classically described as a "bag of worms"
- Present in about 30% of all men diagnosed with infertility

Underlying pathophysiology
- Because of a valvular disorder in the spermatic vein, blood pools in the pampiniform plexus of veins that drain each testis rather than flowing into the venous system
- One function of the pampiniform plexus is to keep the testes slightly cooler than body temperature (optimal for sperm production); incomplete blood flow through the testis therefore interferes with spermatogenesis
- Testicular atrophy may also occur because of reduced blood flow

Causes
- Incompetent or congenitally absent valves in the spermatic veins
- Tumor or thrombus obstructing the inferior vena cava (unilateral [left-sided] varicocele)

Pathophysiologic changes
- Feeling of heaviness on the affected side due to dilated veins
- Testicular pain and tenderness on palpation due to tortuous veins in the spermatic cord

Complications
- Infertility
- Hydrocele
- Metastasis from a renal tumor leading to sudden development of a varicocele in an older man (late sign)

Diagnostic test findings
- Physical examination allows palpation of the "bag of worms" when the patient is upright

Key treatments for varicocele

- Scrotal support
- Surgical repair

Key postoperative nursing considerations for varicocele

- Administer pain medication as ordered.
- Monitor voiding.

TOP 6

Items to study for your next test on the reproductive system

1. Effects of hormones on the male and female reproductive systems
2. Pathophysiologic changes related to menstrual alterations
3. Common diagnostic tests for reproductive system disorders
4. Nursing considerations for the patient undergoing hysterectomy or resection of the prostate
5. Treatments for such reproductive system disorders as abnormal uterine bleeding, endometriosis, herpes simplex type 2, and polycystic ovarian syndrome
6. Pathophysiology of toxic shock syndrome

● **Treatment**
- Conservative treatment with a scrotal support to relieve discomfort (with mild varicocele, if fertility isn't an issue)
- Surgical repair or removal involving ligation of the spermatic cord at the internal inguinal ring (if infertility is an issue)

● **Nursing considerations**
- Promote the patient's comfort before surgery; administer pain medications as ordered
- Provide appropriate postoperative care
  – Administer pain medication, as ordered
  – Monitor voiding
  – Apply an ice bag with a cover to reduce edema and to protect the wound from contamination
  – Allow the patient to perform as many normal daily activities as possible

NCLEX CHECKS

It's never too soon to begin your licensure examination preparation. Now that you've reviewed this chapter, carefully read each of the following questions and choose the best answer. Then compare your responses to the correct answers.

1. A client has been diagnosed with chronic polymenorrhea. Her problem can best be described as:
- ☐ **1.** an episode of vaginal bleeding between menses.
- ☐ **2.** heavy or prolonged menses.
- ☐ **3.** a menstrual cycle lasting less than 18 days.
- ☐ **4.** infrequent menses.

2. Primary amenorrhea is a result of:
- ☐ **1.** Asherman's syndrome.
- ☐ **2.** a dysfunctional hypothalamic-pituitary-ovarian axis.
- ☐ **3.** cervical stenosis.
- ☐ **4.** hypogonadotropic-hypoestrogenic anovulation.

3. A client complains of difficulty starting urination, dribbling, and nocturia. He's diagnosed with mild BPH. Which treatment is the physician likely to recommend?
- ☐ **1.** Excretory urography
- ☐ **2.** PSA test
- ☐ **3.** Suprapubic resection of the prostate
- ☐ **4.** Saw palmetto, evenly spaced intake of fluids, and finasteride

4. A client complains of pelvic pain spreading to her lower back and delayed menstruation with a very heavy flow. Following a pelvic examination and ultrasound, a follicular cyst is discovered. Place an X on the site where the cyst is likely to form.

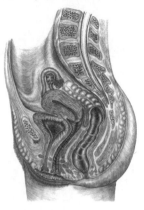

5. A client receives treatment for prostatitis but doesn't respond. A biopsy reveals that the actual diagnosis is granulomatous prostatitis. What causative organism was found on the biopsy?

☐ **1.** *E. coli*
☐ **2.** HSV-2
☐ **3.** *M. tuberculosis*
☐ **4.** *N. gonorrhoeae*

6. An area of swelling in the scrotal area that doesn't transilluminate when a light is shone on it could be indicative of a:

☐ **1.** tumor.
☐ **2.** communicating hydrocele.
☐ **3.** noncommunicating hydrocele.
☐ **4.** varicocele.

7. While caring for a client awaiting surgery for an ovarian cyst, a nurse observes abdominal distention and rigidity without fever. The nurse understands that these are signs of:

☐ **1.** constipation.
☐ **2.** a ruptured cyst.
☐ **3.** peritonitis.
☐ **4.** intraperitoneal hemorrhage.

8. One of the signs and symptoms of TSS is a deep-red rash. Where is this rash most pronounced?

☐ **1.** Face
☐ **2.** Palms and soles
☐ **3.** Trunk
☐ **4.** Arms and legs

9. The classic description "bag of worms" is used to describe which disorder?
- ☐ **1.** Hydrocele
- ☐ **2.** Testicular torsion
- ☐ **3.** Cryptorchidism
- ☐ **4.** Varicocele

10. The classic symptoms of endometriosis are dysmenorrhea, abnormal uterine bleeding, and:
- ☐ **1.** infertility.
- ☐ **2.** dyspareunia.
- ☐ **3.** dysuria.
- ☐ **4.** constipation.

ANSWERS AND RATIONALES

1. CORRECT ANSWER: 3

Chronic polymenorrhea refers to a menstrual cycle lasting less than 18 days. It's related to hormonal imbalances. *Metrorrhagia* is the term describing bleeding between menses; *hypermenorrhea* describes heavy bleeding or bleeding lasting longer than 8 days. Infrequent menses is called *oligomenorrhea*. All of these conditions represent abnormal patterns of menstruation with various causes.

2. CORRECT ANSWER: 2

In primary amenorrhea, the hypothalamic-pituitary-ovarian axis of hormone regulation is dysfunctional. Because of anatomic defects of the CNS, the ovary doesn't receive hormonal signals that normally initiate the development of secondary sex characteristics and the beginning of menstruation. The other answers listed are causes of secondary amenorrhea.

3. CORRECT ANSWER: 4

Mild BPH is treated medically, as with the herb saw palmetto or finasteride to reduce the size of the prostate gland, as well as techniques to avoid straining the bladder, including spacing out fluid intake evenly and limiting nighttime intake of fluids (also prevents nocturia). Suprapubic resection would be done only if the client had significant complications, such as kidney involvement or intractable urinary retention and bladder abnormality. Excretory urography and PSA testing are used to diagnose, not treat, BPH.

4. CORRECT ANSWER:

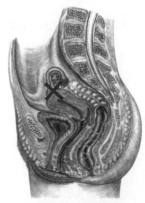

A follicular cyst is one type of ovarian cyst. Follicles that have failed to rupture properly or have sealed off too quickly cause this type of cyst.

5. CORRECT ANSWER: 3

Granulomatous prostatitis is caused by *M. tuberculosis* and is treated with antitubercular drug combinations. *E. coli* is the most common bacterial source of acute prostatitis, although sexually transmitted diseases, such as gonorrhea, may also be culprits. HSV-2 causes genital herpes.

6. CORRECT ANSWER: 1

Transillumination is performed to distinguish fluid-filled from solid masses. A tumor is dense and therefore doesn't transilluminate. Hydroceles and varicoceles contain fluid and would transilluminate.

7. CORRECT ANSWER: 2

Increasing abdominal distention and rigidity as well as the client's report of increased abdominal pain may indicate that an ovarian cyst has ruptured. The presence of fever would indicate possible peritonitis. The findings aren't indicative of constipation or intraperitoneal hemorrhage.

8. CORRECT ANSWER: 2

A deep-red rash, especially on the palms and soles, develops within hours of TSS onset; desquamation occurs later. The rash may spread to the other areas listed in some individuals.

9. CORRECT ANSWER: 4

Varicocele, a mass of dilated and tortuous varicose veins in the spermatic cord, is classically described as a "bag of worms." A hydrocele is the accumulation of fluid between the layers of the tunica vaginalis of the testis or along the spermatic cord. Testicular torsion occurs when the spermatic cord becomes abnormally twisted. Failure of one or both testes to descend into the scrotal sac is known as *cryptorchidism.*

10. CORRECT ANSWER: 1

Endometriosis is the presence of endometrial tissue outside the lining of the uterine cavity. The classic symptoms of this disorder are dysmenorrhea, abnormal uterine bleeding, and infertility due to implantation of ectopic tissues and adhesions. Dyspareunia, dysuria, and constipation may also occur, depending on the spread of the endometrial tissue.

12

Genetic disorders

LEARNING OBJECTIVES

After studying this chapter, you should be able to:

- Identify defects that lead to genetic disorders.
- Discuss the relationship between presenting signs and symptoms and the pathophysiologic changes for any genetic disorder.
- List three probable causes of genetic disorders.
- Write three teaching goals for a patient with a genetic disorder.
- List medications that may improve symptoms of genetic disorders.
- Identify nursing interventions for a patient with a genetic disorder.

CHAPTER OVERVIEW

Genetic disorders are medical conditions that arise from aberrations in the structure, location, or arrangement of chromosomes or from mutations involving individual genes or sets of genes. Many genetic disorders produce anomalies that are apparent at birth, whereas others become recognizable only when symptoms begin to manifest. All genetic disorders can pose significant physical challenges and psychosocial problems for patients, especially children and their parents.

Caring for a patient with a genetic disorder requires special knowledge of the pathophysiologic changes that occur, the signs and symptoms they produce, and the interventions that are necessary to prevent complications and improve the patient's quality of life. The first section of this chapter provides an overview of key pathophysiologic concepts related to genetic disorders. Common genetic disorders are then defined, and underlying pathophysiology, causes, pathophysiologic changes, complications, diagnostic test findings, treatments, and nursing considerations are outlined.

PATHOPHYSIOLOGIC CONCEPTS

● **Chromosomal defects**
- Chromosomal defects include aberrations in the number or structure of chromosomes
- In defects involving the number of chromosomes, the entire chromosome is duplicated or missing
  - Responsible for various congenital anomalies (birth defects) and autosomal (sex-linked) disorders
  - May be inherited, or may occur during meiosis
- Defects in the structure of chromosomes involves the loss or addition of chromosome parts or rearrangement of genetic material
  - May occur through deletion of a section of chromosome during egg or sperm formation
  - May occur through duplication, in which a small portion of chromosome is gained or duplicated somewhere along its length
  - May occur through translocation (shifting or moving of chromosomal material), when chromosomes split apart and rejoin in abnormal arrangement; cells still have the normal amount of genetic material, and commonly there are no visible abnormalities

● **Genetic errors**
- A genetic error is a permanent change in genetic material (mutation) that may occur anywhere in the genome (entire inventory of genes)
- An error may occur spontaneously or after cellular exposure to radiation, certain chemicals, or viruses
- If not identified or repaired, the error may produce a trait different from the original, which can then be transmitted to offspring during reproduction

● **Autosomal disorders**
- These disorders result from an error that occurs at a single gene site on a deoxyribonucleic acid (DNA) strand
- They're inherited in clearly identifiable patterns (as are normal traits)
  - Chance of inheritance depends on whether one or both parents have affected gene
  - Usually, males and females have equal chance of inheriting disorder
- The type of disorder a person has depends on transmission of either a dominant gene (autosomal-dominant inheritance) or a recessive gene (autosomal-recessive inheritance); autosomal-recessive disorders may occur with no family history of disease

● **Multifactorial disorders**
- These disorders commonly result from the effects of several different genes and an environmental component
- They're sometimes apparent at birth (cleft lip, cleft palate, congenital heart disease, anencephaly, clubfoot, myelomeningocele), or they may manifest later (type 2 diabetes mellitus, hypertension, hyperlipidemia, autoimmune disease, cancer)

Key facts about chromosomal defects

Defects in number
- Result if a chromosome is duplicated or missing
- Cause congenital anomalies and autosomal disorders

Defects in structure
- Involve the loss or addition of chromosome parts or rearrangement of genetic material

Key facts about genetic errors
- Permanent mutations that may occur anywhere in the genome
- May occur spontaneously or after cellular exposure to radiation, certain chemicals, or viruses
- Can be transmitted to offspring

Key facts about autosomal disorders
- Result from an error at a single gene site on a DNA strand
- May be autosomal-dominant or autosomal-recessive

Key facts about multifactorial disorders
- Result from the effects of different genes and an environmental component
- May be apparent at birth (such as cleft lip) or may manifest later in life (such as type 2 diabetes)

Key facts about sex-linked disorders

- Caused by a genetic error on one of the sex chromosomes
- Most commonly transmitted from the union of a carrier female and normal male

Key facts about cleft lip and cleft palate

- Abnormalities of the lip and palate
- Result when lip or palate fuses imperfectly in utero
- Caused by a chromosomal abnormality, exposure to teratogens, genetic abnormality, or environmental factors

● **Sex-linked disorders**
- These disorders are caused by a genetic error located on one of the sex chromosomes (most commonly the X chromosome, usually involving transmission of a recessive trait)
- Patterns of transmission differ with males and females
  - With males (only one X chromosome): single X-linked recessive gene can cause disease
  - With females (two X chromosomes): can be homozygous for disease allele (variant), homozygous for normal allele, or heterozygous (carrier)
- A person with an abnormal trait typically has one affected parent; the most common transmission is from the union of a carrier female and normal male
- Inheritance of the dominant or recessive gene is critical (most dominant disorders are lethal in males)
  - When the father is affected (either dominant or recessive gene): all daughters will be affected (dominant gene) or carriers (recessive gene); all sons will be unaffected or noncarriers
  - When the mother is carrier (recessive gene): unaffected sons will not transmit disorder
  - When the mother is affected (dominant gene): each child has a 50% chance of being affected

CLEFT LIP AND CLEFT PALATE

● **Definition**
- Abnormalities involving the lip and palate (may occur separately or in combination) develop in the second month of pregnancy, when the front and sides of the face and the palatine shelves fuse imperfectly
- May occur unilaterally, bilaterally, or in the midline (rarely); may involve only the lip, or the defect may extend into the upper jaw or nasal cavity (see *Types of cleft deformities*)
- Cleft lip (with or without cleft palate) occurs twice as often in males as in females; cleft palate alone (without cleft lip) is more common in females
- Most common among whites

● **Underlying pathophysiology**
- During the second month of pregnancy, the front and sides of the face and the palatine shelves develop; because of a chromosomal abnormality, exposure to teratogens, genetic abnormality, or environmental factors, the lip or palate fuses imperfectly
- Deformity may range from a simple notch to a complete cleft; cleft palate may be partial or complete
- Complete cleft includes the soft palate, the bones of the maxilla, and the alveolus on one or both sides of the premaxilla
- Double cleft is most severe of the deformities
  - Runs from the soft palate forward to either side of the nose
  - Separates the maxilla and premaxilla into freely moving segments
  - May cause tongue and other muscles to displace the segments, enlarging the cleft

Types of cleft deformities

These illustrations show variations of cleft lip and cleft palate.

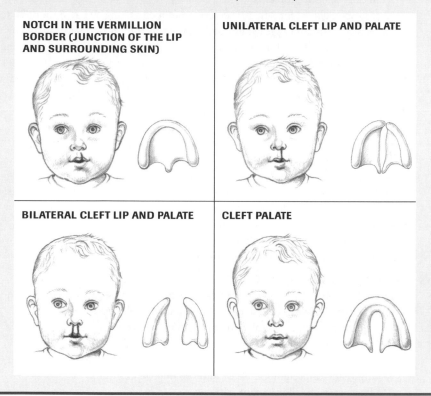

NOTCH IN THE VERMILLION BORDER (JUNCTION OF THE LIP AND SURROUNDING SKIN)

UNILATERAL CLEFT LIP AND PALATE

BILATERAL CLEFT LIP AND PALATE

CLEFT PALATE

● **Causes**
  - Chromosomal or Mendelian syndrome (cleft defects are associated with more than 300 syndromes)
  - Exposure to teratogens during fetal development (environmental factors)
  - Combined genetic and environmental factors

● **Pathophysiologic changes**
  - Obvious cleft lip and/or palate due to imperfect fusion of lip or palate
  - Feeding difficulties due to incomplete fusion of the palate

● **Complications**
  - Malnutrition
  - Hearing impairment
  - Permanent speech impediment
  - Possible aspiration
  - Impaired self-esteem (if cleft isn't repaired during infancy or due to scarring from surgical repair)

● **Diagnostic test findings**
  - Clinical presentation is obvious at birth
  - Prenatal targeted ultrasound reveals the abnormality

Key pathophysiologic changes in cleft lip and cleft palate
● Obvious cleft lip or palate

Key diagnostic test results for cleft lip and cleft palate
● Prenatal targeted ultrasound: Presence of the abnormality, which is also obvious at birth

Key treatments for cleft lip and cleft palate

- Surgical correction
- Orthodontic prosthesis
- Speech and hearing therapy
- Adequate nutrition

Key nursing considerations for cleft lip and cleft palate

- Experiment with feeding devices.
- Teach the parents how to best feed the infant, especially proper positioning to prevent aspiration.

After surgery

- Assess infant for signs of infection.
- Maintain a patent airway.
- Record intake and output.
- Restrain infant as needed to prevent injury.

● Treatment

- Surgical correction of cleft lip
  - Usually done in the first few days of life to permit sucking and prevent or reduce speech problems
  - May be delayed for 8 to 10 weeks (sometimes as long as 6 to 8 months) to allow the infant to grow and mature, thereby minimizing surgical and anesthesia risks, ruling out associated congenital anomalies, and allowing time for parental bonding
- Surgical correction of cleft palate at 12 to 18 months (when child has gained weight and is free from infection)
- Orthodontic prosthesis to improve sucking
- Speech therapy to correct speech patterns
- Speech and hearing therapy (using audiometric evaluation) for hearing loss due to frequent otitis media
- Use of a contoured speech bulb attached to the posterior of a denture to occlude the nasopharynx when a wide horseshoe defect makes surgery impossible (to help the child develop intelligible speech)
- Adequate nutrition for normal growth and development
- Use of a large, soft nipple with large holes, such as a lamb's nipple, to improve feeding patterns and promote nutrition

● Nursing considerations

- Teach the mother that ingestion of 0.4 mg of folic acid twice daily before conception may decrease the risk of isolated cleft defects in future pregnancies
  - Approach subject tactfully and without blame (mother may already have feelings of guilt)
  - Encourage daily multivitamin containing folic acid throughout childbearing years (until menopause or induced end of fertility)
  - Teach same to all pregnant patients
- Place the child with Pierre Robin syndrome (lower jaw abnormally small [micrognathia], tongue displaced downward [glossoptosis], abnormal opening in the roof of the mouth [cleft soft palate]) on his side for sleeping (never place the child on his back because his tongue could fall back and obstruct his airway); most other infants with a cleft palate can sleep on their backs without difficulty
- Maintain adequate nutrition to ensure normal growth and development; experiment with feeding devices (the infant may feed better from a bottle and nipple designed specifically for infants with cleft defects)
- Teach the parents how to best feed the infant
  - Advise them to hold the infant in a near-sitting position, with the flow directed to the side or back of the infant's tongue to prevent aspiration and decrease the amount of air swallowed during feeding
  - Tell them to burp the infant frequently because of swallowed air
  - If the underside of the nasal septum becomes ulcerated and the infant refuses to suck because of the pain, instruct the parents to direct the nipple to the side of the mouth to give the mucosa time to heal; tell them to gently clean the palatal cleft with a cotton-tipped applicator dipped in half-strength hydrogen peroxide or water after each feeding

- If no ulceration is present, instruct the parents to rinse the infant's mouth with water after each feeding to decrease the amount of residual formula in the palate
- Encourage the mother of an infant with cleft lip to breast-feed if the cleft doesn't prevent effective sucking
  - May not be possible in an infant with a cleft palate or one who has just had corrective surgery (postoperatively, the infant can't suck for 6 to 10 weeks)
  - May suggest use of a breast pump to express breast milk, which can be fed to infant from a bottle (specially designed nipples require very little sucking)
- Provide appropriate postoperative care
  - Assess the infant for signs of infection, including redness, swelling, or increased temperature
  - Maintain a patent airway
  - Assist with gentle suction of the nasopharynx to prevent atelectasis and pneumonia (physician usually performs this; may also be necessary before surgery)
  - Restrain the infant to prevent him from hurting himself (elbow restraints allow the infant to move his hands while keeping them away from his mouth); remove restraints frequently to assess for changes in skin integrity and circulation
  - Record intake and output, and maintain good nutrition
  - Keep the suture line clean, and prevent extra tension on the suture line
  - Use an infant seat when necessary to keep the child sitting comfortably; hang toys within reach of restrained hands
  - Provide appropriate care after placement of a curved metal bow over a repaired cleft lip to minimize tension on the suture line; remove the gauze before feedings, replace it often, and moisten it with normal saline solution until the sutures are removed (follow agency protocols)
- Help the parents deal with their feelings about the child's condition
  - Teach them about the condition (answer their questions and reinforce what the physician has told them) and show them their infant as soon as possible
  - Remain calm and provide positive information (stressing that surgical repairs can be made)
  - Help them deal with feelings of guilt and grief
  - Direct their attention to the child's assets
- Include the parents in the care and feeding of the child right from the start to encourage normal bonding (infants with genetic anomalies are at increased risk for neglect or abuse)
- Provide the instructions, emotional support, and reassurance the parents will need to take proper care of the child at home
- Refer the parents to a social worker who can guide them to community resources, if needed, and to a genetic counselor to determine the risk in future offspring

CYSTIC FIBROSIS

● **Definition**
  - Autosomal-recessive disorder resulting in dysfunction of the exocrine glands and chronic airway infection
  - Affects multiple organ systems and is associated with numerous complications; patients have average life expectancy of 32 years

● **Underlying pathophysiology**
  - Most cases arise from a mutation in the genetic coding of a single amino acid, resulting in a dysfunctional protein called *cystic fibrosis transmembrane regulator (CFTR)*; CFTR resembles other transmembrane transport proteins, but it lacks the phenylalanine found in normal genes
  - This regulator interferes with cyclic adenosine monophosphate-regulated chloride channels and transport of other ions by preventing adenosine triphosphate from binding to the protein or by interfering with activation by protein kinase (see *Cystic fibrosis: How it happens*)

● **Causes**
  - Genetic mutation on chromosome 7q
    – May involve as many as 350 alleles within CFTR

 GO WITH THE FLOW

Cystic fibrosis: How it happens

Cystic fibrosis is a chronic, progressive, incurable disease affecting the exocrine glands. It typically arises from a mutation in the genetic coding of a single amino acid found in protein.

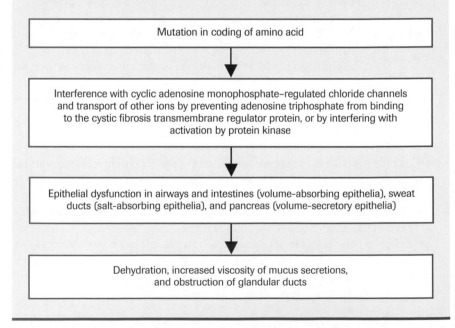

Mutation in coding of amino acid

↓

Interference with cyclic adenosine monophosphate–regulated chloride channels and transport of other ions by preventing adenosine triphosphate from binding to the cystic fibrosis transmembrane regulator protein, or by interfering with activation by protein kinase

↓

Epithelial dysfunction in airways and intestines (volume-absorbing epithelia), sweat ducts (salt-absorbing epithelia), and pancreas (volume-secretory epithelia)

↓

Dehydration, increased viscosity of mucus secretions, and obstruction of glandular ducts

Pathophysiologic changes

- Thick secretions and dehydration due to ionic imbalance
- Chronic airway infections with *Staphylococcus aureus, Pseudomonas aeruginosa,* and *P. cepacea,* possibly due to abnormal airway surface fluids and failure of lung defenses
- Bronchiectasis, bronchiolectasis, exocrine pancreatic insufficiency, intestinal dysfunction, abnormal sweat gland function, and reproductive dysfunction from chronic airway infection
- Dyspnea with dry cough due to accumulation of thick secretions in bronchioles and alveoli
- Paroxysmal cough due to stimulation of the secretion-removal reflex
- Barrel chest, cyanosis, and clubbing of fingers and toes from chronic hypoxia
- Crackles on auscultation due to thick, airway-occluding secretions
- Wheezing on auscultation due to constricted airways
- Bicarbonate and water retention due to an absence of the CFTR chloride channel in the pancreatic ductile epithelia (limits membrane function and leads to retention of pancreatic enzymes, chronic cholecystitis and cholelithiasis, and ultimate destruction of the pancreas)
- Obstruction of the small and large intestine due to inhibited chloride and water secretion and excessive liquid absorption
- Biliary cirrhosis due to biliary secretion retention
- Fatal shock and arrhythmias due to hyponatremia and hypochloremia from sodium lost in sweat
- Failure to thrive (poor weight gain, poor growth, distended abdomen, thin extremities, and sallow skin with poor turgor) due to malabsorption
- Clotting problems, retarded bone growth, and delayed sexual development due to deficiency of fat-soluble vitamins
- Rectal prolapse (in infants and children) due to malnutrition and wasting of perirectal supporting tissues
- Esophageal varices due to cirrhosis and portal hypertension

Complications

- Bronchiectasis
- Pneumonia
- Atelectasis or emphysema
- Dehydration
- Distal intestinal obstruction syndrome
- Diabetes
- Gastroesophageal reflux
- Cor pulmonale
- Biliary disease
- Clotting problems
- Retarded bone growth
- Pancreatitis
- Hepatic failure
- Malnutrition and malabsorption of fat-soluble vitamins (A, D, E, and K)
- Azoospermia
- Secondary amenorrhea
- Electrolyte imbalances

Key pathophysiologic changes in cystic fibrosis

- Thick secretions
- Dehydration
- Chronic airway infections
- Dyspnea
- Cyanosis
- Crackles
- Wheezing

Common complications of cystic fibrosis

- Bronchiectasis
- Pneumonia
- Dehydration
- Malnutrition and malabsorption of fat-soluble vitamins

Key diagnostic test results for cystic fibrosis

- Sweat tests: Elevated sodium chloride levels
- Stool specimen analysis: Absence of trypsin
- DNA testing: Delta F508 deletion on affected gene

Key treatments for cystic fibrosis

- Breathing exercises, postural drainage, and chest percussion
- Bronchodilators
- Oxygen therapy
- Pancreatic enzyme replacement
- Low-fat, high-calorie, high-protein diet

Key nursing considerations for cystic fibrosis

- Perform chest physiotherapy.
- Ensure adequate hydration.
- Teach patient and parents about the disease and its treatments.

- Cardiac arrhythmias
- Potentially fatal shock
- Death

● Diagnostic test findings

- Two sweat tests detect elevated sodium chloride levels; the results may be inaccurate in very young infants because they might not produce enough sweat for a valid test
- Chest X-rays show early signs of obstructive lung disease
- Stool specimen analysis indicates the absence of trypsin, suggesting pancreatic insufficiency
- DNA testing can locate the presence of the delta F508 deletion on the affected gene
- Pulmonary function tests reveal decreased vital capacity, elevated residual volume due to air entrapments, and decreased forced expiratory volume in 1 second
- Sputum culture reveals organisms, such as *Staphylococcus* and *Pseudomonas,* which typically and chronically colonize in patients with cystic fibrosis
- Blood testing reveals a decreased serum albumin level, liver enzyme tests may reveal hepatic insufficiency, and serum electrolyte analysis may show hypochloremia and hyponatremia

● Treatment

- Hypertonic radiocontrast materials delivered by enema to treat acute obstructions resulting from meconium ileus
- Breathing exercises, postural drainage, and chest percussion to clear pulmonary secretions
- Bronchodilators to increase expectoration
- Antibiotics (guided by sputum culture results) to treat lung infection
- Oxygen therapy during exacerbation periods
- Domase alfa, a genetically engineered pulmonary enzyme, to help liquefy mucus and increase clearance
- Inhaled beta-adrenergic agonists to control airway constriction
- Pancreatic enzyme replacement to maintain adequate nutrition
- Sodium-channel blocker to decrease sodium resorption from secretions and to improve viscosity
- Uridine triphosphate to stimulate chloride secretion by non-CFTR protein
- Low-fat, high-calorie, high-protein diet (essential)
- Salt supplements (especially in summer) to replace electrolytes lost through sweat
- Recombinant alpha-antitrypsin to counteract excessive proteolytic activity produced during airway inflammation
- Gene therapy to introduce normal CFTR into affected epithelial cells
- Heart or lung transplantation for severe organ failure

● Nursing considerations

- Perform chest physiotherapy to loosen secretions
- Ensure adequate hydration
- Provide a high-calorie, high-protein diet
- Teach the patient and his parents about the disease and its treatments

TIME-OUT FOR TEACHING

Teaching topics in cystic fibrosis

Include this information in your teaching plan for patients with cystic fibrosis:

- explanation of cystic fibrosis, including signs and symptoms and sequelae
- complications of cystic fibrosis
- the importance of physical activity to improve overall fitness and lung function and to help dislodge mucus
- the need for a high-calorie, high-protein diet
- use of pancreatic enzymes to aid digestion
- other prescribed medications, including purpose, adverse reactions, and precautions

- the importance of chest physiotherapy (postural drainage, percussion, vibration, and coughing)
- self-care, such as self-percussion (including use of a mechanical percussion mask), positive expiratory pressure, and forced expiratory technique
- oxygen therapy, types of aerosol therapy, and care of equipment
- the need to prevent dehydration and ways to do so
- other issues, including sexual concerns, coping techniques, and follow-up care.

- Refer the patient or parents to the Cystic Fibrosis Foundation for educational and support services, and genetic counseling (family planning or prenatal diagnosis options) (see *Teaching topics in cystic fibrosis*)
  - Stress the roles of exercise and special diet in improving overall health
- Stay aware of promising new research developments
  - Lung transplantation to reduce the effects of the disease
  - Aerosol gene therapy to help reduce pulmonary symptoms
  - Identification of genetic defect responsible for cystic fibrosis (also found in patients with some forms of unexplained pancreatitis)

DOWN SYNDROME

● **Definition**
- Spontaneous chromosomal abnormality that causes characteristic facial features, other distinctive physical abnormalities, and mental retardation
- Also known as *trisomy 21*
- Commonly associated with cardiac defects and other congenital disorders
- Median life expectancy of 49 years (significantly increased [from 25 years in 1983] by improved treatment for heart defects, respiratory and other infections, and acute leukemia)

● **Underlying pathophysiology**
- Nearly all cases of Down syndrome result from trisomy 21
  - Produces three copies of chromosome 21 instead of the normal two because of faulty meiosis (nondisjunction) of the ovum or, sometimes, the sperm
  - Results in karyotype of 47 chromosomes instead of the usual 46

Key facts about Down syndrome

- Commonly results from a chromosomal abnormality that produces three copies of chromosome 21 instead of the normal two
- Causes characteristic facial features, other physical abnormalities, and mental retardation
- Has a median life expectancy of 49 years

Key pathophysiologic changes in Down syndrome

- Small head with low nasal bridge, epicanthic folds, protruding tongue, and low-set ears
- Simian crease
- Brushfield's spots

Key diagnostic test results for Down syndrome

- Amniocentesis or chorionic villi sampling: Provision of prenatal diagnosis
- AFP testing: Reduced levels

Key treatments for Down syndrome

- Surgery
- Early intervention programs
- Supportive therapies

- Down syndrome may also result from an unbalanced translocation or chromosomal rearrangement in which the long arm of chromosome 21 breaks and attaches to another chromosome
- Some affected persons and some asymptomatic parents may have chromosomal mosaicism, a mixture of two cell types, some with the normal 46 and some with 47 (an extra chromosome 21)

● Causes

- Advanced parental age (mother age 35 or older at delivery or father age 42 or older)
- Deterioration of the oocyte resulting from cumulative effects of radiation and viruses

● Pathophysiologic changes

- Small head with distinctive facial features (low nasal bridge, epicanthic folds, protruding tongue, and low-set ears); small, open mouth and disproportionately large tongue due to chromosomal aberration
- Small, short, thick fingers and hands; single transverse crease on the palm (Simian crease); small white spots on the iris (Brushfield's spots) due to chromosomal aberration
- Mental retardation (estimated IQ of 30 to 70) and congenital defects (heart defects, duodenal atresia, Hirschsprung's disease, polydactyly, syndactyly) due to chromosomal aberration
- Developmental delay due to hypotonia and decreased cognitive processing
- Impaired reflexes due to decreased muscle tone in limbs

● Complications

- Death
- Leukemia
- Premature senile dementia
- Acute and chronic infections
- Strabismus and cataracts
- Diabetes mellitus
- Thyroid disorders

● Diagnostic test findings

- Karyotype analysis or chromosome mapping shows chromosomal abnormality (confirms diagnosis)
- Amniocentesis or chorionic villi sampling provides prenatal diagnosis
- Prenatal targeted ultrasonography identifies duodenal obstruction or an atrioventricular canal defect (suggestive of Down syndrome)
- Alpha-fetoprotein (AFP) levels are reduced (suggestive of Down syndrome)
- Developmental screening test indicates the severity and progress of retardation

● Treatment

- Surgery to correct heart defects and other related congenital abnormalities
- Plastic surgery to correct characteristic facial traits (especially protruding tongue; may help improve speech, reduce susceptibility to dental caries, and result in fewer orthodontic problems)
- Early intervention programs and supportive therapies to maximize mental and physical capabilities
- Antibiotics for recurrent infections

- Thyroid hormone replacement for hypothyroidism

Nursing considerations

- Establish a trusting relationship with the parents, and encourage communication during the difficult period soon after diagnosis
- Recognize and respond to the signs of grieving (for the "normal" child the parents expected)
- Teach parents the importance of a balanced diet for the child
- Stress the need for patience while feeding the infant, who may have difficulty sucking and may be less demanding and seem less eager to eat than other infants
- Teach parents about the signs and symptoms and ways to prevent infection
- Encourage the parents to hold and nurture their child to reinforce bonding
- Emphasize the importance of adequate exercise and maximal environmental stimulation; refer the parents for infant stimulation classes, which may begin in the early months of life
- Help the parents set realistic goals for their child
  - Mental development may seem normal at first, but this shouldn't be taken as a sign of future progress
  - Development may begin to lag behind that of other children by age 1
- Refer the parents and older siblings for genetic and psychological counseling, as appropriate, to help them evaluate future reproductive risks; discuss options for prenatal testing
- Encourage the parents to remember and meet the emotional needs of other children in the family
- Refer the parents to national or local Down syndrome organizations and support groups for information and support

HEMOPHILIA

Definition

- X-linked (defect with X chromosome), recessive bleeding disorder characterized by prolonged coagulation time
- Severity and prognosis of bleeding vary with degree of deficiency, or nonfunction, and the site of bleeding
- Hemophilia A (classic hemophilia): deficiency of clotting factor VIII; more common than type B, affecting more than 80% of all patients with hemophilia
- Hemophilia B (Christmas disease): affects 15% of all patients with hemophilia and results from a factor IX deficiency
- Hemophilia C (very rare): results from factor XI deficiency and follows an atypical bleeding pattern; commonly triggered by surgery
  - Doesn't follow the typical sex-linked inheritance of the other two types of hemophilia
  - Mainly found in Ashkenazi Jews, although it may affect anyone
- No relationship between factor VIII, factor IX, and factor XI inherited defects

Underlying pathophysiology

- A low level of the blood protein necessary for clotting causes disruption of the normal intrinsic coagulation cascade

- Factors VIII and IX are components of the intrinsic clotting pathway; factor IX is an essential factor, and factor VIII is a critical cofactor (accelerates the activation of factor X by several thousand-fold)
- Excessive bleeding occurs when these clotting factors are reduced by more than 75%; bleeding may be mild, moderate, or severe, depending on the degree of activation of the clotting factors
- A person with hemophilia forms a platelet plug at a bleeding site, but clotting factor deficiency impairs the ability to form a stable fibrin clot
- Delayed bleeding is more common than immediate hemorrhage

Causes
- Defect in a specific gene on the X chromosome that codes for factor VIII synthesis (hemophilia A)
- More than 300 different base-pair substitutions involving factor IX gene on the X chromosome (hemophilia B)
- Autosomal recessive inheritance (hemophilia C)

Pathophysiologic changes
- Spontaneous bleeding in severe hemophilia (prolonged or excessive bleeding after circumcision is commonly the first sign) due to lack of clotting factor
- Excessive or continued bleeding or bruising; hematomas after minor trauma or surgery due to lack of clotting
- Large subcutaneous and deep intramuscular hematomas from mild trauma
- Prolonged bleeding in mild hemophilia after major trauma or surgery, but no spontaneous bleeding after minor trauma due to lack of clotting factor
- Pain, swelling, and tenderness due to bleeding into joints (especially weight-bearing joints)
- Internal bleeding (commonly manifested as abdominal, chest, or flank pain) due to lack of clotting factor
- Hematuria from bleeding into the kidney
- Hematemesis or tarry stools from bleeding into the GI tract

Complications
- Peripheral neuropathy, pain, paresthesia, and muscle atrophy
- Ischemia and gangrene
- Decreased tissue perfusion and hypovolemic shock
- Increased risk of exposure to human immunodeficiency virus (HIV) and other blood-borne diseases through contaminated blood products given during transfusion (currently much less common because of more rigorous screening protocols)

Diagnostic test findings
- Factor VIII assay shows 0% to 30% of normal and prolonged partial thromboplastin time (PTT) (hemophilia A); or deficient factor IX and normal factor VIII levels (hemophilia B)
- Degree of factor deficiency defines severity (hemophilia A and B)
  - Mild hemophilia: factor levels 5% to 25% of normal
  - Moderate hemophilia: factor levels 1% to 5% of normal
  - Severe hemophilia: factor levels less than 1% of normal
- Blood testing reveals normal platelet count and function, bleeding time, and prothrombin time (hemophilia A and B), and prolonged PTT in hemophilia A

Key pathophysiologic changes in hemophilia

- Spontaneous bleeding (severe hemophilia)
- Excessive or continued bleeding or bruising after minor trauma or surgery
- Pain, swelling, and tenderness in joints

Key diagnostic test results for hemophilia

- Factor VIII assay: 0% to 30% of normal and prolonged PTT (hemophilia A); deficient factor IX and normal factor VIII levels (hemophilia B)

Treatment

- Cryoprecipitate (hemophilia A) or lyophilized factor VIII or IX to increase clotting factor levels and permit normal hemostasis levels
- Factor IX concentrate during bleeding episodes (hemophilia B)
- Aminocaproic acid (Amicar) for oral bleeding (inhibits plasminogen activator substances)
- Prophylactic desmopressin (DDAVP) before dental procedures or minor surgery to release stored von Willebrand's factor (vWF) and factor VIII, thereby reducing the risk of bleeding
- Protective clothing (padded patches on knees and elbows of young children) and avoidance of contact sports (older children) to help prevent injury and bleeding episodes

Nursing considerations

- Teach the child to avoid contact sports and to use helmets and knee pads when participating in active pursuits such as biking
- Provide appropriate care during bleeding episodes
  - **Give clotting agents as ordered; repeat infusions as ordered until bleeding stops because the body uses up antihemophilic factor in 48 to 72 hours**
  - Apply cold compresses or ice bags, and keep the injured body part elevated
  - Restrict activity for 48 hours after bleeding is under control (to prevent recurrent bleeding)
  - Control pain with an analgesic, such as acetaminophen (Tylenol), propoxyphene (Darvocet), codeine, or meperidine (Demerol), as ordered
    - Aspirin and aspirin-containing medications are contraindicated (decrease platelet adherence and may increase bleeding)
    - Other nonsteroidal anti-inflammatory drugs, such as ibuprofen (Motrin, Advil) and ketoprofen (Orudis), should be used cautiously
  - Avoid I.M. injections because of possible hematoma formation at the injection site
- Provide appropriate care for the patient who has suffered bleeding into a joint
  - Immediately elevate the joint
  - To restore joint mobility, begin range-of-motion (ROM) exercises, if ordered, at least 48 hours after the bleeding is controlled
  - Instruct the patient to avoid weight bearing until bleeding stops and swelling subsides
- Monitor the patient closely after bleeding episodes and surgery
  - **Watch closely for signs of further bleeding, such as increased pain and swelling, fever, or symptoms of shock**
  - Closely monitor PTT
- Teach parents special precautions to prevent bleeding episodes
- Refer any new patient to a hemophilia treatment center for evaluation; the center will devise a treatment plan for the patient's primary physician and will serve as a resource for other medical and school personnel
- Provide additional medical and emotional support to patients who have been exposed to HIV through contaminated blood products
- Refer patients and carriers for genetic counseling

Key treatments for hemophilia

- Cryoprecipitate (hemophilia A) or lyophilized factor VIII or IX
- Factor IX concentrate during bleeding episodes (hemophilia B)

Key nursing considerations for hemophilia

- Teach parents precautions to prevent bleeding episodes.
- Monitor patient closely after bleeding episodes and surgery.

During bleeding episodes
- Give clotting agents as ordered.
- Control pain with an analgesic.
- Elevate affected joints.
- Avoid I.M. injections.

Key facts about Marfan syndrome

- Degenerative disease of the connective tissue resulting from elastin and collagen defects
- Caused by a mutation in an allele of a gene on chromosome 15
- Causes excessive bone growth, ocular disorders, and cardiac defects

Key pathophysiologic changes in Marfan syndrome

- Increased height
- Long extremities
- Arachnodactyly
- Funnel chest or pigeon breast

Key diagnostic test results for Marfan syndrome

- X-rays: Presence of skeletal abnormalities
- DNA analysis: Identification of defective gene

MARFAN SYNDROME

● Definition
- Rare, degenerative, generalized disease of the connective tissue resulting from elastin and collagen defects
- Autosomal-dominant mutation
- Causes ocular, skeletal, and cardiovascular anomalies
- Death from cardiovascular complications occurring from early infancy to adulthood
- Occurs in 1 out of every 20,000 individuals, affecting males and females equally

● Underlying pathophysiology
- Marfan syndrome is caused by a mutation in a single allele of a gene located on chromosome 15
- The gene codes for fibrillin, a glycoprotein component of connective tissue; these small fibers are abundant in large blood vessels and the suspensory ligaments of the ocular lenses
- The effect on connective tissue is varied and includes excessive bone growth, ocular disorders, and cardiac defects (see *Marfan syndrome: How it happens*)

● Causes
- In 85% of cases, there's a family history
- Advanced paternal age (possible cause in about 15% of patients with no family history of the disease)

● Pathophysiologic changes
- Increased height, long extremities, and arachnodactyly (long, spiderlike fingers) due to effects on long bones and joints and excessive bone growth
- Defects of the sternum (funnel chest or pigeon breast), chest asymmetry, scoliosis, and kyphosis due to excessive bone growth
- Hypermobile joints due to effects on connective tissue
- Nearsightedness due to elongated ocular globe
- Lens displacement due to altered connective tissue (ocular hallmark of syndrome)
- Valvular abnormalities (redundancy of leaflets, stretching of chordae tendineae, and dilation of valvulae annulus) due to altered connective tissue
- Mitral valve prolapse due to weakened connective tissue
- Aortic insufficiency due to dilation of aortic root and ascending aorta

● Complications
- Weak joints and ligaments, predisposing the patient to injury
- Cataracts and retinal tears and detachment
- Severe mitral valve regurgitation
- Spontaneous pneumothorax
- Inguinal and incisional hernias
- Dilation of the dural sac (portion of the dura mater beyond the caudal end of the spinal cord)
- Death due to cardiovascular disease and complications

● Diagnostic test findings
- Skin culture allows detection of fibrillin defects

GO WITH THE FLOW

Marfan syndrome: How it happens

Marfan syndrome is inherited as an autosomal-dominant trait that has been mapped to a specific gene located on chromosome 15. This gene codes for fibrillin (small, abundant fibers found in large blood vessels and the suspensory ligaments of ocular lenses). More than 20 mutations have been identified.

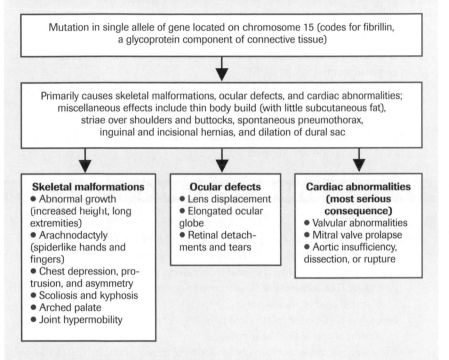

- X-rays confirm skeletal abnormalities
- Echocardiography shows dilation of the aortic root
- DNA analysis identifies the defective gene

● Treatment

- Surgical repair of aneurysms to prevent rupture
- Surgical correction of ocular deformities to improve vision
- Surgical replacement of the aortic and mitral valve for extreme dilation
- Surgical correction of scoliosis if the curvature is greater than 45 degrees
- Steroid and sex hormone therapy to induce early epiphyseal closure and limit adult height
- Beta-adrenergic blockers to delay or prevent aortic dilation
- Mechanical bracing and physical therapy for mild scoliosis if the curvature is greater than 20 degrees

Key treatments for Marfan syndrome

- Surgical repair of cardiac defects
- Steroids
- Sex hormone therapy

Key nursing considerations for Marfan syndrome

- Recommend that high school and college athletes who meet the criteria for Marfan syndrome undergo clinical and cardiac examination.
- Stress the need for frequent checkups.
- Emphasize the importance of taking prescribed drugs.

Key facts about NTDs

- Involve the spine or skull
- Result from failure of neural tube to close at approximately 28 days after conception
- Classified as open (with protrusion of spinal cord or meninges) or closed (without protrusion)
- Include spina bifida, anencephaly, and encephalocele

● **Nursing considerations**
- Recommend that high school and college athletes (particularly basketball players) who meet the criteria for Marfan syndrome undergo a careful clinical and cardiac examination before being allowed to play, to prevent sudden death due to dissecting aortic aneurysm or other cardiac complications
- Provide the patient with supportive care, as appropriate for his clinical status
- Educate the patient and his family about the course of the disease and its potential complications
- Stress the need for frequent checkups to detect and treat degenerative changes early
- Emphasize the importance of taking prescribed medications as ordered and the need to avoid contact sports and isometric exercise
- Provide hormonal therapy, as ordered, to induce early epiphyseal closure and prevent abnormal adult height
- Advise the parents to avoid unrealistic expectations for their child simply because he's tall and looks older than his years (to encourage normal adolescent development)
- Refer the patient and his family to the National Marfan Foundation for additional information and support

NEURAL TUBE DEFECTS

● **Definition**
- Birth defects involving the spine or skull, resulting from failure of the neural tube to close at approximately 28 days after conception
- Classified as open or closed neural tube defects (NTDs)
  - Open NTD: incomplete closure of one or more vertebrae with protrusion of spinal cord or meninges
  - Closed NTD: incomplete closure of one or more vertebrae without protrusion of spinal cord or meninges
- Most common forms are spina bifida (50% of cases), anencephaly (40%), and encephalocele (10%)

● **Underlying pathophysiology**
- Spina bifida occulta (least severe spinal cord defect) is characterized by incomplete closure of one or more vertebrae without protrusion of the spinal cord or meninges
- Spina bifida cystica (more severe form of spina bifida) is characterized by incomplete closure of one or more vertebrae with protrusion of the spinal contents into an external sac or cystic lesion (see *Understanding spina bifida*)
  - Classified as myelomeningocele (meningomyelocele) or meningocele
  - In myelomeningocele, the external sac contains meninges, cerebrospinal fluid (CSF), and a portion of the spinal cord or nerve roots distal to the conus medullaris; when the spinal nerve roots end at the sac, motor and sensory functions below the sac are terminated
  - In meningocele, the sac contains only meninges and CSF; this condition is less severe than myelomeningocele and may produce no neurologic symptoms

Understanding spina bifida

Spina bifida occulta is characterized by a depression or raised area and a tuft of hair over the defect. Spina bifida cystica can take two forms — myelomeningocele or meningocele. In myelomeningocele, an external sac contains meninges, cerebrospinal fluid (CSF), and a portion of the spinal cord or nerve roots. In meningocele, an external sac contains only meninges and CSF.

SPINA BIFIDA OCCULTA   **MYELOMENINGOCELE**   **MENINGOCELE**

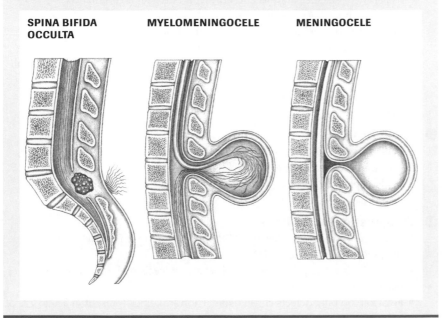

- In encephalocele, a saclike portion of the meninges and brain protrudes through a defective opening in the skull — usually in the occipital area, but sometimes in the parietal, nasopharyngeal, or frontal area
- In anencephaly, the most severe type of NTD, the closure defect occurs at the cranial end of the neuroaxis; consequently, part or the entire top of the skull is missing, severely damaging the brain; portions of the brain stem and spinal cord may be missing as well

⚫ **Causes**
- Lack of folic acid in the mother's diet around the time of conception
- Exposure to a teratogen
- Part of a multiple malformation syndrome (for example, chromosomal abnormalities such as trisomy 18 or 13 syndrome)
- In isolated birth defects, a combination of genetic and environmental factors

⚫ **Pathophysiologic changes**
- Possibly, a depression or dimple, tuft of hair, soft fatty deposits, port wine nevi, or a combination of these abnormalities on the skin over the spinal defect due to incomplete closure of one or more vertebrae without protrusion of spinal cord or meninges (spina bifida occulta)

TOP 2

Causes of NTDs

1. Lack of folic acid in mother's diet at conception
2. Exposure to a teratogen

- Foot weakness or bowel and bladder disturbances, especially likely during rapid growth phases due to incomplete closure of one or more vertebrae without protrusion of spinal cord or meninges (spina bifida occulta)
- Saclike structure that protrudes over the spine, trophic skin disturbances, and ulcerations (myelomeningocele, meningocele) due to incomplete closure of one or more vertebrae with protrusion of spinal contents (spina bifida cystica)
- Depending on the level of the defect, permanent neurologic dysfunction, such as flaccid or spastic paralysis and bowel and bladder incontinence (myelomeningocele) due to spinal nerve root ending at sac
- Paralysis, hydrocephalus, mental retardation, and encephalocele (findings may vary with degree of tissue involvement and location of defect) due to saclike portion of meninges and brain protruding through defective opening in skull
- Exposed neural tissue, skull malformation (anencephaly) — froglike appearance when viewed from front — due to closure defect at cranial end of neuroaxis

Complications

- Paralysis below the level of the defect
- Infection such as meningitis
- Hydrocephalus
- Death

Diagnostic test findings

- Amniocentesis detects elevated AFP levels in amniotic fluid, which indicates the presence of an open NTD
- Acetylcholinesterase analysis reveals elevated levels with open NTDs (not usually effective for closed NTDs)
- Fetal karyotyping detects chromosomal abnormalities (present in 5% to 7% of NTDs)
- Maternal serum AFP screening in combination with other serum markers, such as human chorionic gonadotropin (hCG), free beta-hCG, or unconjugated estriol (for patients with a lower risk of NTDs and women who will be under age 34½ at the time of delivery), allows estimation of fetal risk of an NTD and possible increased risk for perinatal complications, such as premature rupture of the membranes, abruptio placentae, or fetal death
- Ultrasonography may detect an open NTD in utero, suspected on the basis of family history or abnormal serum screening results (not conclusive for closed NTDs or ventral wall defects)
- Other diagnostic tests are conducted on the infant if the NTD isn't diagnosed in utero
  - Spinal X-ray to identify spina bifida occulta
  - Myelography to differentiate spina bifida occulta from other spinal abnormalities, especially spinal cord tumors
  - Transillumination of the protruding sac to distinguish between myelomeningocele (typically doesn't transilluminate) and meningocele (typically transilluminates)
  - Skull X-rays, cephalic measurements, and computed tomography (CT) scan to demonstrate associated hydrocephalus
  - X-rays show a basilar bony skull defect; CT scan and ultrasonography further define the defect in encephalocele

Treatment
- Surgical closure of the protruding sac and continual assessment of growth and development (meningocele)
- Surgical repair of the sac and supportive measures to promote independence and prevent further complications (myelomeningocele)
- Shunt insertion to relieve associated hydrocephalus
- Surgery during infancy to place protruding tissues back in the skull, excise the sac, and correct associated craniofacial abnormalities (encephalocele)

Nursing considerations
- Refer prospective parents to a genetic counselor when an NTD has been diagnosed prenatally
- Encourage all women of childbearing age to take a daily multivitamin containing folic acid until menopause or end of childbearing potential (recent research indicates that the risk of an open NTD may be reduced by 50% to 70% in pregnant women who take such vitamins daily)
- Develop short- and long-term goals to help the parents deal with the child's condition
  - Immediate goals: psychological support to help parents accept the diagnosis; appropriate measures for preoperative and postoperative care
  - Long-term goals: patient and family teaching; measures to prevent contractures, pressure ulcers, urinary tract infections (UTIs), and other complications
- Provide appropriate preoperative care
  - Prevent local infection by cleaning the defect gently with sterile normal saline solution or other solutions as ordered, inspect the defect often for signs of infection, and cover it with sterile dressings moistened with sterile normal saline solution
  - Prevent skin breakdown by placing sheepskin or a foam pad under the infant; keep skin clean and apply lotion to the infant's knees, elbows, chin, and other pressure areas
  - Give antibiotics as ordered
  - Handle the infant carefully without applying pressure to the defect (usually, a diaper or a shirt can't be worn until after surgical correction because they will irritate the sac, so the infant must be kept warm in an Isolette)
  - Hold and cuddle the infant; place him on his abdomen on your lap; teach the parents to do the same
  - Provide adequate time for parent-child bonding, if possible
  - Measure head circumference daily, and watch for signs of hydrocephalus and meningeal irritation (fever or nuchal rigidity); be sure to mark the spot to ensure accurate readings
  - Minimize contractures with passive ROM exercises and casting, as ordered; to prevent hip dislocation, moderately abduct hips with a pad between the knees or with sandbags and ankle rolls
  - Monitor intake and output, and watch for decreased skin turgor, dryness, or other signs of dehydration
  - Provide meticulous skin care to the genitals and buttocks to prevent infection
  - Ensure adequate nutrition

Key treatments for NTDs
- Surgical repair of protruding sac
- Shunt insertion

Key nursing considerations for NTDs
- Prevent local infection by covering the defect with moist, sterile dressings.
- Prevent skin breakdown by placing sheepskin or foam pad under infant.
- Avoid applying pressure to the defect.
- Measure head circumference daily.

After surgery
- Watch for hydrocephalus.
- Monitor infant's vital signs often, watching for signs of shock, infection, and increased ICP.
- Check for and report signs of drainage, wound rupture, and infection.
- Help parents cope with their infant's physical problems.
- Stress the need for stimulation appropriate for the child's age and abilities.

- Provide appropriate postoperative care
  - Watch for hydrocephalus, which commonly occurs after surgery (measure the infant's head circumference as ordered)
  - Monitor the infant's vital signs often, watching for signs of shock, infection, and increased intracranial pressure (ICP), such as projectile vomiting and bulging fontanels
    - Typical signs of increased ICP not shown before age 2 because suture lines aren't fully closed
    - In infants, the most telling sign is bulging fontanels (monitor frequently)
  - Change the dressing regularly as ordered, and check for and report signs of drainage, wound rupture, and infection
  - Place the infant in the prone position to protect and assess the site
  - Watch for signs that the child is outgrowing the cast (when applied to treat deformities); regularly check distal pulses to ensure adequate circulation
- Help parents cope with their infant's physical problems and successfully meet long-term treatment goals
  - Teach the parents to recognize early signs of complications, such as hydrocephalus, decubitus ulcers, and UTIs
  - Provide psychological support and encourage a positive attitude
  - Encourage the parents to begin training their child in a bladder routine by age 3
  - Emphasize the need for increased fluid intake to prevent UTIs; teach intermittent catheterization and conduit hygiene as ordered
  - Stress the need for increased fluid intake, a high-bulk diet, exercise, and a stool softener, as ordered, to prevent constipation and bowel obstruction; if possible, teach parents to help empty their child's bowel by telling him to bear down and giving a glycerin suppository as needed
  - Urge early recognition of developmental lags (a possible result of hydrocephalus); if present, stress the importance of follow-up IQ assessment to help plan realistic educational goals (the child may need to attend a school with special facilities)
  - Stress the need for stimulation to ensure maximum mental development; help parents plan activities appropriate to their child's age and abilities
  - Refer parents for genetic counseling and further support (Spina Bifida Association of America)

SICKLE CELL ANEMIA

- **Definition**
  - Congenital hemolytic anemia that results from structurally defective hemoglobin molecules
  - Results in death by early twenties in half of patients (few live to middle age)
  - Occurs primarily in persons of African and Mediterranean descent
- **Underlying pathophysiology**
  - Sickle cell anemia results from substitution of the amino acid valine for glutamic acid in the hemoglobin S gene encoding the beta chain of hemoglobin

---

Key facts about sickle cell anemia

- Congenital hemolytic anemia
- Results when the amino acid valine substitutes for glutamic acid in the hemoglobin S gene
- Causes rigid, rough, and elongated sickle-shaped cells with reduced oxygen-carrying capacity
- Produces hemolysis and accumulation of altered cells in capillaries
- Leads to obstruction, anoxia, and further sickling and obstruction

- Abnormal hemoglobin S, found in the red blood cells (RBCs) of patients, becomes insoluble during hypoxia; as a result, these cells become rigid, rough, and elongated, forming a characteristic crescent or sickle shape that reduces their oxygen-carrying capacity (see *Characteristics of sickled cells*)
- Sickling produces hemolysis and accumulation of altered cells in the capillaries and smaller blood vessels, making the blood more viscous; this impairs normal circulation, causing pain, tissue infarction, and swelling
- The blockages plug the vascular space, causing anoxic changes that lead to further sickling and obstruction
- Each patient has a different hypoxic threshold and different factors that trigger a sickle cell crisis; usually, a crisis is precipitated by illness, exposure to cold, stress, acidotic states, or a pathophysiologic process that pulls water out of sickled cells (see *Sickle cell crisis*, page 440)

● Causes
- Autosomal-recessive inheritance (homozygous inheritance of hemoglobin S–producing gene)

● Pathophysiologic changes
- Tachycardia, cardiomegaly, chronic fatigue, unexplained dyspnea, hepatomegaly, joint swelling, aching bones, and chest pain due to repeated cycles of deoxygenation from sickling

---

Key pathophysiologic changes in sickle cell anemia

- Severe pain in abdomen, thorax, muscles, or bones
- Tachycardia
- Pale lips, tongue, palms, or nail beds
- Chest pain

Characteristics of sickled cells

Normal red blood cells (RBCs) and sickled cells vary in shape, life span, oxygen-carrying capacity, and the rate at which they're destroyed. These illustrations show normal and sickled cells, and the major differences between them are listed.

NORMAL RBCS
- 120-day life span
- Hemoglobin (Hb) has normal oxygen-carrying capacity
- 12 to 14 g/ml of Hb
- RBCs destroyed at normal rate

SICKLED CELLS
- 30- to 40-day life span
- Hb has decreased oxygen-carrying capacity
- 6 to 9 g/ml of Hb
- RBCs destroyed at accelerated rate

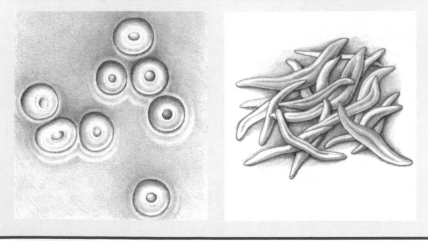

Triggers of sickle cell crisis

1. Infection
2. Overexertion
3. Exposure to cold

Sickle cell crisis

Infection, exposure to cold, high altitude, overexertion, or other situations that cause cellular oxygen deprivation may trigger a sickle cell crisis. The deoxygenated, sickle-shaped red blood cells stick to the capillary wall and to one another, blocking blood flow and causing cellular hypoxia. The crisis worsens as tissue hypoxia and acidic waste products cause more sickling and cell damage. With each new crisis, organs and tissues are slowly destroyed, especially the spleen and kidneys.

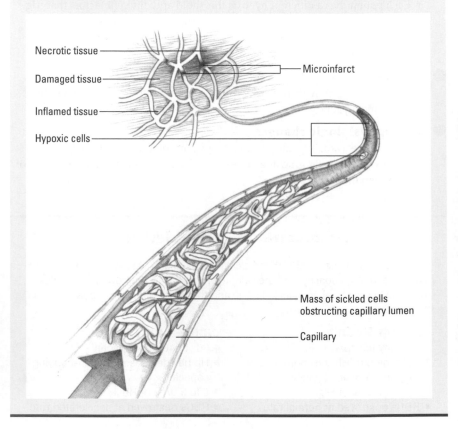

Types of sickle cell crisis

- Aplastic (megaloblastic) crisis
- Acute sequestration crisis
- Hemolytic crisis

- Severe pain in the abdomen, thorax, muscles, or bones (characterizes painful crisis)
- Pale lips, tongue, palms, or nail beds; lethargy; listlessness; sleepiness; irritability; severe pain; and fever due to blood vessel obstruction by rigid, tangled, sickled cells (leading to tissue anoxia and possible necrosis)
- Jaundice and dark urine due to increased bilirubin production
- *Streptococcus pneumoniae* sepsis due to autosplenectomy (splenic damage and scarring in patients with long-term disease)
- Aplastic (megaloblastic) crisis due to bone marrow depression (associated with infection, usually viral, and characterized by pallor, lethargy, sleepiness, dyspnea, possible coma, markedly decreased bone marrow activity, and RBC hemolysis)

- Acute sequestration crisis (rare; affects infants ages 8 months to 2 years; may cause lethargy, pallor, and hypovolemic shock) due to the sudden massive entrapment of cells in the spleen and liver
- Hemolytic crisis (rare); usually affects patients who also have glucose-6-phosphate dehydrogenase deficiency
  - Degenerative changes causing liver congestion and enlargement; chronic jaundice worsens

● **Complications**
  - Retinopathy
  - Nephropathy
  - Cerebrovascular occlusion
  - Hypovolemic shock
  - Necrosis
  - Infection and gangrene
  - Death

● **Diagnostic test findings**
  - Hemoglobin electrophoresis shows hemoglobin S abnormality
  - Electrophoresis of umbilical cord blood provides screening for all neonates at risk
  - Stained blood smear analysis shows sickle cells
  - Additional blood studies reveal a low RBC count and decreased RBC survival, elevated white blood cell and platelet counts, decreased erythrocyte sedimentation rate, increased serum iron level, and reticulocytosis (hemoglobin level may be low or normal)
  - Lateral chest X-ray shows "Lincoln log" deformity (H-shaped appearance of the vertebrae from osteopenia and vascular thrombosis of the spinal artery) in the vertebrae of many adults and some adolescents

● **Treatment**
  - Packed RBC transfusion to correct hypovolemia (if hemoglobin level decreases)
  - Sedatives and analgesics, such as meperidine or morphine sulfate (MSIR, Roxanol), for pain
  - Oxygen administration to correct hypoxia
  - Large amounts of oral or I.V. fluids to correct hypovolemia and prevent dehydration and vessel occlusion
  - Prophylactic penicillin before age 4 months to prevent infection
  - Hydroxyurea administration (interferes with hydrophobic bonds of the hemoglobin S molecules) to reduce painful episodes by increasing fetal hemoglobin production
  - Iron and folic acid supplements to prevent anemia
  - Splenectomy for spleen enlargement caused by hemolysis and phagocytosis

● **Nursing considerations**
  - Provide appropriate care during a painful crisis
    - Apply warm compresses to painful areas, and cover the patient with a blanket (never use cold compresses because they aggravate the condition)
    - Administer an analgesic–antipyretic, such as aspirin or acetaminophen (additional pain relief may be required during an acute crisis)
    - Encourage bed rest, and place the patient in a sitting position

Key diagnostic test results for sickle cell anemia
- Hemoglobin electrophoresis: Hemoglobin S abnormality
- Electrophoresis of umbilical cord blood: Screens neonates at risk

Key treatments for sickle cell anemia
- Packed RBC transfusion
- Analgesics
- Oxygen
- Oral or I.V. fluids

Key nursing considerations for sickle cell anemia
- Advise patient to avoid strenuous exercise, cold temperatures, and high altitudes.
- Stress the need to increase fluid intake.
- Emphasize the need for prompt treatment of infection.
- Teach about special needs related to pregnancy and family planning.

During crises
- Apply warm compresses to painful areas.
- Administer an analgesic–antipyretic.
- Encourage bed rest.

– Give antibiotics as ordered (when indicated by cultures)
• During remissions, focus care on patient (and parent) teaching
  – Advise the patient to avoid tight clothing that restricts circulation
  – Warn against strenuous exercise, vasoconstricting medications, cold temperatures (including drinking large amounts of ice water and swimming), flying in unpressurized aircraft, high altitudes, and other circumstances that provoke hypoxia
  – Keep arms and legs covered to prevent chills
  – Stress the importance of normal childhood immunizations, meticulous wound care, good oral hygiene, regular dental checkups, and a balanced diet as safeguards against infection
  – Emphasize the need for prompt treatment of infection, stressing the importance of reporting a sore throat or cold symptoms
  – Explain the need to increase fluid intake to prevent dehydration due to impaired ability to concentrate urine properly; teach parents to encourage their child to drink more fluids, especially in the summer, by offering such beverages as milkshakes, ice pops, and eggnog
• Teach patients about special needs related to pregnancy and family planning
  – Caution female patients about possible increased obstetrical risks (use of hormonal contraceptives may be risky; refer women of childbearing age to an obstetrician-gynecologist for birth-control counseling)
  – Encourage the patient who becomes pregnant to maintain a balanced diet and to take a folic acid supplement
• Provide appropriate preoperative and postoperative care for patients scheduled for surgery under general anesthesia
  – Make sure that the surgeon and anesthesiologist are aware of the patient's sickle cell anemia diagnosis
  – Provide optimal ventilation to prevent a hypoxic crisis
  – Prepare a preoperative transfusion of packed RBCs, as needed
• Caution parents against being overprotective (to encourage normal mental and social development); although the child must avoid strenuous exercise, he can enjoy most everyday activities
• Refer parents for genetic counseling to answer their questions about the risk to future offspring, and recommend screening other family members to determine if they're heterozygote carriers
• Refer parents for psychological counseling to cope with feelings of guilt, and suggest that they join an appropriate community support group
• Advise adolescent or adult males that they may experience sudden, painful episodes of priapism (such episodes are common and, if prolonged, can have serious reproductive consequences); tell the patient to contact his physician if this occurs

Key facts about Tay-Sachs disease

• Results from an absence or deficiency of the enzyme hexosaminidase A
• Causes lipid pigments to accumulate and destroy CNS cells

TAY-SACHS DISEASE

Definition

• The most common lipid-storage disease that results from congenital enzyme deficiency (hexosaminidase A)
• Also known as GM_2 *gangliosidosis*
• Autosomal-recessive disorder

- Leads to progressive mental and motor deterioration and always is fatal, usually before age 5
- Occurs mostly in those of Eastern European, Jewish descent

Underlying pathophysiology

- The enzyme hexosaminidase A is absent or deficient in patients with Tay-Sachs disease
- This enzyme is necessary to metabolize gangliosides (water-soluble glycolipids found primarily in the central nervous system ([CNS])
- Without hexosaminidase A, lipid pigments accumulate and progressively destroy and demyelinate CNS cells

Causes

- Congenital deficiency of hexosaminidase A

Pathophysiologic changes

- Exaggerated Moro reflex (also called *startle reflex*) at birth, and apathy (response only to loud sounds) by age 3 to 6 months due to demyelination of CNS cells
- Inability to sit up, lift the head, or grasp objects; difficulty turning over; lethargy during infancy (unusually quiet and difficult to arouse); progressive vision loss due to CNS involvement
- Deafness, blindness, seizure activity, paralysis, spasticity, and continued neurologic deterioration by age 18 months due to CNS involvement
- Recurrent bronchopneumonia due to diminished protective reflexes

Complications

- Blindness
- Generalized paralysis
- Recurrent bronchopneumonia
- Dementia
- Seizures
- Death, usually before age 5

Diagnostic test findings

- Serum analysis shows deficient hexosaminidase A
- Amniocentesis or chorionic villus sampling can detect hexosaminidase A deficiency in the fetus

Treatment

- Tube feedings to provide nutritional supplements
- Suctioning and postural drainage to maintain a patent airway
- Skin care to prevent pressure ulcers in a bedridden child
- Laxatives to relieve neurogenic constipation

Nursing considerations

- Monitor the patient's gag reflex to prevent aspiration
- Offer carrier testing to all couples from high-risk ethnic groups
- Refer the parents for genetic counseling; stress the importance of amniocentesis in future pregnancies
- Refer siblings for carrier screening; refer adult sibling carriers for genetic counseling, and reassure them that there's no danger of transmitting the disease to offspring if they don't have a child with another carrier

- Refer the couple to an appropriate preimplantation geneticist if they express an interest in assisted reproductive technology (some in vitro fertilization centers have recently started offering these programs)
- Provide emotional support; if indicated, refer the parents for psychological counseling (many parents feel guilt because of the child's illness and experience stress due to emotional and financial burdens)
- Teach the parents caring for their child at home to perform suctioning, postural drainage, and tube feeding; teach them how to provide good skin care to prevent pressure ulcers
- Refer the parents to the National Tay-Sachs and Allied Diseases Association for additional support and information

VON WILLEBRAND DISEASE

Definition
- Hereditary bleeding disorder characterized by prolonged bleeding time, moderate deficiency of clotting factor VIII (antihemophilic factor), and impaired platelet function from a deficit of von Willebrand factor (vWF)
- Also known as *angiohemophilia, pseudohemophilia,* and *vascular hemophilia*

Underlying pathophysiology
- von Willebrand disease causes mild to moderate deficiency of factor VIII and defective platelet coagulation time
- It results from a deficiency of vWF, which is the carrier protein for the factor VIII molecule and is necessary for the production of factor VIII and proper platelet adhesion and coagulation
- Defective platelet function is characterized by decreased agglutination and adhesion at the bleeding site, reduced platelet retention (when filtered through a column of packed glass beads), and diminished ristocetin-induced platelet aggregation

Causes
- Inherited as autosomal-dominant trait
- Acquired form identified in patients with cancer and immune disorders

Pathophysiologic changes
- Bruising, epistaxis, and bleeding from the gums due to deficiency of vWF and factor VIII and prolonged bleeding time
- Hemorrhage after laceration or surgery, menorrhagia, and GI bleeding (severe forms) due to a factor VIII deficiency

Complications
- Hemorrhage

Diagnostic test findings
- Blood testing reveals normal platelet count and clot retraction; prolonged bleeding time (more than 6 minutes) and slightly prolonged PTT (more than 45 seconds); and absent or reduced factor VIII–related antigen levels and low factor VIII activity
- Ritocetin coagulation factor assay shows defective in vitro platelet aggregation (vWF deficiency)

Key facts about von Willebrand disease
- Hereditary bleeding disorder
- Causes mild to moderate deficiency of factor VIII and defective platelet coagulation time
- Results from a deficiency of vWF

Key pathophysiologic changes in von Willebrand disease
- Bruising
- Epistaxis
- Hemorrhage after laceration or surgery

Key diagnostic test results for von Willebrand disease
- Blood testing: Absent or reduced factor VIII–related antigen levels, low factor VIII activity
- Ritocetin coagulation factor assay: Shows vWF deficiency

Key treatments for von Willebrand disease
- I.V. infusion of cryoprecipitate or fresh frozen plasma
- Desmopressin
- Avoidance of aspirin

Treatment
- Decreasing bleeding time by local measures and by replacing factor VIII
- Avoidance of aspirin
- Altered activities and rest periods if the patient is fatigued after a bleeding episode
- I.V. infusion of cryoprecipitate or fresh frozen plasma (in sufficient quantities to raise factor VIII levels to 50% of normal) during bleeding episodes and before surgery to shorten bleeding time
- Desmopressin given parenterally or intranasally to raise serum levels of vWF

Nursing considerations
- **Monitor the patient's bleeding time for 24 to 48 hours after surgery, and watch for signs of new bleeding**
- Elevate the bleeding site and apply cold compresses and gentle pressure during a bleeding episode
- Advise the patient to consult the physician for even minor trauma and before all surgery to determine if replacement of blood components is necessary
- Teach the patient and his parents ways to prevent bleeding, unnecessary trauma, and complications
    - Caution the patient not to use aspirin and other drugs that impair platelet function
    - Advise the patient with severe disease to avoid contact sports
- Refer parents of affected children for genetic counseling

NCLEX CHECKS

It's never too soon to begin your licensure examination preparation. Now that you've reviewed this chapter, carefully read each of the following questions and choose the best answer. Then compare your responses to the correct answers.

1. The nurse is speaking with parents who are concerned about their child's risk of producing a child with a birth defect. Which defect is an example of a multifactorial disorder?
- ☐ **1.** Cleft lip
- ☐ **2.** Hemophilia
- ☐ **3.** Marfan syndrome
- ☐ **4.** Sickle cell anemia

2. When caring for an infant with cleft palate, which problem should be the nurse's highest priority?
- ☐ **1.** Scarring
- ☐ **2.** Speech difficulties
- ☐ **3.** Malnutrition
- ☐ **4.** Parental bonding

3. Esophageal varices can develop in a client with cystic fibrosis as a result of:
- ☐ **1.** medications.
- ☐ **2.** portal hypertension.
- ☐ **3.** malabsorption.
- ☐ **4.** fat-soluble vitamin deficiencies.

Key nursing considerations for von Willebrand disease
- Monitor bleeding time for 24 to 48 hours after surgery, and watch for signs of new bleeding.
- Teach ways to prevent bleeding.

During a bleeding episode
- Elevate the bleeding site.
- Apply cold compresses and gentle pressure.

TOP 4

Items to study for your next test on genetic disorders

1. Pathophysiology of common genetic disorders, such as sickle cell anemia, cleft lip and palate, cystic fibrosis, and Down syndrome

2. Common diagnostic tests for bleeding disorders such as hemophilia

3. Teaching topics for cystic fibrosis, including its complications and the need for a high-calorie, high-protein diet

4. Nursing considerations for bleeding episodes related to genetic disorders

4. A client with Down syndrome has difficulty speaking clearly and has various dental problems. What's the likely source of these difficulties?

☐ **1.** Repeated lung infections
☐ **2.** Mental retardation
☐ **3.** Vocal cord abnormalities
☐ **4.** A thrusting tongue

5. A client with hemophilia A has frequent bleeding into his joints. The nurse knows that hemophilia A is a deficiency of which factor?

☐ **1.** III
☐ **2.** VIII
☐ **3.** IX
☐ **4.** XI

6. The nurse is speaking with a pregnant client who has expressed concern about preventing birth defects in her child. The nurse advises her about the need for which essential nutrient to help reduce the risk of an NTD?

☐ **1.** Vitamin A
☐ **2.** Vitamin E
☐ **3.** Folic acid
☐ **4.** Calcium

7. A pregnant woman and her husband discuss with the nurse their baby's risk of inheriting Marfan syndrome. The husband reveals that he has the disorder. After assessing the couple's understanding of genetic disorders and transmission principles, the nurse shows them this chart, depicting autosomal inheritance patterns. Based on the chart, what's the child's chance of being born without the disorder?

	A	a
a	Aa	aa
a	Aa	aa

Key:
a = recessive, normal
A = dominant, abnormal

☐ **1.** 0%
☐ **2.** 25%
☐ **3.** 50%
☐ **4.** 75%

8. A child with sickle cell anemia is being discharged after treatment for a crisis. Which instruction to the parents is most important for avoiding future crises?

☐ **1.** "Use cold packs to relieve joint pain."
☐ **2.** "Report a sore throat promptly."
☐ **3.** "Restrict dietary intake of folic acid."
☐ **4.** "Encourage bed rest instead of active games."

9. After surgery, how long should the nurse monitor the bleeding time of a client with von Willebrand disease?

- ☐ **1.** 2 to 4 hours
- ☐ **2.** 8 to 12 hours
- ☐ **3.** 12 to 24 hours
- ☐ **4.** 24 to 48 hours

10. Before participating in sports, high school athletes who meet the criteria for Marfan syndrome should undergo a clinical examination with particular attention to which body system?

- ☐ **1.** Musculoskeletal
- ☐ **2.** Cardiac
- ☐ **3.** Respiratory
- ☐ **4.** Sensory

ANSWERS AND RATIONALES

1. CORRECT ANSWER: 1

Most multifactorial disorders result from the effects of several different genes and an environmental component. Although the exact cause of cleft lip and cleft palate is unknown, they're thought to be caused by combined genetic and environmental factors. The other disorders are not multifactorial.

2. CORRECT ANSWER: 3

Because of an incomplete fusion of the palate, an infant can have feeding difficulties that may lead to malnutrition. Until the palate is surgically corrected, specially designed nipples and bottles should be used to help ensure adequate nutrition. Scarring after surgery, speech difficulties, and parental bonding are all legitimate concerns; however, they aren't the highest priority.

3. CORRECT ANSWER: 2

Cystic fibrosis is a dysfunction of the exocrine glands that affects multiple organ systems. The increased viscosity of mucus secretions can obstruct the biliary system, leading to cirrhosis, portal hypertension and, eventually, esophageal varices. The remaining options are unrelated to this situation.

4. CORRECT ANSWER: 4

Nearly all cases of Down syndrome result from trisomy 21 and are characterized by distinctive head and facial features, including a thrusting or protruding tongue. Surgery can repair this defect and improve speech and dental abnormalities. Repeated lung infections can occur in clients with associated cardiac defects, but they don't affect speech. The mental ability of the patient doesn't generally affect speech, although the characteristic retardation may affect learning. Vocal cord abnormalities aren't characteristic of this disorder.

5. CORRECT ANSWER: 2

Hemophilia A, or classic hemophilia, is a deficiency of factor VIII, a component of the intrinsic clotting pathway that accelerates the activation of factor X. Hemophilia B is a deficiency of factor IX, whereas hemophilia C affects factor XI. There's no factor III deficiency disorder.

6.   CORRECT ANSWER: 3

Recent research sponsored by the March of Dimes indicates that the risk of an open NTD may be reduced 50% to 70% in pregnant women who take a daily multivitamin containing folic acid. Calcium and vitamins A and E, although important during pregnancy, are unrelated to NTDs.

7.   CORRECT ANSWER: 3

Marfan syndrome is an autosomal-dominant trait that results in elastin and collagen defects. The chart shows that any child carrying the dominant gene for Marfan syndrome from either parent would have the disease, but any child with the recessive, normal gene from each parent would be unaffected. Therefore, the child has a 50% chance of being born without the disorder.

8.   CORRECT ANSWER: 2

Because infections can precipitate a sickle cell crisis, parents must take special care to promptly report any sign of a cold or respiratory infection, including a sore throat. Rest, cold packs to affected joints, and restricted folic acid are all indicated during a sickle cell crisis.

9.   CORRECT ANSWER: 4

A client with von Willebrand's disease has a bleeding disorder characterized by prolonged bleeding time and impaired platelet function. Therefore, the nurse should monitor the patient's bleeding time for 24 to 48 hours after surgery.

10.   CORRECT ANSWER: 2

A high school athlete meeting the criteria for Marfan syndrome should undergo a careful clinical and cardiac examination before being allowed to play because of the risk of sudden death due to a dissecting aortic aneurysm or other cardiac complications. Clients with Marfan syndrome may also have ocular defects, musculoskeletal injuries (which aren't life-threatening), and spontaneous pneumothorax, which isn't as immediately life-threatening as cardiac side effects.

13

Fluid and electrolyte disorders

LEARNING OBJECTIVES

After studying this chapter, you should be able to:

- Identify conditions that alter acid-base and electrolyte balance.
- Describe the relationship between presenting signs and symptoms and the pathophysiologic changes for any fluid or electrolyte imbalance.
- List three probable causes for a patient with an acid-base imbalance.
- Identify interventions for a patient with a fluid or electrolyte imbalance.
- Write three teaching goals for a patient with a fluid or electrolyte imbalance.
- Identify medications that may improve acid-base imbalance.

CHAPTER OVERVIEW

The body is primarily composed of water in which various ions of essential elements are dissolved. These ions include the electrolytes most needed for survival: sodium (Na^+), potassium (K^+), chloride (Cl^-), bicarbonate (HCO_3^-), calcium (Ca^{2+}), hydrogen (H^+), magnesium (Mg^+), phosphate (PO_4^{3+}), and sulfate (SO_4^{2+}). Concentrations of these elements must remain in a very narrow range for the body to function properly. The kidneys, skin, and lungs all play a part in maintaining our chemical balance of water and electrolytes.

Caring for a patient with a fluid or electrolyte disorder or an acid-base imbalance requires an understanding of the pathophysiologic changes that occur, the signs and symptoms they produce, and the appropriate ways to intervene. The first section of this chapter provides an overview of key pathophysiologic concepts related to fluid and electrolyte imbalances. Common fluid and electrolyte disorders are defined, and definitions, underlying pathophysiology, causes, pathophysiologic changes, complications, diagnostic test findings, treatments, and nursing considerations are outlined.

PATHOPHYSIOLOGIC CONCEPTS

- **Acidosis**
  - Systemic increase in hydrogen ion concentration may occur in various circumstances
    - Lungs fail to eliminate carbon dioxide (CO_2), and volatile (carbonic) or nonvolatile (lactic) acid products of metabolism accumulate
    - Persistent diarrhea causes loss of alkaline bicarbonate anions, so extra hydrogen is left unbound in the extracellular fluid (ECF)
    - Kidneys fail to reabsorb bicarbonate or to secrete hydrogen ions in the urine

- **Alkalosis**
  - Systemic decrease in hydrogen ion concentration
  - Decreased hydrogen ion concentration may result from
    - Excessive loss of carbon dioxide during hyperventilation
    - Loss of nonvolatile acids during vomiting
    - Excessive ingestion of a base (alkali)

- **Edema**
  - Increased volume of fluid in interstitial spaces; results from abnormal expansion of interstitial fluid or accumulation of fluid in third spaces (the spaces around the organs)
  - May be localized; caused by obstruction of veins or lymphatic system or by increased vascular permeability
  - May be systemic (generalized); due to heart failure or renal disease
  - Anasarca: massive systemic edema

- **Electrolyte imbalances**
  - Too much or too little of any electrolyte will affect most body systems
  - Insufficient or excess potassium, or insufficient calcium or magnesium, can increase excitability of cardiac muscle, causing arrhythmias
  - Insufficient or excessive sodium or excess potassium can cause oliguria
  - GI tract is particularly susceptible to electrolyte imbalance
    - Excess potassium: abdominal cramps, nausea, and diarrhea
    - Insufficient potassium: paralytic ileus
    - Excess magnesium: nausea, vomiting, and diarrhea
    - Excess calcium: nausea, vomiting, and constipation

- **Tonicity**
  - Relative concentration of electrolytes (osmotic pressure) on both sides of a semipermeable membrane (cell wall or capillary wall)
  - Isotonic alterations: Intracellular and extracellular fluids have equal osmotic pressure, but a dramatic change in total-body fluid volume occurs
    - In physiology, "normal" as in "normal saline solution" refers to the isotonic nature of a 0.9% salt solution with the salt content of blood

Key facts about acidosis

- Involves systemic increase in hydrogen ion concentration
- May result from lungs failing to eliminate carbon dioxide, persistent diarrhea, or kidneys failing to reabsorb bicarbonate or to secrete hydrogen ions in the urine

Key facts about alkalosis

- Involves decreased hydrogen ion concentration
- May result from hyperventilation, loss of nonvolatile acids during vomiting, or excessive ingestion of a base (alkali)

Key facts about edema

- Increased fluid volume in interstitial spaces
- Results from abnormal expansion of interstitial fluid or fluid accumulation in third spaces
- Classified as localized, generalized, or anasarca

Key facts about electrolyte imbalances

- Involve too much or too little of any electrolyte
- Affect most body systems, particularly the GI tract

- Hypertonic alterations: ECF is more concentrated than intracellular fluid (ICF); causes water to flow out of cell through the semipermeable cell membrane (cell shrinkage)
- Hypotonic alterations: ECF is less concentrated than ICF; osmotic pressure forces some ECF into cells, causing cells to swell

HYPOVOLEMIA

- ● **Definition**
  - Disorder involving ECF volume
  - Characterized by isotonic loss of body fluids and relatively equal losses of sodium and water
- ● **Underlying pathophysiology**
  - Fluid volume deficit decreases capillary hydrostatic pressure and fluid transport
  - Cells are deprived of normal nutrients that serve as substrates for energy production, metabolism, and other cellular functions
  - Decreased renal blood flow triggers the renin-angiotensin system to increase sodium and water resorption
  - Cardiovascular system compensates by increasing heart rate, cardiac contractility, venous constriction, and systemic vascular resistance, thus increasing cardiac output and mean arterial pressure
  - Hypovolemia also triggers the thirst response, releasing more antidiuretic hormone (ADH) and producing more aldosterone
  - When metabolic compensation fails, hypovolemic shock follows a predictable sequence
    - Decreased intravascular fluid volume
    - Diminished venous return (reduces preload and decreases stroke volume, reduces capillary refill time)
    - Reduced cardiac output
    - Decreased mean arterial pressure
    - Impaired tissue perfusion
    - Decreased oxygen (O_2) and nutrient delivery to cells
    - Multisystem organ failure
- ● **Causes**
  - Causes of fluid loss
    - Hemorrhage
    - Excessive perspiration
    - Renal failure with polyuria
    - Abdominal surgery
    - Vomiting or diarrhea
    - Nasogastric (NG) drainage
    - Diabetes mellitus with polyuria or diabetes insipidus
    - Fistulas
    - Excessive use of laxatives
    - Excessive diuretic therapy
    - Fever
  - Possible causes of reduced fluid intake
    - Dysphagia

Key facts about tonicity

- Refers to osmotic pressure on both sides of a semipermeable membrane

Isotonic alterations
- Involve equal osmotic pressure of ECF and ICF but a change in total-body fluid volume

Hypertonic alterations
- Result when ECF is more concentrated than ICF
- Cause water to flow out of cell

Hypotonic alterations
- Occur when ECF is less concentrated than ICF
- Force some ECF into cells, causing cells to swell

Key facts about hypovolemia

- Results when a fluid volume deficit decreases capillary hydrostatic pressure
- Deprives cells of nutrients
- Leads to decreased renal blood flow, which triggers renin-angiotensin system to increase sodium and water resorption
- Triggers thirst response, releasing ADH and aldosterone
- Can lead to hypovolemic shock

Common causes of hypovolemia

- Hemorrhage
- Excessive perspiration
- Renal failure with polyuria
- Abdominal surgery
- Vomiting or diarrhea
- NG drainage

– Coma
– Environmental conditions preventing fluid intake
– Psychiatric illness
• Factors that may be related to fluid shift
– Burns (during the initial phase)
– Acute intestinal obstruction
– Acute peritonitis
– Pancreatitis
– Crushing injury
– Pleural effusion
– Hip fracture (1.5 to 2 L of blood may accumulate in tissues around the fracture)

Pathophysiologic changes

• Orthostatic hypotension due to increased systemic vascular resistance and decreased cardiac output
• Tachycardia induced by the sympathetic nervous system counteracts decreased cardiac output and mean arterial pressure
• Thirst to prompt ingestion of fluid (increased ECF osmolality stimulates the thirst center in the hypothalamus)
• Flattened jugular veins due to decreased circulating blood volume
• Sunken eyes due to decreased volume of total-body fluid and consequent dehydration of connective tissue and aqueous humor
• Dry mucous membranes due to decreased body fluid volume (glands that produce fluids to moisten and protect the vascular mucous membranes fail, causing rapid drying)
• Diminished skin turgor due to decreased fluid in the dermal layer (making skin less pliant)
• Rapid weight loss due to acute loss of body fluid
• Decreased urine output due to decreased renal perfusion from renal vasoconstriction
• Prolonged capillary refill time due to increased systemic vascular resistance (see *Estimating fluid loss*)

Complications

• Shock
• Acute renal failure
• Death

Diagnostic test findings

• Blood testing shows increased blood urea nitrogen (BUN), an early sign, elevated serum creatinine (late sign), and rising blood glucose level
• Blood testing shows increased serum protein, hemoglobin level, and hematocrit (unless caused by hemorrhage, when loss of blood elements causes subnormal values)
• Serum osmolality is elevated (or low in hyponatremia)
• Serum electrolyte tests and arterial blood gas (ABG) analysis may reflect associated clinical problems due to underlying cause of hypovolemia or treatment regimen
• If the patient has no underlying renal disorder, typical urine testing shows urine specific gravity greater than 1.030, urine sodium level less than 50 mEq/L, and increased urine osmolality

---

Key pathophysiologic changes in hypovolemia

• Orthostatic hypotension
• Tachycardia
• Thirst
• Dry mucous membranes

Key diagnostic test results for hypovolemia

• Blood testing: Increased BUN (early sign), elevated serum creatinine (late sign), elevated blood glucose level
• Serum osmolality: Elevated (or low in hyponatremia)
• Serum electrolyte tests and ABG analysis: Reveal associated clinical problems

Estimating fluid loss

These assessment parameters indicate the severity of fluid loss.

MINIMAL FLUID LOSS
Intravascular volume loss of 10% to 15% is regarded as minimal. Signs and symptoms include:
- slight tachycardia
- normal supine blood pressure
- positive postural vital signs, including a decrease in systolic blood pressure of more than 10 mm Hg or an increase in pulse rate of more than 20 beats/minute
- increased capillary refill time (more than 3 seconds)
- urine output greater than 30 ml/hour
- cool, pale skin on arms and legs
- anxiety.

MODERATE FLUID LOSS
Intravascular volume loss of approximately 25% is regarded as moderate.

Signs and symptoms include:
- rapid, thready pulse
- supine hypotension
- cool truncal skin
- urine output of 10 to 30 ml/hour
- severe thirst
- restlessness, confusion, or irritability.

SEVERE FLUID LOSS
Intravascular volume loss of 40% or more is regarded as severe. Signs and symptoms include:
- marked tachycardia
- marked hypotension
- weak or absent peripheral pulses
- cold, mottled, or cyanotic skin
- urine output less than 10 ml/hour
- loss of consciousness.

● Treatment
- Oral fluids for the patient with mild hypovolemia who's alert enough to swallow and able to tolerate fluids
- Parenteral fluids to supplement or replace oral therapy in the patient with moderate to severe hypovolemia (type of parenteral fluid depends on type of fluids lost, severity of hypovolemia, and the patient's cardiovascular, electrolyte, and acid-base status)
- Resuscitation by rapid I.V. fluid administration to restore intravascular volume and raise blood pressure (for severe volume depletion)
- I.V. dopamine (Intropin) or norepinephrine (Levophed) to increase cardiac contractility and renal perfusion (if the patient remains symptomatic after fluid replacement)
- Blood or blood products for the patient with hemorrhage to restore intravascular volume
- Autotransfusion (for some patients with hypovolemia caused by trauma)
- Antidiarrheals as needed
- Antiemetics as needed
- Oxygen therapy to ensure sufficient tissue perfusion

● Nursing considerations
- Start I.V. infusions with the shortest, largest-bore catheters possible; they offer less resistance to fluid flow than do long, thin catheters
- Monitor the patient's mental status and vital signs closely, including orthostatic blood pressure measurements when appropriate

Levels of fluid loss
- Minimal (intravascular volume loss of 10% to 15%)
- Moderate (intravascular volume loss of 25%)
- Severe (intravascular volume loss of 40% or more)

Key treatments for hypovolemia
- Oral or parenteral fluids
- I.V. dopamine or norepinephrine
- Transfusion of blood or blood products

Key nursing considerations for hypovolemia
- Use the shortest, largest-bore I.V. catheters possible.
- Monitor mental status and vital signs.

- If blood pressure doesn't respond to interventions as expected, reassess the patient for a bleeding site that might have been missed (be aware that a fractured hip or pelvis can result in a large amount of internal blood loss)

HYPONATREMIA

● Definition
- Electrolyte imbalance characterized by cellular edema due to insufficient sodium relative to body water
- Serum sodium less than 135 mEq/L
- If severe, can lead to seizures, coma, and permanent neurologic damage

● Underlying pathophysiology
- Sodium is the major cation (90%) in ECF; potassium, the major cation in ICF
- During repolarization of the cell membrane, the sodium-potassium pump continually shifts sodium into the cells and shifts potassium out of the cells; during depolarization, it does the reverse
- Sodium functions include maintaining tonicity and concentration of ECF, acid-base balance (reabsorption of sodium and excretion of hydrogen), nerve conduction and neuromuscular function, glandular secretion, and water balance
- When serum sodium levels decrease, serum osmolality also decreases (increased water and decreased sodium in blood vessels)
- Fluid is moved by osmosis from the extracellular areas to the more-concentrated intracellular areas, resulting in possible cerebral edema and hypovolemia

● Causes
- Excessive sodium loss caused by GI losses, excessive sweating, burns, adrenal insufficiency, diuretic use, or starvation
- Dilutional hyponatremia from excessive water gain resulting from excessive administration of I.V. fluids, syndrome of inappropriate antidiuretic hormone (SIADH), oxytocin use during labor, water intoxication, or heart failure

● Pathophysiologic changes
- Muscle twitching and weakness due to osmotic swelling of cells
- Lethargy, confusion, seizures, and coma due to altered neurotransmission
- Hypotension and tachycardia due to decreased extracellular circulating volume
- Nausea, vomiting, and abdominal cramps due to edema affecting receptors in the brain or the vomiting center of the brain stem
- Oliguria or anuria due to renal dysfunction

● Complications
- Seizures
- Coma
- Permanent neurologic damage

● Diagnostic test findings
- Blood testing reveals decreased BUN, serum sodium level lower than 135 mEq/L, decreased (usually) serum chloride level, and decreased serum osmolality (less than 280 mOsm/kg)

- Urine testing reveals urine specific gravity less than 1.010
- Urine testing in patients with SIADH reveals increased urine specific gravity and elevated urine sodium (0.20 mEq/L)

Treatment

- Restricted fluid intake and administration of oral sodium supplements to treat mild hyponatremia associated with hypervolemia
- Isotonic I.V. fluids (normal saline solution) for hyponatremia associated with hypovolemia
- High-sodium foods (if able to tolerate oral feedings) when serum sodium levels are below 110 mEq/L
- Infusion of hypertonic (3% or 5% saline) solution slowly and in small volumes to prevent fluid overload
- Administration of loop diuretics (furosemide [Lasix]) to increase water elimination
- Monitoring for signs of circulatory overload or worsening neurologic status to prevent or promptly treat complications
- Steroid therapy, if needed for cerebral edema

Nursing considerations

- Give prescribed I.V. fluids
  - Watch the patient closely for signs of hypervolemia (dyspnea, crackles, engorged jugular or hand veins during administration of isosmolar or hyperosmolar saline solution)
  - Report conditions that may cause excessive sodium loss (diaphoresis or prolonged diarrhea or vomiting)
- Monitor vital signs, serum sodium and chloride levels, urine specific gravity, intake and output, and neurologic status
- Teach the patient about drug therapy and possible adverse reactions, dietary changes and fluid restrictions, and the need to monitor daily weight
- Refer the patient on maintenance diuretics to a dietitian for instruction about dietary sodium intake

HYPERNATREMIA

Definition

- Electrolyte imbalance characterized by excess sodium relative to body water
- Serum sodium greater than 145 mEq/L
- If severe, can lead to seizures, coma, and permanent neurologic damage

Underlying pathophysiology

- Sodium is the major cation (90%) in ECF; potassium, the major cation in ICF
- During repolarization, the sodium-potassium pump continually shifts sodium into the cells and shifts potassium out of the cells; during depolarization, it does the reverse
- Excessive sodium intake or water deficit increases sodium osmolality in ECF (increased saline concentrations in the body)
- Fluid moves by osmosis from ICF to ECF for balance
- Cellular dehydration occurs as fluid leaves cells
- This cellular dehydration results in neurologic impairment and hypervolemia from increased ECF volume in the blood vessels

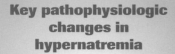

Key pathophysiologic changes in hypernatremia

- Agitation
- Decreased LOC
- Hypertension
- Tachycardia
- Pitting edema
- Excessive weight gain

Key diagnostic test results for hypernatremia

- Blood testing: Serum sodium level greater than 145 mEq/L

Key treatments for hypernatremia

- Oral fluid replacement
- Restricted oral sodium intake
- Diuretics

Key nursing considerations for hypernatremia

- Obtain drug history to check for drugs that promote sodium retention.
- Monitor vital signs for changes, especially rising pulse rate.
- Observe for signs of cerebral edema during fluid replacement therapy.

Causes
- Decreased water intake
- Excess adrenocortical hormones (as in Cushing's syndrome)
- Excess ADH (diabetes insipidus)
- Excessive I.V. administration of sodium solutions
- Use of diuretics, corticosteroids, or vasopressin (Pitressin)
- Salt intoxication (less common)

Pathophysiologic changes
- Agitation, restlessness, fever, decreased level of consciousness (LOC), and possible seizures due to altered cellular metabolism
- Hypertension, tachycardia, pitting edema, and excessive weight gain due to water shift from ICF to ECF
- Involuntary muscle twitches and contractions, progressing to skeletal muscle weakness, from depletion of potassium in muscle fibers
- Thirst, increased viscosity of saliva, and rough tongue due to dehydration from fluid shift
- Dyspnea, respiratory arrest, and death from dramatic increase in osmotic pressure

Complications
- Seizures
- Coma
- Permanent neurologic damage
- Respiratory arrest

Diagnostic test findings
- Blood testing reveals serum sodium level greater than 145 mEq/L
- Urine testing reveals urine sodium level less than 40 mEq/24 hours and high urine osmolality

Treatment
- Oral fluid replacement administered gradually over 48 hours to avoid shifting fluid into brain cells, thus preventing cerebral edema
- I.V. fluid replacement with salt-free solutions (dextrose 5% in water) to return sodium level to normal
- Follow-up of I.V. infusion with half-normal saline solution to prevent hyponatremia and cerebral edema
- Restricted oral sodium intake, and use of diuretics with oral or I.V. fluid replacement to promote sodium loss

Nursing considerations
- Obtain a drug history to check for drugs that promote sodium retention
- Monitor vital signs for changes, especially rising pulse rate
- Assist with oral hygiene
- Observe for signs of cerebral edema during fluid replacement therapy
- Monitor intake and output accurately, checking for fluid loss; weigh the patient daily
- Measure serum sodium levels every 6 hours (or daily as ordered)
- Stress the importance of sodium restriction (low-sodium diet, avoiding over-the-counter [OTC] medications that contain sodium); teach the patient about drug therapy and adverse reactions as well as signs and symptoms of hypernatremia

HYPOKALEMIA

● **Definition**
- Potassium deficiency caused by the body's inability to effectively conserve potassium
- Serum potassium less than 3.5 mEq/L

● **Underlying pathophysiology**
- Potassium facilitates contraction of both skeletal and smooth muscle, including myocardial contraction
- Potassium figures prominently in nerve impulse conduction, acid-base balance, enzyme action, and cell membrane function
- A slight deviation in serum levels can produce profound clinical consequences
- Inadequate intake or excessive loss of potassium (from prolonged suctioning, vomiting, gastric lavage, osmotic diuresis, or magnesium) leads to shift of potassium from ECF to ICF
- Movement of potassium into cells as hydrogen moves out can cause alkalosis

● **Causes**
- Excessive GI or urinary potassium losses, such as by vomiting, gastric suction, diarrhea, dehydration, anorexia, or chronic laxative abuse
- Trauma (injury, burns, or surgery)
- Chronic renal disease with tubular potassium wasting
- Diuretics, steroids, or antibiotics (carbenicillin [Geocillin])
- Acid-base imbalances
- Hyperglycemia
- Cushing's syndrome
- Primary hyperaldosteronism
- Low-potassium diet
- Severe serum magnesium deficiency

● **Pathophysiologic changes**
- Dizziness, hypotension, arrhythmias, electrocardiogram (ECG) changes, and cardiac arrest due to changes in membrane excitability
- Nausea, vomiting, anorexia, diarrhea, decreased peristalsis, and abdominal distention due to decreased bowel motility
- Muscle weakness, fatigue, and leg cramps due to decreased neuromuscular excitability
- Shallow, ineffective respirations due to diminished skeletal muscle activity

● **Complications**
- Cardiac arrhythmias
- Cardiac arrest
- Rhabdomyolysis

● **Diagnostic test findings**
- Blood testing reveals serum potassium levels less than 3.5 mEq/L and slightly elevated serum glucose levels
- ABG analysis shows elevated pH and bicarbonate levels
- ECG reveals flattened T wave and depressed ST segment and U wave

● **Treatment**
- High-potassium diet and oral potassium supplements to treat potassium deficit

Key facts about hypokalemia

- Involves serum potassium less than 3.5 mEq/L
- Results from inadequate intake or excessive loss of potassium, which is involved in nerve impulse conduction, acid-base balance, enzyme action, and cell membrane function
- Causes shift of potassium from ECF to ICF

Key pathophysiologic changes in hypokalemia

- Dizziness
- Hypotension
- Arrhythmias
- Muscle weakness

Key diagnostic test results for hypokalemia

- Blood testing: Serum potassium levels less than 3.5 mEq/L, slightly elevated serum glucose levels

Key treatments for hypokalemia

- Oral or I.V. potassium supplement

- I.V. potassium for rapid replacement (or if unable to tolerate oral potassium supplements)

● **Nursing considerations**
- Give prescribed drugs
- Insert an indwelling urinary catheter, if ordered
- Be alert for signs of hyperkalemia after treatment
- Monitor vital signs, intake and output, serum potassium levels, cardiac rhythm, and respiratory status
- For patients taking cardiac glycosides, closely monitor for hypokalemia, which can potentiate the action of the drug and cause toxicity

HYPERKALEMIA

● **Definition**
- Electrolyte disorder characterized by excess potassium relative to body fluid
- Serum potassium greater than 5 mEq/L
- Most dangerous of the electrolyte disorders

● **Underlying pathophysiology**
- Potassium facilitates contraction of both skeletal and smooth muscles, including myocardial contraction
- Potassium figures prominently in nerve impulse conduction, acid-base balance, enzyme action, and cell membrane function
- Slight deviation in serum potassium levels can produce profound clinical consequences
- Potassium imbalance can lead to muscle weakness and flaccid paralysis because of an ionic imbalance in neuromuscular tissue excitability (see *Hyperkalemia: How it happens*)

● **Causes**
- Renal dysfunction or failure
- Use of potassium-sparing diuretics
- Burns
- Crushing injuries
- Adrenal insufficiency
- Dehydration
- Diabetic acidosis
- Increased intake of potassium
- Decreased urinary excretion of potassium
- Severe infection
- Multiple blood transfusions
- Certain drugs (see *Drugs that can cause hyperkalemia*, page 460)

● **Pathophysiologic changes**
- Tachycardia changing to bradycardia, ECG changes, and cardiac arrest due to hypopolarization and alterations in repolarization
- Nausea, diarrhea, and abdominal cramps due to decreased gastric motility
- Muscle weakness and flaccid paralysis due to inactivation of membrane sodium channels

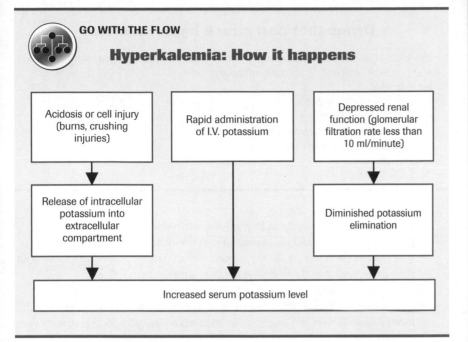

GO WITH THE FLOW

Hyperkalemia: How it happens

| Acidosis or cell injury (burns, crushing injuries) | Rapid administration of I.V. potassium | Depressed renal function (glomerular filtration rate less than 10 ml/minute) |

↓ ↓ ↓

| Release of intracellular potassium into extracellular compartment | | Diminished potassium elimination |

↓ ↓ ↓

Increased serum potassium level

Complications
- Cardiac arrhythmias
- Metabolic acidosis
- Cardiac arrest

Diagnostic test findings
- Blood testing reveals serum potassium levels greater than 5 mEq/L
- ABG analysis reveals decreased arterial pH
- ECG shows a tall, tented T wave; widened QRS complex; prolonged PR interval; flattened or absent P waves; and depressed ST segment

Treatment
- Restricted potassium intake to decrease levels or absorption
- Medication evaluation and adjustment to eliminate drugs or readjust dosages that may be contributing to elevated potassium levels
- Polystyrene sulfonate (Kayexalate) orally, via NG tube, or rectally (enema) to exchange sodium for potassium in the intestine
- Regular insulin and I.V. hypertonic dextrose to move potassium into cells and to monitor for hypoglycemia
- Sodium bicarbonate (in cases of acidosis) to shift potassium into cells
- Calcium gluconate (10% solution) to counteract myocardial effects of hyperkalemia

Nursing considerations
- Administer polystyrene sulfonate orally or rectally (by retention enema)
- Be alert for signs of hypokalemia after treatment
- Monitor serum potassium and other electrolyte levels, cardiac rhythm, and intake and output

Key diagnostic test results for hyperkalemia
- Blood testing: Serum potassium levels greater than 5 mEq/L

Key treatments for hyperkalemia
- Restricted potassium intake
- Oral polystyrene sulfonate

Key nursing considerations for hyperkalemia

- Be alert for signs of hypo-kalemia after treatment.
- Monitor serum potassium and other electrolyte levels, cardiac rhythm, and intake and output.
- Watch for clinical effects of hypoglycemia with repeated insulin and glucose treatments.
- Teach patient about prescribed drugs and dietary restrictions.

Key facts about hypochloremia

- Results when serum chloride is less than 98 mEq/L
- Leads to sodium and bicarbonate retention by kidneys, which can cause potassium and calcium ion changes
- May lead to hypochloremic metabolic alkalosis

Drugs that can cause hyperkalemia

Drugs that can increase potassium levels and cause hyperkalemia include:
- angiotensin-converting enzyme inhibitors
- antibiotics
- beta-adrenergic blockers
- chemotherapeutic drugs
- nonsteroidal anti-inflammatory drugs
- potassium (in excessive amounts)
- spironolactone.

- Watch for clinical effects of hypoglycemia (muscle weakness, syncope, hunger, diaphoresis) with repeated insulin and glucose treatments
- Watch for signs of hyperkalemia in predisposed patients, especially those with poor urine output or those receiving potassium orally or I.V.
- Teach the patient about prescribed drugs and potential adverse reactions
- Discuss the need for a potassium-restricted diet, and teach the patient which foods should be avoided (such as bananas, oranges, and dark green, leafy vegetables)
- Teach the patient how to prevent a future episode of hyperkalemia

HYPOCHLOREMIA

Definition
- Electrolyte imbalance characterized by deficiency of chloride in ECF
- Serum chloride less than 98 mEq/L

Underlying pathophysiology
- Chloride is secreted by the stomach's mucosa as hydrochloric acid; it provides an acid medium that aids digestion and activation of enzymes
- Chloride helps to maintain acid-base and body water balances, influences the osmolality or tonicity of ECF, plays a role in the exchange of oxygen and carbon dioxide in red blood cells (RBCs), and helps activate salivary amylase
- Decreased chloride intake or absorption, or increased loss of chloride, leads to retention of sodium and bicarbonate ions by the kidneys, which can cause potassium and calcium ion changes
- Bicarbonate ions accumulate in ECF
- Excess bicarbonate increases blood pH levels and may cause hypochloremic metabolic alkalosis

Causes
- Untreated diabetic ketoacidosis
- Addison's disease
- Chloride-deficient formula (infants)
- Salt-restricted diets
- Prolonged use of mercurial diuretics
- Administration of dextrose I.V. without electrolytes
- Chronic respiratory acidosis

- Prolonged diarrhea or diaphoresis
- Loss of hydrochloric acid secretion due to vomiting, gastric suctioning, or gastric surgery
- Diuretics (loop, osmotic, thiazide)

Pathophysiologic changes
- Muscle twitching and weakness due to osmotic swelling of cells
- Muscular hypertonicity and tetany due to altered neurotransmission
- Shallow, depressed breathing due to alkalosis
- Oliguria or anuria due to renal dysfunction

Complications
- Respiratory arrest
- Seizures
- Coma

Diagnostic test findings
- Blood testing reveals serum chloride level less than 98 mEq/L, serum sodium level below 135 mEq/L, and serum carbon dioxide level of about 32 mEq/L
- ABG analysis reveals serum pH above 7.45

Treatment
- Increased dietary intake of chloride, fluid administration (I.V. normal saline solution), or drug therapy to replace chloride loss
- Treatment of associated metabolic alkalosis or electrolyte imbalance to correct abnormalities

Nursing considerations
- Monitor serum chloride levels frequently, particularly during I.V. therapy
- Offer foods high in chloride, such as salty broths and snacks
- Monitor the patient's LOC, muscle strength and movement, and cardiac rhythm
- Monitor ABG levels and serum electrolytes for metabolic alkalosis and signs of electrolyte imbalance
- Monitor fluid intake and output in patients who are vulnerable to chloride imbalance, particularly those recovering from gastric surgery; report excessive or continuous loss of gastric secretions
- Teach the patient about drug therapy and possible adverse reactions as well as signs and symptoms of electrolyte imbalance

HYPOCALCEMIA

Definition
- Electrolyte imbalance that occurs when calcium levels fall below normal range (serum calcium less than 8.5 mg/dl and ionized serum calcium less than 4.5 mg/dl)

Underlying pathophysiology
- Together with phosphorus, calcium is responsible for the formation and structure of bones and teeth
- Calcium helps maintain cell structure and function
- Calcium plays a role in cell membrane permeability and impulse transmission

Signs of tetany

1. Chvostek's sign
2. Trousseau's sign

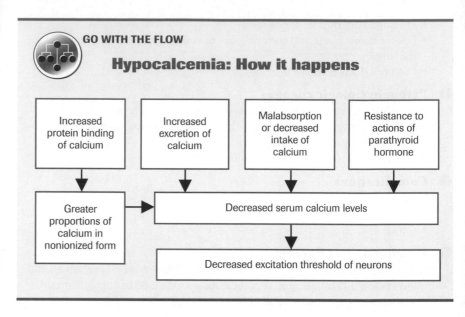

GO WITH THE FLOW

Hypocalcemia: How it happens

| Increased protein binding of calcium | Increased excretion of calcium | Malabsorption or decreased intake of calcium | Resistance to actions of parathyroid hormone |

Greater proportions of calcium in nonionized form

→ Decreased serum calcium levels

↓

Decreased excitation threshold of neurons

- Calcium affects the contraction of cardiac muscle, smooth muscle, and skeletal muscle, and also plays a role in the blood-clotting process (see *Hypocalcemia: How it happens*)

Causes
- Inadequate intake of calcium and vitamin D (needed for calcium absorption)
- Hypoparathyroidism
- Surgical removal of thyroid or parathyroid glands
- Malabsorption or loss of calcium from the GI tract
- Severe infections or burns
- Overcorrection of hypercalcemia
- Low serum albumin levels
- Alcohol addiction
- Pancreatic insufficiency
- Renal failure
- Hypomagnesemia

Pathophysiologic changes
- Mental changes (depression, confusion, delirium, anxiety, and irritability), mouth twitching, hyperactive deep tendon reflexes, laryngospasm, seizures, tetany, and positive Chvostek's and Trousseau's signs due to enhanced neuro-muscular irritability (see *Eliciting signs of hypocalcemia*)
- Hypotension, ECG changes, and arrhythmias due to decreased calcium influx

Complications
- Laryngeal spasm
- Seizures
- Cardiac arrhythmia
- Respiratory arrest

Key pathophysiologic changes in hypocalcemia

- Anxiety
- Irritability
- Mouth twitching
- Laryngospasm
- Seizures

Eliciting signs of hypocalcemia

When the patient complains of muscle spasms and paresthesia in his limbs, try eliciting Chvostek's and Trousseau's signs (indications of tetany associated with calcium deficiency).

Follow the procedures described here, keeping in mind the discomfort they typically cause. During these tests, watch the patient for laryngospasm, monitor his cardiac status, and have resuscitation equipment nearby. If you detect these signs, notify the physician immediately.

CHVOSTEK'S SIGN

To elicit Chvostek's sign, tap the patient's facial nerve just in front of the earlobe and below the zygomatic arch, or between the zygomatic arch and the corner of the mouth, as shown here.

A positive response (indicating tetany) ranges from simple mouth-corner twitching to twitching of all facial muscles on the side tested. Simple twitching may be normal in some patients. However, a more pronounced response usually confirms Chvostek's sign.

TROUSSEAU'S SIGN

In this test, occlude the brachial artery by inflating a blood pressure cuff on the patient's upper arm to a level between diastolic and systolic blood pressure. Maintain this inflation for 3 minutes while observing the patient for carpal spasm (shown here), which is Trousseau's sign.

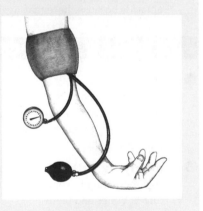

Key diagnostic test results for hypocalcemia

● Blood testing: Serum calcium levels less than 8.5 mg/dl and ionized calcium levels less than 4.5 mg/dl

Key treatments for hypocalcemia

● Administration of I.V. calcium gluconate or calcium chloride
● Vitamin D supplementation (in chronic cases)

● **Diagnostic test findings**
  • Blood testing reveals serum calcium levels less than 8.5 mg/dl and ionized calcium levels less than 4.5 mg/dl
  • ECG shows lengthened QT interval, prolonged ST segment, and arrhythmias

● **Treatment**
  • Immediate calcium replacement with administration of I.V. calcium gluconate or calcium chloride for acute hypocalcemia
  • Magnesium replacement to enhance calcium therapy (hypocalcemia doesn't respond to calcium therapy alone)
  • Vitamin D supplementation (in chronic cases) to facilitate calcium absorption
  • Dietary adjustments to increase intake of calcium, vitamin D, and protein

- Phosphate binders to lower elevated phosphorus levels (if needed)

● **Nursing considerations**
- Monitor blood pressure
- Keep the patient in bed for I.V. calcium replacement (to prevent orthostatic hypotension)
- Provide safety measures; institute seizure precautions, if appropriate
- Give prescribed calcium replacement
- Assess I.V. sites if administering calcium I.V. (infiltration causes sloughing)
- Monitor cardiac rhythms and serum calcium levels
- Watch for hypocalcemia in patients receiving massive transfusions of citrated blood; in those with chronic diarrhea, severe infections, and insufficient dietary intake of calcium and protein (especially elderly patients); and in those who are hyperventilating
- Monitor closely for a possible drug interaction in patients receiving a cardiac glycoside with large doses of oral calcium supplements; watch for signs of digoxin (Digitek, Lanoxin) toxicity (anorexia, nausea, vomiting, yellow vision, cardiac arrhythmias)
- Administer oral calcium supplements 1 to 1 ½ hours after meals or with milk to reduce GI upset
- Teach the patient about calcium supplements and the need to follow a high-calcium diet
- Discourage chronic use of laxatives, and caution the patient not to overuse antacids because these may aggravate the condition

HYPERCALCEMIA

● **Definition**
- Electrolyte imbalance that occurs when serum calcium is greater than 10.5 mg/dl and serum ionized calcium is greater than 5.3 mg/dl
- Becomes life-threatening when serum calcium reaches critical value (greater than 13 mg/dl)

● **Underlying pathophysiology**
- Together with phosphorus, calcium is responsible for the formation and structure of bones and teeth
- Calcium helps to maintain cell structure and function, and plays a role in cell membrane permeability and impulse transmission
- Calcium affects the contraction of cardiac muscle, smooth muscle, and skeletal muscle, and plays a role in the blood-clotting process
- Increased resorption of calcium from bone leads to increased rate of calcium entry into ECF
- This increased resorption results in more calcium in ECF than that excreted by the kidneys

● **Causes**
- Hyperparathyroidism
- Hypervitaminosis D
- Certain cancers
- Multiple fractures and prolonged immobilization

- Drugs, such as antacids that contain calcium, calcium preparations (oral or I.V.), lithium (Eskalith), vitamin A, and vitamin D

Pathophysiologic changes
- Drowsiness, lethargy, headaches, irritability, confusion, depression, apathy, and heart block due to decreased neuromuscular irritability (increased threshold)
- Weakness and muscle flaccidity due to depressed neuromuscular irritability and release of acetylcholine at myoneural junction
- Bone pain and pathologic fractures due to calcium loss from bone
- Anorexia, nausea, vomiting, constipation, and dehydration due to hyperosmolarity
- Excessive urination due to altered renal tubular function
- Flank pain due to kidney stone formation

Complications
- Renal calculi
- Coma
- Cardiac arrest
- Respiratory failure

Diagnostic test findings
- Blood testing reveals serum calcium levels greater than 10.5 mg/dl and ionized calcium levels less than 5.3 mg/dl
- ECG shows a shortened QT interval and ventricular arrhythmias

Treatment
- Limited dietary intake of calcium
- Discontinuation of medications or infusions containing calcium
- Hydration with normal saline solution to prevent volume depletion, encourage diuresis, and increase urinary excretion of calcium
- Loop diuretics to promote calcium excretion (avoid thiazide diuretics, which inhibit calcium excretion)
- Dialysis (if condition is life-threatening) to eliminate excess calcium
- Corticosteroids to block bone resorption of calcium and decrease absorption in GI tract
- Etidronate disodium (Didronel) to inhibit action of osteoclasts in bone
- Plicamycin (Mithracin) for hypercalcemia resulting from cancer
- Calcitonin (Miacalcin) to inhibit bone resorption (effects are short-lived)
- I.V. phosphorus to promote reduced calcium levels

Nursing considerations
- Provide safety measures and institute seizure precautions, if appropriate
- Watch for signs of heart failure in patients receiving normal saline diuresis
- Monitor serum calcium levels frequently; watch for cardiac arrhythmias if serum calcium level exceeds 5.7 mg/dl
- Increase fluid intake to dilute calcium in serum and urine and to prevent renal damage and dehydration
- Administer loop diuretics (not thiazide diuretics) as ordered, monitor intake and output and check urine for renal calculi and acidity, and provide acid-ash

---

Key pathophysiologic changes in hypercalcemia

- Drowsiness
- Lethargy
- Headaches
- Irritability
- Heart block
- Anorexia
- Nausea

Key diagnostic test results for hypercalcemia

- Blood testing: Serum calcium levels greater than 10.5 mg/dl, ionized calcium levels less than 5.3 mg/dl

Key treatments for hypercalcemia

- Limited dietary intake of calcium
- Hydration
- Loop diuretics

drinks, such as cranberry or prune juice (calcium salts are more soluble in acid than in alkali)
- Check ECG and vital signs frequently
- In the patient receiving cardiac glycosides, watch for signs of toxicity, such as anorexia, nausea, vomiting, and bradycardia (commonly with arrhythmia)
- Ambulate the patient as soon as possible, and handle the patient with chronic hypercalcemia gently to prevent pathologic fractures
- If the patient is bedridden, reposition him frequently and encourage range-of-motion (ROM) exercises to promote circulation and prevent urinary stasis and calcium loss from bone
- Teach the patient to avoid OTC drugs that are high in calcium and to follow a low-calcium diet

HYPOMAGNESEMIA

● **Definition**
- Electrolyte imbalance that occurs when serum magnesium levels are low (less than 1.8 mg/dl)
- Typically accompanied by hypokalemia and hypocalcemia

● **Underlying pathophysiology**
- Magnesium enhances neuromuscular integration and stimulates parathyroid hormone secretion, thus regulating ICF calcium levels
- Magnesium may also regulate skeletal muscles through its influence on calcium utilization, by depressing acetylcholine release at synaptic junctions
- Magnesium activates many enzymes for proper carbohydrate and protein metabolism and aids in cell metabolism and the transport of sodium and potassium, calcium, and protein
- About one-third of the magnesium taken into the body is absorbed through the small intestine and eventually excreted in urine; the remaining unabsorbed magnesium is excreted in stool
- Poor dietary intake or excessive loss of magnesium from the GI or urinary tract leads to impaired magnesium regulation
- This impaired regulation may result in transient hypoparathyroidism, or interference with the peripheral action of parathyroid hormone

● **Causes**
- Malabsorption syndrome
- Chronic diarrhea or excessive laxative use
- Postoperative complications after bowel resection
- Chronic alcoholism
- Prolonged diuretic therapy
- NG suctioning
- Burns, sepsis, or pancreatitis
- Exchange transfusion
- Protein-calorie malnutrition
- Diabetic acidosis
- Cardiac dysfunction
- Hyperaldosteronism

- Use of osmotic diuretics or antibiotics
- Hypercalcemia

● Pathophysiologic changes

- Hyperirritability, tetany, leg and foot cramps, positive Chvostek's and Trousseau's signs, confusion, delusions, and seizures due to altered neuro-muscular transmission
- Arrhythmias, vasodilation, and hypotension due to enhanced inward sodium current or concurrent effects of calcium and potassium imbalance

● Complications

- Laryngeal stridor
- Seizures
- Respiratory depression
- Cardiac arrhythmia
- Cardiac arrest

● Diagnostic test findings

- Blood testing reveals serum magnesium levels less than 1.8 mg/dl and below-normal serum potassium or calcium levels
- Urine testing shows 24-hour quantitative magnesium level below 75 mg or 3 mEq (urinary magnesium decreases before serum magnesium and is a bet-ter indicator of depleted magnesium stores)
- ECG shows abnormalities, such as prolonged QT interval and atrioventricular block

● Treatment

- Dietary replacement or oral magnesium supplements (in mild cases) to re-place magnesium (takes several days)
- I.V. or I.M. doses of magnesium in more severe cases (requires careful assess-ment of renal function)

● Nursing considerations

- Institute seizure precautions
- Report abnormal serum electrolyte levels immediately
- Be aware that a low magnesium level may increase retention of cardiac glycosides; in the patient taking digoxin, be alert for signs of digoxin tox-icity, such as nausea and vomiting and visual changes
- Monitor vital signs during I.V. therapy; infuse magnesium slowly, and watch for bradycardia, heart block, and decreased respiratory rate; keep calcium gluconate I.V. available to reverse hypermagnesemia from over-correction
- Measure intake and output frequently (urine output shouldn't fall below 25 ml/hour or 600 ml/day); be aware that the kidneys excrete excess magne-sium and that hypermagnesemia could occur with renal insufficiency
- Watch for and report signs of hypomagnesemia in patients with predisposing diseases or conditions, especially those not permitted anything by mouth and those receiving I.V. fluids without magnesium
- Teach the patient to avoid drugs that deplete magnesium (such as diuretics and laxatives), and stress the need to adhere to a high-magnesium diet (in-cluding such foods as fish and green vegetables)

Key diagnostic test results for hypomagnesemia

- Blood testing: Serum magne-sium levels less than 1.8 mg/dl, below-normal serum potassium or calcium levels

Key treatments for hypomagnesemia

- Oral, I.V. or I.M. magnesium supplements

Key nursing considerations for hypomagnesemia

- Institute seizure precautions.
- Be aware that a low magnesium level may increase retention of cardiac glycosides.
- Measure intake and output fre-quently.
- Teach patient to avoid drugs that deplete magnesium and encourage high-magnesium diet.

During I.V. therapy
- Monitor vital signs.
- Infuse magnesium slowly.
- Watch for bradycardia, heart block, and decreased respiratory rate.
- Keep I.V. calcium gluconate available.

Key facts about hyperphosphatemia

- Involves serum phosphorus levels greater than 4.5 mg/dl
- Occurs when kidneys are unable to excrete excess phosphorus, causing phosphorus to shift from ICF to ECF
- Results from imbalance between phosphate and calcium (renal tubular reabsorption of phosphate is inversely regulated by calcium levels)
- Causes phosphorus to bind with calcium, forming insoluble compounds that deposit in lungs, heart, kidneys, eyes, skin, and other soft tissues

Key pathophysiologic changes in hyperphosphatemia

- Irritability
- Anxiety
- Laryngospasm
- Tetany

Key diagnostic test results for hyperphosphatemia

- Blood testing: Serum phosphate level over 4.5 mg/dl, serum calcium level below 8.9 mg/dl, increased BUN and creatinine levels

HYPERPHOSPHATEMIA

- **Definition**
  - Electrolyte imbalance that occurs when the kidneys are unable to excrete excess phosphorus, and serum levels rise (greater than 4.5 mg/dl)
  - Usually asymptomatic, unless condition leads to hypocalcemia

- **Underlying pathophysiology**
  - Phosphorus exists primarily in inorganic combination with calcium in teeth and bones
  - In ECF, the phosphate ion supports several metabolic functions: utilization of B vitamins, acid-base homeostasis, bone formation, nerve and muscle activity, cell division, transmission of hereditary traits, and metabolism of carbohydrates, proteins, and fats
  - Renal tubular reabsorption of phosphate is inversely regulated by calcium levels; an increase in phosphorus causes a decrease in calcium
  - An imbalance between phosphate and calcium causes hypophosphatemia or hyperphosphatemia
  - Excessive intake of phosphorus or vitamin D, or renal insult or failure, can drop the glomerular filtration rate below 30 ml/minute
  - Inability of the kidneys to filter excess phosphorus adequately leads to shifting of phosphorus from intracellular to extracellular fluid, resulting in an increased serum phosphorus level
  - Binding of phosphorus with calcium forms insoluble compounds
  - The insoluble compounds are deposited in the lungs, hearts, kidneys, eyes, skin, and other soft tissues

- **Causes**
  - Acid-base disorders (metabolic acidosis, respiratory acidosis)
  - Chemotherapy
  - Hypocalcemia
  - Hypervitaminosis D
  - Hypoparathyroidism
  - Renal failure
  - Overuse of laxatives with phosphates or phosphate enemas

- **Pathophysiologic changes**
  - Irritability, anxiety, mouth twitching, laryngospasm, tetany, and positive Chvostek's and Trousseau's signs due to enhanced neuromuscular irritability
  - Hypotension, ECG changes, and arrhythmias due to decreased calcium influx

- **Complications**
  - Soft-tissue calcifications
  - Hypocalcemia
  - Bone fractures

- **Diagnostic test findings**
  - Blood testing reveals a serum phosphate level over 4.5 mg/dl, a serum calcium level below 8.9 mg/dl, and increased BUN and creatinine levels
  - X-ray studies may reveal skeletal changes caused by osteodystrophy in chronic hyperphosphatemia
  - ECG may show changes characteristic of hypercalcemia

Treatment

- Limited dietary intake of phosphorus or use of phosphorus-containing medications
- Use of aluminum, magnesium, or calcium gel or phosphate-binding agents to decrease GI absorption of phosphorus
- Administration of I.V. saline solution (in severe cases) to promote renal excretion (ineffective in patients with renal insufficiency)
- Dialysis to reduce phosphate levels, if hyperphosphatemia is related to renal failure

Nursing considerations

- Be alert for signs of hypocalcemia, such as muscle twitching and tetany, which commonly accompany hyperphosphatemia
- Give antacids with meals to increase their effectiveness
- Help the patient select a low-phosphorus diet (see *Sources of phosphorus*)
- Monitor vital signs as well as serum phosphorus and calcium levels, and conduct renal studies
- Monitor intake and output, and notify the physician immediately if urine output falls below 25 ml/hour or 600 ml/day (decreased output can seriously affect renal clearance of excess serum phosphorus)
- Teach the patient about prescribed medications and avoidance of foods that contain phosphorus; obtain a dietary consultation if the condition results from chronic renal insufficiency

TIME-OUT FOR TEACHING

Sources of phosphorus

Most patients know little about which foods and drugs contain phosphorus. When caring for a patient on a restricted phosphorus diet, teach him to avoid the items listed here. When caring for a patient who needs to increase his phosphorus intake, encourage him to eat more of these foods and to consider some of these supplemental sources of phosphorus.

DIETARY SOURCES
- Beans
- Bran
- Cheese
- Chocolate
- Dark-colored sodas
- Ice cream
- Lentils
- Milk
- Nuts
- Peanut butter
- Seeds
- Yogurt

SUPPLEMENTAL SOURCES
- Enemas (such as Fleet)
- Laxatives containing phosphorus or phosphate
- Oral phosphorus supplements
- Parenteral phosphorus supplements (sodium phosphate, potassium phosphate)
- Vitamin D supplements

Key treatments for hyperphosphatemia
- Limited dietary phosphorus intake
- Aluminum, magnesium, or calcium gel or phosphate-binding agents
- Dialysis

Key nursing considerations for hyperphosphatemia
- Be alert for signs of hypocalcemia.
- Teach patient about prescribed medications and dietary restrictions.
- Monitor intake and output; report urine output below 25 ml/hour or 600 ml/day.

METABOLIC ACIDOSIS

Definition
- Acid-base disorder characterized by excess acid and deficient bicarbonate; caused by an underlying nonrespiratory disorder
- Primary decrease in plasma bicarbonate causes hydrogen to increase and pH to fall
- Can occur with increased production of a nonvolatile acid (such as lactic acid), decreased renal clearance of a nonvolatile acid (as in renal failure), or loss of bicarbonate (as in chronic diarrhea)
- Symptoms result from action of compensatory mechanisms in the lungs, kidneys, and cells
- Severe or untreated metabolic acidosis can be fatal

Underlying pathophysiology
- As acid (hydrogen) starts to accumulate in the body, chemical buffers (plasma bicarbonate and proteins) in the cells and ECF bind the excess hydrogen ions
- Excess hydrogen that the buffers can't bind decreases blood pH and stimulates chemoreceptors in the medulla to increase respiration
- The consequent fall of partial pressure of arterial carbon dioxide ($PaCO_2$) frees hydrogen to bind with bicarbonate; respiratory compensation occurs in minutes but isn't sufficient to correct the acidosis
- Healthy kidneys try to compensate by secreting excess hydrogen into the renal tubules
- These ions are buffered by either phosphate or ammonia and are excreted into the urine in the form of weak acid; for each hydrogen ion secreted into the renal tubules, the tubules resorb and return to the blood one sodium and one bicarbonate ion
- The excess hydrogen in ECF passively diffuses into cells
- To maintain the balance of charge across the membranes, the cells release potassium; excess hydrogen changes the normal balance of potassium, sodium, and calcium ions, thereby impairing neural excitability

Causes
- Usually results from excessive fat metabolism in the absence of usable carbohydrates and can be caused by:
  - Diabetic ketoacidosis
  - Chronic alcoholism
  - Malnutrition
  - Low-carbohydrate, high-fat diet
- Other causes
  - Anaerobic carbohydrate metabolism (forces a shift from aerobic to anaerobic metabolism, causing a corresponding increase in lactic acid level), as in:
    - Cardiac pump failure after myocardial infarction
    - Pulmonary or hepatic disease
    - Shock
    - Anemia
  - Underexcretion of metabolized acids or inability to conserve bicarbonate (alkali) due to renal insufficiency and failure (renal acidosis)

– Diarrhea, intestinal malabsorption, or loss of sodium bicarbonate from the intestines, causing bicarbonate buffer system to shift to the acidic side (for example, ureteroenterostomy and Crohn's disease can induce metabolic acidosis)

– Salicylate intoxication (overuse of aspirin), exogenous poisoning or, less frequently, Addison's disease (increased excretion of sodium and chloride, and retention of potassium)

– Inhibited secretion of acid due to hypoaldosteronism or the use of potassium-sparing diuretics

● **Pathophysiologic changes**

• Headache, malaise, and lethargy progressing to drowsiness, due to changes in pH level

• Central nervous system (CNS) depression due to a change in electrolyte balance from excess hydrogen ions (results in impaired neural excitability)

• Kussmaul's respirations due to compensatory mechanism of the lungs to blow off carbon dioxide

• Hypotension due to decreased cardiac output resulting from increasing pH

• Anorexia, nausea, vomiting, diarrhea and, possibly, dehydration due to GI distress

• Warm, flushed skin due to a pH-sensitive decrease in vascular response to sympathetic stimuli

• Fruity-smelling breath from fat catabolism and excretion of accumulated acetone through the lungs due to underlying diabetes mellitus

● **Complications**

• Weakness and flaccid paralysis

• Coma

• Ventricular arrhythmias and, possibly, cardiac arrest

• Growth retardation in children

• Bone disorders such as renal osteodystrophy

● **Diagnostic test findings**

• ABG analysis reveals arterial pH less than 7.35 (as low as 7.10 in severe acidosis), a $Paco_2$ value that's normal or less than 34 mm Hg, and bicarbonate levels less than 22 mEq/L (see *Interpreting ABG values,* pages 472 and 473)

• ECG shows arrhythmias from abnormal potassium levels

• Urinalysis reveals urine pH less than 4.5 in the absence of renal disease (as the kidneys excrete acid to raise blood pH)

• Blood testing shows serum potassium greater than 5.5 mEq/L (from chemical buffering), serum glucose greater than 150 mg/dl, serum ketone bodies (in diabetes), and elevated plasma lactic acid (in lactic acidosis)

• Blood chemistry reveals an anion gap greater than 14 mEq/L in high-anion gap metabolic acidosis, lactic acidosis, ketoacidosis, aspirin overdose, alcohol poisoning, renal failure, or other conditions characterized by accumulation of organic acids, sulfates, or phosphates

• Blood chemistry reveals an anion gap of 12 mEq/L or less in normal-anion gap metabolic acidosis from bicarbonate loss, GI or renal loss, increased acid load (hyperalimentation fluids), rapid I.V. saline administration, or other conditions characterized by loss of bicarbonate (see *Finding the anion gap,* page 473)

Key pathophysiologic changes in metabolic acidosis

● Malaise
● Lethargy progressing to drowsiness
● Kussmaul's respirations
● Hypotension
● Fruity-smelling breath

Key diagnostic test results for metabolic acidosis

● ABG analysis: Arterial pH less than 7.35, $Paco_2$ that's normal or less than 34 mm Hg, bicarbonate levels less than 22 mEq/L

● Blood testing: Serum potassium greater than 5.5 mEq/L, serum glucose greater than 150 mg/dl, serum ketone bodies (in diabetes), elevated plasma lactic acid (in lactic acidosis)

Interpreting ABG values

This chart compares abnormal arterial blood gas (ABG) values and outlines their significance for patient care.

DISORDER	pH	Paco$_2$ (mm HG)	BICARBONATE (mEq/L)
Normal	**7.35 to 7.45**	**35 to 45**	**22 to 26**
Respiratory acidosis	< 7.35	> 45	• Acute: may be normal • Chronic: > 26
Respiratory alkalosis	> 7.45	< 35	• Acute: may be normal • Chronic: < 22
Metabolic acidosis	< 7.35	< 35	< 22
Metabolic alkalosis	> 7.45	> 45	> 26

Key treatments for metabolic acidosis

- I.V. sodium bicarbonate
- I.V. lactated Ringer's solution
- Correction of underlying cause

Key nursing considerations for metabolic acidosis

- Keep sodium bicarbonate ampules handy for emergency administration.
- Frequently monitor vital signs and LOC.
- Monitor plasma electrolytes during sodium bicarbonate therapy (potassium level may fall as pH rises).
- Record intake and output.
- Watch for signs of excessive serum potassium, possibly leading to cardiac arrest.
- Position patient to prevent aspiration.
- Prepare to observe seizure precautions.

● Treatment

- Sodium bicarbonate I.V. for severe high-anion gap to neutralize blood acidity in patients with pH less than 7.20 and bicarbonate loss
- I.V. lactated Ringer's solution to correct normal-anion gap metabolic acidosis and ECF volume deficit
- Evaluation and correction of electrolyte imbalances
- Correction of the underlying cause
- Mechanical ventilation, if needed to maintain respiratory compensation
- Antibiotic therapy to treat infection
- Dialysis for patients with renal failure or certain drug toxicities
- Antidiarrheal agents for diarrhea-induced bicarbonate loss

● Nursing considerations

- Keep sodium bicarbonate ampules handy for emergency administration
  - Frequently monitor vital signs and LOC because changes can occur rapidly
  - Monitor plasma electrolytes, especially potassium, during sodium bicarbonate therapy (potassium level may fall as pH rises)
- Watch for secondary changes due to hypovolemia (such as decreasing blood pressure) in patients with diabetic acidosis
- Record intake and output accurately to monitor renal function
  - Watch for signs of excessive serum potassium (weakness, flaccid paralysis, and arrhythmias), possibly leading to cardiac arrest
  - After treatment, check for overcorrection, which can cause hypokalemia
- Position the patient to prevent aspiration because metabolic acidosis commonly causes vomiting
- Prepare to observe seizure precautions, if needed
- Provide good oral hygiene; use sodium bicarbonate washes to neutralize mouth acids, and lubricate the patient's lips with lemon-glycerin swabs

COMPENSATION

- Renal: Increased secretion and excretion of acid; compensation takes 24 hours to begin
- Respiratory: Rate increases to expel carbon dioxide

- Renal: Decreased hydrogen secretion and active secretion of bicarbonate into urine

- Respiratory: Lungs expel more carbon dioxide by increasing rate and depth of respirations

- Respiratory: Hypoventilation is immediate but limited because of ensuing hypoxemia
- Renal: More effective than respiratory compensation but slow to excrete less acid and more base

- To prevent metabolic acidosis, carefully observe patients receiving I.V. therapy, those with intestinal tubes, and patients suffering from shock, hyperthyroidism, hepatic disease, circulatory failure, or dehydration
- Teach the patient with diabetes how to routinely test urine for glucose and acetone, and encourage strict adherence to insulin or oral hypoglycemic therapy

Finding the anion gap

The anion gap is the difference between concentrations of serum cations and anions, determined by measuring one cation (sodium) and two anions (chloride and bicarbonate). Here are some important related facts:

- The normal concentration of sodium is 140 mEq/L.
- The normal concentration of chloride is 102 mEq/L.
- The normal concentration of bicarbonate is 26 mEq/L.
- Thus, the anion gap between measured cations (actually, sodium alone) and measured anions is about 12 mEq/L (140 minus 128).

Concentrations of potassium, calcium, and magnesium (unmeasured cations), or of proteins, phosphate, sulfate, and organic acids (unmeasured anions), aren't needed to measure the anion gap. Added together:

- The concentration of unmeasured cations would be about 11 mEq/L.
- The concentration of unmeasured anions would be about 23 mEq/L.
- Thus, the normal anion gap between unmeasured cations and anions is about 12 mEq/L (23 minus 11) ± 2 mEq/L for normal variation.

An anion gap greater than 14 mEq/L indicates metabolic acidosis. It may result from accumulation of excess organic acids or from retention of hydrogen ions, which chemically bond with bicarbonate and decrease bicarbonate levels.

Cations and ions used in anion gap

- Sodium (cation)
- Chloride (anion)
- Bicarbonate (anion)

Key facts about metabolic alkalosis

- Occurs when low levels of acid or high bicarbonate levels cause metabolic, respiratory, and renal responses
- Involves decreased intracellular hydrogen levels, decreased calcium ionization, and increased permeability of nerve cells to sodium
- Triggers neural impulses in peripheral nervous system and CNS as sodium moves into cells

TOP 2

Causes of critical acid loss

1. Chronic vomiting
2. NG tube drainage

METABOLIC ALKALOSIS

● **Definition**
- Acid-base disturbance that occurs when low levels of acid or high bicarbonate cause metabolic, respiratory, and renal responses, producing characteristic symptoms (most notably, hypoventilation)
- Always occurs secondary to an underlying condition

● **Underlying pathophysiology**
- Chemical buffers in the ECF and ICF bind bicarbonate that accumulates in the body
- Excess, unbound bicarbonate raises blood pH, which depresses chemoreceptors in the medulla, inhibiting respiration and raising $PaCO_2$
  - Carbon dioxide combines with water to form carbonic acid
  - Low oxygen levels limit respiratory compensation
- When bicarbonate rises to 28 mEq/L or more, the amount filtered by the renal glomeruli exceeds the reabsorptive capacity of the renal tubules; excess bicarbonate is excreted in the urine, and hydrogen is retained
- To maintain electrochemical balance, sodium and water are excreted with the bicarbonate
- When hydrogen levels in ECF are low, hydrogen diffuses passively out of the cells and, to maintain the balance of charge across the cell membrane, extracellular potassium moves into the cells
- As intracellular hydrogen levels continue to fall, calcium ionization decreases and nerve cells become more permeable to sodium
- As sodium moves into the cells, they trigger neural impulses, first in the peripheral nervous system and then in the CNS

● **Causes**
- Loss of acid, retention of base, or renal mechanisms associated with low serum levels of potassium and chloride
- Critical acid loss
  - Chronic vomiting
  - NG tube drainage or lavage without adequate electrolyte replacement
  - Fistulas
  - Use of steroids and certain diuretics (furosemide, thiazides, and ethacrynic acid [Edecrin])
  - Massive blood transfusions
  - Cushing's disease, primary hyperaldosteronism, and Bartter's syndrome
- Excessive bicarbonate retention causing chronic hypercapnia
  - Excessive intake of bicarbonate of soda (baking soda) or other antacids
  - Excessive intake of absorbable alkali (as in milk-alkali syndrome)
  - Excessive amounts of I.V. fluids with high concentrations of bicarbonate or lactate
  - Respiratory insufficiency
- Alterations in extracellular electrolyte levels, including low chloride (as chloride diffuses out of the cell, hydrogen diffuses into the cell) and low plasma potassium (causes increased hydrogen excretion by the kidneys)

Pathophysiologic changes

- Irritability, picking at bedclothes (carphology), twitching, and confusion due to decreased cerebral perfusion
- Cardiovascular abnormalities due to hypokalemia
- Respiratory disturbances (such as cyanosis and apnea) and slow, shallow respirations due to compensatory response when severe respiratory alkalosis leads to respiratory failure
- Diminished peripheral blood flow during repeated blood pressure checks (may provoke carpopedal spasm in the hand [Trousseau's sign, a possible sign of impending tetany])

Complications

- Seizures
- Coma

Diagnostic test findings

- ABG analysis shows blood pH greater than 7.45 and bicarbonate greater than 26 mEq/L (confirm diagnosis), and $PaCO_2$ greater than 45 mm Hg (indicates attempts at respiratory compensation)
- Blood chemistry reveals low levels of potassium (less than 3.5 mEq/L), calcium (less than 8.9 mg/dl), and chloride (less than 98 mEq/L)
- Urinalysis reveals urine pH of approximately 7 (alkaline urine after the renal compensatory mechanism begins to excrete bicarbonate)
- ECG may show a low T wave merging with a P wave, and atrial or sinus tachycardia

Treatment

- *Cautious* use of ammonium chloride I.V. (rarely) or hydrochloric acid to restore ECF hydrogen and chloride levels
- Potassium chloride (KCl) and normal saline solution (except in heart failure); usually sufficient to replace losses from gastric drainage
- Discontinuation of diuretics, followed by discontinuation of supplementary potassium chloride to prevent metabolic alkalosis from potent diuretic therapy
- Oral or I.V. acetazolamide ([Diamox] enhances renal bicarbonate excretion) to correct metabolic alkalosis without rapid volume expansion (acetazolamide also enhances potassium excretion, so potassium may be given first)

Nursing considerations

- Administer I.V. therapy cautiously (observe carefully), and strictly monitor the patient's status
- Dilute potassium when giving I.V. fluids containing potassium salts, and monitor the infusion rate to prevent damage to blood vessels; watch for signs of phlebitis
- Limit ammonium chloride 0.9% infusion rate to 1 L/4 hours; more rapid infusion may cause hemolysis of (RBCs); don't give ammonium chloride with signs of hepatic or renal disease (instead, use hydrochloric acid)
- Watch closely for signs of muscle weakness, tetany, or decreased activity
- Monitor vital signs frequently, and record intake and output to evaluate respiratory, fluid, and electrolyte status
  - Watch for decreased respiratory rate (usually occurs in an effort to compensate for alkalosis)

Key pathophysiologic changes in metabolic alkalosis

- Irritability
- Twitching
- Confusion
- Cardiovascular abnormalities
- Cyanosis
- Apnea

Key diagnostic test results for metabolic alkalosis

- ABG analysis: Blood pH greater than 7.45, bicarbonate greater than 26 mEq/L, $PaCO_2$ greater than 45 mm Hg
- Blood studies: Potassium level less than 3.5 mEq/L, calcium level less than 8.9 mg/dl, chloride level less than 98 mEq/L

Key treatments for metabolic alkalosis

- Potassium chloride and normal saline solution
- Discontinuation of diuretics

Key nursing considerations for metabolic alkalosis

- Watch for signs of muscle weakness, tetany, or decreased activity.
- Monitor vital signs frequently.
- Record intake and output.
- Watch for decreased respiratory rate.
- Be aware that hypotension and tachycardia may indicate electrolyte imbalance.

– Be aware that hypotension and tachycardia may indicate electrolyte imbalance, especially hypokalemia
• Observe seizure precautions
• To prevent metabolic alkalosis, caution patients not to overuse alkaline agents; irrigate NG tubes with isotonic saline solution instead of plain water to prevent loss of gastric electrolytes; monitor I.V. fluid concentrations of bicarbonate or lactate; and teach patients with ulcers to recognize signs of milk-alkali syndrome (distaste for milk, anorexia, weakness, and lethargy)

RESPIRATORY ACIDOSIS

Definition
• Acid-base disturbance characterized by reduced alveolar ventilation (pulmonary system can't clear enough carbon dioxide from the body)
• Leads to hypercapnia ($PaCO_2$ greater than 45 mm Hg) and acidosis (pH less than 7.35)
• Can be acute (due to a sudden failure in ventilation) or chronic (in long-term pulmonary disease)
• May result from any compromise in the essential components of breathing (ventilation, perfusion, and diffusion)

Underlying pathophysiology
• When pulmonary ventilation decreases, $PaCO_2$ is increased and the carbon dioxide level rises in all tissues and fluids, including the medulla and cerebrospinal fluid
• Retained carbon dioxide combines with water to form carbonic acid, which dissociates to release free hydrogen and bicarbonate ions
• Increased $PaCO_2$ and free hydrogen stimulate the medulla to increase respiratory drive and expel carbon dioxide
• As pH falls, 2,3-diphosphoglycerate (2,3-DPG) accumulates in RBCs, where it alters hemoglobin to release oxygen
• This reduced hemoglobin, which is strongly alkaline, picks up hydrogen ions and carbon dioxide and removes them from the serum
• As respiratory mechanisms fail, rising $PaCO_2$ stimulates the kidneys to retain bicarbonate and sodium and to excrete hydrogen
• As a result, more sodium bicarbonate is available to buffer free hydrogen; some hydrogen is excreted in the form of ammonium ion, neutralizing ammonia, which is an important CNS toxin
• As the hydrogen concentration overwhelms compensatory mechanisms, hydrogen moves into the cells and potassium moves out
• Without enough oxygen, anaerobic metabolism produces lactic acid; electrolyte imbalances and acidosis critically depress neurologic and cardiac functions

Causes
• Drugs (opioids, general anesthesia, hypnotics, alcohol, sedatives, and some of the new "designer" drugs, such as MCMA [or "ecstasy"]) that decrease the sensitivity of the respiratory center
• CNS trauma (injury to the medulla may impair ventilatory drive)
• Cardiac arrest (acute)

Key facts about respiratory acidosis
• Characterized by reduced alveolar ventilation
• Causes carbon dioxide level to rise in all tissues and fluids, releasing hydrogen and stimulating medulla to increase respiratory drive
• Leads to electrolyte imbalances and acidosis that depress neurologic and cardiac function

Common causes of respiratory acidosis
• Drugs
• CNS trauma
• Cardiac arrest

- Sleep apnea
- Chronic metabolic alkalosis as respiratory compensatory mechanisms try to normalize pH by decreasing alveolar ventilation
- Ventilation therapy
    - High-flow oxygen in patients with chronic respiratory disorders (suppresses hypoxic drive to breathe)
    - High positive end-expiratory pressure (PEEP) in the presence of reduced cardiac output (may cause hypercapnia)
- Neuromuscular diseases in which respiratory muscles can't respond properly to respiratory drive (such as myasthenia gravis, Guillain-Barré syndrome, and poliomyelitis)
- Airway obstruction or parenchymal lung disease (interferes with alveolar ventilation)
- Chronic obstructive pulmonary disease (COPD) or asthma
- Severe adult respiratory distress syndrome (reduced pulmonary blood flow and poor exchange of carbon dioxide and oxygen between the lungs and blood)
- Chronic bronchitis
- Large pneumothorax
- Extensive pneumonia
- Pulmonary edema

Pathophysiologic changes

- Restlessness, confusion, apprehension, somnolence, fine or flapping tremor (asterixis), coma, or headaches; dyspnea and tachypnea; papilledema; depressed reflexes; hypoxemia, unless the patient is receiving oxygen; tachycardia; atrial and ventricular arrhythmias; hypertension; hypotension with vasodilation (bounding pulses and warm periphery, in severe acidosis) due to cerebral edema and depressed CNS activity (from dilation of cerebral blood vessels and increased blood flow to brain)

Complications

- Profound CNS and cardiovascular deterioration
- Myocardial depression (leading to shock and cardiac arrest)
- Elevated $PaCO_2$ despite optimal treatment (in chronic lung disease)

Diagnostic test findings

- ABG analysis shows $PaCO_2$ greater than 45 mm Hg; pH less than 7.35; and normal bicarbonate in the acute stage and elevated bicarbonate in the chronic stage (confirm the diagnosis)
- Additional blood testing reveals serum potassium greater than 5 mEq/L and low serum chloride
- Chest X-ray detects such causes as heart failure, pneumonia, COPD, and pneumothorax
- Urinalysis reveals acidic urine pH (as the kidneys excrete hydrogen to return blood pH to normal)
- Drug screening may confirm suspected drug overdose

Treatment

- Removal of a foreign body from the airway
- Artificial airway through endotracheal intubation or tracheotomy and mechanical ventilation (if unable to breathe spontaneously)

Key treatments for respiratory acidosis

- Artificial airway
- I.V. sodium bicarbonate with oxygen
- Bronchodilators
- PEEP

Key nursing considerations for respiratory acidosis

- Stay alert for changes in respiratory, CNS, and cardiovascular function.
- Maintain patent airway and provide adequate humidification if acidosis requires mechanical ventilation.
- Closely monitor patients with COPD and chronic carbon dioxide retention for signs of acidosis.
- Closely monitor all patients receiving opioids and sedatives.

- Careful use of sodium bicarbonate I.V. with oxygen or mechanical ventilation to increase the partial pressure of arterial oxygen (PaO_2) to at least 60 mm Hg and to increase pH above 7.2 to avoid cardiac arrhythmias
- Aerosolized or I.V. bronchodilators to open constricted airways
- Antibiotics to treat pneumonia
- Chest tubes to correct pneumothorax
- PEEP to prevent alveolar collapse
- Thrombolytic or anticoagulant therapy for massive pulmonary emboli
- Bronchoscopy to remove excessive retained secretions
- Treatment for COPD
    - Bronchodilators
    - Oxygen at low flow rates, generally 2 L/minute or less (increasing oxygen supplementation higher than the patient's prescribed rate may remove the hypoxic drive, further reducing alveolar ventilation)
    - Corticosteroids
    - Gradual reduction in $PaCO_2$ to baseline to provide sufficient chloride and potassium ions to enhance renal excretion of bicarbonate (in chronic respiratory acidosis)
- Other treatments
    - Drug therapy for such conditions as myasthenia gravis
    - Dialysis or charcoal to remove toxic drugs
    - Correction of metabolic alkalosis
    - Careful administration of I.V. sodium bicarbonate

Nursing considerations
- Stay alert for critical changes in the patient's respiratory, CNS, and cardiovascular functions; immediately report such changes as well as any variations in ABG levels or electrolyte status
- Maintain adequate hydration
- **Maintain a patent airway and provide adequate humidification if acidosis requires mechanical ventilation**
    - Perform tracheal suctioning regularly and vigorous chest physiotherapy if ordered
    - Continuously monitor ventilator settings and respiratory status
- Closely monitor patients with COPD and chronic carbon dioxide retention for signs of acidosis (to prevent respiratory acidosis); administer oxygen at low flow rates
- Closely monitor all patients receiving opioids and sedatives
- Instruct the patient who has received general anesthesia to turn, cough, and perform deep-breathing exercises frequently to prevent the onset of respiratory acidosis

RESPIRATORY ALKALOSIS

Definition
- Acid-base disturbance characterized by a $PaCO_2$ less than 35 mm Hg and blood pH greater than 7.45
- Most common acid-base disturbance in critically ill patients
- Caused by alveolar hyperventilation

- Hypocapnia (below-normal $PaCO_2$) occurs when the lungs eliminate more carbon dioxide than the cells produce

● Underlying pathophysiology

- When pulmonary ventilation increases more than needed to maintain normal carbon dioxide levels, excessive amounts of carbon dioxide are exhaled
- The consequent hypocapnia leads to a chemical reduction of carbonic acid, excretion of hydrogen and bicarbonate, and a rising pH
- In defense against the increasing serum pH, the hydrogen-potassium buffer system pulls hydrogen out of the cells and into the blood in exchange for potassium
- The hydrogen entering the blood combines with available bicarbonate to form carbonic acid, and the pH falls
- Hypocapnia stimulates the carotid and aortic bodies as well as the medulla, increasing the heart rate (which hypokalemia can further aggravate) but not elevating blood pressure
- At the same time, hypocapnia causes cerebral vasoconstriction and decreased cerebral blood flow; it also overexcites the medulla, pons, and other parts of the autonomic nervous system
- When hypocapnia lasts longer than 6 hours, the kidneys secrete more bicarbonate and less hydrogen; full renal adaptation to respiratory alkalosis requires normal volume status and renal function (may take several days)
- Continued low $PaCO_2$ and the vasoconstriction it causes increases cerebral and peripheral hypoxia
- Severe alkalosis inhibits calcium ionization; as calcium becomes unavailable, nerves and muscles become progressively more excitable
- Eventually, alkalosis overwhelms the CNS and heart, leading to tetany, seizures, and cardiac arrhythmias

● Causes

- Pulmonary
  - Severe hypoxemia
  - Pneumonia
  - Interstitial lung disease
  - Pulmonary vascular disease
  - Acute asthma
  - Hyperventilation
- Nonpulmonary
  - Anxiety
  - Fever
  - Aspirin toxicity
  - Metabolic acidosis
  - CNS disease (inflammation or tumor)
  - Sepsis
  - Hepatic failure
  - Pregnancy

● Pathophysiologic changes

- Deep, rapid breathing (possibly more than 40 breaths/minute and much like the Kussmaul's respirations that characterize diabetic acidosis), usually caus-

---

Key facts about respiratory alkalosis

- Characterized by $PaCO_2$ less than 35 mm Hg and blood pH greater than 7.45
- Caused by alveolar hyperventilation
- Leads to hypocapnia, which stimulates carotid and aortic bodies and medulla to increase heart rate and causes cerebral vasoconstriction and decreased cerebral blood flow
- Leads to tetany, seizures, and cardiac arrhythmias

Common causes of respiratory alkalosis

- Severe hypoxemia
- Fever
- Aspirin toxicity
- CNS disease

Key pathophysiologic changes in respiratory alkalosis

- Deep, rapid breathing
- Light-headedness or dizziness
- Agitation

ing CNS and neuromuscular disturbances (cardinal sign of respiratory alkalosis) due to hypoxemia
- Light-headedness or dizziness due to decreased cerebral blood flow
- Agitation; circumoral and peripheral paresthesias; carpopedal spasms, twitching (possibly progressing to tetany), and muscle weakness due to decreased cerebral blood flow and CNS excitability

● Complications
- Cardiac arrhythmias that may not respond to conventional treatment as the hemoglobin-oxygen buffer system becomes overwhelmed
- Hypocalcemic tetany; seizures
- Periods of apnea if pH remains high and $Paco_2$ remains low

● Diagnostic test findings
- ABG analysis shows $Paco_2$ less than 35 mm Hg; elevated pH in proportion to the decrease in $Paco_2$ in the acute stage (but decreasing toward normal in the chronic stage); normal bicarbonate in the acute stage but less than normal in the chronic stage (confirms respiratory alkalosis and rules out respiratory compensation for metabolic acidosis)
- Serum electrolyte studies detect metabolic disorders causing compensatory respiratory alkalosis, such as a low serum chloride level
- ECG may indicate cardiac arrhythmias
- Toxicology screening may reveal salicylate poisoning
- Urinalysis reveals alkaline urine pH as kidneys excrete bicarbonate to raise blood pH

● Treatment
- Removal of ingested toxins, such as salicylates, by inducing emesis or using gastric lavage
- Treatment of fever or sepsis
- Oxygen for acute hypoxemia
- Treatment of CNS disease
- Having patient breathe into a paper bag to increase carbon dioxide and help relieve anxiety (for hyperventilation caused by severe anxiety)
- Adjustment of tidal volume and minute ventilation (according to ABG results) in patients on mechanical ventilation to prevent hyperventilation

● Nursing considerations
- Watch for and report changes in neurologic, neuromuscular, or cardiovascular function
- Watch for twitching and cardiac arrhythmias (may be associated with alkalemia and electrolyte imbalances)
- Monitor ABG and serum electrolyte levels closely, reporting any variations immediately
- Explain diagnostic tests and procedures to reduce anxiety

NCLEX CHECKS

It's never too soon to begin your licensure examination preparation. Now that you've reviewed this chapter, carefully read each of the following questions and choose the best answer. Then compare your responses to the correct answers.

1. One cause of fluid shift that leads to hypovolemia is:
- [ ] **1.** excessive diuretic therapy.
- [x] **2.** hip fracture.
- [ ] **3.** excessive laxative use.
- [ ] **4.** dysphagia.

2. The best indicator for ECF volume excess is:
- [x] **1.** acute weight gain.
- [ ] **2.** edema.
- [ ] **3.** moist skin.
- [ ] **4.** dyspnea.

3. A patient reports to the emergency department complaining of anorexia for 3 days that has now progressed to nausea and vomiting. She states she has been taking an antibiotic for 5 days and drinking 12 glasses of water a day because of a urinary tract infection. The nurse would expect to see which result of electrolyte testing?
- [ ] **1.** A serum chloride level of 102 mEq/L
- [ ] **2.** A serum potassium level of 4.2 mEq/L
- [x] **3.** A serum sodium level of less than 135 mEq/L
- [ ] **4.** A serum carbon dioxide level of 26 mEq/L

4. A patient is taking digoxin (Digitek, Lanoxin) daily for chronic atrial fibrillation. For what disorder should he be closely monitored?
- [ ] **1.** Hyponatremia
- [ ] **2.** Hypernatremia
- [x] **3.** Hypokalemia
- [ ] **4.** Hyperkalemia

5. An ECG showing a tall, tented T wave and widened QRS complex could be an indication of:
- [ ] **1.** hypokalemia.
- [ ] **2.** hyperkalemia.
- [ ] **3.** hypocalcemia.
- [ ] **4.** hypercalcemia.

6. The electrolyte that plays a major role in cell membrane permeability is:
- [ ] **1.** sodium.
- [ ] **2.** potassium.
- [ ] **3.** chloride.
- [ ] **4.** calcium.

7. A patient admitted to the hospital has low blood pressure, positive Chvostek's and Trousseau's signs, slightly elevated calcium and a low magnesium level, confusion, leg and foot cramping, and hyperreflexia. I.V. magnesium replacement is ordered. How should the nurse intervene?

TOP 4

Items to study for your next test on fluid and electrolyte disorders

1. Common diagnostic tests for fluid and electrolyte disorders, such as ABG analysis and serum electrolytes

2. Pathophysiologic changes involved in fluid and electrolyte imbalances

3. Treatments and nursing considerations for disorders such as metabolic alkalosis, respiratory acidosis, hypovolemia, and hypokalemia

4. Key facts about acidosis and alkalosis

☐ **1.** Monitor for bradycardia, heart block, and decreased respiratory rate.
☐ **2.** Have I.V. phosphate on hand to reverse an overreplacement of magnesium.
☐ **3.** Restrict fluids to decrease urine output.
☐ **4.** Monitor for muscle weakness and flaccidity.

8. A patient in the emergency department reports that he has been vomiting excessively for the past 2 days. His ABG analysis shows a pH of 7.49, $PaCO_2$ of 42 mm Hg, PaO_2 of 75 mm Hg, and bicarbonate of 40 mEq/L. Place these steps in the correct order to show the pathophysiologic pathway of metabolic alkalosis.

Unordered options:

1. As serum bicarbonate rises to 28 mEq/L or more, the kidneys are unable to reabsorb the excess ion produced in filtration and it is excreted in the urine while hydrogen ions are retained.

2. Hydrogen ions are lost as stomach acid is vomited.

3. Sodium and water are excreted in the urine to maintain electrochemical balance.

4. Excess bicarbonate is neutralized by chemical buffers in the extracellular and intracellular fluid.

5. Intracellular hydrogen ions diffuse back into the ECF with resultant calcium ion decrease, so nerve cells become permeable to sodium, triggering nerve impulses and resulting in muscle twitching and confusion.

6. Bicarbonate begins to accumulate again, causing chemoreceptors for respiration to depress breathing rate in an effort to retain more carbon dioxide that will combine with water to neutralize the bicarbonate ion into weak carbonic acid.

7. Extracellular potassium moves into cells to maintain the balance of positive charge across the cell membrane caused by decreased hydrogen in the ECF, with resultant cardiac irritability.

Ordered responses:

9. A patient with excessive, prolonged vomiting and metabolic alkalosis will demonstrate many electrolyte disturbances. What change would you expect in the serum potassium level?

- ☐ **1.** Decrease
- ☐ **2.** Increase
- ☐ **3.** Normal
- ☐ **4.** Unchanged

10. Treatment of respiratory acidosis for a patient with COPD includes:

- ☐ **1.** increased oxygen flow rate.
- ☐ **2.** decreased oxygen flow rate.
- ☐ **3.** sedation.
- ☐ **4.** restricting fluid intake.

ANSWERS AND RATIONALES

1. CORRECT ANSWER: 2

A patient with a hip fracture may have a fluid shift of 1.5 to 2 L of blood that accumulates in tissues around the fracture, which can lead to hypovolemia. The excessive diuretic therapy, excessive laxative use, and dysphagia with decreased fluid intake are all causes of loss of fluid but not of internal shifting of fluids.

2. CORRECT ANSWER: 1

Acute weight gain due to increased volume of total-body fluid from circulatory overload is the best indicator of ECF excess. Edema represents fluid shifting from the plasma to the interstitial spaces. Moist skin indicates the body's attempt to rid itself of excess fluid, and dyspnea is found as fluid accumulates in the pleural spaces.

3. CORRECT ANSWER: 3

Serum sodium levels less than 135 mEq/L indicate hyponatremia — in this patient's case, from probable overhydration. All of the other laboratory values are within the reference range.

4. CORRECT ANSWER: 3

Patients taking a cardiac glycoside should be closely monitored for hypokalemia, which can potentiate the action of the cardiac glycoside and cause toxicity. Sodium balance and excess potassium levels don't affect the action of cardiac glycosides.

5. CORRECT ANSWER: 2

An ECG showing a tall, tented T wave and a widened QRS complex (as well as a prolonged PR interval, flattened or absent P waves, or a depressed ST segment) indicates potassium levels greater than 5 mEq/L. Low potassium levels are characterized by a flattened T wave and a depressed ST segment and U wave. Changes in calcium levels are associated with neuromuscular excitability when the level is high, and with neuromuscular depression when the level is low.

6. CORRECT ANSWER: 4

Calcium helps to maintain cell structure and function and plays a role in cell membrane permeability and impulse transmission. Potassium is primarily found outside the cells; sodium and chloride, inside the cells.

7. CORRECT ANSWER: 1

Adverse effects of excessively rapid magnesium infusion include bradycardia, heart block, and hypoventilation. The antidote is calcium gluconate I.V., not phosphate. Intake and output should be monitored, but fluids shouldn't be restricted because renal insufficiency could lead to overretention of magnesium. Tetany and muscular hyperirritability, not flaccidity and weakness, are hallmarks of hypomagnesemia.

8. CORRECT ANSWER:

2. Hydrogen ions are lost as stomach acid is vomited.

4. Excess bicarbonate is neutralized by chemical buffers in the extracellular and intracellular fluid.

6. Bicarbonate begins to accumulate again, causing chemoreceptors for respiration to depress breathing rate in an effort to retain more carbon dioxide that will combine with water to neutralize the bicarbonate ion into weak carbonic acid.

1. As serum bicarbonate rises to 28 mEq/L or more, the kidneys are unable to reabsorb the excess ion produced in filtration and it is excreted in the urine while hydrogen ions are retained.

3. Sodium and water are excreted in the urine to maintain electrochemical balance.

7. Extracellular potassium moves into cells to maintain the balance of positive charge across the cell membrane caused by decreased hydrogen in the ECF, with resultant cardiac irritability.

5. Intracellular hydrogen ions diffuse back into the ECF with resultant calcium ion decrease, so nerve cells become permeable to sodium, triggering nerve impulses and resulting in muscle twitching and confusion.

Metabolic alkalosis develops as listed above in the presence of excessive vomiting. It is caused by the failure of the kidneys and lungs to compensate for excessive hydrogen loss.

9. CORRECT ANSWER: 1

In patients with metabolic alkalosis, serum potassium levels are low, as are serum calcium and chloride levels. Serum potassium levels are low as a result of potassium ions moving into cells as hydrogen ions diffuse passively out of cells in response to low hydrogen levels in ECF.

10. CORRECT ANSWER: 2

Oxygen should be delivered at low flow rates because increasing oxygen beyond the COPD patient's normal oxygen level removes the hypoxic drive, or brain signals stimulating breathing. This stimulation further reduces alveolar ventilation. Sedation may cause hypoventilation, a contributing factor to respiratory acidosis. Fluid restriction has no effect on COPD.

14

Neoplasms

LEARNING OBJECTIVES

After studying this chapter, you should be able to:

- Describe the relationship between presenting signs and symptoms, and the pathophysiologic changes for any type of neoplasm.
- List three probable causes of neoplasm development.
- Describe interventions for a patient with a neoplasm.
- Write three teaching goals for a patient with a neoplasm.
- Identify classes of medications that may improve or control neoplasms.

CHAPTER OVERVIEW

Neoplasms refer to a group of more than 100 different diseases that are characterized by deoxyribonucleic acid (DNA) damage that causes abnormal cell growth and development. Malignant cells have two defining characteristics: they can no longer divide and differentiate normally, and they have acquired the ability to invade surrounding tissues and travel to distant sites.

Caring for a patient with a neoplasm requires an understanding of the pathophysiologic changes that occur, the signs and symptoms these changes display, and the appropriate ways to intervene. The first section of this chapter provides an overview of key pathophysiologic concepts related to neoplasms. Common neoplasms are then defined, and underlying pathophysiology, causes, pathophysiologic changes, complications, diagnostic test findings, treatments, and nursing considerations are outlined.

PATHOPHYSIOLOGIC CONCEPTS

● Abnormal cell growth
- Controls for cell growth are absent in cancer cells; cell production exceeds cell loss
- Cancer cells enter the cell cycle more frequently and at different rates than do normal cells; they're most commonly found in the synthesis and mitosis phases of the cell cycle, and they spend little time in the resting phase
- Chemical mediators (called *cytokines*) released by injured or infected nearby cells also affect cellular reproduction
  - Interleukin stimulates production of natural killer cells
  - Interferon may affect cell reproduction rate
- Cells in close proximity communicate with one another through gap junctions (channels through which ions and other small molecules pass)
  - Allows for density-dependent growth inhibition (formation of only a single layer of cells) in healthy tissue
- Control genes fail to function normally; imbalance of growth factors may occur, or the cells may fail to respond to the suppressive action of the growth factors
- Control genes fail to recognize signals (about available tissue space) emitted by nearby cells

● Anaplasia
- Anaplasia is the lost ability of a cell to differentiate, resemble the original cell, function, and die like the original cell
- It occurs in varying degrees; some cancer cells begin functioning as other types of cells, possibly becoming sites for hormone production
- Cancer cells look like other cancer cells, not the tissue from which they arose
- Cell mitosis is abnormal, and chromosome defects are common

● Intracellular changes
- Abnormal and uncontrolled proliferation of cancer cells is associated with numerous changes within the cancer cell itself
  - Cell membrane fibronectin (large glycoproteins that normally hold cells in place) is defective or broken down as it's produced
    - Affects cell organization, structure, adhesion, and migration, leading to metastasis
    - Affects the density of the receptors on the cell membrane and the cell's shape; communication between cells becomes impaired, resulting in uncontrolled growth
    - Permeability of the cell membrane is altered
  - Functions of cytoskeleton components are altered
    - Cytoskeleton is composed of protein filament networks, including actin and microtubules
    - Microtubules control cell shape, movement, and division
    - Microtubules become abnormally shaped and can no longer support the structure of the cell
  - Cytoplasmic components are fewer in number and abnormally shaped
    - Less cellular work occurs because of a decrease in endoplasmic reticulum and mitochondria

Key facts about abnormal cell growth
- May result from absence of cell growth controls, failure of control genes to function normally, or failure of control genes to recognize signals about available tissue space
- May involve cytokines, which are released by injured or infected nearby cells and affect cellular reproduction

Key facts about anaplasia
- Refers to cell's inability to differentiate, resemble the original cell, function, and die like the original cell
- Causes abnormal cell mitosis and chromosome defects

Key facts about intracellular changes
- Refer to changes within a cancer cell

TOP 4
Intracellular changes
1. Cell membrane fibronectin is defective
2. Functions of cytoskeleton components are altered
3. Cytoplasmic components are fewer in number and abnormally shaped
4. Nuclei in cancer cells are pleomorphic

- Nuclei in cancer cells are pleomorphic (enlarged and of various shapes and sizes)
    - Nuclear membrane is irregular and has projections, pouches or blebs, and fewer pores
    - Chromatin (uncoiled chromosomes) may clump along the outer areas of the nucleus
    - Chromosome defects stem from increased mitotic rate

● **Tumor growth**

- Tumor growth depends on specific characteristics of the tumor and the host; initiating events include exposure to chemicals, viruses, radiation, smoking, and ultraviolet (UV) rays
    - Conditions needed for tumor growth
        - Initiating event causes DNA mutation that will transform normal cell to cancer cell
        - Tumor continues to grow if available nutrients, oxygen, and blood supply are adequate and if immune system fails to recognize or respond to tumor
    - Effect of tumor characteristics
        - Tumor location determines cell cycle time
        - Degree of anaplasia affects tumor growth; the more anaplastic the tumor's cells, the less differentiated the cells and the more rapidly they divide
    - Host characteristics
        - Advanced age
        - Gender
        - Early sexual activity (cervical cancer)
        - Overall health and nutritional status
        - Immune system function
        - Ethnicity

● **Tumor promotion**
- Factors that enhance cancer cell growth
    - Hormones such as estrogen, which affects breast cancer cells exposed to it

---

GO WITH THE FLOW

How cancer metastasizes

Metastasis usually occurs through the bloodstream to other organs and tissues, as described here.

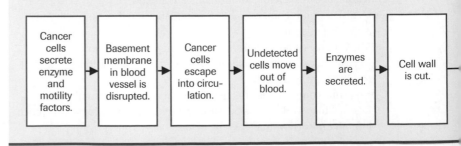

| Cancer cells secrete enzyme and motility factors. | Basement membrane in blood vessel is disrupted. | Cancer cells escape into circulation. | Undetected cells move out of blood. | Enzymes are secreted. | Cell wall is cut. |

- Food additives, such as nitrates in processed meats and soots and tars in smoked meats
- Drugs, such as nicotine in cigarettes and diethylstilbestrol (DES)
- Industrial agents, such as asbestos, benzene, carbon tetrachloride, vinyl chloride, and many insecticides and pesticides

● Tumor spread

- Dysplasia (changes in the size, shape, and organization of the cells)
  - Caused by exposure to chemicals, viruses, radiation, or chronic inflammation
  - May be reversed by removing the initiating stimulus or treating its effects
- Localized tumor
  - Initially remains localized
  - Cancer cells communicate poorly with nearby cells
  - Tumor angiogenesis factor secreted by macrophages: Stimulates neovascularization in the stroma of tumors but not in healthy cells nearby
  - Tumor continues to grow, exerting pressure on neighboring cells, blocking blood supply, and subsequently causing the normal cells' death
- Invasive tumor
  - Growth of tumor into surrounding tissue
  - Five mechanisms linked to invasion
    - Cellular multiplication
    - Mechanical pressure
    - Lysis of nearby cells
    - Reduced cell adhesions
    - Increased motility
- Metastatic tumor
  - Tumors in which cancer cells have traveled from the original or primary site to a second or more distant site
  - Occurs through the blood vessels and lymphatic system
  - Also can be transported from one body location to another by external means, such as by instruments or gloves during surgery (see *How cancer metastasizes*)

Key facts about tumor spread

- Dysplasia: Changes in size, shape, and organization of cells
- Localized: Tumor grows, exerts pressure on, and kills neighboring normal cells
- Invasive: Tumor grows into surrounding tissue
- Metastatic: Cancer cells travel from primary site to more distant site through blood vessels and lymphatic system or by external means

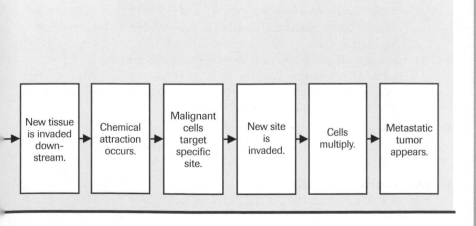

New tissue is invaded downstream. → Chemical attraction occurs. → Malignant cells target specific site. → New site is invaded. → Cells multiply. → Metastatic tumor appears.

Key facts about basal cell carcinoma

- Is a slow-growing, destructive skin tumor
- May develop from undifferentiated basal cells that become carcinomatous instead of differentiating into sweat glands, sebum, and hair

Key pathophysiologic changes in basal cell carcinoma

- Small, smooth, pinkish or darkly pigmented lesions (nodular ulcerative lesions)
- Oval or irregularly shaped, lightly pigmented plaques (superficial form)
- Waxy, sclerotic, yellow-to-white plaques (sclerosing form)

Key diagnostic test results for basal cell carcinoma

- Biopsy and histology: May determine the tumor type and histologic subtype

BASAL CELL CARCINOMA

- ● **Definition**
  - Slow-growing, destructive skin tumor; also called *basal cell epithelioma*
  - Accounts for more than 75% of all nonmelanoma skin cancers and 50% of all cancers
  - Changes in epidermal basal cells can diminish maturation and normal keratinization; continuing division of basal cells leads to mass formation

- ● **Underlying pathophysiology**
  - Although the pathogenesis is uncertain, some experts hypothesize that basal cell carcinoma originates from undifferentiated basal cells becoming carcinomatous instead of differentiating into sweat glands, sebum, and hair

- ● **Causes**
  - Prolonged sun exposure (most common)
  - Arsenic, radiation exposure, burns, immunosuppression, vaccinations (rare)

- ● **Pathophysiologic changes**
  - Nodular ulcerative lesions
  - Appear most commonly on the face (forehead, eyelid margins, nasolabial folds)
    - Early stages: Lesions are small, smooth, pinkish or darkly pigmented (in dark-skinned people), translucent papules; telangiectatic vessels cross skin surface; lesions are occasionally pigmented (due to unrepaired mutations in skin cells)
    - As lesions enlarge: Depressed center with firm, elevated borders due to unrepaired mutations in skin cells
    - Ulcerations and local invasion: Rodent ulcers (chronic, persisting ulcers that spread locally) eventually appear due to unrepaired mutations in skin cells; rarely metastasize, but if untreated can spread to other nearby tissues and become infected, possibly causing massive hemorrhage if large blood vessels are invaded
  - Superficial basal cell carcinoma
    - Can be numerous; commonly occur on chest and back
    - Oval or irregularly shaped, lightly pigmented plaques with sharply defined, slightly elevated, threadlike borders (due to unrepaired mutations in skin cells)
    - Superficial erosion: lesions appear red and scaly and have small, atrophic areas in center, resembling psoriasis or eczema (due to unrepaired mutation in skin cells)
  - Sclerosing basal cell carcinoma (morphea-like epitheliomas)
    - Occur on head and neck
    - Lesions: Waxy, sclerotic, yellow-to-white plaques without distinct borders (due to unrepaired mutations in skin cells)

- ● **Complications**
  - Disfigurement of eye, nose, and other structures around tumor site
  - Possible enucleation

- ● **Diagnostic test findings**
  - Incisional or excisional biopsy and histology may help to determine the tumor type and histologic subtype

Treatment
- Curettage and electrodesiccation to remove small lesions (offers good cosmetic results)
- Mohs' micrographic surgery (formerly known as *Mohs' chemosurgery*) to excise horizontal layers of the tumor and examine them microscopically, identifying cancer-free borders until all cancer cells are removed
    - Highest cure rate with least amount of damage to normal skin
    - Skin grafting may be needed after removal of large lesions
- Irradiation to eradicate the tumor; use depends on tumor location and patient status (if elderly, debilitated, or unable to withstand surgery, may be better candidate for irradiation)
- Cryotherapy (with liquid nitrogen) to freeze and kill cancerous cells
- Localized chemotherapy for persistent or recurrent lesions or for those not amenable to other treatments, such as application of topical imiquimod (Aldara) or fluorouracil (Efudex, Carac) for superficial lesions, and injection of nodular lesions with interferon alfa-2b (Intron A)

Nursing considerations
- Instruct the patient to avoid excessive sun exposure and to use a sunscreen or sunshade with a sun protection factor (SPF) of 15 or higher to protect skin from damage by UV rays
- Advise the patient to relieve local inflammation from topical fluorouracil with cool compresses or corticosteroid ointment
- Teach the patient to wash the skin gently if ulcerations and crusting occur; scrubbing too vigorously may cause bleeding
- Encourage the patient to have a dermatologist check all skin at least once per year to detect other areas of skin cancer

MALIGNANT MELANOMA

Definition
- Neoplasm that arises from melanocytes; up to 70% arise from a preexisting nevus (circumscribed deformity of the skin with either increased pigmentation or increased vascularity)
- Characterized by enlargement of skin lesion or nevus accompanied by changes in color or texture, or by inflammation, soreness, itching, ulceration, or bleeding
- Common sites: head and neck (men), legs (women), and back (those exposed to excessive sunlight)
- Classified as superficial spreading melanoma, nodular malignant melanoma, lentigo maligna melanoma, and acral-lentiginous melanoma

Underlying pathophysiology
- Melanomas arise as a result of malignant degeneration of melanocytes located either along the basal layer of the epidermis or in a benign melanocytic nevus
- The melanoma spreads through the lymphatic and vascular systems and metastasizes to the regional lymph nodes, skin, liver, lungs, and central nervous system (CNS)
- Malignant melanoma follows an unpredictable course; recurrence and metastasis may not appear for more than 5 years after resection of the primary lesion

Key pathophysiologic changes in malignant melanoma

- Superficial spreading: Red, white, and blue color over brown or black background
- Nodular: Polyplike nodule with uniformly dark discoloration
- Lentigo: Large, flat freckle of tan, brown, black, whitish, or slate color, with black nodules
- Acral-lentiginous: Irregular, enlarging black macule on palms and soles

Key diagnostic test results for malignant melanoma

- Excisional biopsy and full-depth punch biopsy with histologic examination: Determine tumor thickness and disease type

Key treatments for malignant melanoma

- Surgical resection
- Chemotherapy or immunotherapy
- Radiation therapy

● **Causes**
- UV rays damage skin and can cause malignant melanoma
- Risk factors
  - Excessive exposure to sunlight
  - Fair complexion
  - Personal or family history of melanoma
  - Increased age, particularly older than age 60
  - Preexisting multiple moles, atypical nevi, or a changing nevus

● **Pathophysiologic changes**
- Superficial spreading melanoma
  - Most common type
  - Red, white, and blue color over a brown or black background; irregular, notched margin; larger than 6 mm
- Nodular melanoma
  - Polyplike nodule with uniformly dark discoloration appearing as a blackberry, but possibly flesh colored with flecks of pigment around base (due to mutation in melanin-producing cells of skin)
- Lentigo maligna melanoma
  - Large, flat freckle of tan, brown, black, whitish, or slate color, with irregularly scattered black nodules on surface (due to mutation in melanin-producing cells of skin)
- Acral-lentiginous melanoma
  - Develops as irregular, enlarging black macule occurring mainly on palms and soles (due to mutation in melanin-producing cells of skin)

● **Complications**
- Metastasis to the lungs, liver, or brain

● **Diagnostic test findings**
- Complete blood count (CBC) with differential may reveal anemia if bone metastasis has occurred
- Platelet count and liver function studies are abnormal if metastasis to the liver has occurred
- Serum S-100 protein level may serve as tumor marker in patients with metastasis
- Chest X-rays, computed tomography (CT) and positron emission tomography (PET) scanning, and magnetic resonance imaging (MRI) assist in staging if metastasis is suspected (otherwise, not routinely ordered)
- Excisional biopsy and full-depth punch biopsy with histologic examination show tumor thickness and reveal disease type

● **Treatment**
- Surgical resection to remove tumor (extent of resection depends on size and location of primary tumor; may require skin graft)
- Regional lymphadenectomy to help prevent metastasis and check for spread
- Chemotherapy or immunotherapy to eliminate or reduce number of tumor cells in deeper lesions
- Radiation therapy or gene therapy for metastatic disease
- Long-term follow-up to detect metastasis and recurrences
- Patient teaching with recommended use of sunscreen with SPF of 15 or higher to help prevent recurrence

Nursing considerations

- Tell the patient what to expect before and after surgery
  - Tell him what the wound will look like and what type of dressing he'll have
  - Prepare him for donor site pain (for skin grafting), which may be as painful as the tumor excision site, if not more so
- Take steps to prevent infection after surgery
  - Check dressings often for excessive drainage, foul odor, redness, or swelling
  - If surgery included lymphadenectomy, minimize lymphedema by applying a compression stocking and instructing the patient to keep the extremity elevated
- Prepare for adverse effects of chemotherapy, and take appropriate measures to minimize them
- Prevent and control pain in the patient with advanced metastatic disease
  - Maintain consistent administration of regularly scheduled analgesics
  - Make referrals for home care and social services as needed

Key nursing considerations for malignant melanoma

- Take steps to prevent infection after surgery.
- Prevent and control pain in patient.

SQUAMOUS CELL CARCINOMA

Definition

- Invasive tumor with metastatic potential that arises from keratinizing epidermal cells
- Occurs most commonly in fair-skinned, white men over age 60

Underlying pathophysiology

- Transformation from a premalignant lesion to squamous cell carcinoma may begin with induration and inflammation of an existing lesion
- When squamous cell carcinoma arises from normal skin, the nodule grows slowly on a firm, indurated base; if untreated, this nodule eventually ulcerates and invades underlying tissues

Causes

- Unknown in some cases
- Damage from solar UV (actinic) radiation
- Ionizing radiation
- Chemical carcinogens (pesticides, benzene, rubber by-products)
- Risk factors
  - Overexposure to UV rays
  - Radiation therapy
  - Ingestion of herbicides containing arsenic
  - Chronic skin irritation and inflammation
  - Exposure to local carcinogens (such as tar and oil)
  - Hereditary diseases (such as xeroderma pigmentosum and albinism)

Pathophysiologic changes

- Nodule with firm, indurated base (due to mutation in keratinizing epidermal cells of skin)
- Early lesions: scaling and ulceration of opaque, firm nodules with indistinct borders; may appear on face, ear, dorsa of hand and forehead, or other sun-damaged area (resulting from inflammation and induration of lesion)

Key facts about squamous cell carcinoma

- Is invasive and potentially metastatic
- Begins with induration and inflammation of existing lesion
- Grows slowly

Key pathophysiologic changes in squamous cell carcinoma

- Nodule with firm, indurated base
- Scaling and ulceration of opaque, firm nodules (early lesions)

Key diagnostic test results for squamous cell carcinoma

- Excisional biopsy: Definitive diagnosis

Key treatments for squamous cell carcinoma

- Surgical excision
- Electrodesiccation and curettage

Key nursing considerations for squamous cell carcinoma

- Keep wound dry and clean.
- Teach patient to avoid excessive sun exposure, wear protective clothing, and use sunscreen.

Key facts about Hodgkin's disease

- Characterized by painless, progressive enlargement of lymph nodes, spleen, and other lymphoid tissue
- Results from proliferation of lymphocytes, histocytes, eosinophils, and Reed-Sternberg cells

- Later lesions: scaly; most common on face and hands (sun-exposed areas); lesion on lower lip or ear may indicate invasive metastasis (generally poor prognosis) caused by keratinization
- Metastatic disease: pain, malaise, fatigue, weakness, and anorexia due to metastasis to regional lymph nodes

● **Complications**
- Lymph node involvement
- Visceral metastasis

● **Diagnostic test findings**
- Excisional biopsy provides a definitive diagnosis

● **Treatment**
- Surgical excision to remove lesion
- Electrodesiccation and curettage to remove lesion (good cosmetic results for smaller lesions)
- Radiation therapy to reduce lesion (generally for elderly or debilitated patients who may be poor surgical candidates)
- Mohs' micrographic surgery to systematically remove cancer cells using identification of cancer-free borders
- Topical or systemic antibiotics to alter the lesion's bacterial flora and temporarily control odor

● **Nursing considerations**
- Keep the wound dry and clean
- Prepare for problems that accompany metastatic disease (pain, fatigue, weakness, anorexia)
- Teach the patient to avoid excessive sun exposure, wear protective clothing, and use sunscreen (containing para-aminobenzoic acid, benzophenone, and zinc) and lip balm to minimize the risk of future sun damage
- Help the patient deal with disfiguring lesions; encourage him to express his feelings and concerns

HODGKIN'S DISEASE

● **Definition**
- Neoplastic disorder characterized by painless, progressive enlargement of lymph nodes, spleen, and other lymphoid tissue from proliferation of various blood cells
- Typically occurs between ages 15 and 34 or in people age 55 and older; affects more men than women

● **Underlying pathophysiology**
- Enlarged lymphoid tissue results from proliferation of lymphocytes, histocytes, eosinophils, and Reed-Sternberg cells
- Untreated Hodgkin's disease follows a variable but relentlessly progressive and ultimately fatal course (see *Teaching about coping with cancer*)
- When treated, the prognosis is usually excellent for long-term remission or cure

● **Causes**
- Cause commonly unknown

TIME-OUT FOR TEACHING

Teaching about coping with cancer

Cancer is a scary word. Even though cancer survival rates are higher than ever, patients need psychological support to channel their anxiety into useful coping skills to help them through the recovery process. For those whose cancer can't be effectively treated, support is aimed at helping the patient come to terms with the prognosis and, ultimately, to experience a death that's as comfortable and dignified as possible. Nurses are commonly on the front lines of providing this support and can do much to teach patients about their fears and help them find effective ways to deal with them.

Whether or not your patient will be a survivor, most patients will go through some of the five stages of dying, first outlined by Dr. Elisabeth Kübler Ross:

- denial
- bargaining
- anger
- depression
- acceptance.

Your first step will typically be to teach patients that the feelings they're experiencing are normal. Introduce patients to other cancer patients (particularly survivors, if possible) through one-on-one visits or a support group. Reinforce that whatever emotions they feel are acceptable and "right" for that time.

If the patient has intense anxiety, teach relaxation skills, such as deep breathing or the use of positive imagery while listening to relaxing music. Distraction is also useful: Encourage patients to read, watch movies, go for a massage, visit with friends and loved ones, bake — whatever activities have been useful to them in the past when they've been anxious. Remind them

that some anxiety is normal, but encourage them to share their fears with the physician so they can get accurate information about their disease and treatment process.

If the patient is angry, again, teach relaxation skills first. Also instruct the patient on ways to displace the anger usefully. You can illustrate how imagery can be used to characterize the cancer as the object of anger and visualize ways to "shoot it down" or fight it in some way that's meaningful to the patient. Physical activity (within each patient's capability) can also relieve anger — even just designating a certain pillow to hit when the feelings are overwhelming, instead of lashing out at a loved one, can help patients feel more in control. Researching their disease or ways to maximize their health, such as through nutrition, can also be encouraged as ways to empower them and to channel their anger-related energy into a more useful form.

If the patient is depressed, emphasize activities that have brought the patient relief in the past when life has been tough. Encourage patients to journal their feelings, especially if they regret showing a "down" face to loved ones. Relaxation techniques are also useful to help patients remove themselves for a while from the burden of sadness and to access sources of inner strength. Encourage activity and exercise (within tolerance) as another way to break through the depression. Tell patients not to hesitate to express their feelings to a supportive counselor, friend, or staff person, which can help them move through the depression and develop other coping skills.

Kübler-Ross's five stages of dying

- Denial
- Bargaining
- Anger
- Depression
- Acceptance

- Linked to Epstein-Barr virus (causes infectious mononucleosis) in about half the cases, but relationship between them is unknown
- Evidence of a genetic link in some cases

● **Pathophysiologic changes**
- Symptoms are classified according to stages I, II, III, and IV and a letter designation, A or B (see *Staging lymphomas*)
- Painless swelling in one of the lymph nodes (usually the cervical region) with a history of upper respiratory infection
- Persistent fever, night sweats, fatigue, weight loss, susceptibility to infection, and malaise related to hypermetabolic state of cellular proliferation and defective immune function
- Pruritus that becomes acute as a result of disease progression
- Extremity pain, nerve irritation, or absence of pulse due to rapid enlargement of lymph nodes
- Pericardial friction rub, pericardial effusion, and jugular vein engorgement secondary to direct invasion from mediastinal lymph nodes
- Enlargement of retroperitoneal nodes, spleen, and liver related to progression of disease and cellular infiltration

● **Complications**
- Multiple organ failure

● **Diagnostic test findings**
- Hematologic tests show mild to severe normocytic anemia; normochromic anemia in 50% of patients; elevated, normal, or reduced white blood cell (WBC) count and differential; and any combination of neutrophilia, lymphocytopenia, monocytosis, and eosinophilia
- Elevated serum alkaline phosphatase levels indicate liver or bone involvement
- CT scanning or MRI identifies sites of lymph node enlargement or metastasis to internal organs
- Lymph node biopsy is used to determine lymph node involvement; it confirms the presence of Reed-Sternberg cells, abnormal histocyte proliferation, and nodular fibrosis and necrosis
- Staging laparotomy is performed as an alternative to organ biopsy in patients younger than age 55, and in those without obvious stage III or IV disease, lymphocyte predominance subtype histology, or medical contraindications

● **Treatment**
- Determined by patient's overall health and stage of disease
  - Number of nodes involved
  - Whether involved nodes are unilateral or bilateral, and above or below the diaphragm
  - Whether the liver, bone marrow, or other organs are involved
- Radiation therapy to kill cancer cells and shrink lymphomas in stage I or II disease
- Combined radiation therapy and chemotherapy to kill cancer cells and shrink lymphomas in stage III
- Chemotherapy alone (or chemotherapy and radiation therapy to involved sites) to kill cancer cells and shrink lymphomas in stage IV disease (sometimes induces complete remission)

Staging lymphomas

Hodgkin's disease and non-Hodgkin's lymphoma are classified into stages so that treatment protocols can be established and outcomes predicted. The Ann Arbor classification system is used.

STAGES

Stage I
- Involvement of a single lymph node region

OR
- Localized involvement of a single extranodal organ or site

Stage II
- Involvement of two or more lymph node regions on the same side of the diaphragm

OR
- Localized involvement to a single associated extranodal organ or site and its regional lymph nodes with or without other lymph node regions on the same side of the diaphragm

Stage III
- Involvement of lymph node regions on both sides of the diaphragm that may also be accompanied by localized involvement of an extranodal organ or site, by involvement of the spleen, or by both

Stage IV
- Disseminated involvement of one or more extralymphatic sites with or without associated lymph node involvement

OR
- Isolated extralymphatic organ involvement with distant (nonregional) nodal involvement
  Extralymphatic sites include the liver, lungs, bone marrow, pleurae, bone, and skin as well as tissues separate from but near to major lymphatic clusters. The spleen is considered a lymphatic site.

LETTER DESIGNATION

The stages are also accompanied be a letter designation that refers to patient symptoms as follows:
- **A** means absence of the specific symptoms listed in **B** but may include other common symptoms such as pruritus.
- **B** includes the presence of at least one of the following three symptoms:
– temperature greater than 100.4° F (38° C)
– unexplained loss of more than 10% of body weight in the preceding 6 months
– drenching night sweats.

- Autologous bone marrow transplantation or autologous peripheral blood sternal transfusions and immunotherapy to treat Hodgkin's disease that's resistant to standard treatment
- Well-balanced diet to promote adequate nutritional intake (crucial during radiation and chemotherapy)
- Frequent rest periods to fight fatigue

- Psychological support to promote communication and trust and to help the patient and his family deal effectively with the diagnosis, prognosis, and treatments

● Nursing considerations

- Teach the patient to watch for and report adverse effects of radiation and chemotherapy (particularly anorexia, nausea, vomiting, diarrhea, fever, and bleeding)
- Minimize adverse effects of radiation by maintaining good nutrition (aided by eating small, frequent meals of favorite foods), drinking plenty of fluids, pacing activities to counteract therapy-induced fatigue, and keeping skin dry in irradiated areas
- Control pain and bleeding of stomatitis by using a soft toothbrush, cotton swab, or anesthetic mouthwash such as viscous lidocaine (as prescribed, not to be swallowed); applying petroleum jelly to the lips; and avoiding astringent mouthwashes
- If a female patient is of childbearing age, advise her to delay pregnancy until prolonged remission is achieved (radiation and chemotherapy can cause genetic mutations and spontaneous abortions)
- Provide emotional support
- Refer the patient and his family to the American Cancer Society for information and supportive counseling

NON-HODGKIN'S LYMPHOMA

● Definition

- One of many different subtypes of malignant lymphoma originating in lymph glands and other lymphoid tissue
- Usually found in adults over age 50; exceptions are two highly aggressive subtypes generally found in children or young adults
- Five times more common than Hodgkin's lymphoma
- Seventh most common cancer in the world
- Usually classified according to histologic, anatomic, and immunomorphic characteristics developed by the National Cancer Institute
- New, recently identified subtypes of non-Hodgkin's lymphoma, called *mantle zone lymphoma* and *marginal zone lymphoma* (see *Non-Hodgkin's lymphoma: How it happens*)

● Underlying pathophysiology

- Overproliferation of abnormal lymph cells or failure of previously normal lymph cells to die, caused by genetic mutations within the cells, many of which have been identified
- Prognosis depends on the subtype and stage and on the overall age and health of the patient
- Median survival is 5 to 10 years for patients with lowest-grade lymphomas, 2 to 5 years for intermediate-grade lymphomas, and less than 2 years for those with high-grade, aggressive lymphomas

● Causes

- Exact cause unknown
- Risk factors

- Genetic factors
- Viral factors (some subtypes linked to Epstein-Barr virus, others to hepatitis B virus, some to herpesvirus)
- Exposure to ionizing radiation and chemicals (herbicides, pesticides, benzene)

● Pathophysiologic changes
- Swollen lymph glands; enlarged tonsils and adenoids; painless, rubbery nodes in cervical supraclavicular areas due to cellular proliferation
- Dyspnea and coughing due to lymphocytic infiltration of oropharynx and thorax
- Abdominal pain and constipation due to mechanical obstruction of abdominal tissues
- Fatigue, malaise, fever, weight loss, and night sweats due to disseminated disease, and extensive tumor growth and spread to organs

● Complications
- Hypercalcemia
- Hyperuricemia
- Lymphomatosis
- Meningitis
- Anemia
- Liver, kidney, and lung problems from impingement by lymphatic tumor growth

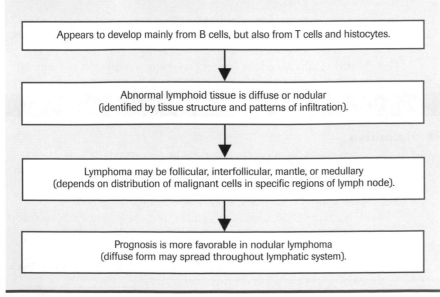

GO WITH THE FLOW

Non-Hodgkin's lymphoma: How it happens

The pathophysiology of non-Hodgkin's lymphoma is similar to that of Hodgkin's disease, but Reed-Sternberg cells aren't present.

Appears to develop mainly from B cells, but also from T cells and histocytes.

↓

Abnormal lymphoid tissue is diffuse or nodular (identified by tissue structure and patterns of infiltration).

↓

Lymphoma may be follicular, interfollicular, mantle, or medullary (depends on distribution of malignant cells in specific regions of lymph node).

↓

Prognosis is more favorable in nodular lymphoma (diffuse form may spread throughout lymphatic system).

Key diagnostic test results for non-Hodgkin's lymphoma

- CBC: Anemia, thrombocytopenia, leukopenia, and lymphocytosis
- Lymph node biopsy: Cell type
- Biopsy of tonsils, bone marrow, liver, bowel, or skin: Presence of malignant cells

Key treatments for non-Hodgkin's lymphoma

- Radiation therapy
- Chemotherapy

Key nursing considerations for non-Hodgkin's lymphoma

- Plan small, frequent meals scheduled around treatment.
- Instruct patient to keep irradiated skin dry.
- Provide emotional support.

Key facts about leukemia

- Group of malignant disorders
- Characterized by abnormal proliferation and maturation of lymphocytes and nonlymphocytic cells
- Suppresses normal cells
- Classified as acute or chronic and as lymphocytic or myelogenous

- Possible increased intracranial pressure (ICP) resulting from CNS lymphatic involvement

● **Diagnostic test findings**
- CBC shows anemia, thrombocytopenia, leukopenia, and lymphocytosis
- Blood testing shows normal or elevated uric acid levels, elevated liver function and lactic dehydrogenase (with liver involvement and chronic inflammation), elevated serum calcium level (from bone lesions in some subtypes), and abnormal serum protein levels
- Lymph node biopsy reveals the cell type
- Biopsy of tonsils, bone marrow, liver, bowel, or skin reveals malignant cells
- Bone and chest X-rays, lymphangiography, liver and spleen scans, and abdominal CT scanning show evidence of metastasis

● **Treatment**
- Radiation therapy to kill cancer cells and shrink lymphomas (mainly in early, localized disease)
- Chemotherapy to kill cancer cells (most effective with multiple combinations of antineoplastics)
- Bone marrow and stem cell transplants to treat disease that's resistant to standard treatment (especially following relapse after initial chemotherapy)
- Psychological support to promote communication and trust and to help the patient and his family deal effectively with the diagnosis, prognosis, and treatments

● **Nursing considerations**
- Observe the patient who's receiving radiation or chemotherapy for anorexia, nausea, vomiting, or diarrhea
  - Plan small, frequent meals scheduled around treatment, or maintain nothing-by-mouth status if ordered
  - Give I.V. fluids, antiemetics, and sedatives (as ordered) for the patient who can't tolerate oral feedings
- Instruct the patient to keep irradiated skin dry
- Provide emotional support
  - Explain all diagnostic tests and procedures
  - Keep the patient and his family informed about prognosis and diagnosis, and listen to their concerns
  - Refer them to the American Cancer Society for information and support

LEUKEMIA

● **Definition**
- Group of malignant disorders characterized by abnormal proliferation and maturation of lymphocytes and nonlymphocytic cells, leading to suppression of normal cells
- Classified as acute or chronic and as lymphocytic or myelogenous
  - Acute lymphocytic leukemia: Abnormal growth of lymphocytic precursors (lymphoblasts)—most common type in young children and adults age 65 and older
  - Acute myelogenous leukemia: Rapid accumulation of myeloid precursors (myeloblasts)—can affect children and adults

– Chronic myelogenous leukemia: Abnormal overgrowth of granulocytic precursors (myeloblasts, promyelocytes, metamyelocytes, and myelocytes) in bone marrow, blood, and body tissues — occurs mainly in adults (rare in children)

– Chronic lymphocytic leukemia: Uncontrollable spread of small, abnormal lymphocytes in lymphoid tissue, blood, and bone marrow — occurs mainly in adults older than age 55 (rare in children)

• More common in males than females, and in Whites than Blacks

• Acute forms can typically be cured; chronic forms can't be cured but can commonly be controlled (remission) for long periods

Underlying pathophysiology

• Immature, nonfunctioning WBCs appear to accumulate first in the tissue where they originate, such as lymphocytes in lymph tissue and granulocytes in bone marrow

• Immature, nonfunctioning WBCs spill into the bloodstream and overwhelm red blood cells (RBCs) and platelets; from there, they infiltrate other tissues

• Because of possible relapse, it commonly takes years to determine whether a patient is cured or is just in long-term remission

Causes

• Unknown

• Risk factors
   – Radiation (especially prolonged exposure)
   – Certain chemicals and drugs, such as benzene, and some chemotherapeutic agents
   – Viruses
   – Genetic abnormalities (increased incidence in people with Down syndrome)

Pathophysiologic changes

• Acute leukemia
   – Sudden onset of high fever resulting from bone marrow invasion and cellular proliferation within bone marrow
   – Thrombocytopenia and abnormal bleeding secondary to bone marrow suppression
   – Weakness and lassitude related to anemia from bone marrow invasion
   – Pallor and weakness related to anemia
   – Chills and recurrent infections related to proliferation of immature, nonfunctioning WBCs
   – Bone pain from leukemic infiltration of bone
   – Neurologic manifestations, including headache, papilledema, facial palsy, blurred vision, and meningeal irritation secondary to leukemic infiltration or cerebral bleeding
   – Liver, spleen, and lymph node enlargement related to leukemic cell infiltration

• Chronic leukemia
   – Slow onset of fatigue related to anemia
   – Splenomegaly secondary to increased numbers of lysed RBCs being filtered
   – Hepatomegaly and lymph node enlargement from infiltration by leukemic cells

Types of leukemia

• Acute lymphocytic leukemia – abnormal growth of lymphoblasts

• Acute myelogenous leukemia – rapid accumulation of myeloblasts

• Chronic myelogenous leukemia – abnormal overgrowth of granulocytic precursors

• Chronic lymphocytic leukemia – uncontrollable spread of small, abnormal lymphocytes

Key pathophysiologic changes in leukemia

Acute
• Sudden onset of high fever
• Thrombocytopenia
• Weakness
• Recurrent infections

Chronic
• Slow onset of fatigue
• Lymph node enlargement
• Infections

Key diagnostic test results for leukemia

- Blood counts: Thrombocytopenia and neutropenia, WBC differential showing the cell type, serum hemoglobin below 11 g/dl
- Bone marrow aspiration: Proliferation of immature WBCs (acute leukemia)

Key treatments for leukemia

- Chemotherapy
- Bone marrow or stem cell transplantation
- Antibiotic, antifungal, and antiviral therapies
- Platelet and RBC transfusions

Key nursing considerations for leukemia

- Watch for symptoms of meningeal leukemia and provide appropriate care after intrathecal chemotherapy.
- Teach patient about adverse effects of radiation.
- Watch for early signs of cardiotoxicity if patient receives daunorubicin or doxorubicin.
- Control infection by instituting neutropenic precautions.
- Monitor patient's temperature every 4 hours.
- Watch for bleeding.
- Minimize stress and promote rest.

- – Bleeding tendencies secondary to thrombocytopenia
- – Infections related to deficient humoral immunity

● **Complications**
- Infection
- Organ malfunction through tumor spread or hemorrhage

● **Diagnostic test findings**
- Blood counts reveal thrombocytopenia and neutropenia, a WBC differential showing the cell type, and serum hemoglobin below 11 g/dl (anemia)
- Serum globulin level is decreased, indicating cell breakdown
- CT scan shows the affected organs
- Lumbar puncture detects meningeal involvement; cerebrospinal fluid (CSF) analysis shows abnormal WBC invasion of the CNS
- Bone marrow aspiration shows a proliferation of immature WBCs, confirming acute leukemia; if the aspirate is dry or free from leukemic cells but the patient has other typical signs of leukemia, a bone marrow biopsy, usually of the posterior superior iliac spine, is performed

● **Treatment**
- Chemotherapy (varies according to type of leukemia) to eradicate leukemic cells and induce remission
- Bone marrow or stem cell transplantation (in some cases) to eradicate leukemic cells and induce remission
- Antibiotic, antifungal, and antiviral therapies to prevent or control secondary infection
- Platelet and RBC transfusions to treat anemia and prevent bleeding
- Local radiation to reduce organ size (when chronic lymphocytic leukemia causes obstruction or organ impairment)
- Psychological support to promote communication and trust and to help the patient and his family deal effectively with the diagnosis, prognosis, and treatments
- Palliative and supportive care for patients with disease that's refractory to chemotherapy, or for those in the terminal phase of disease

● **Nursing considerations**
- Watch for symptoms of meningeal leukemia (confusion, lethargy, headache); if these occur, provide appropriate care after intrathecal chemotherapy
  - – Place the patient in Trendelenburg's position for 30 minutes; then force fluids and keep the patient supine for 4 to 6 hours
- Check the lumbar puncture site often for bleeding
- If the patient receives radiation, teach him about potential adverse effects
- Take appropriate steps to prevent hyperuricemia, a possible result of chemotherapy-induced leukemic cell lysis
  - – Force fluids to about 2 L/day
  - – Prepare to give acetazolamide (Diamox), sodium bicarbonate tablets, and allopurinol (Zyloprim); watch for rash or other hypersensitivity reaction to allopurinol
  - – Check frequently to ensure urine pH is above 7.5
- Watch for early signs of cardiotoxicity, such as arrhythmias and signs of heart failure, if the patient receives daunorubicin (Cerubidine) or doxorubicin (Adriamycin)

- Control infection by placing the patient in a private room and instituting neutropenic precautions
    - Avoid indwelling urinary catheters and I.M. injections
    - Screen staff and visitors (watch for and report any signs of infection)
    - Don't allow fresh flowers or fresh, unpeeled fruit
- Provide thorough skin care by keeping the patient's skin and perineal area clean and dry
- Monitor the patient's temperature every 4 hours; a patient with a temperature over 99° F (37.2° C) and decreased WBC counts should receive prompt antibiotic therapy
- Watch for bleeding; if it occurs, apply ice compresses and pressure and elevate the affected extremity; regularly check for pallor, petechiae, and bruising
- Prevent constipation by providing adequate hydration, a high-residue diet, stool softeners, and mild laxatives
- Control mouth ulceration by checking often for obvious ulcers and gum swelling and by providing frequent mouth care and saline rinses
- Plan care to help prevent exhaustion, if the patient has anemia
- Provide emotional support; establish a trusting relationship, explain all diagnostic tests and procedures, keep the patient and his family informed about the diagnosis and prognosis, and listen to concerns
- Minimize stress by providing a calm, quiet atmosphere that promotes rest and relaxation

BONE CANCER

Definition
- Osseous bone tumors
    - Arise from bony structure itself
    - Include osteogenic sarcoma (most common), parosteal osteogenic sarcoma, chondrosarcoma (chondroblastic sarcoma), and malignant giant cell tumor
- Nonosseous bone tumors
    - Arise from hematopoietic, vascular, and neural tissues
    - Include Ewing's sarcoma, fibrosarcoma (fibroblastic sarcoma), and chordoma (see *Types of primary malignant bone tumors*, page 504)
- Rare as primary cancer; more common as metastatic disease

Underlying pathophysiology
- Cancerous cells clump to form a tumor
- The cells proliferate and are able to spread beyond the original site
- Osteogenic sarcoma (the most common form of bone cancer) arises in osteoid or immature bone, typically involving the long bones of the arms or legs (especially around the knee)
- Parosteal osteogenic sarcoma arises on the surface of the bone, commonly on the femur near the knee
- Chondrosarcoma, which originates in cartilage cells, usually occurs in bones of the pelvis, hip, shoulder, or ribs
- Malignant giant cell tumors originate in the epiphyses of the long bones, with most tumors developing in the femur and tibia (some in the humerus and radius)

Key facts about bone cancer
- May be osseous (arising from bony structure) or nonosseous (arising from hematopoietic, vascular, and neural tissues)
- Develops when cancerous cells clump to form tumor
- Progresses when cells proliferate and spread beyond original site

Types of primary malignant bone tumors

This chart lists types of primary malignant bone tumors and their clinical features and outlines treatments.

TYPE	CLINICAL FEATURES	TREATMENT
Osseous origin		
Chondro-sarcoma (chondro-blastic sarcoma)	• Develops from cartilage • Painless; grows slowly but is locally recurrent and invasive • Occurs most commonly in pelvis, proximal femur, ribs, and shoulder girdle • Usually in men ages 30 to 50	• Hemipelvectomy, surgical resection (ribs) • Radiation (palliative) • Chemotherapy
Malignant giant cell tumor	• Arises from benign giant cell tumor • Found most commonly in long bones, especially in the knee area • Usually in women ages 18 to 50	• Curettage • Total excision • Radiation for recurrent disease
Osteogenic sarcoma	• Osteoid tumor present in biopsy specimen • Tumor arises from bone-forming osteoblast and bone-digesting osteoclast • Occurs most commonly in femur but also in tibia and humerus; occurs occasionally in fibula, ileum, vertebra, or mandible • Usually in males ages 10 to 30	• Surgery (tumor resection, high thigh amputation, hemipelvectomy, interscapulothoracic surgery) • Chemotherapy
Parosteal osteogenic sarcoma	• Develops on surface of bone instead of interior • Progresses slowly • Occurs most commonly in distal femur but also in tibia, humerus, and ulna • Usually in women ages 30 to 40	• Surgery (tumor resection, possible amputation, interscapulothoracic surgery, hemipelvectomy) • Chemotherapy • Combination of the above
Nonosseous origin		
Chordoma	• Derived from embryonic remnants of notochord • Progresses slowly • Usually found at end of spinal column and in spheno-occipital, sacrococcygeal, and vertebral areas • Characterized by constipation and visual disturbances • Usually in men ages 50 to 60	• Surgical resection (commonly resulting in neural defects) • Radiation (palliative or when surgery not applicable, as in occipital area)
Ewing's sarcoma	• Originates in bone marrow and invades shafts of long and flat bones • Usually affects lower extremities; most commonly, femur, innominate bones, ribs, tibia, humerus, vertebra, and fibula; may metastasize to lungs • Pain increasingly severe and persistent • Usually in males ages 10 to 20 • Prognosis poor	• High-voltage radiation (tumor is radiosensitive) • Chemotherapy to slow growth • Amputation only if there's no evidence of metastasis
Fibrosarcoma (fibroblastic sarcoma)	• Relatively rare • Originates in fibrous tissue of bone • Invades long or flat bones (femur, tibia, mandible) but also involves periosteum and overlying muscle • Usually in men ages 30 to 40	• Amputation • Radiation • Chemotherapy • Bone grafts (with low-grade fibrosarcoma)

Causes

- No immediately apparent cause in most cases
- Genetic abnormalities (retinoblastoma, Rothmund-Thomson syndrome)
- Chemical carcinogen exposure
- Heredity
- Bone trauma
- Excessive radiation therapy

Pathophysiologic changes

- Pain due to inflammation within bone and surrounding tissues related to the vascular content of bone, and due to pressure within the bone
- Palpable mass resulting from tumor growth
- Fractures caused by weakened bone structure
- Metastasis to the lung due to vascular spread to susceptible tissues

Complications

- Infection
- Hemorrhage
- Local recurrence
- Amputation

Diagnostic test findings

- Blood testing reveals elevated serum alkaline phosphatase levels (with sarcoma)
- Bone X-rays and radioisotope bone and CT scans show the tumor size
- Bone scans and CT scans of the lungs reveal metastatic disease
- Incision or aspiration biopsy confirms primary malignancy

Treatment

- Tumor excision (along with 1" [2.5-cm] margin of bone) and bone grafting or insertion of metal plate to remove tumor and maintain function
- External beam radiation, chemotherapy, or brachytherapy (placement of small radioactive pellets directly into tumor) to eradicate tumor or reduce size
- Amputation when other treatments fail
- Physical therapy when assistive devices are needed
- Emotional support to help the patient and his family cope with diagnosis, prognosis, and treatments

Nursing considerations

- Encourage communication, and help the patient set realistic goals
- Give prescribed I.V. infusions and drugs, give pain medications prior to activities of daily living (ADLs) and therapy sessions if needed
- Elevate the foot of the bed or place the stump on a pillow for the first 24 hours after amputation; be careful not to leave the stump elevated for more than 48 hours because doing so can lead to contractures
- Monitor vital signs and circulation to the affected extremity when wrappings allow
- Monitor wound dressings for drainage
- Teach the patient about wound care, how to use assistive devices, and to report new pain or masses
- Promote referral to physical or occupational therapy as needed
- Explain the need for antibiotic prophylaxis when undergoing dental procedures (with bone grafts or prosthetic implants)

• Provide emotional support; prepare the patient for diagnostic tests and procedures, answer questions and listen to concerns, and refer the patient to the American Cancer Society for additional information and support

Key facts about brain tumor

• Involves abnormal growth among cells within intracranial space
• Causes destruction of intracranial tissues
• Results in CNS changes

Key pathophysiologic changes in brain tumor

• Headache, dizziness
• Motor deficits
• Personality or behavioral changes
• Vision or hearing disturbances

BRAIN TUMOR

● Definition
• Abnormal growth among cells within the intracranial space
• May affect brain tissue, meninges, pituitary gland, and blood vessels
• In adults, most common tumor types are gliomas, meningiomas (usually occur above the covering of the cerebellum or supratentorially), and schwannoma
• In children, most common tumor types are astrocytomas, medulloblastomas, ependymomas, and brain stem gliomas
• Classified according to histology or grade of cell malignancy

● Underlying pathophysiology
• Cancer cells invade and destroy intracranial tissues
• Invasion of the cancer cells, tissue destruction, and secondary effects result in CNS changes (mainly compression of the brain, cranial nerves, and cerebral vessels; cerebral edema; and increased ICP)

● Causes
• Exact cause unknown
• Possible link to radiation, chemical exposure, or viruses

● Pathophysiologic changes
• Headache, dizziness, vertigo, nausea and vomiting, and papilledema secondary to increased ICP from tumor invasion and compression of surrounding tissues
• Cranial nerve dysfunction secondary to tumor invasion or compression of cranial nerves
• Focal deficits, including motor deficits (weakness, paralysis, or gait disorders) and sensory disturbances (anesthesia, paresthesia, or disturbances of vision or hearing) secondary to tumor invasion or compression of motor or sensory control areas of the brain
• Disturbances of higher function, including deficits in cognition, learning, and memory
• Dementia, personality or behavioral changes, gait disturbances, ataxia, hemiparesis, seizures, and language impairments (depending on location of tumor within the brain)
• Sensory loss, hemianopsia, pupillary abnormalities, nystagmus, cranial nerve dysfunction, and autonomic dysfunction (depending on specific nerves affected by tumor)

● Complications
• Radiation encephalopathy
• Coma
• Respiratory or cardiac arrest
• Brain herniation

Diagnostic test findings
- Skull X-rays confirm the presence of the tumor
- Brain scan confirms the presence and size of the tumor
- CT scans and MRI provide detailed images of the tumor and some of its characteristics
- Cerebral angiography shows vascularity of the tumor and involvement or proximity to large vessels
- PET scans confirm the presence of bony tumors
- Tissue biopsy confirms tumor type
- Lumbar puncture reveals increased CSF pressure, which reflects ICP, increased protein levels, decreased glucose levels and, occasionally, tumor cells in the CSF

Treatment
- Treatments vary with tumor's histologic type, radiosensitivity, and location
  - Glioma: Resection by craniotomy, followed by radiation therapy and chemotherapy
  - Low-grade, cystic cerebellar astrocytoma: Surgical resection
  - Astrocytoma: Repeated surgeries, radiation therapy, and shunting of fluid from obstructed CSF pathways
  - Oligodendroglioma and ependymoma: Surgical resection and radiation therapy
  - Medulloblastoma: Surgical resection and (possibly) intrathecal methotrexate (Trexall) or other antineoplastic
  - Meningioma: Surgical resection, including dura mater and bone
  - Schwannoma: Microsurgical technique
- Emotional support to help the patient and his family cope effectively with the diagnosis, prognosis, and treatments

Nursing considerations
- Maintain a patent airway
- Prepare to take seizure precautions (high risk)
- Give prescribed medications, including chemotherapy drugs, steroids, antacids and histamine-receptor antagonists, and anticonvulsants
- Elevate the head of the bed about 30 degrees to prevent increased ICP and to promote venous return after supratentorial craniotomy
- Keep the patient flat for 48 hours after infratentorial craniotomy to prevent brain stem herniation into the spinal canal from increased ICP
- Instruct the patient to avoid Valsalva's maneuver and isometric muscle contractions when moving or sitting up in bed (as appropriate) to prevent increased ICP
- Consult with occupational, speech, and physical therapists for rehabilitation of any neurologic deficits
- Monitor neurologic status, vital signs, and the wound site; be alert for postoperative complications, such as infection and increased ICP
- Teach the patient about signs of infection or bleeding that may result from chemotherapy
- Teach the patient how to recognize early signs of tumor recurrence (similar to original signs or any other neurologic changes)

Key facts about laryngeal cancer

- Involves malignant cells in tissues of larynx or voice box
- May be intrinsic (located on true vocal cords) or extrinsic (located on another part of larynx)
- Classified as supraglottic, glottic, or subglottic (rare)

Key pathophysiologic changes in laryngeal cancer

- Hoarseness lasting longer than 3 weeks
- Lump in throat
- Pain or burning
- Dysphagia

- Provide emotional support; teach the patient about the disease process; explain all diagnostic tests, procedures, and treatments; keep the patient and his family informed; answer questions and listen to concerns; and refer the patient to the American Cancer Society for additional information and support

LARYNGEAL CANCER

- **Definition**
  - Malignant cells in the tissues of the larynx or voice box
  - Squamous cell carcinoma: most common form

- **Underlying pathophysiology**
  - The tumor is intrinsic (located on the true vocal cords; tends not to spread because underlying connective tissue lack lymph nodes) or extrinsic (located on another part of the larynx; tends to spread easily)
  - Malignant cells that proliferate can cause swallowing and breathing impairment
  - Tumor can decrease mobility of the vocal cords
  - Laryngeal cancer is classified by its location
    - Supraglottic (on the false vocal cords)
    - Glottic (on the true vocal cords)
    - Subglottic (rare downward extension from the vocal cords)

- **Causes**
  - Unknown

- **Risk factors**
  - Alcoholism
  - Chronic inhalation of noxious fumes
  - Familial disposition
  - History of gastroesophageal reflux disease
  - Smoking

- **Pathophysiologic changes**
  - Hoarseness longer than 3 weeks related to encroachment on the true vocal cord
  - Lump in the throat or pain or burning when drinking citrus juice or hot liquids related to tumor growth
  - Dysphagia secondary to increasing pressure and obstruction with tumor growth
  - Dyspnea and cough related to progressive tumor growth and metastasis
  - Enlargement of cervical lymph nodes and pain radiating to ear related to invasion of lymphatic and subsequent pressure

- **Complications**
  - Increased difficulty swallowing
  - Increased pain
  - Metastasis

- **Diagnostic test findings**
  - Xeroradiography, laryngeal tomography, CT scan, and laryngography confirm the presence of a mass

- Chest X-ray rules out or confirms metastasis
- Laryngoscopy allows definitive staging by obtaining multiple biopsy specimens to establish a primary diagnosis, to determine the extent of the disease, and to identify additional premalignant lesions or second primaries
- Biopsy identifies cancer cells

Treatment
- Goal: Speech preservation (if not possible, speech rehabilitation may include esophageal speech or prosthetic devices or experimental surgical reconstruction of the voice box)
- Diet based on treatment options (may require enteral feeding)
- Frequent rest periods
- Precancerous lesions
  - Laser surgery
- Early lesions
  - Laser surgery
  - Radiation therapy
- Advanced lesions
  - Radiation therapy
  - Chemotherapy

Nursing considerations
- Reassure the patient that speech rehabilitation may help him speak again
- Support the patient through the grieving process, as needed; if his depression seems severe, consider a psychiatric referral
- Before surgery
  - Teach the patient about laryngeal structures and the areas affected by the cancer (see *Teaching about laryngeal structures,* page 510)
  - Instruct the patient to maintain good oral care
  - If appropriate, instruct a male patient to shave off his beard
  - Encourage the patient to express his concerns; help him choose a temporary nonspeaking communication method such as writing
- After partial laryngectomy surgery
  - Give I.V. fluids and, usually, tube feedings for the first 2 days postoperatively; then resume oral feedings
  - Keep the tracheostomy tube (inserted during surgery) in place until edema subsides
  - Keep the patient from using his voice until he has medical permission (usually 2 to 3 days postoperatively); then caution him to whisper until healing is complete
- After total laryngectomy surgery
  - Place the patient on his side and elevate his head 30 to 45 degrees
  - When moving the patient, remember to support his neck
  - If applicable, provide laryngectomy tube care (requires same care as tracheostomy)
  - If applicable, watch for crusting and skin breakdown around the laryngectomy tube; remove crusting with petroleum jelly, antimicrobial ointment, and moist gauze
  - Provide adequate room humidification
  - Teach stoma care

Teaching about laryngeal structures

To help your patient understand his laryngeal cancer, start by taking a few minutes to explain how normal laryngeal structures look and work. Explain to the patient that the larynx is a boxy, tubelike structure that lies in the neck between the base of the tongue and the trachea. The epiglottis seals off the trachea from the esophagus so that food and fluids can't enter the lungs.

Lining the larynx are two sets of fold, known as the *vocal cords.* One set, the true vocal cords, vibrate to make speech as air moves through a passageway called the *glottis.* The second set, the false vocal cords, are located directly above the true vocal cords. They're also involved in sound production.

After teaching the patient about the location and function of the laryngeal structures, discuss the areas affected by his type of cancer.

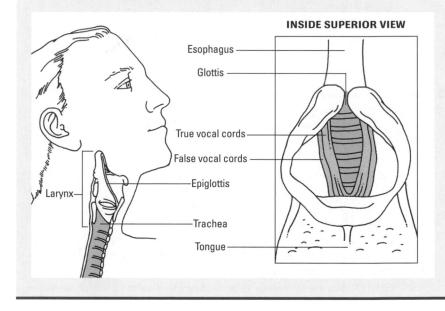

INSIDE SUPERIOR VIEW

Esophagus

Glottis

True vocal cords

False vocal cords

Epiglottis

Larynx

Trachea

Tongue

— Watch for and report complications, including signs and symptoms of fistula formation (redness, swelling, and secretions on suture line), carotid artery rupture (bleeding), and tracheostomy stenosis (constant shortness of breath)
— If the patient has a fistula, feed him through a nasogastric (NG) tube; otherwise food will leak through the fistula and delay healing
— Monitor vital signs
— Be alert for fever, which indicates infection
— Record fluid intake and output, and watch for dehydration
— Give frequent mouth care
— Suction gently; unless otherwise ordered, don't attempt deep suctioning because it could penetrate the suture line
— Suction through the tube and the patient's nose because the patient can longer blow air through his nose

– After insertion of a drainage catheter (usually connected to a blood drainage system or a GI drainage system), don't stop suction without the physician's consent
– After catheter removal, check the dressings for drainage
– Give analgesics as ordered
– If the patient has an NG feeding tube, check the placement of the tube and elevate the patient's head to prevent aspiration

THYROID CANCER

● Definition
- Proliferation of cancer cells in the thyroid gland
- Most common endocrine malignancy
- Papillary carcinomas: 50% of all cases
- Medullary cancer: may be associated with pheochromocytoma (curable when detected before it causes symptoms)

● Underlying pathophysiology
- Papillary cancer is usually multifocal and bilateral
  - Metastasizes slowly into regional nodes of the neck, mediastinum, lungs, and other distant organs
  - Least virulent form of thyroid cancer
- Follicular cancer is less common but is more likely to recur, metastasize to the regional lymph nodes, and spread through blood vessels into the bones, liver, and lungs
- Medullary (solid) carcinoma originates in the parafollicular cells derived from the last bronchial pouch
  - Contains amyloid and calcium deposits
  - Can produce calcitonin, histaminase, corticotropins (producing Cushing's syndrome), and prostaglandin E2 and F3 (producing diarrhea)
  - When untreated, grows rapidly, commonly metastasizing to bones, liver, and kidneys
- Anaplastic carcinoma (giant, squamoid, and spindle cell subtypes) resists radiation and is almost never curable by resection
  - Metastasizes rapidly, causing death by invading the trachea and compressing adjacent structures

● Causes
- Previous exposure to radiation treatment in the neck area
- Prolonged secretion of thyroid-stimulating hormone (TSH) (radiation or hereditary)

● Pathophysiologic changes
- Painless, hard nodule or swelling in the thyroid gland, or palpable lymph nodes with thyroid enlargement (reflecting tumor growth)
- Hoarseness, dysphagia, and dyspnea or constant wheezing from increased tumor growth and pressure on surrounding structures
- Hyperthyroidism due to excess thyroid hormone production from tumor
- Hypothyroidism secondary to destruction of thyroid gland by tumor

● Complications
- Dysphagia

Key facts about thyroid cancer
- Involves cancer cells in thyroid gland
- Papillary cancer — usually multifocal and bilateral
- Follicular cancer — metastasizes to regional lymph nodes and spreads through blood vessels into bones, liver, and lungs
- Medullary carcinoma — originates in parafollicular cells
- Anaplastic carcinoma — resists radiation; rarely curable by resection

Key pathophysiologic changes in thyroid cancer
- Painless, hard nodule in thyroid gland
- Hoarseness
- Dysphagia
- Constant wheezing

Key diagnostic test results for thyroid cancer

- MRI and CT scans: Extent of disease
- Fine-needle aspiration biopsy: Differentiates benign from malignant thyroid nodules

Key treatments for thyroid cancer

- Total or subtotal thyroidectomy
- ^{131}I therapy
- External radiation

Key postoperative nursing considerations for thyroid cancer

- Keep patient in semi-Fowler's position after he regains consciousness.
- Monitor vital signs.
- Check patient's dressing, neck, and back for bleeding.
- Loosen dressing and call physician if patient says dressing feels tight.
- Watch for signs of hemorrhage, tetany, thyroid storm, and respiratory obstruction.
- Keep tracheostomy set and oxygen equipment readily available.
- Maintain adequate nutrition.

- Stridor
- Hormone alterations
- Distant metastasis

● **Diagnostic test findings**
- Calcitonin assay reveals the levels of calcitonin and identifies silent medullary carcinoma
- Thyroid scan differentiates functional nodes (which are rarely malignant) from hypofunctional nodes, which are commonly malignant
- Ultrasonography shows changes in the size of the thyroid nodules after thyroxine suppression therapy
- MRI and CT scanning show the extent of the disease in the thyroid and surrounding structures
- Fine-needle aspiration biopsy differentiates benign from malignant thyroid nodules
- Histologic analysis stages the disease

● **Treatment**
- Total or subtotal thyroidectomy with modified node dissection (bilateral or unilateral) on the side of the primary cancer (papillary or follicular)
- Total thyroidectomy and radical neck excision for medullary, anaplastic cancers
- Radioactive iodine (^{131}I) therapy to treat metastasis
- ^{131}I therapy with external radiation to treat inoperable cancer (sometimes used postoperatively in lieu of radical neck excision)
- Adjunctive thyroid suppression with exogenous thyroid hormones to suppress TSH production
  - Simultaneous administration of an adrenergic-blocking agent, such as propanolol (Inderal), increasing tolerance to surgery and radiation
- Chemotherapy for symptomatic, widespread metastasis
  - Limited use, but doxorubicin is sometimes beneficial

● **Nursing considerations**
- Before surgery, tell the patient to expect hoarseness (but not voice loss) lasting several days after surgery
- After surgery, provide appropriate postoperative care
  - Keep the patient in semi-Fowler's position after he regains consciousness; make sure his head is neither hyperextended nor flexed, to avoid pressure on the suture line
  - **Monitor vital signs, and then check the patient's dressing, neck, and back for bleeding; loosen the dressing and call the physician immediately if the patient complains that the dressing feels tight**
  - Check serum calcium levels every 12 hours because hypocalcemia may develop if the parathyroid glands have been removed
  - Watch for and report other complications: hemorrhage and shock (elevated pulse rate and hypotension), tetany (carpopedal spasm, twitching, and seizures), thyroid storm (high fever, severe tachycardia, delirium, dehydration, and extreme irritability), and respiratory obstruction (dyspnea, crowing respirations, retraction of neck tissues) (see *What happens in thyroid storm*)

What happens in thyroid storm

Normally, the hypothalamus stimulates the release of thyrotropin-releasing hormone (TRH), which causes the anterior pituitary gland to release thyroid-stimulating hormone (TSH). The thyroid gland then secretes triiodothyronine (T_3) and thyroxine (T_4).

In thyroid storm, however, the thyroid overproduces T_3 and T_4, and systemic adrenergic activity increases. This increase causes epinephrine overproduction and severe hypermetabolism, leading to GI, cardiovascular, and sympathetic nervous system decompensation.

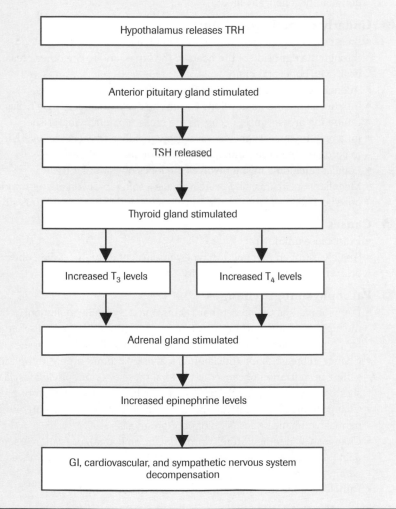

- Keep a tracheostomy set and oxygen equipment handy in case of respiratory obstruction
- Prepare for I.V. fluids or a soft diet, although many patients can tolerate a regular diet within 24 hours after surgery

Key facts about breast cancer

- Results from malignant proliferation of epithelial cells lining breast ducts or lobules
- Spreads by way of lymphatic system
- If infiltrating, occurs in parenchymal tissue
- If adenocarcinoma, arises from epithelium

Key pathophysiologic changes in breast cancer

- Lump or mass in breast
- Change in nipple
- Change in breast shape

- Explain all diagnostic tests, procedures, and treatments; answer the patient's questions and listen to his concerns; and refer the patient to the American Cancer Society for additional information and support

BREAST CANCER

● **Definition**
- Malignant proliferation of epithelial cells lining the ducts or lobules of the breast
- Most common cancer affecting women
- May develop anytime after puberty; most common after age 50
- One percent of all breast cancers in the United States occur in males (predominantly genetically linked)

● **Underlying pathophysiology**
- Breast cancer spreads by way of the lymphatic system and the bloodstream, through the right side of the heart to the lungs, and to the other breast, chest wall, liver, bone, and brain
- Adenocarcinoma (ductal) arises from the epithelium
- Intraductal carcinoma develops within the ducts (includes Paget's disease)
- Infiltrating breast cancer occurs in the breast's parenchymal tissue
- Inflammatory breast cancers (rare) grow rapidly and cause the overlying skin to become edematous, inflamed, and indurated
- Lobular carcinoma in situ involves the lobes of glandular tissue
- Medullary or circumscribed carcinoma is a soft, rapidly enlarging tumor composed of sheets of large epithelial cells surrounded by scant fibrous stroma

● **Causes**
- Exact cause unknown
- Possibly estrogen therapy, antihypertensive agents, high-fat diet, obesity, fibrocystic breast disease, or heredity

● **Pathophysiologic changes**
- Lump or mass in the breast (hard, stony mass is usually malignant); change in the nipple (itching, burning, erosion, or retraction) and nipple discharge (watery, serous, creamy, bloody) due to mutation in cells of breast tissue
- Change in breast shape (thickening, scaly skin around nipple, dimpling) resulting from fixation of cancer to pectoral muscles or underlying fascia or shortening of the ligaments supporting the breast caused by tumor pressure
- Change in breast skin texture (peau d'orange) caused by invasion of the subdermal lymphatic nodes (sign of poor prognosis)
- Change in skin temperature (warm, hot, or pink area), ulceration, edema, or pain (not usually present; should be investigated) caused by advanced spread within the breast
- Pathologic bone fractures; edema of the arm due to metastasis

● **Complications**
- Distant metastasis
- Infection
- CNS effects
- Respiratory effects

Diagnostic test findings

- Blood chemistry reveals distant metastases (alkaline phosphatase levels and liver function)
- Hormonal receptor assay determines whether the tumor is estrogen- or progesterone-dependent; it also guides decisions to use therapy that blocks the action of the estrogen hormone that supports tumor growth
- Mammography can reveal a tumor that's too small to palpate
- Ultrasonography can distinguish between a fluid-filled cyst and a solid mass
- Chest X-ray can pinpoint metastases in the chest
- Scans of the bone, brain, liver, and other organs can detect distant metastases
- Fine-needle aspiration and excisional biopsy provide cells for histologic examination that may confirm the diagnosis

Treatment

- Choice of treatment usually depends on stage and type of disease, woman's age and menopausal status, and the disfiguring effects of surgery
  - May include any combination of surgery, radiation, chemotherapy, and hormone therapy
- Primary radiation therapy to kill cancer cells in tumor
- Preoperative breast irradiation to shrink tumor size prior to excision
- Chemotherapy, such as a combination of drugs, including cyclophosphamide (Cytoxan), fluorouracil (Adrucil), methotrexate (Trexall), doxorubicin, vincristine (Vincasar), paclitaxel (Taxol), and prednisone (Orasone); given as sole treatment or in combination with surgery or radiation or both
- Antiestrogen, antiprogesterone therapy, with such drugs as tamoxifen (Nolvadex) to prevent growth and spread of hormone-dependent tumors
- Hormonal therapy, including estrogen, progesterone, androgen, or antiandrogen aminoglutethimide therapy to stop further spread by changing hormone balance
- Monoclonal antibody drug treatment to manage non-hormone-receptive tumors
- Lumpectomy to remove localized malignancy
- Partial, total, or modified radical mastectomy to remove tumor and, possibly, lymph nodes and surrounding muscle tissue

Nursing considerations

- Provide information about the disease process, diagnostic tests, and treatments
- Give prescribed drugs
- Provide patient teaching and emotional support before surgery
  - Advise the patient to ask her physician about reconstructive surgery (may be planned prior to mastectomy)
  - Teach the patient about breast prostheses, and refer her to a support group such as Reach to Recovery
  - Prepare the patient for surgery, including postoperative appearance of mastectomy site
  - Encourage patient to express fears and concerns
- Provide appropriate postoperative care
  - Monitor the wound site, vital signs, and intake and output (for at least 48 hours after general anesthesia); watch for postoperative complications

— Prevent lymphedema of the arm (may be early complication of any breast cancer treatment that involves lymph node manipulation)
  • Instruct patient to exercise her hand and arm regularly
  • Caution her to avoid activities that might cause infection or impairment in the hand or arm (increases chance of lymphedema development)
— Provide continued emotional support; refer the patient and his family to a support group as needed

LUNG CANCER

● **Definition**
• Development of neoplasm, usually within wall or epithelium of bronchial tree
• Most common types: epidermoid (squamous cell) carcinoma, small-cell (oat cell) carcinoma, adenocarcinoma, and large-cell (anaplastic) carcinoma

● **Underlying pathophysiology**
• Lung cancer usually begins with the transformation of one epithelial cell within the airway
• Although the exact cause of such changes remains unclear, some lung cancers originate in the bronchi, which may be more vulnerable to injuries from carcinogens
• As the tumor grows, it can partially or completely obstruct the airway, resulting in lobar collapse distal to the tumor
• Early metastasis may occur to other thoracic structures

● **Causes**
• Exact cause unknown
• Risk factors
  — Smoking
  — Exposure to carcinogenic and industrial air pollutants (asbestos, arsenic, chromium, coal dust, iron oxides, nickel, radioactive dust, and uranium)
  — Genetic predisposition

● **Pathophysiologic changes**
• Cough, hoarseness, wheezing, dyspnea, hemoptysis, and chest pain related to local infiltration of pulmonary membranes and vasculature
• Fever, weight loss, weakness, and anorexia related to increased tumor growth needs from hypermetabolic state of cellular proliferation
• Bone and joint pain from cartilage erosion due to abnormal production of growth hormone
• Cushing's syndrome related to abnormal production of adrenocorticotropic hormone
• Hypercalcemia related to abnormal production of parathyroid hormone or bone metastasis
• Hemoptysis, atelectasis, pneumonitis, and dyspnea from bronchial obstruction related to increasing growth
• Shoulder pain and unilateral paralysis of diaphragm due to phrenic nerve involvement
• Dysphagia related to esophageal compression

Key facts about lung cancer

● Develops within bronchial tree's wall or epithelium
● Usually begins with transformation of one epithelial cell within airway
● May originate in bronchi

Key pathophysiologic changes in lung cancer

● Cough
● Hoarseness
● Wheezing
● Dyspnea
● Weakness
● Weight loss
● Hemoptysis

- Venous distention and facial, neck, and chest edema secondary to obstruction of vena cava
- Piercing chest pain, increasing dyspnea, and severe arm pain secondary to invasion of the chest wall

Complications
- Metastasis to intrathoracic structures
- Tracheal obstruction
- Sympathetic nerve paralysis with Horner syndrome
- Spinal cord compression
- Hypoxemia
- Neoplastic and paraneoplastic syndromes, including Pancoast's syndrome and syndrome of inappropriate secretion of antidiuretic hormone

Diagnostic test findings
- Cytologic sputum analysis shows diagnostic evidence of pulmonary malignancy
- Liver function tests are abnormal, especially with metastasis
- Chest X-rays show advanced lesions and can detect a lesion up to 2 years before signs and symptoms appear; also may reveal tumor size and location
- Contrast studies of the bronchial tree (chest tomography, bronchography) demonstrate size and location as well as spread of lesions
- Bone scanning is used to detect metastasis
- CT scanning of the chest detects malignant pleural effusion
- CT scanning of the brain detects metastasis
- PET scanning aids in diagnosis of primary and metastatic sites
- Bronchoscopy can be used to identify the tumor site; washings provide material for cytologic and histologic study
- Needle biopsy of the lungs provides firm diagnosis in 80% of patients by detecting tumors in the outer lung portions
- Tissue biopsy of metastatic sites is used to assess disease extent
- Thoracentesis allows chemical and cytologic examination of pleural fluid
- Exploratory thoracotomy is used to obtain biopsy specimen

Treatment
- Surgical excision of carcinoma; may include partial removal of lung (wedge resection, segmental resection, lobectomy, radical lobectomy) or total removal (pneumonectomy, radical pneumonectomy)
- Radiation therapy to destroy cancer cells when surgery is contraindicated
- Preoperative radiation therapy to destroy cancer cells (recommended for stage I and stage II lesions; for stage III lesions when disease is confined to involved hemithorax and ipsilateral supraclavicular lymph nodes)
- Postoperative radiation therapy to destroy any remaining cancer cells (delayed until 1 month after surgery to allow wound to heal, then directed to part of the chest most likely to develop metastasis)
- Chemotherapy to induce regression of tumor or prevent metastasis
- Laser therapy (through bronchoscope) to destroy local tumors

Nursing considerations
- Provide appropriate preoperative care

Key diagnostic test results for lung cancer
- Cytologic sputum analysis: Evidence of pulmonary malignancy
- Chest X-rays: Presence of advanced lesions; possibly tumor size and location
- Needle biopsy of the lungs: Detection of tumors in outer lung portion (provides firm diagnosis)

Key treatments for lung cancer
- Surgical excision of carcinoma
- Radiation therapy
- Chemotherapy
- Laser therapy

Key nursing considerations for lung cancer

- Explain expected postoperative procedures.
- Teach patient how to perform coughing, deep-breathing, and ROM exercises.

After surgery

- Maintain patent airway.
- Monitor chest tubes and closed chest drainage; report air leaks.
- Position patient on surgical side.
- Monitor vital signs and report abnormal respiration and other changes.
- Encourage coughing and deep breathing.
- Monitor intake and output.
- Maintain adequate hydration.

Key facts about liver cancer

- Usually originates in parenchymal cells
- Commonly results from metastasis from other primary cancers

- – Explain expected postoperative procedures, such as insertion of an indwelling catheter, use of an endotracheal tube or chest tube, dressing changes, and I.V. therapy
    - – Teach the patient how to perform coughing, deep-breathing, and range-of-motion (ROM) exercises
- Provide appropriate care after thoracic surgery
    - – Maintain a patent airway, and monitor chest tubes to reestablish normal intrathoracic pressure and prevent postoperative and pulmonary complications
    - – Monitor vital signs and report abnormal respiration and other changes
    - – Suction patient often and encourage coughing and deep breathing
    - – Monitor closed chest drainage; keep chest tubes patent and draining effectively; watch for air leaks and report them immediately; position the patient on surgical side to promote drainage and lung reexpansion
    - – Monitor intake and output
    - – Maintain adequate hydration
    - – Apply antiembolism stockings and encourage ROM exercises to prevent pulmonary embolus
    - – Watch for and treat infection, shock, hemorrhage, atelectasis, dyspnea, mediastinal shift, and pulmonary embolus
- Provide appropriate care for the patient receiving chemotherapy and radiation
    - – Explain possible adverse reactions; watch for, treat and, when possible, take steps to prevent them
    - – Provide soft, nonirritating, protein-rich foods, and encourage high-calorie, between-meal snacks
    - – During radiation therapy, provide good skin care to minimize breakdown
- Provide emotional support; encourage the patient to express fears and concerns

LIVER CANCER

- ● **Definition**
    - Malignant cells growing in the tissues of the liver
    - Rapidly fatal, usually within 6 months
    - After cirrhosis, the leading cause of fatal hepatic disease
    - Liver metastasis occurring as a solitary lesion (the first sign of recurrence after remission)

- ● **Underlying pathophysiology**
    - Most (90%) primary liver tumors originate in the parenchymal cells and are hepatomas; others originate in the intrahepatic bile ducts (cholangiomas)
    - Approximately 30% to 70% of patients with hepatomas also have cirrhosis
    - The liver is one of the most common sites of metastasis from other primary cancers; cells metastasize to the gallbladder, mesentery, peritoneum, and diaphragm by direct extension

- ● **Causes**
    - Immediate cause unknown
    - Environmental exposure to carcinogens

- Possibly androgens and oral estrogens
- Hepatitis B and C viruses

Pathophysiologic changes

- Mass in the right upper quadrant with a tender, nodular liver on palpation secondary to tumor cell growth
- Severe pain in epigastrium or right upper quadrant related to tumor size and increased pressure on surrounding tissue
- Bruit, hum, or rubbing sound if tumor involves a large part of the liver
- Weight loss, weakness, and anorexia related to increased tumor growth needs
- Dependent edema secondary to tumor invasion and obstruction of portal vein

Complications

- GI hemorrhage
- Progressive cachexia
- Liver failure

Diagnostic test findings

- Needle or open biopsy of the liver confirms the cell type
- Blood chemistry reveals elevated serum glutamic-oxaloacetic transaminase, alkaline phosphatase, lactic dehydrogenase, and bilirubin, indicating abnormal liver function
- Alpha-fetoprotein analysis reveals elevated levels
- Chest X-ray reveals possible metastasis
- Serum electrolyte studies reveal hypernatremia and hypercalcemia
- Serum laboratory studies reveal hypoglycemia, leukocytosis, or hypocholesterolemia

Treatment

- Resection by lobectomy or partial hepatectomy
- Radiation therapy for unresectable tumors (palliative)
- Chemotherapy with I.V. fluorouracil, methotrexate, streptozocin (Zanosar), lomustine (CeeNU), or doxorubicin, or with regional infusion of fluorouracil or floxuridine (FUDR) (catheters are placed directly into the hepatic artery or left brachial artery for continuous infusion for 7 to 21 days, or permanent implantable pumps are used on an outpatient basis)
- Liver transplantation (for a small subset of patients)

Nursing considerations

- Control edema and ascites
  - Monitor the patient's diet; restrict sodium, fluids (no alcohol), and protein
  - Weigh the patient daily and record intake and output
  - Watch for signs of ascites (peripheral edema, orthopnea, or dyspnea on exertion); if present, measure and record abdominal girth daily
- Monitor respiratory function, noting any increase in respiratory rate or shortness of breath; watch for signs of hypoxemia
- Administer aspirin suppositories to relieve fever (avoid acetaminophen, which can't be metabolized by the diseased liver)
- Administer antibiotics for infection
- Provide meticulous skin care; turn the patient frequently to prevent pressure ulcers
- Watch for signs of encephalopathy (confusion, restlessness, irritability, agitation, delirium, asterixis, lethargy, and coma)

Key pathophysiologic changes in liver cancer

- Mass in right upper quadrant
- Pain in epigastrium or right upper quadrant
- Anorexia
- Weight loss

Key diagnostic test results for liver cancer

- Needle or open biopsy: Confirmation of cell type
- Blood chemistry: Elevated serum glutamic-oxaloacetic transaminase, alkaline phosphatase, lactic dehydrogenase, and bilirubin

Key treatments for liver cancer

- Surgical resection
- Radiation therapy
- Chemotherapy

Key nursing considerations for liver cancer

- Control edema and ascites.
- Monitor respiratory function.
- Watch for signs of encephalopathy.
- Monitor serum ammonia levels and vital signs.

After surgery
- Watch for intraperitoneal bleeding and sepsis.
- Check urine output, BUN, and creatinine levels hourly.

- Monitor serum ammonia levels, vital signs, and neurologic status; be prepared to administer sorbitol (Lactulose) to control ammonia accumulation, neomycin (Neo-fradin) to control bacterial elaboration of ammonia, and sodium polystyrene sulfonate (Kayexalate) to lower potassium levels
- Frequently irrigate the transhepatic catheter (if used to relieve obstructive jaundice) with prescribed solution; monitor vital signs frequently for any indication of bleeding or infection
- After surgery, watch for intraperitoneal bleeding and sepsis, which may precipitate coma; monitor for renal failure by checking urine output, blood urea nitrogen (BUN), and creatinine levels hourly
- When all treatments have failed, concentrate on keeping the patient comfortable and free from pain; provide as much psychological support as possible

PANCREATIC CANCER

Definition
- Proliferation of cancer cells in the pancreas
- Poor prognosis; most patients die within 1 year

Underlying pathophysiology
- Pancreatic cancer is almost always adenocarcinoma
- Nearly two-thirds of tumors appear in the head of the pancreas; islet cell tumors and tumors found mostly in the tail of the pancreas (which are responsible for insulin, glucagon, and somatostatin production and release) are rare. (see *Islet cell tumors*)
- Two main tissue types form fibrotic nodes
  - Cylinder cells arise in ducts and degenerate into cysts
  - Large, fatty, granular cells arise in the parenchyma
- A high-fat or excessively high-protein diet induces chronic hyperplasia of the pancreas, with increased cell turnover

Causes
- Possible link to inhalation or absorption of carcinogens (such as cigarette smoke, excessive fat and protein, food additives, and industrial chemicals), which the pancreas then excretes
- Risk factors
  - Chronic pancreatitis
  - Diabetes
  - Chronic alcohol abuse
  - Smoking
  - Occupational exposure to chemicals
  - High-fat diet

Pathophysiologic changes
- Jaundice with clay-colored stools and dark urine secondary to obstruction of bile flow from tumor in head of pancreas
- Recurrent thrombophlebitis from tumor cytokines acting as platelet aggregation factors
- Nausea and vomiting secondary to duodenal obstruction
- Weight loss, anorexia, and malaise secondary to effects of increased tumor growth needs

Islet cell tumors

Relatively uncommon, islet cell tumors (insulinomas) affect insulin, glucagon, and somatostatin production and release. Tumors may be benign or malignant, and they produce signs and symptoms in three stages:

1. Slight hypoglycemia — fatigue, restlessness, malaise, and excessive weight gain
2. Compensatory secretions of epinephrine — pallor, clamminess, perspiration, palpitations, finger tremors, hunger, decreased temperature, and increased pulse and blood pressure
3. Severe hypoglycemia — ataxia, clouds sensorium, diplopia, episodes of violence, and hysteria

Usually, insulinomas metastasize only to the liver, but they may metastasize to bone, the brain, and the lungs. Death results from a combination of hypoglycemic reactions and widespread metastasis. Treatment consists of enucleation of the tumor (if benign) and chemotherapy with streptozocin (Zanosar) or resection that includes pancreatic tissue (if malignant).

- Abdominal or back pain secondary to tumor pressure
- Blood in the stool from ulceration of GI tract or ampulla of Vater

Complications
- Nutrient malabsorption
- Type 1 diabetes
- Liver and GI problems
- Mental status changes
- Hemorrhage
- Pulmonary congestion

Diagnostic test findings
- Blood testing shows an absence of pancreatic enzymes
- Prolonged prothrombin time
- Blood chemistry reveals increased serum bilirubin, possibly increased serum lipase and amylase levels, and markedly elevated alkaline phosphatase levels (in biliary obstruction)
- Analysis reveals elevated levels of aspartate aminotransferase and alanine aminotransferase (if liver cell necrosis present)
- Plasma insulin immunoassay shows measurable serum insulin in the presence of islet cell tumors
- Fasting blood glucose test may reveal hypoglycemia or hyperglycemia
- Blood testing reveals specific tumor markers for pancreatic cancer are elevated, including carcinoembryonic antigen, pancreatic oncofetal antigen, alpha-fetoprotein, and serum immunoreactive elastase I
- Barium swallow, retroperitoneal insufflation, cholangiography, and scintigraphy locate the neoplasm and detect changes in the duodenum or stomach
- Ultrasonography and CT scans identify masses
- MRI discloses tumor location and size

Key diagnostic test results for pancreatic cancer
- Blood testing: Specific tumor markers for pancreatic cancer are elevated, including carcinoembryonic antigen, pancreatic oncofetal antigen, alpha-fetoprotein, and serum immunoreactive elastase I
- Ultrasonography and CT scans: Presence of masses
- MRI: Tumor location and size
- Endoscopic retrograde cholangiopancreatography: Tumor visualization

Key treatments for pancreatic cancer

- Palliative care
- Radiation therapy
- Chemotherapy
- Surgery
- Anticholinergics

Key nursing considerations for pancreatic cancer

Before surgery
- Maintain adequate nutrition and positive nitrogen balance.

After surgery
- Monitor fluid balance, abdominal girth, metabolic state, and weight daily.
- Watch for signs of hypoglycemia or hyperglycemia.
- Watch for signs of upper GI bleeding.
- Provide meticulous skin care.
- Ensure adequate rest and sleep.

- Angiography reveals tumor vascularity
- Endoscopic retrograde cholangiopancreatography allows tumor visualization and specimen biopsy
- Percutaneous fine-needle aspiration biopsy may detect tumor cells
- Laparotomy with biopsy allows definitive diagnosis

Treatment
- Mainly palliative
- May involve radiation therapy as adjunct to fluorouracil chemotherapy
- Standard chemotherapy for patients with locally unresectable cancer includes gemcitabine (Gemzar)
- Other medications
  - Antibiotics to prevent infection and relieve symptoms
  - Anticholinergics to decrease GI tract spasm and motility and to reduce pain and secretions
  - Antacids to decrease secretion of pancreatic enzymes and to suppress peptic activity, thereby reducing stress-induced damage to gastric mucosa
  - Diuretics to mobilize extracellular fluid from ascites
  - Insulin to provide adequate exogenous insulin supply after pancreatic resection
  - Opioids to relieve pain, but only after other analgesics fail (morphine, meperidine [Demerol], and codeine can lead to biliary tract spasm and increase common bile duct pressure)
  - Pancreatic enzymes to assist in digestion of proteins, carbohydrates, and fats when pancreatic juices are insufficient because of surgery or obstruction
- Surgical procedures
  - Total pancreatectomy
  - Cholecystojejunostomy, choledochoduodenostomy, and choledochojejunostomy
  - Whipple's operation or pancreatoduodenectomy
  - Gastrojejunostomy

Nursing considerations
- Provide appropriate preoperative care
  - Make sure that the patient is medically stable, particularly regarding nutrition; if he can't tolerate oral feedings, provide total parental nutrition and I.V. fat emulsions to correct deficiencies and to maintain positive nitrogen balance
  - Give blood transfusions (to combat anemia), vitamin K (to overcome prothrombin deficiency), antibiotics (to prevent postoperative complications), and gastric lavage (to maintain gastric decompression), as ordered
- Provide appropriate postoperative care
  - Report complications, such as fistula, pancreatitis, fluid and electrolyte imbalance, infection, hemorrhage, skin breakdown, nutritional deficiency, hepatic failure, renal insufficiency, and diabetes
  - If the patient is receiving chemotherapy, treat adverse effects symptomatically
- Monitor fluid balance, abdominal girth, metabolic state, and weight daily
  - For weight loss, replace nutrients

  – For weight gain (due to ascites), impose dietary restrictions, such as low-sodium or a fluid-retention diet, as ordered
  – Maintain a 2,500-calorie diet; provide small, frequent meals
- Prevent constipation; administer laxatives, stool softeners, and cathartics, as ordered, and increase fluid intake
- Ensure adequate rest and sleep
- Assist with ROM and isometric exercises as appropriate
- Watch for signs of hypoglycemia or hyperglycemia; administer glucose or antidiabetic agent as ordered (monitor blood glucose and urine glucose levels)
- Provide meticulous skin care to avoid pruritus and necrosis
- Watch for signs of upper GI bleeding; test stools and vomitus for occult blood and monitor hemoglobin and hematocrit
  – Promote gastric vasoconstriction with prescribed medications to control active bleeding
- Apply antiembolism stockings to prevent thrombosis
- Provide psychological support

GASTRIC CANCER

Definition
- Cancer of the GI tract
- Classified according to gross appearance
  – Polypoid
  – Ulcerating
  – Ulcerating and infiltrating
  – Diffuse
- Prognosis depends on stage of disease at time of diagnosis

Underlying pathophysiology
- Develops in the epithelial cells of the stomach's innermost walls (when confined to this layer, it's typically curable)
- Develops in the stomach, most commonly in the pylorus (see *Sites of gastric cancer,* page 524)
- Rapidly metastasizes to the regional lymph nodes, omentum, liver, and lungs

Causes
- Unknown

Risk factors
- Alcohol consumption
- Family history of gastric cancer
- Gastritis with gastric atrophy
- Consumption of smoked foods, pickled vegetables, and salted fish and meat
- Smoking
- Type A blood (10% increased risk)

Pathophysiologic changes
- Chronic dyspepsia and epigastric discomfort related to tumor growth in gastric cells and destruction of mucosal barrier
- Weight loss, anorexia, feeling of fullness after eating, anemia, and fatigue secondary to increased tumor growth needs

Key facts about gastric cancer
- Develops in epithelial cells of stomach's innermost walls
- Classified as polypoid, ulcerating, ulcerating and infiltrating, or diffuse

Key pathophysiologic changes in gastric cancer
- Chronic dyspepsia
- Weight loss
- Anorexia
- Blood in stools

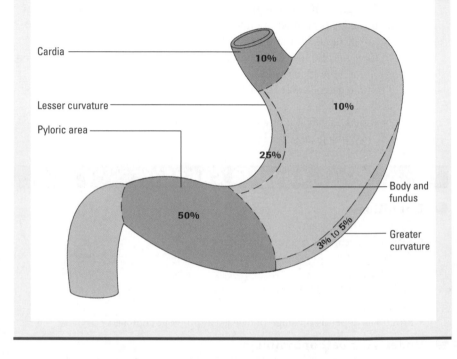

Sites of gastric cancer

The most common site of gastric cancer is the pyloric area, accounting for approximately 50% of cases. The next most common site is the lesser curvature of the stomach, which accounts for approximately 25% of cases.

Cardia

Lesser curvature

Pyloric area

10%

10%

25%

50%

3% to 5%

Body and fundus

Greater curvature

- Blood in stools resulting from erosion of the gastric mucosa caused by tumors

● Complications
- Malnutrition
- GI obstruction
- Iron-deficiency anemia
- Metastasis

● Diagnostic test findings
- CBC shows iron-deficiency anemia
- Liver function studies are elevated with metastatic spread of the tumor to the liver
- Carcinoembryonic antigen radioimmunoassay level is elevated
- Barium X-rays of the GI tract with fluoroscopy shows changes that suggest gastric cancer, including a tumor or filling defect in the outline of the stomach, loss of flexibility and distensibility, and abnormal gastric mucosa with or without ulceration
- Gastroscopy with fiber-optic endoscopy allowing direct visualization, which helps to rule out other diffuse gastric mucosal abnormalities
- Gastroscopic biopsy permits evaluation of gastric mucosal lesions

- Gastric acids stimulation test discloses whether the stomach is able to properly secrete acid

Treatment

- Radiation therapy combined with chemotherapy (not indicated preoperatively because it may damage viscera and impede healing)
- Diet based on the extent of the disorder and clinical condition
- Parenteral feeding if patient is unable to consume adequate calories
- Drug therapy
  - Vitamin and iron supplements to treat anemia
  - Antacids and histamine-2 receptor antagonists to treat GI ulcers
  - Analgesics to relieve pain
  - Chemotherapy to shrink the tumor and halt its spread
- Excision of lesion with appropriate margins (in more than one-third of patients)
- Surgical procedures
  - Gastroduodenostomy
  - Gastrojejunostomy
  - Partial gastric resection
  - Total gastrectomy
  - If metastasis has occurred, removal of omentum and spleen

Nursing considerations

- Provide a high-protein, high-calorie diet with dietary supplements
- Provide parenteral nutrition as appropriate
- After surgery
  - Encourage the patient to gradually increase his activity level
  - Advise the patient to rest often and to avoid stress
  - Monitor NG tube function and drainage
  - Monitor vital signs, pain control, and effects of medication
  - Monitor intake and output, hydration, and nutritional status
  - Provide modified diets, as ordered
- After gastrectomy, provide a special diet to patients who experience poor digestion and absorption: frequent feedings of small amounts of clear liquids, increasing to small, frequent feedings of bland food
- After total gastrectomy, instruct patients to eat small amounts of clear liquid, advancing to full liquid, and then 6 small feedings
- Monitor the wound site for wound dehiscence and delayed healing caused by decreased protein, anemia, and avitaminosis
- Teach the patient about his dietary plan
- Instruct the patient to avoid of crowds and people known to have infections
- Teach the patient relaxation techniques
- Inform the patient about his medications, including possible adverse effects

COLORECTAL CANCER

Definition

- Slow-growing cancer that usually starts in inner layer of intestinal tract
- Commonly begins as polyp

Key treatments for gastric cancer

- Combination radiation therapy and chemotherapy
- Surgery

Key nursing considerations for gastric cancer

- Monitor NG tube function and drainage.
- Monitor wound site for dehiscence.
- Monitor vital signs and pain control.
- Teach patient about dietary plan.

Key facts about colorectal cancer

- Tends to grow slowly
- Usually starts in inner layer of intestinal tract
- Commonly involves moderately differentiated adenocarcinomas

- Signs and symptoms depend on location of tumor
- Potentially curable if diagnosed early

● **Underlying pathophysiology**
- Most lesions of the large bowel are moderately differentiated adenocarcinomas
- Tumors tend to grow slowly and remain asymptomatic for long periods
- Tumors in the sigmoid and descending colon undergo circumferential growth and constrict the intestinal lumen
- Tumors in the ascending colon are usually large at diagnosis and are palpable on physical examination

● **Causes**
- Unknown
- Risk factors
    - Inherited gene mutations
    - Family or personal history of colorectal cancer
    - History of intestinal polyps
    - History of chronic inflammatory bowel disease
    - Aging
    - High-fat diet
    - Obesity and physical inactivity
    - Diabetes
    - Smoking
    - Heavy alcohol intake

● **Pathophysiologic changes**
- Right side of colon
    - Early signs
        · Black, tarry stool; anemia due to GI bleeding
        · Abdominal aching, pressure, or dull cramps caused by bowel irritation
    - Late signs
        · Weakness, fatigue, and exertional dyspnea due to anemia
        · Diarrhea, obstipation, anorexia, weight loss, and vomiting due to intestinal obstruction
- Left side of colon and rectum
    - Early signs
        · Black, tarry stool or rectal bleeding due to GI bleeding
        · Intermittent abdominal fullness or cramping; rectal pressure due to intestinal obstruction
    - Late signs
        · Obstipation, diarrhea, or ribbon- or pencil-shaped stool due to intestinal obstruction
        · Dark or bright red blood in stool and mucus (in or on stool) due to GI bleeding

● **Complications**
- Abdominal distention and intestinal obstruction as tumor growth encroaches on abdominal organs
- Anemia

Common risk factors for colorectal cancer

- History of chronic inflammatory bowel disease
- History of intestinal polyps
- Family history of colorectal cancer

Key pathophysiologic changes in colorectal cancer

Right side of colon
- Black, tarry stool
- Weakness
- Weight loss
- Vomiting

Left side of colon and rectum
- Black, tarry stool
- Rectal bleeding
- Abdominal cramping
- Ribbon-shaped stool

Diagnostic test findings

- Fecal occult blood test shows blood in stools, a warning sign of colorectal cancer
- Carcinoembryonic antigen testing provides monitoring before and after treatment to detect metastasis or recurrence
- Excretory urography verifies bilateral renal function and allows inspection for displacement of the kidneys, ureters, or bladder by a tumor pressing against these structures
- Barium enema studies reveal the location of lesions
- CT scans allow better visualization if a barium enema yields inconclusive results or if metastasis to the pelvic lymph nodes is suspected
- Proctoscopy or sigmoidoscopy permits visualization of the lower GI tract; can detect up to 66% of colorectal cancers
- Colonoscopy permits visualization of the colon up to the ileocecal valve and provides access for polypectomies and biopsies of suspected lesions
- Digital rectal examination can be used to detect almost 15% of colorectal cancers

Treatment

- Surgery to remove tumor
  - Cecum and ascending colon: right hemicolectomy
  - Proximal and middle transverse colon: right colectomy
  - Sigmoid colon: typically limited to sigmoid colon and mesentery
  - Upper rectum: anterior or low anterior resection
  - Lower rectum: abdominoperineal resection and permanent sigmoid colostomy
- Chemotherapy for patients with metastasis, residual disease, or recurrent inoperable tumor
- Radiation therapy (may be used before or after surgery or in combination with chemotherapy) to induce tumor regression
- Referral to enterostomal therapist (if appropriate) for stoma management

Nursing considerations

- Provide appropriate preoperative care
  - Monitor the patient's dietary modifications, laxatives, enemas, and antibiotics — all of which are used to clean the bowel and decrease abdominal and perineal cavity contamination during surgery
  - Teach the patient and his family about the colostomy (if applicable)
  - Prepare the patient for postoperative I.V. infusions, NG tube, and indwelling urinary catheter
- Provide appropriate postoperative care
  - Encourage the patient to look at the stoma and participate in its care as soon as possible; teach good hygiene and skin care
    - After several months, many ostomates establish control with irrigation and no longer need to wear a pouch; a stoma cap or gauze sponge placed over the stoma protects it and absorbs mucoid secretions
  - Teach the patient when physical activities may be resumed, but caution against heavy lifting because herniation or prolapse may occur through weakened muscles in the abdominal wall

---

Key diagnostic test results for colorectal cancer

- Fecal occult blood test: Presence of blood in stools
- Proctoscopy or sigmoidoscopy: Visualization of lower GI tract
- Colonoscopy: Visualization of colon up to ileocecal valve; also provides access for polypectomy and biopsy

Key treatments for colorectal cancer

- Surgery
- Chemotherapy
- Radiation therapy

Key nursing considerations for colorectal cancer

- Prepare patient for postoperative procedures.
- Encourage patient to participate in stoma care.
- Teach patient when physical activities may be resumed.

– Encourage the patient to get annual screening and testing (anyone who's had colorectal cancer is at increased risk for recurrence)

BLADDER CANCER

Key facts about bladder cancer

- Can develop on or within bladder wall
- Usually involves transitional cell carcinomas, which arise from transitional epithelium of mucous membranes
- Invades underlying muscle quickly

Key pathophysiologic changes in bladder cancer

- Hematuria
- Urinary frequency

Key diagnostic test results for bladder cancer

- Excretory urography: Large, early stage tumor or infiltrating tumor; functional problems in upper urinary tract; presence of hydronephrosis; bladder wall deformity
- Retrograde cystography: Bladder structure and integrity; confirmation of diagnosis
- Cystoscopy and biopsy: Cancer cells

● Definition
- Can develop on bladder wall surface (benign or malignant papillomas) or grow within bladder wall (generally more virulent)
- Quickly invades underlying muscles (see *Understanding bladder structures and function*)
- Most common type: transitional cell carcinoma, arising from transitional epithelium of mucous membranes
- Less common types: adenocarcinoma, epidermoid carcinoma, squamous cell carcinoma, sarcoma, tumor in bladder diverticula, and carcinoma in situ

● Underlying pathophysiology
- About 90% of bladder cancers are transitional cell carcinomas, arising from the transitional epithelium of mucous membranes (may result from malignant transformation of benign papillomas)

● Causes
- Exact cause unknown
- Associated with chronic bladder irritation and infection in patients with renal calculi, indwelling urinary catheters, chemical cystitis caused by cyclophosphamide, or pelvic irradiation

● Pathophysiologic changes
- Early stages commonly produce no symptoms
- Gross, painless, intermittent hematuria due to tumor invasion
- Suprapubic pain after voiding caused by pressure exerted by tumor or obstruction
- Bladder irritability, urinary frequency, nocturia, and dribbling caused by tumor compression and invasion

● Complications
- Bone metastasis
- Problems resulting from tumor invasion of contiguous viscera

● Diagnostic test findings
- CBC helps to detect anemia
- Urinalysis detects blood and malignant cells in urine
- Excretory urography identifies a large, early stage tumor or an infiltrating tumor, delineates functional problems in the upper urinary tract, indicates the presence of hydronephrosis, and detects rigid deformity of the bladder wall
- Retrograde cystography is used to evaluate the bladder structure and integrity; helps confirm a bladder cancer diagnosis
- Bone scan can be used to detect metastasis
- CT scan defines the thickness of the involved bladder wall and discloses enlarged retroperitoneal lymph nodes
- Ultrasonography reveals metastases in tissues beyond the bladder and can distinguish a bladder cyst from a bladder tumor

Understanding bladder structures and function

The bladder lies in the front portion of the pelvic cavity and is composed of an inner mucosal lining, several layers of muscle, and outer perivesical fat. The ureters transport urine from the kidneys into the bladder. After the bladder fills, the urine leaves the body through another tubelike structure called the *urethra*. Tumors can form in any of the layers of the bladder or in related structures.

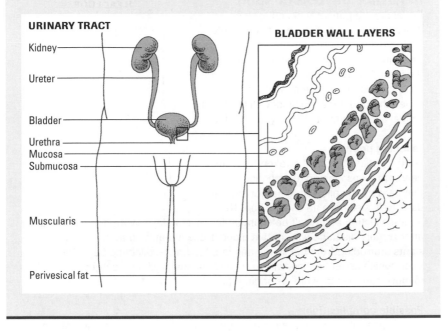

URINARY TRACT
- Kidney
- Ureter
- Bladder
- Urethra
- Mucosa
- Submucosa
- Muscularis
- Perivesical fat

BLADDER WALL LAYERS

- Cystoscopy and biopsy confirm bladder cancer diagnosis; if the test results show cancer cells, further studies are used to determine the cancer stage and treatment

● Treatment
- For a superficial bladder tumor
  - Transurethral (cystoscopic) resection and fulguration (electrical destruction) to remove the tumor
  - Intravesicular chemotherapy (for multiple tumors) to kill cancer cells
  - Fulguration if additional tumors develop (may be repeated every 3 months for years) to remove the tumor
- For a large tumor
  - Segmental bladder resection to remove a full-thickness section of the bladder (only if the tumor isn't near the bladder neck or ureteral orifices)
  - Bladder instillation of thiotepa (TESPA) after transurethral resection to slow or stop growth of cancer cells
- For infiltrating bladder tumors
  - Radical cystectomy (treatment of choice), which requires urinary diversion, usually an ileal conduit (see *Teaching about urinary diversions,* pages 530 and 531)

Key treatments for bladder cancer
- Resection or cystectomy (depending on tumor type)
- Chemotherapy

Types of urinary diversions

- Ileal loop or ileal conduit
- Continent urinary diversion
- Ureterostomy

TOP 4

Possible complications of ileal loop or ileal conduit

1. Anuria
2. Urine or fecal leakage
3. Stomal stenosis
4. Stomal ulceration

TIME-OUT FOR TEACHING

Teaching about urinary diversions

If your patient is scheduled for a simple or radical cystectomy, he'll need a urinary diversion to substitute for his bladder. Teach him about the diversion he'll receive.

ILEAL LOOP OR ILEAL CONDUIT

Explain to the patient that an ileal loop or ileal conduit is one of the most commonly performed supravesicular-urinary diversions. In this procedure, about 6″ (15 cm) of the ileum is sutured and closed, the ureters are attached to the ileum, the ileum is pulled through the abdominal wall to form a stoma, and then the bowel is reconnected.

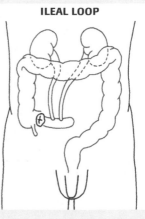

ILEAL LOOP

Teaching points

Tell the patient that he'll awaken from surgery with a nasogastric tube in place and that he won't be allowed to eat for several days. He'll also have an ostomy bag. This urine-collecting bag won't be changed for several days. Warn him that initially after surgery his urine will contain blood. Explain that he may see catheters or stents protruding from the stoma and into the urine-collecting bag. These devices, which assist healing, will be removed a few days after surgery. Urge him to move carefully to avoid dislodging them.

Possible complications

Review possible problems, such as anuria from edema or obstruction at the ureterointestinal anastomosis, urine or fecal leakage at the anastomosis, abdominal distention or a dusky stoma from vascular infarction of the conduit site, stomal stenosis, pyelonephritis, renal calculi, and skin problems — for example, stomal ulceration.

CONTINENT URINARY DIVERSION

If a continent urinary diversion procedure is performed, tell the patient that his ureters will be diverted into his sigmoid colon so that he'll void through his anus. He won't need to wear an ostomy bag. This procedure is done only if the patient has good anal sphincter tone.

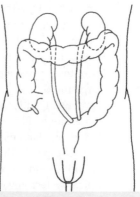

CONTINENT URINARY DIVERSION

Teaching points

Advise the patient to sit or stand frequently after surgery to avoid urine reflux. Also warn him that this diversion may produce urinary incontinence when he passes flatus. Explain that choosing a diet low in gas-forming foods may help to allay this problem. Teach the patient to avoid possible electrolyte imbalances related to this diversion by following a diet low in chloride and salt and by taking potassium supplements.

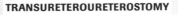

Teaching about urinary diversions *(continued)*

Possible complications
Explain that anuria, resulting from ureteral obstruction, stricture, edema, or fecal matter and mucus, can lead to kidney failure. Other potential complications include urine leakage from the anastomosis, pyelonephritis, electrolyte imbalances, and renal calculi formation.

URETEROSTOMY
Teach the patient that ureterostomy involves diverting the ureters through an opening in the abdominal wall. Depending on the procedure, one or more stomas will be created. For example, for a transureteroureterostomy, one ureter is directed into the other so that only one tube opens to the outside, thereby requiring only one stoma. Two stomas are required for a double-barrel ureterostomy, which brings the two ureters side by side to the abdominal surface. Because this procedure can be completed quickly, it may be done with a patient who has a low tolerance for anesthesia.

Teaching points
Tell the patient that he'll need to wear an ostomy bag after surgery. However, because the stoma created by this diversion rises very little above skin level, the ostomy bag may adhere poorly. Recommend using an adhesive-backed ostomy bag for better results.

Possible complications
Warn the patient that a dusky (cyanotic) stoma may signal vascular insufficiency, which can lead to stenosis.

TRANSURETEROURETEROSTOMY

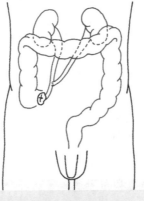

DOUBLE-BARREL URETEROSTOMY

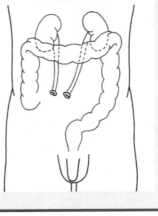

TOP 3
Possible complications of continent urinary diversion

1. Anuria
2. Urine leakage from anastomosis
3. Electrolyte imbalance

TOP 2
Possible complications of ureterostomy

1. Vascular insufficiency
2. Stenosis

- Possible penile implant (later) to treat erectile dysfunction
- Referral to the American Cancer Society and, if the patient received an ostomy, the United Ostomy Association for information and support
- For advanced bladder cancer
  - Cystectomy to remove the tumor
  - Radiation therapy to destroy cancer cells
  - Systemic chemotherapy (cisplatin, cyclophosphamide, fluorouracil, doxorubicin) to destroy cancer cells
  - Investigational treatments (clinical trials currently being conducted)
  - Photodynamic therapy and intravesicular administration of interferon alfa and tumor necrosis factor to destroy cancer cells

– Bacillus Calmette-Guérin (BCG), intravesical (immunomodulating agent) to treat superficial bladder cancer after surgery to remove the tumor
– Biologic response modifiers (interferons, interleukins, colony-stimulating factors, monoclonal antibodies, vaccines) to destroy cancer cells

● **Nursing considerations**
• Before surgery, assist in selecting a stoma site that the patient can see (usually in the rectus muscle to minimize the risk of herniation)
• Teach the patient about the type of diversion planned
• After surgery, encourage the patient to look at the stoma; provide a mirror to make viewing easier
• When a patient with a urinary diversion is discharged, arrange for follow-up care or provide a referral to an enterostomal therapist, who will coordinate the patient's care
• Teach the patient about the urinary stoma; encourage the spouse, other relatives, and friends to attend the teaching session
• All high-risk people (for example, people who work with chemicals and those with a history of benign bladder tumors or persistent cystitis) should have periodic cytologic examinations and learn about the danger of disease-causing agents

PROSTATE CANCER

● **Definition**
• Slow-growing, most common neoplasm in men older than age 50
• Commonly forms as adenocarcinoma (derived from glandular tissue); sarcomas rarely occur
• Usually originates in posterior prostate gland; sometimes originates near urethra
• Seldom results from benign hyperplastic enlargement (common with aging)
• Clinical manifestations typically associated with later stages of disease

● **Underlying pathophysiology**
• Typically, when a primary prostatic lesion spreads beyond the prostate gland, it invades the prostatic capsule and spreads along ejaculatory ducts in the space between the seminal vesicles or perivesicular fascia
• Endocrine factors may play a role, leading researchers to suspect that androgens speed tumor growth

● **Causes**
• Exact cause unknown
• Risk factors
– Older than age 40
– Infection
– Vasectomy
– Family history
– Heavy metal exposure

Key nursing considerations for bladder cancer

• Teach patient about the urinary stoma.
• Arrange for follow-up care or provide referral to enterostomal therapist.

Key facts about prostate cancer

• Usually originates in posterior prostate gland
• Grows slowly
• May spread beyond prostate gland and invade prostatic capsule and ejaculatory ducts

Pathophysiologic changes
- Difficulty initiating urinary stream, dribbling, urine retention, and unexplained cystitis due to obstruction of urinary tract by tumor
- Hematuria due to infiltration of bladder tumor
- Back pain caused by bone metastasis

Complications
- Spinal cord compression
- Deep vein thrombosis
- Pulmonary emboli
- Myelophthisis
- Death

Diagnostic test findings
- Serum prostate-specific antigen level is elevated (may indicate cancer with or without metastasis)
- Transrectal prostatic ultrasonography shows prostate size and presence of abnormal growths
- Bone scan and excretory urography determines extent of disease
- MRI and CT scanning define extent of tumor
- Direct rectal (digital) examination reveals a small, hard nodule
- Blood testing reveals elevated serum acid phosphatase levels
- Biopsy confirms the cell type

Treatment
- Radiation therapy to treat locally invasive lesions (may also relieve bone pain associated with metastasis)
- Radioactive seed implants into prostate (brachytherapy) to enhance radiation of cancerous area with minimal exposure to surrounding tissue
- Hormonal therapy (flutamide [Eulexin]) to treat androgen-dependent prostate cancer
- Radical prostatectomy to remove prostate gland and tumor
- Transurethral resection of prostate (TURP) to relieve obstruction
- Orchiectomy to decrease androgen production
- Cryoablation to remove tumor by freezing
- Pain management to alleviate pain associated with bone metastasis

Nursing considerations
- Provide appropriate care before prostatectomy
  - Explain the expected aftereffects of surgery (such as impotence and incontinence) and radiation
  - Teach the patient to do perineal exercises 1 to 10 times per hour; have him squeeze his buttocks together, hold this position for a few seconds, and then relax
- Provide appropriate care after prostatectomy or suprapubic prostatectomy
  - Regularly check the dressing, incision, and drainage system for excessive bleeding; watch the patient for signs of bleeding (pallor, falling blood pressure, rising pulse rate) and infection
  - Maintain adequate fluid intake
  - Give antispasmodics, as ordered, to control postoperative bladder spasms; give analgesics as needed

---

Key pathophysiologic changes in prostate cancer
- Difficulty initiating urinary stream
- Urine retention
- Hematuria

Key diagnostic test results for prostate cancer
- Serum prostate-specific antigen: Elevated
- Transrectal prostatic ultrasonography: Presence of abnormal growths
- Direct rectal examination: Presence of small, hard nodule

Key treatments for prostate cancer
- Radiation therapy
- Brachytherapy
- Hormonal therapy
- Surgery

Key nursing considerations for prostate cancer

After surgery
- Monitor dressings and incision site.
- Provide meticulous catheter care.
- Give antispasmodics as ordered.

After radiation therapy
- Urge patient to drink at least 2 qt (2 L) of fluid daily.
- Give analgesics as ordered.

– Provide meticulous catheter care (especially if a three-way catheter with a continuous irrigation system is in place); check the tubing for kinks and blockages, especially if the patient reports pain, and caution him not to pull on the catheter
- Provide appropriate care after TURP
  – Watch for signs of urethral stricture (dysuria, decreased force and caliber of urine stream, and straining to urinate) and abdominal distention (from urethral stricture or catheter blockage); irrigate the catheter as ordered
- Provide appropriate care after perineal prostatectomy
  – Avoid taking a rectal temperature or inserting any kind of rectal tube
  – Provide pads to absorb urine leakage, a rubber ring for the patient to sit on, and sitz baths for pain and inflammation
- Provide appropriate care after perineal and retropubic prostatectomy
  – Explain that urine leakage after catheter removal is normal and will subside
  – When a patient receives hormonal therapy, watch for adverse effects (gynecomastia, fluid retention, nausea, and vomiting are common)
- Watch for common adverse reactions after radiation therapy (proctitis, diarrhea, bladder spasms, and urinary frequency)
  – Be aware that internal radiation usually results in cystitis in the first 2 to 3 weeks
  – Urge the patient to drink at least 2 qt (2 L) of fluid daily
  – Give analgesics and antispasmodics as ordered

TESTICULAR CANCER

● **Definition**
- Proliferation of cancerous cells in the testicles
- Most originate from germinal cells, and about 40% become seminomas

● **Underlying pathophysiology**
- Testicular cancer spreads through the lymphatic system to the iliac, para-aortic, and mediastinal nodes
- Metastasis affects the lungs, liver, viscera, and bone

● **Causes**
- Exact cause unknown
- Risk factors
  – Cryptorchidism (see *Cryptorchidism and testicular cancer*)
  – Mumps orchitis
  – Inguinal hernia in childhood
  – Maternal use of DES or other estrogen-progestin combinations during pregnancy

● **Pathophysiologic changes**
- Firm, painless, smooth testicular mass and occasional complaints of heaviness secondary to tumor growth
- Gynecomastia and nipple tenderness related to tumor production of chorionic gonadotropin or estrogen
- Urinary complaints related to ureteral obstruction

Key facts about testicular cancer

- Usually originates from germinal cells
- Spreads through the lymphatic system to iliac, para-aortic, and mediastinal nodes

Key pathophysiologic changes in testicular cancer

- Firm, painless, smooth testicular mass
- Complaints of testicular heaviness

Cryptorchidism and testicular cancer

In men with cryptorchidism (the failure of a testicle to descend into the scrotum), testicular tumors are about 50 times more common than in men with normal anatomic structure. A simple surgical procedure called *orchiopexy* can bring the testicle to its normal position in the scrotum and reduce the testicular cancer risk. Nevertheless, testicular tumors occur more commonly in a surgically descended testicle than in a naturally descended one.

WHAT HAPPENS IN ORCHIOPEXY
In orchiopexy, the surgeon incises the groin area and separates the testicle and its blood supply from surrounding abdominal structures. Then he creates a "tunnel" into the scrotum to accommodate the descent of the testicle.

FURTHER REDUCING THE RISK
After orchiopexy, the patient should be urged to examine his testicles monthly, allowing detection of a tumor at its earliest stage.

- Cough, hemoptysis, and shortness of breath from invasion of the pulmonary system

● **Complications**
- Back or abdominal pain from retroperitoneal adenopathy
- Metastasis
- Ureteral obstruction

● **Diagnostic test findings**
- Testicular palpation reveals detectable mass
- Transillumination of the testicles reveals an opaque mass
- Surgical excision and biopsy reveal cell type; inguinal exploration determines the extent of nodal involvement
- Excretory urography detects ureteral deviation from para-aortic node involvement
- Serum alpha-fetoprotein and beta human chorionic gonadotropin levels are elevated (tumor markers)
- Lymphangiography, ultrasonography, and abdominal CT scanning are used to detect the mass and reveal possible metastasis

● **Treatment**
- Orchidectomy and retroperitoneal node dissection
- Hormone replacement surgery after bilateral orchiectomy
- Radiation therapy
- Chemotherapy
- Autologous bone marrow transplantation for patients nonresponsive to standard therapy

● **Nursing considerations**
- Explain the procedure and reassure the patient before orchiectomy
  - Reassure him that sterility and impotence need not follow unilateral orchiectomy, that synthetic hormones can restore hormonal balance, and

Key diagnostic test results for testicular cancer
- Testicular palpation: Presence of mass
- Surgical excision and biopsy: Cell type; extent of nodal involvement

Key treatments for testicular cancer
- Surgery
- Radiation therapy
- Chemotherapy

that most surgeons don't remove the scrotum; a testicular prosthesis can correct anatomic disfigurement
- Provide appropriate care after orchiectomy
    - Apply an ice pack to the scrotum and provide analgesics as ordered for the first day after surgery
    - Check for excessive bleeding, swelling, and signs of infection
    - Provide a scrotal athletic supporter to minimize pain during ambulation
- Give antiemetics as needed during chemotherapy
    - Encourage small, frequent meals to maintain oral intake despite anorexia
    - Establish a mouth care regimen and check for stomatitis
- Watch for signs of myelosuppression

OVARIAN CANCER

⬤ **Definition**
- Malignancy arising from the ovary
- Rapidly progressing cancer that's difficult to diagnose
- 90% primary epithelial tumors; stromal and germ cell tumors also important types

⬤ **Underlying pathophysiology**
- Ovarian cancer spreads rapidly intraperitoneally by local extension or surface seeding and, occasionally, through the lymphatics and the bloodstream
- Metastasis to the ovary can originate as breast, colon, gastric, and pancreatic cancer

⬤ **Causes**
- Exact cause unknown
- Risk factors
    - Infertility problems or nulliparity
    - Celibacy
    - Exposure to asbestos and talc
    - History of breast or uterine cancer
    - Family history of ovarian cancer
    - Diet high in saturated fat

⬤ **Pathophysiologic changes**
- Vague abdominal discomfort, dyspepsia, and other mild GI complaints from increasing size of tumor exerting pressure on nearby tissues
- Urinary frequency and constipation from obstruction due to increased tumor size
- Pain from tumor rupture, torsion, or infection
- Feminizing or masculinizing effects secondary to cellular type
- Ascites related to invasion and infiltration of the peritoneum
- Pleural effusions related to pulmonary metastasis

⬤ **Complications**
- Fluid and electrolyte imbalance
- Leg edema
- Ascites
- Intestinal obstruction

- Profound cachexia
- Recurrent malignant effusions

● Diagnostic test findings

- Laboratory tumor marker studies (such as ovarian carcinoma antigen, carcino-embryonic antigen, and human chorionic gonadotropin) shows abnormalities that may indicate complications
- Abdominal ultrasonography, CT scans, or X-rays delineate tumor size
- Mammography (when normal) rules out breast cancer as the primary site
- Aspiration of ascitic fluid reveals atypical cells
- Exploratory laparotomy, including lymph node evaluation and tumor resection, is required for accurate diagnosis and staging

● Treatment

- In girls or young women with a unilateral encapsulated tumor who wish to maintain fertility
  - Resection of the involved ovary
  - Biopsies of the omentum and the uninvolved ovary
  - Peritoneal washings for cytologic examination of pelvic fluid
  - Careful follow-up, including periodic chest X-rays to rule out lung metastasis
- More aggressive treatment
  - Total abdominal hysterectomy and bilateral salpingo-oophorectomy with tumor resection
  - Omentectomy, appendectomy, lymph node palpation with probable lymphadenectomy, tissue biopsies, and peritoneal washings
  - Chemotherapy after surgery
  - Immunotherapy (under investigation)
  - Hormone replacement therapy in prepubertal girls who had bilateral salpingo-oophorectomy (to induce the development of secondary sex characteristics)
  - Radiation therapy (not commonly used because it causes myelosuppression, which limits effectiveness of chemotherapy)
  - Radioisotopes as adjuvant therapy
  - High-protein diet with small, frequent meals

● Nursing considerations

- Prepare the patient for surgery by explaining the procedure and telling her what to expect after surgery
  - Explain all preoperative tests, course of treatment, and surgical and postoperative procedures
  - For premenopausal women, explain that bilateral oophorectomy artificially induces early menopause; explain that they may experience hot flashes, headaches, palpitations, insomnia, depression, and excessive perspiration (discuss treatment options)
- Provide appropriate postoperative care
  - Frequently monitor vital signs, intake and output, and effectiveness of pain control
  - Check the dressing regularly for excessive drainage or bleeding, and watch for signs of infection

Key diagnostic test results for ovarian cancer

- Exploratory laparotomy: Evaluation of lymph node and tumor resection; tumor stage

Key treatments for ovarian cancer

- Surgery
- Chemotherapy after surgery
- Radioisotopes

Key nursing considerations for ovarian cancer

Before surgery
- For premenopausal women, explain that bilateral oophorectomy artificially induces early menopause.

After surgery
- Monitor vital signs, intake and output, and effectiveness of pain control.
- Watch for abdominal distention.
- Provide emotional support.

– Watch for abdominal distention; encourage coughing and deep breathing, reposition the patient often, and encourage her to ambulate
– Monitor and treat adverse effects of radiation and chemotherapy
– Provide psychological support
  • Encourage open communication by answering questions and listening to concerns
  • Enlist the support of a social worker, chaplain, and other members of the health care team
  • Encourage participation in a local support group for additional information and support

UTERINE CANCER

● **Definition**
  • Proliferation of cancer cells in the endometrium
  • Most common gynecologic cancer
  • Also known as *endometrial cancer*

● **Underlying pathophysiology**
  • Uterine cancer is usually adenocarcinoma
  • Metastasis occurs late (usually from the endometrium to the cervix, ovaries, fallopian tubes, and other peritoneal structures)
    – It may spread to distant organs, such as the lungs and the brain, by way of the blood or the lymphatic system
    – Lymph node involvement can also occur
  • Less common uterine tumors include adenoacanthoma, endometrial stromal sarcoma, lymphosarcoma, mixed mesodermal tumors (including carcinosarcoma), and leiomyosarcoma

● **Causes**
  • Exact cause unknown
  • Risk factors
    – Low fertility index and anovulation
    – Nulliparity
    – History of infertility or failure of ovulation
    – Abnormal uterine bleeding
    – Obesity
    – Hypertension
    – Diabetes
    – Familial tendency
    – History of uterine polyps or endometrial hyperplasia
    – Prolonged estrogen therapy (unopposed by progesterone)
    – Tamoxifen therapy

● **Pathophysiologic changes**
  • Uterine enlargement secondary to tumor growth
  • Postmenopausal bleeding or persistent and unusual premenopausal bleeding from erosive effects of tumor growth
  • Pain and weight loss related to progressive infiltration and invasion of tumor cells and continued cellular proliferation

---

Key facts about uterine cancer

• Involves cancer cells in endometrium
• Usually is adenocarcinoma
• May spread to distant organs by way of blood or lymphatic system

Key pathophysiologic changes in uterine cancer

• Postmenopausal bleeding
• Persistent and unusual premenopausal bleeding

Complications
- Anemia
- Intestinal obstruction
- Ascites
- Increasing pain
- Hemorrhage

Diagnostic test findings
- Endometrial, cervical, or endocervical biopsy confirms the presence of cancer cells
- Fractional dilation and curettage is used to identify the problem when the disease is suspected but the endometrial biopsy is negative
- Multiple cervical biopsies and endocervical curettage pinpoint cervical involvement
- Papanicolaou test result may be normal or may show abnormal cells
- Schiller's test (staining the cervix and vagina with an iodine solution) identifies cancerous tissues (healthy tissues turn brown, and cancerous tissues resist the stain)

Treatment
- Surgery (rarely curative)
  - Generally involves total abdominal hysterectomy, bilateral salpingo-oophorectomy, or possible omentectomy with or without pelvic or para-aortic lymphadenectomy
  - Total exenteration (removal of all pelvic organs, including the vagina): Done only when the disease is sufficiently contained to allow surgical removal of diseased portions (see *Managing pelvic exenteration,* page 540)
- Radiation therapy
  - When the tumor isn't well differentiated, intracavity or external radiation (or both) given 6 weeks before surgery may inhibit recurrence and lengthen survival time
- Hormonal therapy
  - Synthetic progesterones, such as medroxyprogesterone or megestrol, may be administered for systemic disease; tamoxifen (which produces a 20% to 40% response rate) may be given as a second-line treatment
- Chemotherapy
  - Varying combinations of cisplatin (Platinol-AQ), doxorubicin, etoposide (Toposar), and dactinomycin (Cosmegen) (usually when other treatments have failed)

Nursing considerations
- Prepare the patient for surgery by explaining all procedures and postoperative care; if she's premenopausal, explain that removal of both her ovaries will induce menopause (reassure her about treatments for menopause-related symptoms)
- Provide appropriate postoperative care
  - Measure fluid contents of the blood drainage system every shift; notify the physician immediately if drainage exceeds 400 ml
  - Give prophylactic antibiotics as ordered, and provide good indwelling urinary catheter care

---

Key diagnostic test results for uterine cancer
- Endometrial, cervical, or endocervical biopsy: Presence of cancer cells
- Schiller's test: Presence of cancerous tissues

Key treatments for uterine cancer
- Surgery
- Radiation therapy
- Hormonal therapy
- Chemotherapy

Key nursing considerations for uterine cancer

After surgery
- Measure fluid contents of blood drainage system; report drainage that exceeds 400 ml.
- Provide analgesics as ordered.
- Check vital signs every 4 hours.

Radiation therapy
- Explain procedure to patient.
- Prepare to implement safety precautions.

Managing pelvic exenteration

Follow these steps when caring for a patient undergoing pelvic exenteration.

BEFORE PELVIC EXENTERATION
- Teach the patient about ileal conduit and possible colostomy, and make sure she understands that her vagina will be removed.
- To minimize the risk of infection, supervise a rigorous bowel and skin preparation procedure; decrease the residue in the patient's diet for 48 to 72 hours, and then maintain a diet ranging from clear liquids to nothing by mouth.
- Administer oral or I.V. therapy, and assist with insertion of a central venous pressure catheter and blood drainage system.
- Pack an unsutured perineal wound with gauze packing.

AFTER PELVIC EXENTERATION
- Check the stoma, incision, and perineal wound for drainage; be especially careful to check the perineal wound for bleeding after the packing is removed.
- Expect red or serosanguinous drainage, but notify the physician immediately if drainage is excessive; continuously bright red, foul-smelling, or purulent, or if there's bleeding from the conduit.
- Provide excellent skin care to prevent skin irritation or breakdown because of draining urine and stool; use warm water and saline solution to clean the skin, because soap may be too drying and may increase skin breakdown.

- Check vital signs every 4 hours; watch for and report any sign of complications, such as bleeding, abdominal distention, severe pain, wheezing, or other breathing difficulties
- Provide analgesics as ordered
- Regularly encourage the patient to breathe deeply and cough; promote the use of an incentive spirometer several times every waking hour to keep the lungs expanded
- Provide appropriate care for patients undergoing internal radiation therapy
  - Explain the internal radiation procedure and answer the patient's questions
  - Explain that internal radiation usually requires a 2- to 3-day hospital stay, bowel preparation, a povidone-iodine vaginal douche, a clear-liquid diet, and nothing by mouth the night before implantation (if done in the operating room, general anesthesia is used)
  - Prepare to implement safety precautions, including time, distance, and shielding, immediately after the patient's radioactive source has been implanted (a private room is required)
  - Encourage the patient to limit movement; check her vital signs every 4 hours; and watch for skin reaction, vaginal bleeding, abdominal discomfort, and evidence of dehydration
- Administer diphenoxylate with atropine, as ordered, to minimize possible adverse effect of pelvic radiation (in patients receiving external radiation)

- Explain external radiation to the patient receiving this treatment
  - Tell the patient that treatment is usually given 5 days per week for 6 weeks; caution her not to scrub body areas marked with indelible ink for treatment because it's important to direct treatment exactly to the same area each time
  - Instruct the patient to maintain a high-protein, high-carbohydrate, low-residue diet to reduce bulk and still maintain calories
  - Teach the patient how to use a vaginal dilator to prevent vaginal stenosis and to facilitate vaginal examinations and sexual intercourse
- Give antiemetics as needed during chemotherapy
  - Encourage small, frequent meals to maintain oral intake despite anorexia
  - Establish a mouth care regimen and check for stomatitis

NCLEX CHECKS

It's never too soon to begin your licensure examination preparation. Now that you've reviewed this chapter, carefully read each of the following questions and choose the best answer. Then compare your responses to the correct answers.

1. When cancer cells lose the ability to differentiate and they no longer appear or function like the original cell, this is known as:
- ☐ **1.** *the cytoskeleton.*
- ☐ **2.** *abnormal cell growth.*
- ☐ **3.** *intracellular changes.*
- ☐ **4.** *anaplasia.*

2. You're caring for a patient admitted to the facility with bone pain. A bone scan is ordered to determine any abnormalities, and osteolytic lesions are seen in the femur. Osseous bone tumors arise from:
- ☐ **1.** the bony structure itself.
- ☐ **2.** hematopoietic tissues.
- ☐ **3.** bone marrow.
- ☐ **4.** neural tissues.

3. The physician orders 25 mg/m^2 of doxorubicin (Adriamycin) to be given I.V. to a patient with Hodgkin's disease. The chart shows that the patient is 68″ (172.8 cm) tall and weighs 170 lb (77.1 kg) with a body surface area (BSA) of 2 m^2. You look up the drug before preparing it and find these parameters for patients with an elevated serum bilirubin: Bilirubin 1.2 to 3 mg/dl, reduce the normal dose by 50%; serum bilirubin 3.1 to 5 mg/dl, reduce the normal dose by 75%. The chart reveals that your patient has a serum bilirubin of 3.6 mg/dl. Before calling the physician, you determine that your patient should receive how many total milligrams of doxorubicin?

TOP 6

Items to study for your next test on neoplasms

1. Factors that affect or promote tumor growth
2. Treatments for various neoplasms
3. Types of medications used to control neoplasms
4. Postoperative care for procedures such as TURP and pelvic exenteration
5. Nursing considerations for radiation therapy and chemotherapy
6. Proper stoma care

4. A patient is diagnosed with a glioma in the parietal lobe on the left side. Following supratentorial craniotomy for the tumor, the nurse should:

- ☐ **1.** keep the patient flat for 48 hours.
- ☐ **2.** keep the patient flat for 24 hours.
- ☐ **3.** elevate the head of the bed about 30 degrees.
- ☐ **4.** elevate the head of the bed about 45 degrees.

5. A 62-year-old woman complains to her physician of dull abdominal cramps and a pressure sensation in the abdomen. She notes that her stools are darker than normal and that she's fatigued all the time. The physician orders a workup, suspecting what type of cancer?

- ☐ **1.** Ascending colon
- ☐ **2.** Stomach
- ☐ **3.** Descending or sigmoid colon
- ☐ **4.** Rectal

6. The treatment of choice for stage III Hodgkin's disease is:

- ☐ **1.** chemotherapy.
- ☐ **2.** radiation therapy.
- ☐ **3.** radiation therapy and chemotherapy.
- ☐ **4.** surgery.

7. A patient is being treated for a severe respiratory infection accompanied by high fever, chills, weakness, headache, lymph node and spleen enlargement, and bone pain. Diagnostic testing reveals acute lymphocytic leukemia. Which finding would you expect on the diagnostic workup?

- ☐ **1.** Hemoglobin 12.8 g/dl
- ☐ **2.** Platelet count $350 \times 10^3/\mu l$
- ☐ **3.** Segmented neutrophils 60%, bands 4%
- ☐ **4.** Bone marrow aspirate with many immature WBCs

8. A large, flat, tan or brown freckle with irregularly scattered black nodules is what type of malignant melanoma?

- ☐ **1.** Superficial spreading
- ☐ **2.** Nodular malignant
- ☐ **3.** Lentigo maligna
- ☐ **4.** Acral-lentiginous

9. The nurse should be alert for signs of urethral stricture after which surgical procedure for prostate cancer?

- ☐ **1.** Suprapubic prostatectomy
- ☐ **2.** TURP
- ☐ **3.** Perineal prostatectomy
- ☐ **4.** Retropubic prostatectomy

10. After surgery for thyroid cancer, which electrolyte imbalance may occur?

- ☐ **1.** Hyperchloridemia
- ☐ **2.** Hypernatremia
- ☐ **3.** Hypokalemia
- ☐ **4.** Hypocalcemia

ANSWERS AND RATIONALES

1. CORRECT ANSWER: 4

Anaplasia occurs in varying degrees and some cells begin functioning as another type of cell, possibly becoming a site for hormone production. Abnormal cell growth is a characteristic of cancer cells, which also exhibit intracellular changes such as in the cytoskeleton. The protein filaments that serve to stiffen cells and help organize movement and division are called the *cytoskeleton.*

2. CORRECT ANSWER: 1

Osseous bone tumors arise from bony structure itself and include chondrosarcoma, malignant giant cell tumor, osteogenic sarcoma, and parosteal osteogenic sarcoma. Nonosseous bone tumors arise from hematopoietic tissues, bone marrow, and neural tissues; examples of these are chordomas, Ewing's sarcoma, and fibrosarcoma.

3. CORRECT ANSWER: 30

The patient's bilirubin is within the range for a 75% reduction of dose. Calculate 25% of the dose (the amount you will actually give) using cross multiplication of proportions as follows:

$$\frac{X\ mg}{60\ mg} = \frac{25}{100}$$

Cross multiply the fractions:

$$X\ mg \times 100 = 60\ mg \times 25$$

Solve for X:

$$100X\ mg = 1{,}500\ mg$$
$$100X\ mg\ /\ 100\ mg = 1{,}500\ mg\ /\ 100\ mg$$
$$X = 15$$

Now, multiply the 15 mg/m^2 dose by the BSA to obtain the total dosage to give the patient: 15 mg $\times$ 2 = 30 mg.

4. CORRECT ANSWER: 3

To promote venous drainage and reduce cerebral edema after supratentorial craniotomy, elevate the head of the patient's bed about 30 degrees. After infratentorial craniotomy, keep the head of the bed flat for 48 hours to prevent prolapse of the midbrain into the spinal canal.

5. CORRECT ANSWER: 1

Dull abdominal cramps and abdominal aching and pressure are caused by bowel irritation by cancer tumors localized to the ascending colon that may lead to obstruction and bleeding. Pain with gastric cancer is more localized to the stomach. Descending, sigmoid, and rectal cancers cause increased rectal pressure and intermittent abdominal fullness and cramping.

6. CORRECT ANSWER: 3

Hodgkin's disease, a neoplastic disease of lymph nodes and tissues, occurs in four stages. Combined radiation therapy and chemotherapy is used to kill cancer cells and shrink lymphomas in stage III.

7. CORRECT ANSWER: 4

Bone marrow aspiration will show the characteristic abnormal WBCs of acute lymphoblastic leukemia. Hemoglobin, platelet count, and segmented and banded neutrophils will all be decreased, not normal. A hemoglobin level less than 11 g/dl is diagnostic.

8. CORRECT ANSWER: 3

Lentigo maligna melanoma is a large, flat freckle of tan, brown, black, whitish, or slate color with irregularly scattered black nodules on the surface due to mutations in melanin-producing cells of skin. Superficial spreading melanoma is a red, white, and blue–colored lesion over brown with irregularly notched margins. Nodular malignant melanoma is a polyplike nodule that's flesh- or blackberry-colored. Acral-lentiginous melanoma is an irregular, enlarging black macule.

9. CORRECT ANSWER: 2

After a TURP, be alert for signs of urethral stricture, which include dysuria, decreased force and caliber of the urine stream, and straining to urinate. The other three procedures don't transect the urethra, so they wouldn't cause this type of complication.

10. CORRECT ANSWER: 4

After thyroid surgery, hypocalcemia may develop if the parathyroid glands are removed. Check serum calcium levels daily. Sodium, potassium, and chloride levels aren't affected by the thyroid or parathyroid glands.

NANDA nursing diagnoses
Glossary
Selected references
Index

NANDA nursing diagnoses

Here's a list of the 2005-2006 North American Nursing Diagnosis Association (NANDA) nursing diagnoses according to their domains.

DOMAIN: *Health promotion*
- Effective therapeutic regimen management
- Health-seeking behaviors (specify)
- Impaired home maintenance
- Ineffective community therapeutic regimen management
- Ineffective family therapeutic regimen management
- Ineffective health maintenance
- Ineffective therapeutic regimen management
- Readiness for enhanced management of therapeutic regimen
- Readiness for enhanced nutrition

DOMAIN: *Nutrition*
- Deficient fluid volume
- Excess fluid volume
- Imbalanced nutrition: Less than body requirements
- Imbalanced nutrition: More than body requirements
- Impaired swallowing
- Ineffective infant feeding pattern
- Readiness for enhanced fluid balance
- Risk for deficient fluid volume
- Risk for imbalanced fluid volume
- Risk for imbalanced nutrition: More than body requirements

DOMAIN: *Elimination/Exchange*
- Bowel incontinence
- Constipation
- Diarrhea
- Functional urinary incontinence
- Impaired gas exchange

- Impaired urinary elimination
- Perceived constipation
- Readiness for enhanced urinary elimination
- Reflex urinary incontinence
- Risk for constipation
- Risk for urge urinary incontinence
- Stress urinary incontinence
- Total urinary incontinence
- Urge urinary incontinence
- Urinary retention

DOMAIN: *Activity/Rest*
- Activity intolerance
- Bathing or hygiene self-care deficit
- Decreased cardiac output
- Deficient diversional activity
- Delayed surgical recovery
- Disturbed energy field
- Disturbed sleep pattern
- Dressing or grooming self-care deficit
- Dysfunctional ventilatory weaning response
- Fatigue
- Feeding self-care deficit
- Impaired bed mobility
- Impaired physical mobility
- Impaired spontaneous ventilation
- Impaired transfer ability
- Impaired walking
- Impaired wheelchair mobility
- Ineffective breathing pattern
- Ineffective tissue perfusion (specify type: renal, cerebral, cardiopulmonary, gastrointestinal, peripheral)

- Readiness for enhanced sleep
- Risk for activity intolerance
- Risk for disuse syndrome
- Sedentary lifestyle
- Sleep deprivation
- Toileting self-care deficit

DOMAIN: *Perception/Cognition*

- Disturbed sensory perception (specify: visual, auditory, kinesthetic, gustatory, tactile, olfactory)
- Impaired environmental interpretation syndrome
- Impaired verbal communication
- Readiness for enhanced communication
- Unilateral neglect
- Wandering

DOMAIN: *Self-perception*

- Chronic low self-esteem
- Disturbed body image
- Disturbed personal identity
- Hopelessness
- Powerlessness
- Readiness for enhanced self-concept
- Risk for loneliness
- Risk for powerlessness
- Risk for situational low self-esteem
- Situational low self-esteem

DOMAIN: *Role relationships*

- Caregiver role strain
- Dysfunctional family processes: Alcoholism
- Effective breast-feeding
- Impaired parenting
- Impaired social interaction
- Ineffective breast-feeding
- Ineffective role performance
- Interrupted breast-feeding
- Interrupted family processes
- Parental role conflict
- Readiness for enhanced family processes
- Readiness for enhanced parenting

- Risk for caregiver role strain
- Risk for impaired parent/infant/child attachment
- Risk for impaired parenting

DOMAIN: *Sexuality*

- Ineffective sexuality patterns
- Sexual dysfunction

DOMAIN: *Coping/Stress tolerance*

- Anticipatory grieving
- Anxiety
- Autonomic dysreflexia
- Chronic sorrow
- Compromised family coping
- Death anxiety
- Decreased intracranial adaptive capacity
- Defensive coping
- Disabled family coping
- Disorganized infant behavior
- Dysfunctional grieving
- Fear
- Impaired adjustment
- Ineffective community coping
- Ineffective coping
- Ineffective denial
- Posttrauma syndrome
- Rape-trauma syndrome
- Rape-trauma syndrome: Compound reaction
- Rape-trauma syndrome: Silent reaction
- Readiness for enhanced community coping
- Readiness for enhanced coping
- Readiness for enhanced family coping
- Readiness for enhanced organized infant behavior
- Relocation stress syndrome
- Risk for autonomic dysreflexia
- Risk for disorganized infant behavior
- Risk for dysfunctional grieving
- Risk for posttrauma syndrome
- Risk for relocation stress syndrome

DOMAIN: *Life principles*
- Decisional conflict (specify)
- Impaired religiosity
- Noncompliance (specify)
- Readiness for enhanced religiosity
- Readiness for enhanced spiritual well-being
- Risk for impaired religiosity
- Risk for spiritual distress
- Spiritual distress

DOMAIN: *Safety/Protection*
- Hyperthermia
- Hypothermia
- Impaired dentition
- Impaired oral mucous membrane
- Impaired skin integrity
- Impaired tissue integrity
- Ineffective airway clearance
- Ineffective protection
- Ineffective thermoregulation
- Latex allergy response
- Risk for aspiration
- Risk for falls
- Risk for imbalanced body temperature
- Risk for impaired skin integrity
- Risk for infection
- Risk for injury
- Risk for latex allergy response
- Risk for other-directed violence
- Risk for perioperative-positioning injury
- Risk for peripheral neurovascular dysfunction
- Risk for poisoning
- Risk for self-directed violence
- Risk for self-mutilation
- Risk for sudden infant death syndrome
- Risk for suffocation
- Risk for suicide
- Risk for trauma
- Self-mutilation

DOMAIN: *Comfort*
- Acute pain
- Chronic pain
- Nausea
- Social isolation

DOMAIN: *Growth/Development*
- Adult failure to thrive
- Delayed growth and development
- Risk for delayed development
- Risk for disproportionate growth

Glossary

acid: hydrogen-containing molecule or ion that's able to give up a proton to an alkaline ion or molecule; pH below 7.0

acute illness: illness having severe symptoms and a short course

agranulocyte: leukocyte (white blood cell) not made up of granules or grains; includes lymphocytes, monocytes, and plasma cells

allele: one of two or more different genes that occupy a corresponding position (locus) on matched chromosomes; allows for different forms of the same inheritable characteristic

allergen: substance that induces an allergy or a hypersensitivity reaction

anaphylaxis: severe allergic reaction to a foreign substance

androgen: steroid hormone that stimulates male characteristics; two main androgens are androsterone and testosterone

anemia: reduction in the number and volume of red blood cells, the amount of hemoglobin, or the volume of packed red cells

aneurysm: sac formed by the dilation of the wall of an artery, a vein, or the heart

angiography: radiographic visualization of blood vessels after injection of radiopaque contrast material

anoxia: absence of oxygen in the tissues

antibody: immunoglobulin molecule that reacts only with the specific antigen that induced its formation in the lymph system

anticholinergic: opposing the actions of the parasympathetic system and cholinergic nerve fibers; for example, atropine

antigen: foreign substance, such as a bacterium or toxin, that induces antibody formation

antitoxin: antibody produced in response to a toxin that's capable of neutralizing the toxin's effects

atrophy: decrease in size or wasting away of a cell, tissue, organ, or body part

autoimmune disorder: disorder in which the body launches an immunologic response against itself

autosome: any chromosome other than the sex chromosomes; twenty-two of the human chromosome pairs are autosomes

bacterium: one-celled microorganism that breaks down dead tissue, has no true nucleus, and reproduces by cell division

baroreceptor: receptor that responds to changes in pressure

base: an alkali; a molecule or compound that's able to give up a hydroxyl ion; pH greater than 7.0

benign: not malignant or recurrent; favorable for recovery

bone marrow: soft organic material that fills the cavities of bones

bruit: harsh or musical sound that can be auscultated and is generally considered abnormal

bursa: fluid-filled sac or cavity found in connecting tissue in the vicinity of joints that acts as a cushion

calculus: any abnormal concentration, usually made up of mineral salts, within the body; for example, gallstones and renal calculi

carcinogen: substance that causes cancer

carcinoma: malignant growth made up of epithelial cells that can infiltrate surrounding tissues and metastasize

cardiac output: volume of blood ejected from the heart per minute

cartilage: dense connective tissue made up of fibers embedded in a strong, gel-like substance that supports, cushions, and shapes body structures

cell: smallest living component of an organism; has the ability to assimilate, grow, reproduce, and respond to stimuli

cholestasis: an arrest in the flow of bile

cholinergic: related to nerves that use acetylcholine as their neurotransmitter and are part of the parasympathetic nervous system

chondrocyte: cartilage cell

chromosome: linear thread in a cell's nucleus that contains deoxyribonucleic acid; occurs in pairs in humans

chronic illness: illness of long duration that includes remission and exacerbation

clearance: complete removal of a substance by the kidneys from a specific volume of blood per unit of time

coagulant: substance that promotes, accelerates, or permits blood clotting

collagen: main supportive protein of skin, tendon, bone, cartilage, and connective tissue

colonoscopy: examination of the upper portion of the rectum with an elongated speculum or colonoscope to visualize the colon, remove polyps, or biopsy suspicious growths

compensation: the counterbalancing of any defect in structure or function; measure of how long the heart takes to adapt to increased blood in ventricles

complement system: major mediator of inflammatory response; a functionally related system made up of 20 proteins circulating as functionally inactive molecules

cytoplasm: aqueous mass within a cell that contains organelles, is surrounded by the cell membrane, and excludes the nucleus

cytotoxic: destructive to cells

degeneration: retrogressive cell damage occurring in the cell's cytoplasm that can progress to the nucleus and cause cell death

demyelination: destruction of a nerve's myelin sheath that interferes with normal nerve conduction

deoxyribonucleic acid (DNA): complex protein in the cell's nucleus that carries genetic material and is responsible for cellular reproduction

depolarization: change in direction from positive to negative or vice versa

differentiation: process of cells maturing into specific types

disease: pathologic condition that occurs when the body can't maintain homeostasis

disjunction: separation of chromosomes that occurs during cell division

distal: farthest away

diverticulitis: inflammation of one or more diverticula in the muscular layer of the colon

dominant gene: gene that expresses itself even if it's carried on only one homologous (matched) chromosome

Dressler syndrome: condition characterized by recurrent episodes of pericarditis after myocardial infarction

dyscrasia: condition related to a disease, usually referring to an imbalance of component elements; for example, blood dyscrasia is a disorder of cellular elements of the blood

dysphagia: difficulty swallowing

dysplasia: abnormal development of tissue

ectopic: out of place; aberrant

electrophoresis: movement of particles in an electric field toward an anode (positively charged pole) or cathode (negatively charged pole)

embolism: sudden obstruction of a blood vessel by foreign substances or a blood clot

endemic: disease of low morbidity that occurs continuously in a particular patient population or geographic area

endochondral ossification: process by which cartilage hardens into bone

endocrine: pertaining to internal hormone secretion by glands; endocrine glands, including the pineal gland, the islets of Langerhans in the pancreas, the gonads, the thymus, and the adrenal, pituitary, thyroid, and parathyroid glands secrete hormones directly into circulation

endogenous: occurring inside the body

erythrocyte: red blood cell; a cell that carries oxygen to tissues and removes carbon dioxide from them

erythropoiesis: production of erythrocytes

estrogen: female sex hormone produced by the ovaries that's responsible for producing female characteristics

etiology: cause of a disease

exacerbation: increase in the severity of a disease or any of its symptoms

exocrine: external or outward secretion of a gland; exocrine glands discharge through ducts opening on an external or internal surface of the body; they include the liver, the pancreas, the prostate, and the salivary, sebaceous, sweat, gastric, intestinal, mammary, and lacrimal glands

exogenous: occurring outside the body

fasciculation: involuntary twitching or contraction of a muscle

fungus: nonphotosynthetic microorganism that reproduces asexually by cell division

gland: specialized cell cluster that produces a secretion used in some other body part

glomerulus: a network of twisted capillaries that bring blood and waste products carried by blood to the nephron

glucagon: hormone released during the fasting state that increases blood glucose concentration

glucocorticoid: any steroidlike compound able to promote glycogen retention within the liver and exert an anti-inflammatory effect; for example, cortisol

granulocyte: any cell containing granules, especially a granular leukocyte

hematopoiesis: production of red blood cells in the bone marrow

hemoglobin: iron-containing pigment in red blood cells that carries oxygen from the lungs to the tissues

hemolysis: red blood cell destruction

hemorrhage: escape of blood from a ruptured vessel

hemostasis: complex process whereby platelets, plasma, and coagulation factors interact to control bleeding

heterozygous genes: genes having different alleles at the same site (locus); if each gene in a chromosome pair produces a different effect, the genes are heterozygous

histocyte: macrophage found in connective tissue

homeostasis: dynamic, steady state of internal balance in the body

homologous genes: gene pairs sharing a corresponding structure and position

homozygous genes: genes that have identical alleles for a given trait; when each gene at a corresponding locus produces the same effect, the genes are homozygous

hormone: chemical substance produced in the body that has a specific regulatory effect on the activity of specific cells or organs

host defense system: elaborate network of safeguards that protects the body from infectious organisms and other harmful invaders

hyperplasia: excessive growth of normal cells that causes an increase in the volume of a tissue or organ

hypersensitivity disorder: state in which the body produces an exaggerated immune response to a foreign antigen

hypertension: abnormally high blood pressure

hypotension: abnormally low blood pressure

hypoxia: reduction of oxygen in body tissues to below-normal levels

iatrogenic: response to surgical or medical treatment caused by the treatment alone

idiopathic: characterizing a disease with no known cause

immunocompetence: ability of cells to distinguish antigens from substances that belong to the body and to launch an immune response

immunodeficiency disorder: disorder caused by a deficiency of the immune response due to hypoactivity or a decreased numbers of lymphoid cells

immunoglobulin: serum protein synthesized by lymphocytes and plasma cells that has known antibody activity; main component of humoral immune response

immunosurveillance: defense mechanism by which the immune system continuously recognizes abnormal cells as foreign and destroys them; for example, an interruption in immunosurveillance can lead to overproduction of cancer cells

inotropic: affecting the contractility of muscle tissue

insulin: hormone secreted into the blood by the islets of Langerhans of the pancreas that promotes the storage of glucose, among other functions

ischemia: decreased blood supply to a body organ or tissue

joint: site of the union of two or more bones; provides motion and flexibility

karyotype: chromosomal arrangement of the cell nucleus

leaflets: cusps in the heart valves that open and close in response to pressure gradients to let blood flow into the chambers

leukocyte: white blood cell that protects the body against disease-producing microorganisms

leukocytosis: increase in the number of leukocytes in the blood; generally caused by infection

leukopenia: reduction in the number of leukocytes in the blood

ligament: band of fibrous tissue that connects bones or cartilage, strengthens joints, provides stability, and limits or facilitates movement

lymphedema: chronic swelling of a body part from accumulation of interstitial fluid secondary to obstruction of lymphatic vessels or lymph nodes

lymph node: structure that filters the lymphatic fluid that drains from body tissues and is later returned to the blood as plasma; removes noxious agents from the blood

lymphocyte: leukocyte produced by lymphoid tissue that participates in immunity

macrophage: highly phagocytic cells that are stimulated by inflammation

malabsorption: insufficient intestinal absorption of nutrients

malignant: condition that endangers health or life; for example, a progressively growing tumor that can spread and result in death if left untreated

megakaryocytes: giant bone marrow cells

meiosis: process of cell division by which reproductive cells (gametes) are formed

melanin: dark skin pigment that filters ultraviolet radiation and is produced and dispersed by specialized cells called melanocytes

metastasis: transfer of disease via pathogenic microorganisms or cells from one organ or body part to another not directly connected with it

mineralocorticoid: one of the steroids of the adrenal gland that affects salt metabolism (sodium and potassium salts); for example, aldosterone

mitosis: process of cell division by which the nucleus and cytoplasm split into two cells

multifactorial disorder: disorder caused by genetic and environmental factors

myelin: lipidlike substance that surrounds the axon of myelinated nerve fibers to permit normal neurologic conduction

myelitis: inflammation of the spinal cord or bone marrow

necrosis: cell or tissue death

neoplasm: abnormal growth in which cell multiplication is uncontrolled and progressive

nephron: structural and functional unit of the kidney; responsible for urine formation

neuritic plaques: areas of nerve inflammation; found on autopsy examination of the brain tissue of people with Alzheimer's disease

neuron: highly specialized conductor cell that receives and transmits electrochemical nerve impulses

nevus: circumscribed, stable malformation of the skin and oral mucosa

nondisjunction: failure of chromosomes to separate properly during cell division; causes an unequal distribution of chromosomes between the two resulting cells

obstipation: intestinal obstruction

oncotic: caused by edema or swelling; in oncology, relating to tumors

opportunistic infection: infection that strikes people with altered, weakened immune systems; caused by a microorganism that doesn't usually cause disease but becomes pathogenic under certain conditions

organ: body part made up of tissues that performs a specific function

organelle: structure of a cell found in the cytoplasm that performs a specific function; for example, the nucleus, mitochondria, and lysosomes

osmolality: concentration of a solution expressed in terms of osmoles of solute per kilogram of solvent

osmoreceptors: specialized neurons located in the thalamus that are stimulated by increased extracellular fluid osmolality to cause release of antidiuretic hormone, thereby helping to control fluid balance

osteoblasts: bone-forming cells whose activity results in bone formation

osteoclasts: giant, multinuclear cells that reabsorb material from previously formed bones, tear down old or excess bone structure, and allow osteoblasts to rebuild new bone

pancytopenia: abnormal depression of all the cellular elements of blood

parasite: single-celled or multi-celled organism that depends on a host for food and a protective environment

parenchyma: essential or functional elements of an organ as distinguished from its framework

pathogen: disease-producing agent or microorganism

pathogenesis: origin and development of a disease

peristalsis: intestinal contractions, or waves, that propel food toward the stomach and into and through the intestine

phagocyte: cell that ingests microorganisms, other cells, and foreign particles

phagocytosis: engulfing of microorganisms, other cells, and foreign particles by a phagocyte

plasma: liquid part of the blood that carries antibodies and nutrients to tissues and carries wastes away from tissues

platelet: disk-shaped structure in blood that plays a crucial role in blood coagulation

polymorphonuclear: having lobular nuclei; for example, a neutrophil

polypeptide chains: chains of amino acids linked by a peptide bond that make up hemoglobin

proximal: nearest to

pulmonary alveoli: grapelike clusters found at the ends of the respiratory passages in the lungs; sites for the exchange of carbon dioxide and oxygen

pulsus paradoxus: pulse marked by a greater than 10 mm Hg drop in systolic blood pressure during inspiration

pyrosis: heartburn

recessive gene: gene that doesn't express itself in the presence of its dominant allele (corresponding gene)

remission: abatement of a disease's symptoms

remyelination: healing of demyelinated nerves

renin: enzyme produced by the kidneys in response to an actual or perceived decline in extracellular fluid volume; an important part of blood pressure regulation

resistance: opposition to airflow in the lung tissue, chest wall, or airways

sepsis: pathologic state resulting from microorganisms or their poisonous products in the bloodstream

sigmoidoscopy: inspection of the rectum and sigmoid colon using a sigmoidoscope

stasis: stagnation of the normal flow of fluids, such as blood and urine, or within the intestinal mechanism

stenosis: constriction or narrowing of a passage or orifice

subchondral: below the cartilage

surfactant: lipid-type substance that coats the alveoli, allowing them to expand uniformly during inspiration and preventing them from collapsing during expiration

synovial fluid: viscous, lubricating substance secreted by the synovial membrane that lines the cavity between the bones of free-moving joints

synovitis: inflammation of the synovial membrane

tendon: fibrous cord of connective tissue that attaches muscle to bone or cartilage and enables bones to move when skeletal muscles contract

thrombolytic: clot dissolving

thrombosis: obstruction of blood vessels by a blood clot

tissue: large group of individual cells that perform a certain function

tophi: clusters of urate crystals surrounded by inflamed tissue

toxin: poison produced by animals, certain plants, or pathogenic bacteria

toxoid: toxin treated to destroy its toxicity without destroying its ability to stimulate antibody production

trabeculae: needlelike, bony structures that form a supportive meshwork of interconnecting spaces filled with bone marrow

transferrin: trace protein in blood that binds and transports iron

translocation: alteration of a chromosome by attachment of a fragment to another chromosome or a different portion of the same chromosome

trisomy 21: aberration in which chromosome 21 has three homologous chromosomes per cell instead of two; another name for Down syndrome

tubercle: a tiny, rounded nodule produced by the tuberculosis bacillus

tubules: small tubes; in the kidney, minute, reabsorptive canals that secrete, collect, and conduct urine

uremic frost: white, flaky deposits of urea on the skin of patients with advanced uremia

urate: salt of uric acid found in urine

urticaria: wheals associated with itching; another name for hives

vasopressor: drug that stimulates contraction of the muscular tissue of the capillaries and arteries

virus: microscopic, infectious parasite that contains genetic material and needs a host cell to replicate

V̇/Q̇ ratio: ratio of ventilation (amount of air in the alveoli) to perfusion (amount of blood in the pulmonary capillaries); expresses the effectiveness of gas exchange

X-linked inheritance: inheritance pattern in which single gene disorders are passed through sex chromosomes; varies according to whether a male or female carries the gene (because the male has only one X chromosome, a trait determined by a gene on that chromosome is always expressed in a male)

Selected references

AIDSMeds.com. (9/2/2003). "Understanding Your T-cell Test" [Online]. Available: *www.aidsmeds.com/lessons/tcelltest.htm* [12/15/2004].

Bell, D. "Heart Failure: A Serious and Common Comorbidity of Diabetes," *Clinical Diabetes* 22(2):61-65, Spring 2004.

Bleeding Disorders Info Center. "Factor XI Deficiency" [Online]. Available: *www.hemophilia.org/bdi/bdi_types9.htm* [2/25/2005].

Brick, W., and Burgess, R. (10/27/2004). "Malignant Melanoma" [Online]. Available: *www.emedicine.com/med/topic1386.htm* [7/20/2005].

Choe, J.M., and Mardovin, W. (1/14/2005). "Neurogenic bladder" [Online]. Available: *www.emedicine.com/med/topic3176.htm* [3/8/2005].

Eastern, J.S. (10/18/2004). "Herpes Zoster" [Online]. Available: *www.emedicine.com/derm/topic180.htm* [4/7/2005].

Guido, M., and Rugge, M. "Liver Biopsy Sampling in Chronic Viral Hepatitis," *Seminars in Liver Disease. Issues in Hepatic Pathology* 24(1):89-97, February 2004.

Harum, P. (8/2004) "Diet and Nutrition for the Pre-ESRD Patient" [Online]. Available: *http://www.ikidney.com/iKidney/Lifestyles/NutritionalTips/JustDiagnosed/DietandNutritionforPreESRDPatient.htm* [2/7/2005].

Huether, S.E., and McCance, K.L. *Understanding Pathophysiology*, 3rd ed. Philadelphia: Mosby–Year Book, Inc., 2004.

Hughes, B.W., et al. "Pathophysiology of Myasthenia Gravis," *Seminars in Neurology* 24(1):21-30, March 2004.

Jiang, S.B. (10/27/2004). "Mohs Surgery" [Online]. Available: *www.emedicine.com/ent/topic29.htm* [3/4/2005].

Kenny, P.E. "The Changing Face of AIDS," *Nursing* 34(8):56-63, August 2004.

Koennecke, H.C. "Secondary Prevention of Stroke: A Practical Guide to Drug Treatment," *CNS Drugs* 18(4):221-41, March 2004.

Kuwabara, S. "Guillain-Barré Syndrome: Epidemiology, Pathophysiology and Management," *Drugs* 64(6):597-610, 2004.

Levi, M., et al. "New Treatment Strategies for Disseminated Intravascular Coagulation Based on Current Understanding of the Pathophysiology," *Annals of Medicine* 36(1):41-49, 2004.

McPhee, S.J., et al. *Pathophysiology of Disease,* 4th ed. New York: McGraw-Hill/Appleton & Lange, 2003.

Meduri, G.U., and Yates, C.R. "Systemic Inflammation-Associated Glucocorticoid Resistance and Outcome of ARDS," *Annals of the New York Academy of Sciences* 1024:24-53, June 2004.

"Methylprednisolone Life-Saving in SARS?" *Inpharma Weekly* 1444:11, July 2004.

National Guideline Clearinghouse. (6/16/2005). "Symptom Management in Cancer: Pain, Depression, and Fatigue" [Online]. Available: *www.guideline.gov/summary/summary.aspx?doc_id=6108&nbr=3963&string=%22Symptom+Management+in+Cancer%3a+Pain%2c+Depression%2c%22+and+Fatigue* [7/20/2005].

Pathophysiology: A 2-in-1 Reference for Nurses. Philadelphia: Lippincott Williams & Wilkins, 2004.

Porth, C. *Essentials of Pathophysiology: Concepts of Altered Health States,* 7th ed. Philadelphia: Lippincott Williams & Wilkins, 2005.

Price, S.A., and Wilson, L.M. *Pathophysiology: Clinical Concepts of Disease Processes,* 6th ed. Philadelphia: Mosby–Year Book, Inc., 2003.

"SARS Coronavirus in Tears," *Journal of Clinical Pathology* 57(9):979, September 2004.

Truscott, M. "Caregiving Challenges: Looks Can Be Deceiving — Dementia, the Invisible Disease," *Alzheimer's Care Quarterly* 5(4):274-77, October-December 2004.

Index

---

i refers to an illustration; t refers to a table; **boldface** indicates color page.

i refers to an illustration; t refers to a table; **boldface** indicates color page.

i refers to an illustration; t refers to a table; **boldface** indicates color page.

---

i refers to an illustration; t refers to a table; **boldface** indicates color page.

---

i refers to an illustration; t refers to a table; **boldface** indicates color page.

i refers to an illustration; t refers to a table; **boldface** indicates color page.

i refers to an illustration; t refers to a table; **boldface** indicates color page.

i refers to an illustration; t refers to a table; **boldface** indicates color page.

i refers to an illustration; t refers to a table; **boldface** indicates color page.

The enclosed CD-ROM is just one more reason why the *Straight A's* series is at the head of its class. The more than 250 additional NCLEX-style questions contained on the CD provide you with another opportunity to review the material and gauge your knowledge. The program allows you to:

- take tests of varying lengths on subject areas of your choice
- learn the rationales for correct and incorrect answers
- print the results of your tests to measure progress over time.

Minimum system requirements

To operate the *Straight A's* CD-ROM, we recommend that you have the following minimum computer equipment:

- Windows 98
- Pentium 166
- 128 MB RAM
- 8 MB of free hard-disk space
- SVGA monitor with High Color (16-bit)
- CD-ROM drive
- mouse.

Installation

Before installing the CD-ROM, make sure that your monitor is set to High Color (16-bit) and your display area is set to 800 × 600. If it isn't, consult your monitor's user's manual for instructions about changing the display settings. (The display settings are typically found in Start/Settings/Control Panel/Display/Settings tab.)

To run this program, you must install it onto the hard drive of your computer, following these three steps:

1. Start Windows 98 (minimum).
2. Place the CD in your CD-ROM drive. After a few moments, the install process will automatically begin. *Note:* If the install process doesn't automatically begin, click the Start menu and select Run. Type *D:\setup.exe* (where *D:* is the letter of your CD-ROM drive) and then click OK.
3. Follow the on-screen instructions for installation.

Technical support

For technical support, call toll-free 1-800-638-3030, Monday through Friday, 8:30 a.m. to 5 p.m. Eastern Time. You may also write to Lippincott Williams & Wilkins Technical Support, 351 W. Camden Street, Baltimore, MD 21201-2436, or e-mail us at *techsupp@lww.com*.